Drug Discovery and Pharmaceutical Formulation

Drug Discovery and Pharmaceutical Formulation

Edited by **Reginald Thornburg**

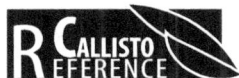

R CALLISTO REFERENCE

New York

Published by Callisto Reference,
106 Park Avenue, Suite 200,
New York, NY 10016, USA
www.callistoreference.com

Drug Discovery and Pharmaceutical Formulation
Edited by Reginald Thornburg

International Standard Book Number: 978-1-63239-743-0 (Hardback)

Contents

Preface

The world is advancing at a fast pace like never before. Therefore, the need is to keep up with the latest developments. This book was an idea that came to fruition when the specialists in the area realized the need to coordinate together and document essential themes in the subject. That's when I was requested to be the editor. Editing this book has been an honour as it brings together diverse authors researching on different streams of the field. The book collates essential materials contributed by veterans in the area which can be utilized by students and researchers alike.

This book contains some path-breaking studies related to drug discovery and pharmaceutical formulation. It unravels the recent discoveries related to this field. Pharmaceutical formulation refers to the science of using present drugs in order to formulate new improved medications. The aim of this field is to discover drugs which are stable, harmless, and adequate for the patient and do not cause any side effects. It incorporates formulation of different forms of drugs like tablets, capsules, lyophilized and liquid, etc. This book will provide interesting topics for research which students, doctors, practitioners and others related to this field can take up Some of the diverse aspects covered herein address the varied branches that fall under this category. It is an essential guide for both academicians and those who wish to pursue this discipline further.

Each chapter is a sole-standing publication that reflects each author's interpretation. Thus, the book displays a multi-facetted picture of our current understanding of applications and diverse aspects of the field. I would like to thank the contributors of this book and my family for their endless support.

Editor

Pandanus odoratissimus (Kewda): A Review on Ethnopharmacology, Phytochemistry, and Nutritional Aspects

Prafulla P. Adkar[1,2] and V. H. Bhaskar[3]

[1]*Department of Pharmacology, JSPM's Jayawantrao Sawant College of Pharmacy and Research, University of Pune, Pune, Maharashtra 411028, India*
[2]*Vinayaka Missions University, Sankari Main Road, NH-47, Ariyanoor, Salem, Tamil Nadu 636308, India*
[3]*Department of Pharmaceutical Medicinal Chemistry, Gahlot Institute of Pharmacy, Plot No. 59, Sector No. 14, Kopar khairane, Navi Mumbai, Maharashtra 400709, India*

Correspondence should be addressed to Prafulla P. Adkar; prafi.phd@gmail.com

Academic Editor: Berend Olivier

Pandanus odoratissimus Linn. (family: Pandanaceae) is traditionally recommended by the Indian Ayurvedic medicines for treatment of headache, rheumatism, spasm, cold/flu, epilepsy, wounds, boils, scabies, leucoderma, ulcers, colic, hepatitis, smallpox, leprosy, syphilis, and cancer and as a cardiotonic, antioxidant, dysuric, and aphrodisiac. It contains phytochemicals, namely, lignans and isoflavones, coumestrol, alkaloids, steroids, carbohydrates, phenolic compounds, glycosides, proteins, amino acids as well as vitamins and nutrients, and so forth. It is having immense importance in nutrition. A 100 g edible *Pandanus* pericarp is mainly comprised of water and carbohydrate (80 and 17 g, resp.) and protein (1.3 mg), fat (0.7 mg), and fiber (3.5 g). *Pandanus* fruits paste provides 321 kilocalories, protein (2.2 g), calcium (134 mg), phosphorus (108 mg), iron (5.7 mg), thiamin (0.04 mg), vitamin C (5 mg), and beta-carotene (19 to 19,000 μg) (a carotenoid that is a precursor to vitamin A). *Pandanus* fruit is an important source of vitamins C, B_1, B_2, B_3, and so forth, usually prepared as a *Pandanus* floured drink. Traditional claims were scientifically evaluated by the various authors and the phytochemical profile of plant parts was well established. The methods for analytical estimations were developed. However, there is paucity of systematic compilation of scientifically important information about this plant. In the present review we have systematically reviewed and compiled information of pharmacognostic, ethnopharmacology, phytochemistry, pharmacology, nutritional aspects, and analytical methods. This review will enrich knowledge leading the way into the discovery of new therapeutic agents with improved and intriguing pharmacological properties.

1. Introduction

The Indian Ayurvedic plant (kewda) *Pandanus odoratissimus* Lam. belonging to the family Pandanaceae (Figure 1) [1]. The overall *Pandanus* genus contains about 600 species distributed mainly in subtropical and tropical regions; there are around 30 to 40 species of *Pandanus* in India. It is widely distributed in India over coastal districts of Orissa (especially in Ganjam), Andhra Pradesh, Tamil Nadu, and to some extent in parts of Uttar Pradesh [2]. *P. odoratissimus* is said to be a restore health, strength, or well-being, promoting a feeling of well-being in tropical climates. Ayurvedic science has found the medicinal action of essential oil yielded by the screw pine's

highly scented flowers to be useful in headaches, earaches and as a liniment for rheumatic pains. It may be chewed as a breath sweetener or used as a preservative in rice made foods. *Pandanus* has antiviral, antiallergy, antiplatelet, anti-inflammatory, antioxidant, and anticancer action [3, 4]. *P. odoratissimus* naturally occurs in high water marking the very edge of the sea and near coastal forests in Southeast Asia, including the Philippines and Indonesia, extending eastward through Papua New Guinea and northern Australia, and throughout the pacific ocean beaches, including Melanesia (Solomon Islands, Vanuatu, New Caledonia, and Fiji), Micronesia (Palau, Northern Marianas, Guam, Federated States of Micronesia, Marshall lands, Kiribati, Tuvalu, and

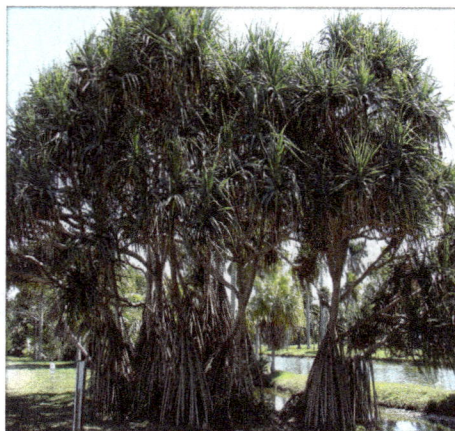

FIGURE 1: Whole plant; *Pandanus odoratissimus* Linn. (Family: Pandanaceae).

Nauru), and Polynesia (Wallis and Futuna, Tokelau, Samoa, American Samoa, Tonga, Niue, Cook Islands, French Polynesia, and Hawaii) [4].

2. Historical Perspectives

P. odoratissimus Linn. is native to South Asia and India has the tradition of alternative therapies; there are no procedures to test the safety and efficacy of traditional remedies and to standardize their effective cure. For these reasons it is essential to increase our efforts in the area of medicinal plant research and exploit it efficiently for the benefit of humanity.

3. Habitat

P. odoratissimus Linn. forest habitat [5] and usually elevations of sea level to 20 m (66 ft), but can grow at elevations of 600 m (1970 ft) or higher [6]. Kewda plants are found growing along seashores, banks of rivers, ponds, canals, and so forth [7]. It grows in tropical climate, where it can withstand drought salty spray and strong wind. It propagates readily from seed but it is also propagated from branch cutting for farm or for garden. It grows fairly quickly [8].

Pandanus plant is also called "pandan" and it is native to Asia and even tropical parts of Australia. *Pandanus* leaves are mostly used in the Southeast Asian cooking (Thomson et al., 2007).

4. Cultivation and Collection

Cultivation of *P. odoratissimus* is too little in India, precisely, the Ganjam district in southern Orissa. The plant can be propagated by off sets or division of the suckers. For raising scented types, a fertile, well-drained-soil is preferable. The tree begins to flower 3 to 4 years after planting. The flowering period is rainy season (July–October). The flowers are harvested early in the morning, and the spa dices take a fortnight to mature, depending upon the weather conditions. In India and Burma, the male flowers are valued for their fragrance

and some kewda products. Highly prized by Indian perfumer a fully mature tree bears 30–40 spadices in a year. It is estimated that there are about 30–40 thousand trees in Ganjam district and nearly to a million spa dices are annually used for the production of kewda attar, kewda water, and kewda oil [9].

5. Pharmacognosy [17]

See Tables 1 and 2.

6. Microscopic Characteristics [17]

6.1. Transverse Section of Leaf (Surface View). Transverse section of leaf showed the presence of single layered upper and lower thin walled epidermal cells, with a moderately thick cuticle, and cells are more or less rectangular. Covering type, unicellular, thick walled, lignified Trichomes, pointed at one end and has a base like that of a hockey stick are emerge from the epidermal layers. Stomata are also seen in the epidermal layer. Mesophyll forms the bulk and is differentiated into thin walled, large, polyhedral, colorless parenchyma with intercellular spaces and 3 to 4 layered, tightly arranged spongy parenchyma (Chlorenchyma). Numerous bundles of acicular rap hides and calcium oxalate crystals as prisms were seen in the parenchymatous cells of mesophyll. Collateral vascular bundles were seen at regular intervals and have protoxylem followed by metaxylem towards upper epidermis and phloem followed by bundle sheath extension (sclerenchyma) towards lower epidermis. The whole vascular bundle is covered by border parenchyma. The TS of the leaf when treated with safranin vascular bundles have stained with pink color and when treated with Sudan red lignified cell wall produced red color.

6.2. Organoleptic Characteristics. Coarsely powdered shade dried leaf of *P. odoratissimus* Linn. is light green in color with characteristic odor and acrid taste.

6.3. Powder Microscopy. It primarily consists of Scalariform and annular xylem vessels; covering type, unicellular, thick walled Trichomes which are lignified and pointed at one end and has a base like that of a hockey stick; paracytic stomata with straight walled epidermal cells surrounding it. Calcium oxalate crystals as prism and acicular raphids scattered in parenchyma.

6.4. Leaf Surface Data. Stomata number and stomata index of leaf of *P. odoratissimus* Linn. were carried out. The value of stomata index of upper epidermis is 23 and lower epidermis is 56.

6.5. Growth Response. Stem growth is slow to moderate, 2–80 cm (0.8–31 in) per year. Growth and development vary with sex of plant (male or female), variety, and types of planting stock (seedling or branch cutting). For seedling plants, there is a 4–9-year semiprostrate juvenile phase, followed by an erect trunk growth phase of 5–12 years, and then a sexual/flowering phase of 40 or more years. Male plants are usually more branched, up to about 30 branches (maximum 60), than

TABLE 1: Synonyms of *Pandanus odoratissimus*.

Botanical	*Pandanus odoratissimus* Lam. or *Pandanus fascicularis* Lamk. and *P. tectorius* [3]
Bengali	Keora, keya, and ketaki
English	Umbrella tree, screw pine, and screw tree
Gujarati	Kevda, ketak
Hawaiian	Hala (*P. tectorius*)
Hindi	केवड़ा, पुष्पचामर, केओड़ा, पांशुका Kewra, kewda, pushpa-chamar, keora, panshuka
Kannada	Kedige, ketake, and tale hu
Malayalam	Kaitha, kainari
Marathi	केतकी, केवड़ा, केगद Ketaki, kewda, kegad
Nepali	केउरा, केराडा, तारीका, Keura, kerada, and tarika Kiora, keura, and kevra
Sanskrit	Ketaka
Tamil	தாழை, தாழம்பூ, கேதகை Tazhai, talai, tazhambu, talambu, and ketakai
Telugu	Mogheli, mogil, gedaga, ketaki, and gojjangi
Urdu	کیتکی, پانشکا, جمبول, جمبالا, کیوڑہ Kiura, kevara, jambala, jambul, panshuka, and ketaki
Russian	Pandanus aromatnejshi
Japanese	Adan, takonoki

females, up to about 15 branches (maximum 30). The rate of stem growth varies from very slow to moderate (2–80 cm (0.8–31 in) per year). Branch diameter is usually reduced by 10–30% at each branching, and branching ceases when branch diameter is less than about 3.5 cm (1.4 in) in males and 4.5 cm (1.8 in) in females. The life span of established *Pandanus* plants is typically about 50–80 years (but longevity may be much greater, as long as 100–150 years in some environments). The productive fruiting life of vegetatively propagated plants may be only 20–25 years. Senescence is associated with a gradual decline in branch diameter, leaf size, and number of live branches. Branch death is due to the death of the apical meristem, mainly due to insect damage or breakage. Plants developed from branch cuttings usually grow much faster in earlier years than seedling-derived plants, for example, elongating about 50–80 cm (20–31 in) per year, and branch from a lower height [6].

7. Phytochemistry [17]

7.1. Phytochemical Extracts. Percentage yield and physical characteristics of various extracts of leaf *Pandanus* are shown in Table 3.

7.2. Chemical Constituents. Phytochemical structures in *Pandanus odoratissimus* Linn. are included in Table 4.

The principle constituent is the kewda oil, isolated from the inflorescences of *Pandanus*. The chemical composition of this essential oil, obtained by hydrodistillation of staminate inflorescences of kewda (*P. odoratissimus*), when subjected to high resolution GC (gas chromatography) and GC-MS (gas chromatography and mass spectrometry) has been shown to yield ether (37.7%), terpene-4-ol (18.6%), α-terpineol (8.3%) and 2-phenylethyl alcohol (7.5%), benzyl benzoate (11%), viridine (8.8%), and germacrene-B (8.3%) along with a small amount of benzyl salicylate, benzyl acetate, benzyl alcohol, and so forth; ethnobotanically kewda oil is used in earache, headache, arthritis, debility, giddiness, laxative, rheumatism, small pox, and spasms. The methanol and aqueous extracts of the leaves of *Pandanus* were subjected to preliminary phytochemical screening and they were tested for the presence of alkaloids, carbohydrates, proteins, steroids, sterols, phenols, tannins, terpenes, flavonoids, gums and mucilage, saponins, and glycosides [10]. The total phenolic content in the aqueous extract was ranged from 3.5 to 10.8% w/w phenolic which are the largest groups of phytochemicals and have been said to account for most of the antioxidants activity of plant extracts [21, 35]. Physcion, cirsilineol, n-triacontanol, β-sitosterol, camphosterol, daucosterol and palmitic acid, and steric acid in rhizomes have been reported [24].

Phytochemicals chemical analysis of the root extracts of *P. odoratissimus* led to the isolation of phenolic compounds, lignans type compounds, and some benzofuran derivative. α-terpineol, β-carotene, β-sitosterol, benzyl-benzoate, pinoresinol germacrene-B, vitamin C, viridine. tangeterine, 5,8-hydroxy-7 methoxy-flavone, vanidine. Among them,

TABLE 2: Plant monograph.

Biogeography and ecology
Plant name: *Pandanus odoratissimus* Linn
Kingdom: Plantae-plants
Subkingdom: Tracheobionta
Family: Pandanaceae
Genus: *Pandanus* L. F.
Species: *Pandanus odoratissimus*
[9, 10]
Botanical description
Flowers
Male flowers
A large, terminal, pendulous, compound, leafy, raceme, the leaves of which are white, linear-oblong, pointed, and concave; in the axill of each, there is a single thyrsus of simple, small racemes, of long-pointed, depending anthers; they are not sessile, but raised from the rachis of the raceme by tapering filaments.
Female flowers
A different plant, terminal and solitary, having no other calyx or corol than the termination of the three rows of leaves forming three imbricate fascicles of white floral leaves, like those of the male raceme, which stand at equal distances, round the base of the young fruit. Germs numerous, collected in firm wedge-shape angular bundles from six to ten or more (these form the compound germs of the future drupes), closely impacted round the receptacle.
Fruit
compound; oval, from five to eight inches in diameter, and from six to ten long, weighing from four to eight pounds; rough, rich orange-colour, composed of drupes numerous, wedge-shape, angular; when ripe, their large or exterior ends are detached from one another and covered with a firm, deeper orange-colored skin; apices flat, consisting of as many angular, somewhat convex, tubercles, as there are cells in the drupe, each crowned with the withered stigma, internally; the exterior half of these drupes (next the apex) consists of dry spongy cavities, their lower part next to the core or common receptacle is yellow, consisting of a rich-looking, yellow pulp, intermixed with strong fibres; here the nut is lodged.
Nut
Each drupe compound, top-shape, exceedingly hard, angular, containing as many cells as there are divisions on the apex of the drupe; each cell is perforated above and below.
Seed
Single, oblong, smooth, adhering lengthways to a small fascicle of strong, white fibers, which pass through the perforation of the cell. By far the greatest numbers of these cells are barren. It is a native of the warmer parts of Asia. All soils and situations seem to suit it equally well; it flowers chiefly during the rainy season. It grows readily from branches, whence it is rare to find the full grown ripe fruit. The male is by far the most common, a circumstance merely accidental; for I have seen some old extensive hedges entirely female, owing to their having been originally a female plant or plants nearest to these places.
Trunk
A plant may be found with a single, pretty v erect one, often feet in height, and a ramous round head; but this is seldom, for it is generally in form of a very large, ramous, spreading bush. From the stems or larger branches issue large carrot-shape, obtuse-pointed, roots, descending till they come to the ground, into which they enter and then divide. The substance of the most solid wood is something like that of a cabbage stem and by age acquires a woody hardness on the outside.
Leaves
confluent, stem-clasping, closely imbricated in three spiral rows, round the extremities of the branches, bowing; from three to five feet long, tapering to a very long fine triangular point, very smooth and glossy, margins and back armed with very fine sharp spines; those on the margins point forward, those of the back point sometimes one way, sometimes the other style.
Stigma
Single, oval, grooved lengthwise, yellow, affixed to the outside of a two-lipped umbilicus on the apex of the germ. It is the tender white leaves of the flowers (chiefly those of the male) that yield that most delightful fragrance, for which they are so universally and deservedly esteemed; and of all the perfumes that I know, it is by far the richest and most powerful. The lower yellow pulpy part of the drupe is sometimes eaten by the natives in times of scarcity and famine, and the tender white base of the leaves are also eaten raw or boiled, at such melancholy times. The taste of the pulpy part of the drupe is to me very disagreeable. The fusiform roots, already mentioned, are composed of tough fibers; they are so soft and spongy as to serve the natives for corks; the leaves also are composed of longitudinal, tough, useful fibers.

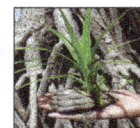

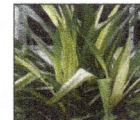

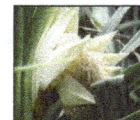

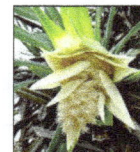

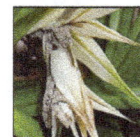

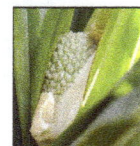

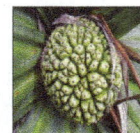

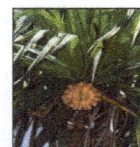

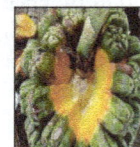

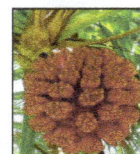

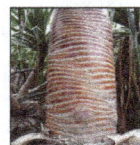

TABLE 2: Continued.

Root
The subterranean root system is concentrated in the surface soil layers. Apart from the aerial and prop roots, the tree's root system is unlikely to interfere with maintenance or recreational activities, lawns, or structures such as sidewalks or foundations [1].

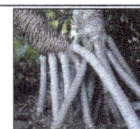

TABLE 3: Phytochemical extracts and their characteristics.

Extracts	% dry wt. in g.	Colour	Odour	Consistency
Alcoholic	11.43	Blackish green	Own characteristic	Sticky
		Successive extraction		
Petroleum Ether (40–60°C)	2.08	Dark brown	Own characteristic	Waxy
Chloroform	2.66	Dark Green	Own characteristic	Powder
Ethyl acetate	1.91	Brownish yellow	Own characteristic	Sticky
n-Butanol	2.11	Brown	Own characteristic	Sticky
Methanol	8.24	Reddish Brown	Own characteristic	Sticky

pinoresinol and 3,4-bis(4-hydroxy-3-methoxybenzyl)tetrahydrofuran showed strong antioxidative activities when BHA was used as a standard in the thiocyanate method. The new compounds were identified as 4-hydroxy-3-(2′,3′-dihydroxy-3′-methylbutyl)-benzoic acid methyl ester and 3-hydroxy-2-isopropenyl-dihydro-benzofuran-5-carboxylic acid methyl ester, by spectroscopic analysis.

The methanol extract of *P. odoratissimus* was subjected to column chromatography to isolate a total of 15 compounds. Steroids, including phytosteroid mixtures; a-spin sterol and stigmast-7-en-3b-ol mixture; a-spinasterol caproate; stigmast-4-en-6b-ol-3-one and three phenolic compounds; vanillin (1); 2 (E)-3-(3′-methoxy-4-hydroxyphenyl)-prop-2-enal (2); 4-hydroxy-3-(2′,3′-dihydroxy-3′-methyl-butyl)-benzoic acid methyl ester (3) and a new benzofuran derivative, 3-hydroxy-2-isopropenyl-dihydrobenzofuran-5-carboxylic acid methyl ester (4); plus six lignans; eudesmin (5); kobusin (6); pinoresinol (7); epipinoresinol (8); de-4′-O-methyleudesmin (9); and 3,4-bis(4-hydroxy-3-methoxy-benzyl)-tetrahydrofuran (10), were isolated and identified by comparing their data with authentic materials on the basis of their mass, UV, IR, and 1H and 13C NMR spectra [36]. And total synthesis of four *Pandanus* alkaloid: Pandamarilactonine-A, and B, and their chemical precursors non Pandamarilactonine-A and B [37].

8. Nutritional Aspects and Staple Food (Figure 2 and Table 5)

8.1. Staple Food. Pandanus fruits are a staple food in parts of Micronesia including the Marshall Islands, Federated States of Micronesia, and Kiribati providing up to 50% of energy intake [11, 15]. They are also widely consumed on Tokelau and Tuvalu [11]. In some places the consumption of *Pandanus* has decreased in recent decades due to the availability of imported foods; for example, *Pandanus* was formerly a major staple food in Nauru [38]. In Micronesia adults may commonly consume 20 fresh keys or about 1 kg (2.2 lb) of fruit per day. The fruit pulp is preserved in several different ways. A paste, which is compared to dates in taste, texture, and appearance, is made by boiling and baking the keys, followed by extracting, processing, and drying the pulp. Cultivars with large amounts of pulp are preferred, and the taste differs among cultivars. On average, 100 g *Pandanus* paste provides 321 kilocalories, 2.2 g protein, 134 mg calcium, 108 mg phosphorus, 5.7 mg iron, 0.04 mg thiamin, 2 mg vitamin C [14–16], and from 390 to 724 μg/100 g beta-carotene (a carotenoid that is a precursor to vitamin A), depending on variety and coloration [12, 13]. Fresh *Pandanus* is an important source of vitamin C. Preserved *Pandanus* pulp mixed with coconut cream makes a tasty, sweet food item. *Pandanus* can also be made into flour that is consumed in different ways, usually prepared as a drink (Figure 2).

8.2. Fruit. The keys of selected edible cultivated varieties, those with low amounts of calcium oxalate crystals, are consume draw or cooked. Juice and jam may also be prepared from the fruit. In parts of Micronesia, chewing *Pandanus* keys is usually done outside of meal times and is a pleasurable, highly social activity. Adults may typically consume 20–50 keys daily during the main fruiting seasons [11].

A 100 g portion of edible pericarp is mainly comprised of water (80 g) and carbohydrates (17 g). There are also significant levels of beta-carotene (19 to 19,000 μg) and vitamin C (5 mg), and small amounts of protein (1.3 mg), fat (0.7 mg), and fiber (3.5 g) [11–13]. The edible flesh of deeper yellow- and orange-colored varieties contain higher provitamin A carotenoid levels. The fruit of these varieties has considerable potential for alleviating vitamin A deficiency in Micronesia [11]. As carotenoid-rich food may protect against diabetes, heart disease, and cancer, the consumption of *Pandanus* may also alleviate these serious emerging problems of the Pacific. *Pandanus* fruit is also a useful source of vitamin C (ascorbic acid), thiamine, riboflavin, and niacin (vitamin B-3) [14, 15]. The fruit of wild forms of *Pandanus* contains oxalate crystals that irritate the mouth unless broken down by cooking.

TABLE 4: Phytochemical structures in *Pandanus*.

Chemical name	Chemical structures
Norpandamarilactonine-A	
Pandamarilacton-32	
Norpandamarilactonine-A	
Norpandamarilactonine-B	
Pandamarilactone-1 ($C_{18}H_{25}NO_4$)	
Pandamarilactonine-A ($C_{18}H_{25}NO_4$)	
Pandanamine ($C_{18}H_{23}NO_4$)	
Pandamarilactonine-C, -D	

TABLE 4: Continued.

Chemical name	Chemical structures
Norpandamarilactonine-A	
Pandanamine	
Pandamarilactone-31	
Artifact	
A compound which is a not "Natural product" ($C_{18}H_{23}NO_4$)	
Pandamarine	

TABLE 4: Continued.

Chemical name	Chemical structures
Pandamarilactam-3y	
Ascorbic acid (vitamin C)	
Riboflavin (vitamin B$_2$)	
Thiamine (vitamin B$_1$)	
Nicotinic acid/niacin (vitamin B$_3$)	

The ripe fruit of wild forms may be consumed following cooking and straining the pericarp, but they are not especially palatable or sweet (Table 5).

8.3. Nut/Seed. The small seeds of a few varieties of *P. tectorius* are eaten. A similar species, *P. dubius*, has larger seeds that are eaten.

8.4. Beverage/Drink/Tea. Juice pressed from the fruits is sweet and slightly acid with a pungent flavor [15]. It is being produced commercially in the Marshall Islands.

9. Traditional Uses and Products

Different parts of the *Pandanus* plant are used to provide a myriad of end products throughout the Pacific Islands, especially on atolls. The trunk and large branches are commonly used for building materials in house construction and for ladders. They are also used to make headrests/hard pillows, vases, and fish traps, as sources of glue or caulking for canoes, to extract cream from grated coconuts, and as an aid in making string. Trunks and branches may be burnt for fuel wood or used to make compost. Prop or aerial roots are used in fabrication of house walls and as supports, basket handles,

Leaves
Fruit

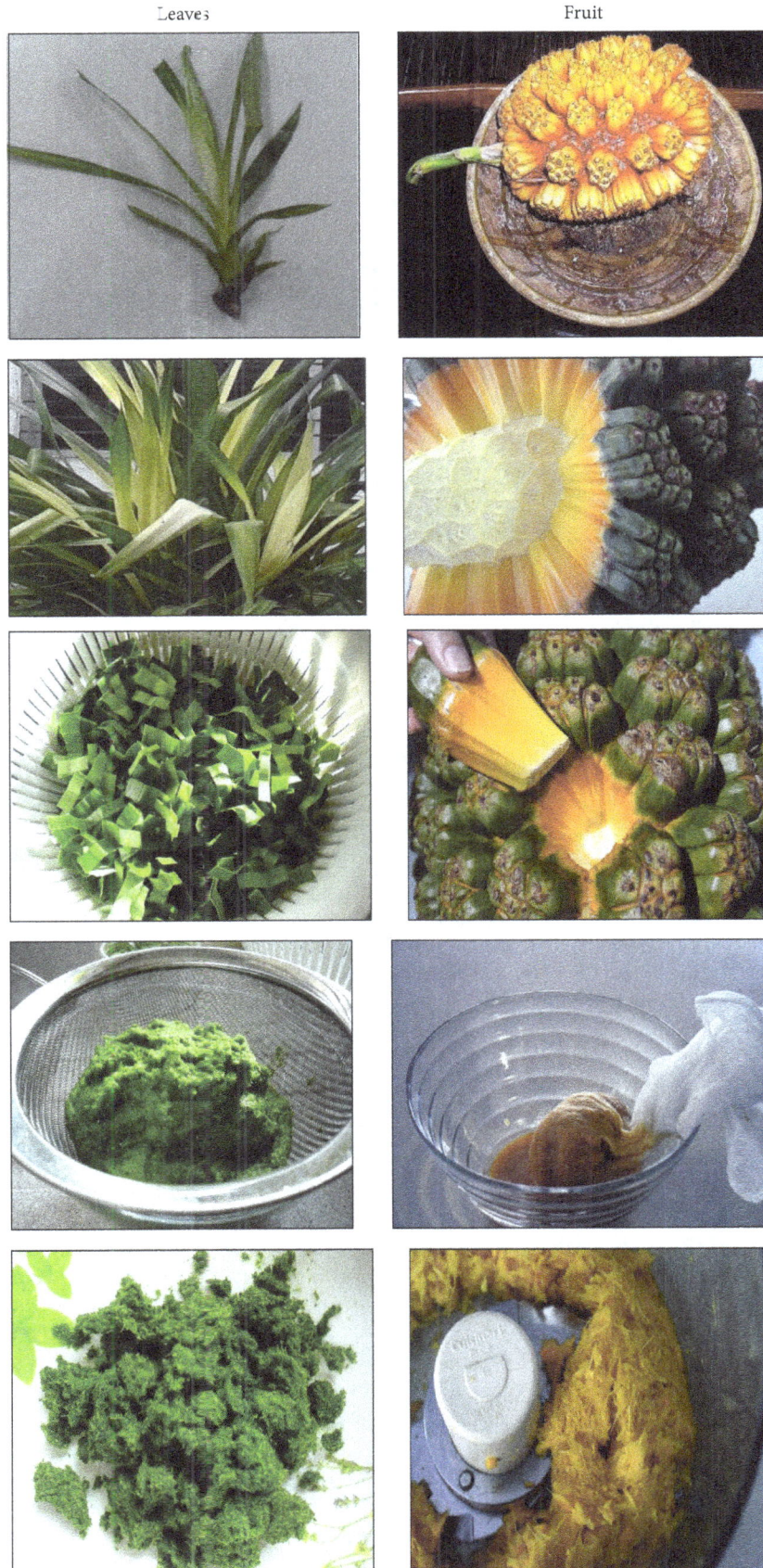

Figure 2: Continued.

Leaves   Fruit

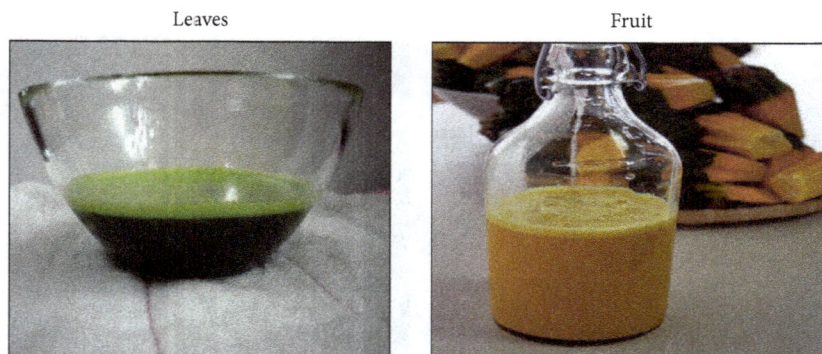

FIGURE 2: Nutritional aspects and staple food of *Pandanus*.

TABLE 5: Nutritional aspects of *Pandanus* or screw pines.

	Edible pericarp*	*Pandanus* paste#	References
Per 100 g of it Contents of pandan	228 kilocalories, water (80 g), carbohydrates (17 g), beta-carotene (19 to 19,000 µg) vitamin C (5 mg), protein (1.3 mg), fat (0.7 mg), fiber (3.5 g)	321 kilocalories, 2.2 g protein, 134 mg calcium, 103 mg phosphorus, 5.7 mg iron, 0.04 mg thiamin, 2 mg vitamin C, 390 to 724 µg beta-carotene (vitamin A)	([11–13])* ([14–16])# [12, 13]
Pandanus pulp	Usually prepared as a drink; mixed with coconut cream makes a tasty, sweet food item		[12, 13]
Flesh of deeper yellow- and orange-colored pandan keys	Adults may consume 20–50 keys typically; highly pleasurable, 50% of energy intake		[11]
	As carotenoid (provitamin-A) rich food may protect against diabetes, heart disease, and cancer and alleviate these serious emerging problems		[11]
Fresh *Pandanus* fruit	Vitamin C (ascorbic acid), thiamine, riboflavin, and niacin (vitamin B-3)		[14, 15]
	Juice and jam In parts of Micronesia, chewing		[11, 15]

paintbrushes, and skipping ropes. They are also used to produce dyes and in production of traditional medicines. The leaves of selected varieties are treated by soaking in the sea and/or boiling or heating and dying and are then used to make mats, baskets (for ladies and to keep valuables), hats, fans, pillows, canoe sails (formerly), toys, and other plaited wares. The leaves are also used for thatching (both walls and roofs) and for making compost, including special composting baskets woven around the base of giant swamp taro, cigarette wrappers, balls for children's games, and ornaments. They are used for traditional medicines and as a cooking aid in some recipes. The young leaves are used in traditional medicine and for lancing boils, making fans, decoration, and pig feed. Throughout the atoll island countries of the central/northern Pacific, the fleshy keys of the fruits of many traditionally selected, named, and cultivated varieties are consumed fresh

or made into various preserved foods. The fruits are also consumed in Solomon Islands and Papua New Guinea. In Polynesia the fragrant, ornamental fruits of different varieties are strung into leis or garlands and used to make perfume. The fibrous, dried, mature drupes are used as paint brushes for painting tapa, for fuel, and for compost, and as fishing line floats. In Kiribati the fruit may also be used as bait for catching lobster. The fragrant male flowers are used to scent coconut oil, perfume tapa cloth, and make garlands.

9.1. Animal Fodder. Leaves, particularly young leaves, are recorded as providing fodder for domestic animals such as pigs and horses.

9.2. Masticant/Stimulant. Male *Pandanus* flowers have been credited with aphrodisiac properties in Marshall Islands.

9.3. Beautiful/Fragrant Flowers. The highly fragrant male flowers are widely used for decoration.

9.4. Timber. The stems are used in house construction and also for making ladders, especially on atoll islands. Male trees have hard, solid trunks with a yellow interior containing dark brown fiber bundles. The male wood is very strong, but brittle, meaning that it can suddenly break under a heavy load. It is also a difficult wood to split. Trunks of female trees are hard on the outside, but soft, pithy, or juicy in the interior [39]. Slats made from the clean, dried aerial/prop roots are used for walls of houses and food cupboards.

9.5. Fuel Wood. In the northern Pacific, the discarded, dried keys are highly prized as fuel wood for cooking because they are slow burning and therefore preferred for barbecues. The trunk and branches are occasionally used as fuel wood where other fuel wood is scarce, such as on atolls.

9.6. Craft Wood/Tools. The wood has many craft uses, such as headrests/pillows, vases, and as an aid for string making and extracting coconut cream. It was formerly used to make weapons (lances and batons). When the flesh is removed from the inner end of a dried key, fibrous bristles are exposed. The bristle end can be used as a brush for decorating tapa, with the hard, woody outer end acting as a handle. Fish traps are made out of the aerial roots in Kiribati.

9.7. Canoe/Boat/Raft Making. The trunk of one variety in the Marshall Islands is used to make the masts of traditional canoes. In Hawaii *Pandanus* leaves were the traditionally main material for making canoes ails [40].

9.8. Fiber/Weaving/Clothing. In many Pacific countries *Pandanus* leaves are used to weave traditional items of attire, including mats for wearing around the waist in Tonga, as well as hats and various types of baskets.

9.9. Rope/Cordage/String. The roots are made into skipping ropes and basket handles. String or cordage is made from the cleaned and dried prop roots.

9.10. Wrapping/Parcelization. The leaves are used to wrap tobacco/cigarettes in Micronesia.

9.11. Thatch/Roofing/Mats. *Pandanus* leaves are used to weave traditional floor mats in many Pacific countries, as well as in the construction of traditional houses (thatch for walls and roofing). A roof made from *Pandanus* leaves is said to last about 15 years, while one of coconut leaves may last only 3 years [39].

9.12. Resin/Gum/Glue/Latex. The trunk is a source of glue or caulking for canoes.

9.13. Body Ornamentation/Garlands. Leaves, often neatly cut, fragrant fruits, and flowers are used in making garlands or leis.

9.14. Ceremonial/Religious Importance. *Pandanus* is sometimes considered to have supernatural and magical properties in parts of Micronesia and Hawaii. In Kiribati it may be used as a ceremonial food, while in Indonesia the male flowers are used in ceremonies.

9.15. Other Uses. In Kiribati and the Marshall Islands the leaves are formed into a ball for use in a kicking game. The trunks of female trees are hard on the outside but soft or juicy in the interior. The female trunks have been used as water pipes after removing the soft interior [39].

In the Philippines, pandan *leaves* are being cooked along with rice to incorporate the flavor and smell to it. As can be observed, the uses of the pandan tree are not limited to cooking uses. Its leaves and *roots* are found to have medicinal benefits. Such parts of the plant have been found to have essential oils, tannin, alkaloids, and glycosides, which are the reasons for the effective treatment of various health concerns. It functions as a pain reliever, mostly for headaches and pain caused by arthritis, and even hangover. It can also be used as antiseptic and antibacterial, which makes it ideal for healing wounds.

In the same manner, a preparation derived from the *bark* of this plant may be used to address skin problems. Many people have also discovered that it is an effective remedy for cough. In India, pandan leaves are being used to treat skin disorders like leprosy and smallpox. The bitter tasting quality of the leaves makes it ideal for health problems which include, but are not limited to, diabetes fever, ulcer, and wounds.

In Hawaii, pandan *flowers* are being chewed by mothers who later give the chewed flowers to their children, as laxative. The juice extracted from pounded roots of this tree are issued and mixed with other ingredients to ease chest pains. Also, it is used as tonic for women who have just given birth and who are still in weak states. Pandan flowers have also been traced with characteristics that function as aphrodisiac. Pandan also manifests anticancer activities, and that is why modern researches in the United States have subjected this plant for further experiments and investigation [41].

Sometimes it is oven dried and kept in bottles for preservation until it is used. This product is mostly available in western countries in dried form. Other than that there are many recipes. To impart its aroma into chicken, pieces of marinated chicken are enclosed in a clever wrapping of "*Pandanus*" leaves and grilled or deep fried. The leaves which are pounded and strained (or blended with a little water) impart flavor and color into cakes and sweets. This flavor is a delicacy to Asians and is as important as vanilla to Westerners. These leaves are used to make small containers for sweets, jelly, and puddings. Some people wrap their hot foods using these leaves as they produce aroma when the food is still warm. These plants can be easily propagated by side shoot cuttings taken from the base of the plant. The higher the maturity of the cutting is, the easier the establishment is [41].

TABLE 6: Ethnomedicinal uses of *P. odoratissimus*.

Plant parts	Medicinal uses
Leaves	Leprosy, aphrodisiac, scabies, anxiety and heart disease, leucoderma, tumors, leprosy, antiepileptic, anticonvulsions, and skin disease Female rats fertility regulator [17]
Flower	Headaches, earaches, antispasmodic, and aphrodisiac [17]
Root	Antidiabetics, antidote, abortifacient; skin diseases, leprosy, scabies, and syphilis [18]
Oil	Rheumatoid arthritis, skin disease, earache, headache, arthritis, debility, depurative, giddiness, laxative, leprosy, small *Pandanus odoratissimus*, and spasms
Fruit	Vat, kaph, urinary discharge, and leprosy, male aphrodisiac [17]

Supercritical carbon dioxide (SC-CO2) and Soxhlet extraction using hexane as solvent were used to extract 2-acetyl-1-pyrroline (2-AP) from pandan leaves. The effect of different extraction pretreatments such as particle size and drying on the extraction yield and concentration of 2-AP were investigated. The identification and quantification of 2-AP were carried out by gas chromatography-mass spectrometry and gas chromatography-flame ionization detector, respectively. This work aims to provide an understanding of the phenomena that occur during cooking and storage, typically on the changes of 2-AP absorption when cooking rice grains with pandan leaves. The parameters investigated were cooking method of excess and optimal water conditions. Even though low in yield and the fact that the 2-AP concentration was obtained from supercritical carbon dioxide extraction, the extracts were pure without any contamination. The grinding and freeze-drying method revealed the best pretreatments for supercritical extraction. The absorption of 2-AP during the cooking of rice grains did not smoothly increase with time. This unexpected result indicated that the phenomena occurring during cooking are quite complex. This work also quantified the potential of pandan leaves to enhance the flavour of cooked rice, particularly under excess water conditions. Storage for 15 min at 24.0 ± 1.0°C is considered as the optimum time for obtaining cooked rice with a high quality of flavor [42].

10. Ethnomedicinal Uses

Pandanus is a very important medicinal plant, with certain varieties sometimes preferred for particular treatments. Leaves, especially the basal white section of young leaves, and roots are used. In Kiribati, *Pandanus* leaves are used in treatments for cold/flu, hepatitis, dysuria, asthma, boils, and cancer, while the roots are used in a decoction to treat hemorrhoids. In Hawaii the main parts used in making traditional medicines are the fruits, male flowers, and aerial roots [40]. These are used individually or in combination with other ingredients to treat a wide range of illnesses, including digestive and respiratory disorders. The root is used in Palauto to make a drink that alleviates stomach cramps, and the leaves are used to alleviate vomiting [43]. The root is also known for its use in traditional medicine in Pohnpei for STD'S, namely, syphilis [17, 18, 44] (Table 6).

11. Pharmacology

A summary of reported pharmacological activity of *Pandanus odoratissimus* is shown in Table 7.

11.1. Acute Oral Toxicity Study

11.1.1. In Mice. Selected animals both female and male mice administered with the extract at a dose of 2000 mg/kg showed no toxicity during the experimentation period. In both sexes of mice, body weight gain of treatment rats was not changed significantly relative to that of control. While conducting the toxicity studies, animals were observed continuously for any general behavioral changes. A significant reduction in spontaneous locomotors motility, drowsiness, and remarkably quiet behaviors were observed. Thus, the extract of *P. odoratissimus* with an LD_{50} > 2000 mg/kg is considered nontoxic through acute exposure in mice [8, 24].

11.1.2. In Rats. Administration of hydroethanol leaf extract of *P. odoratissimus* Linn. 2000 mg/kg/p.o. dose did not show behavioral change (Erwin's test) at continuous observation for 4 h and intermittent of 48 h. No mortality was observed during total observation period of 14 days. LD_{50} was found to be more than 2000 mg/kg calculated by AOT425 *statpgm* (Version: 1.0), Acute Oral Toxicity (OECD Test Guideline 425) Statistical Program (AOT Report) on the basis of AOT425 report 200 and 300 mg/kg doses were selected for evaluating effect as antiepileptic and for fertility effect of *P. odoratissimus* Linn. [19].

11.2. Antioxidant Activity. The antioxidant activity of methanolic extracts of leaves of *P. odoratissimus* by four different *in vitro* models. The lipid peroxidation was assayed by estimating the thiobarbituric acid reactive substances (TBARS) in normal rat by liver homogenates. The reduced glutathione (GSH) was assayed in liver homogenates of different concentrations of *Pandanus* methanol extract using the method of Ellman et al. The nitric oxide (NO) scavenging activity and 1,1-diphenyl, 2-picryl hydrazyl (DPPH) radical scavenging activity were measured using the methods of Sreejayan et al. and Shimada et al., respectively, using spectrophotometer. Vitamin E and normal saline were used as reference standard and control for all four by *in vitro* type of bioassy methods

TABLE 7: A summary of reported pharmacological activity of *P. odoratissimus* [17].

Species/method used	Property	Source
	Antiepileptic and anticonversant	[19]
	Antioxidant	[20, 21]
	Anti-inflammatory	[22]
	Acute anti-inflammatory	[10]
	Analgesic	[23]
Wistar rats	Antidiabetic	[24–26]
	Diuretic activity	[25]
	Hepatotoxic	[27]
	Hepatoprotective & hepatocurative activity	[27, 28]
	Fertility enhancer and regulation activity, in female rats	[17]
	Sex stimulant activity, in male rats	
	Aphrodisiac	[17]
Swiss albino mice	Antidiabetic	[24–26]
	CNS depressant activity	[8]
Bacillus subtilis, *Escherichia coli*, *Staphylococcus aureus*, and *Candida albicans*	Antimicrobial activity	[29–31]
Aspergillus flavus, *Microsporum nanum*, *Epidermophyton floccosum*, *Trichophyton tonsurans*, Mentagrophytes, and Trichophyton verrucosum	Antifungal activity	[32]
Human viruses, herpes simplex, type I (HSV-1), and influenza virus (H1N1)	Antiviral activity	[33]
Inhibition of hydroxyl radicals	Free scavenging activity	[21]
Adult Indian earthworms, *Pheretima posthuma*	Anthelmintic activity	[34]

antioxidant measurement assays. The results showed significant antioxidant activity of *Pandarus* methanol extract in all four by *in vitro* type of bioassay methods used in this study and the IC_{50} (the half maximal inhibitory concentration of an inhibitor that is required for 50% inhibition of antioxidant activity) of plant extract was comparable to that of vitamin E, the reference standard compound used in this study. It is concluded that the methanolic extract of leaves of *P. odoratissimus* has significant antioxidant activity [20, 21].

11.3. Anti-Inflammatory Activity. The anti-inflammatory activity was estimated by carrageenan-induced acute and formalin-induced chronic paw edema models in rats. The methanolic extract of *P. odoratissimus* was given in the doses of 25, 25, and 100 mg/kg^{-1}. The plant extract at the dose of 100 mg kg^{-1} showed significant anti-inflammatory activity at 3 h observation where, it caused increase in inhibition of paw edema by carrageenan-induced acute (68%) and the

formalin-induced chronic (64.2%) paw edema models with standard drug diclofenac sodium in rats [22].

11.4. Acute Anti-Inflammatory Activity. Plants are widely used in the various traditional systems of medicine like Ayurveda, Siddha, and Unani for their analgesic, anti-inflammatory, and antipyretic activity. *P. odoratissimus* (kewda) has been used in rheumatic fever, rheumatism, and rheumatoid arthritis. The chemical composition of this essential oil, obtained by hydrodistillation of staminate inflorescences of kewda includes more than sixty components. The major components of the hydrodistilled kewda oil are 2-phenyl ethyl methyl ether terpene-4-ol, α-terpineol, 2-phenyl ethyl alcohol benzyl benzoate, and so forth. Kewda oil is traditionally used in earache, headache, arthritis, debility, giddiness, laxative, and rheumatism. Both methanolic and hydroalcoholic extracts were tested in rodent models by carrageenan-induced paw edema, albumin induced plantar edema, acetic acid induced vascular permeability, and castor induced diarrhoea. In all these animal models both extracts have shown significant anti-inflammatory activity [10].

11.5. Analgesic Activity. Analgesic activity of aqueous extract of *P. fascicularis* Lam. at doses (400 and 800 mg/kg) by using hot plate models, tail-flick method in rats. and the writhing model of mouse and compared with the analgesic action of codeine and aspirin. *Pandanus* aqueous extract revealed significant analgesic activity by both central ($P < 0.001$) and peripheral ($P < 0.001$) mechanisms in this study, which is comparable to that of codeine and aspirin, and this favors the use of *Pandanus* aqueous extract in rheumatism and rheumatoid arthritis in traditional medicine [23].

11.6. Antidiabetic Activity. The roots of *P. odoratissimus* aqueous extract were tested for its effect on blood glucose levels in normal and diabetic rats. Hypoglycemia was observed in basal condition when tested at an oral dose of 75, 150, and 300 mg/kg body weight. The ethanolic extract has displayed a significant dose-dependent antihyperglycemic activity in oral glucose tolerance test and also found to reduce the increased blood glucose in alloxan-induced diabetic rats (31% at 150 mg/kg and 51% at 300 mg/kg body weight). Chronic administration (10 days) of the ethanolic extract of extract of root significantly reduced the blood glucose in alloxan-induced diabetic rats. The extract was also found to reduce the increased blood urea and inhibit the body weight reduction and leucopenia induced by alloxan administration. The ethanolic extract was also found to effectively scavenge the DPPH and lipid peroxide free radicals by *in vitro* type of bioassay methods with an IC_{50} value of 10 and 8 μg/mL, respectively. The preliminary phytochemical examination reveals the presence of flavanoids and tannins, which may be attributed to observed antioxidant and significant antihyperglycemic properties [24–26, 45].

11.7. Antimicrobial Activity. The antimicrobial effects of petroleum ether, chloroform, and hydroalcoholic extracts of *P. odoratissimus* leaf against *Bacillus subtilis*, *Escherichia coli*, *Staphlococcus aureus*, and *Candida albicans*. In terms of antimicrobial effects, all the three extracts exhibited effective inhibition zones against gram-positive bacteria, that is, *S. aureus*, *B. subtilis*. However, they were ineffective against gram-negative bacteria (*E. coli* and *P. aeruginosa*) and fungi (*C. albicans*). The minimum inhibitory concentration (MIC) of hydroalcoholic, chloroform, and petroleum ether extracts was found to be 25, 50, and 50 mg/mL, respectively, against gram-positive bacteria. Out of three extracts, hydroalcoholic extract showed good antimicrobial activity. The phytochemical study showed the presence of alkaloids and flavonoids in hydroalcoholic extract, which might be responsible for its good antimicrobial activity [29, 30].

11.8. Antifungal Activity. Keratophilic fungi, a type of dermatophytes, cause infection to hair, glabrous skin, and nails of human beings and animals. Soil is well known to be supporting the transient existence of them. The volatile plant oils

have been of concern recently to develop a new antifungal agent. Four different commercially available Itra-Bella (*Lonicera x bella zabel*), kewda (*Pandanus odoratissimus*), Rajnigandha (*Polianthes tuberosa*), and Mogra (*Jasminum sambac*) for their antifungal activity against the *Aspergillus flavus*, *Trichophyton mentagrophytes*, *Trichophyton tonsurans*, *Trichophyton verrucosum*, *Epidermophyton floccosum*, and *Microsporum nanum* were isolated from soil.

The diameters of zone of inhibition formed by Bella, Rajnigandha, kewda, and Mogra against *T. tonsurans* were observed to be 47 mm, 34 mm, 17 mm, and 30 mm, respectively, while it was 30 mm, 22 mm, 15 mm, and 17 mm against the *M. nanum*. The activity was observed quite low against the *Aspergillus flavus* with 17 mm, 15 mm, 11 mm, and 13 mm inhibitory zone shown by Bella, Rajnigandha, kewda, and Mogra, respectively, while it was intermediate against the *Epidermophyton floccosum* with 27 mm, 20 mm, 21 mm, and 15 mm of zone inhibition. Thus, the maximum antifungal effect was shown by Bella with 47 mm inhibitory zone against the *T. tonsurans*, and the minimum was 11 mm shown by kewda against the *Aspergillus flavus*. Significantly, the antifungal activity shown by few Itra was comparatively better than control (antifungal drugs, Terbinafine, Itraconazole, and Fluconazole) [32].

11.9. Antiviral Activity. A lectin, designated Pandanin, was isolated from the saline extract of the leaves of *P. amaryllifolius*, using ammonium sulfate precipitation, affinity chromatography on mannose-agarose, and molecular size exclusion by gel filtration. Pandanin is an unglycosylated protein with a molecular mass of 8.0 kDa both after gel filtration and on sodium dodecyl sulfate-polyacrylamide gel electrophoresis, indicating that it is a single polypeptide chain. These first isolated 10 residues of the N-terminal amino acid sequence are DNILFSDSTL. An analysis of the sequence of first 30 amino acids at the N-terminal region shows that Pandanin has about 50–60% the quality of being similar or corresponding in position or value or structure or function (homology) to those of mannose-specific lectins reported from monocot plants. Pandanin exhibits hemagglutinating activity toward rabbit erythrocytes, and its activity could be reversed exclusively by mannose and mannan. Pandanin also possesses antiviral activities against human viruses, herpes simplex virus type-1 (HSV-1), and influenza virus (H1N1) with 3 days of EC_{50} of 2.94 and 15.63 μM, respectively [33].

11.10. Hepatoprotective and Hepatocurative Activity. In developing countries like India, hepatic disorders are steadily increasing. *Ketaki* (*P. odoratissimus* Roxb) is an important traditional medicine used in northern Karnataka (India) for jaundice. The experimental model was adopted by Watanabe and Takita (1973) to evaluate the hepatoprotective and hepatocurative activities of a *Pandanus* root decoction on CCl_4 induced liver damage in albino rats. The degree of protective and curative activity was determined by measuring the levels of serum glutamate oxaloacetate transaminase (SGOT), serum glutamate pyruvate transaminase (SGPT), alkaline phosphatase (ALP), total serum bilirubin, and serum albumin. Histological studies and all haematological parameters have promoted the hepatocurative activity. *Pandanus* root decoction was found to be hepatocurative but not hepatoprotective [27, 28].

11.11. Hepatotoxic Activity.

The antioxidant effect of methanol extract of *P. odoratissimus* leaf in Wistar albino rats administered with carbon tetrachloride (CCl_4) at $1.5/kg^{-1}$ CCl_4 $1 mL/kg^{-1}$ in liquid paraffin 3 doses (i.p.) at 72 h interval. The extracts at the doses of 50 and 100 mg/kg^{-1} and (Liv-52) 25 mg/kg^{-1} were administered to the CCl_4 treated rats. The effect of extract and Liv-52 on serum transaminase (GOT, GPT), alkaline phosphatase (ALP), bilirubin, and total protein were measured in the rat induced by CCl_4. The effects of extract on lipid peroxidation (LPO), superoxide dismutase (SOD), catalase (CAT), glutathione (GSH), and vitamin E were estimated. The extract and Liv-52 produced significant ($P < 0.05$) effect by decreasing the activity of serum enzymes, bilirubin, uric acid, and lipid peroxidation and significantly ($P < 0.05$) increased in the level of SOD, CAT, GSH, vitamin E, and protein. Hence these results suggest that methanolic extract of *P. odoratissimus* has potent antioxidant properties [27].

11.12. Free Radicals Scavenging Activity.

Pandanus is used in traditional use as a Ayurvedic medicines and it is also famous for its frequency. The antioxidant activity of methanolic extract of *Pandanus* was studied by its ability to scavenge DPPH, nitric acid, superoxide radicals, and hydroxyl radicals. The plant extract shows antioxidant activity by 87.52% reducing the DPPH and 73.55% inhibition of nitric acid. The result also indicates maximum inhibition of superoxide radical's inhibition 74.12% and 78.14% inhibition of hydroxyl radicals. The butylated hydroxytoluene (BHT) was used as standard antioxidant [21].

11.13. Antidiuretic Activity.

The ethanol and aqueous extracts of *Pandanus* are claimed as an antidiuretic by some traditional practitioners. Furosemide was used as a diuretic agent to induce diuresis. Vasopressin (antidiuretic hormone; ADH) was used as a standard. The results demonstrated both the ethanol and aqueous extracts of *Pandanus* and ADH significantly impaired the total urine output. However, antidiuretic potential of ethanol extract was similar to that of ADH. The extracts caused a significant decrease in natriuresis and kaliuresis. It has the potential to impart therapeutic effect in diuretic [25].

11.14. Helminthic Activity.

P. odoratissimus Linn. is found in the tribal area of Koraput district and extensively used traditionally by the tribal people as anthelmintic, rheumatism, stimulant, headache, and antispasmodic. The preliminary investigation of phytochemical constituents of ethyl acetate and ethanol extracts of leaves of plant *P. odoratissimus*. The two doses (25 and 50 mg/mL) of extracts were evaluated for their anthelmintic activities on adult Indian earthworms, *Pheretima posthuma*. The activities are comparable with the standard drugs, piperazine citrate and albendazole. All the doses of ethyl acetate and ethanol extracts of *Pandanus*

showed better anthelmintic activity than the standard drug albendazole except ethyl acetate extract at 25 mg/mL of concentration. The extracts of ethyl acetate at concentration of 25 and 50 mg/mL showed lesser anthelmintic activity than the standard drug piperazine citrate. When the dose of the extract is increased, a gradual increase in anthelmintic activity was observed [34].

11.15. Antitumour Activity.

Antitumour activity of ethanol extract *Pandanus* was evaluated against Dalton's ascitic lymphoma (DAL) tumour model on dose-dependent manner. The activity was assessed using survival time, average increase in body weight haematological parameters, and solid tumour volume. Oral administration of alcoholic *Pandanus* extract increased the survival time and decreased the average body weight of the tumour bearing mice. After 14 days of inoculation, EPF was able to reverse the changes in the haematological parameters, protein and PCV consequent to tumour inoculation. Oral administration of EPF was effective in reducing solid tumour mass development induced by DAL cells. The results showed that EPF possess significant activity in dose-dependent manner [46].

11.16. CNS-Depressant Action.

The effect of methanolic extract of *P. odoratissimus* leaf on the CNS was studied by using different neuropharmacological paradigms including spontaneous motor activity, rota-rod performance, and potentiation of Pentobarbital sodium sleeping time in albino mice. Preliminary phytochemical evaluation and acute toxicity studies were also carried out where $LD_{50} > 2000$ mg/kg was considered nontoxic through acute exposure in rats by the oral route. The *Pandanus* extract (50, 100, and 200 mg/kg i.p.) produced a reduction in spontaneous motor activity, motor coordination and prolonged Pentobarbital sodium sleeping time. These observations suggest that the leaf of *P. odoratissimus* contains some active principles which possess potential CNS-depressant action [8].

11.17. Antiepileptic/Anticonvulsant Activity.

Increase in latency to seizures as well as reduction in duration and frequency of seizures indicated anticonvulsant activity. The selected extract was more effective in all models used except the strychnine-induced convulsions. *P. odoratissimus* ethanol extract (100 and 200 mg/kg body wt.) significantly ($P < 0.05$ to 0.01) shortened the duration of convulsions in maximum electroshock and picrotoxin induced seizures. Delay in the onset of convulsions in the two tests was significant ($P < 0.01$). Reduction in the frequency of seizures was also significant ($P < 0.05, 0.01$) in both tests. *P. odoratissimus* further delayed the onset of seizures in picrotoxin induced seizures model while producing (66.7 and 83.33%) protection against death in mice [19].

12. Pharmaceutical Uses

12.1. Tannin/Dye.

A black dye used in weaving is prepared from the roots in Kiribati. Charcoal from *Pandanus* was used in various mixtures to dye and waterproof canoes.

12.2. Cosmetic/Soap/Perfume. Male flowers picked from uncultivated *Pandanus* are used alone or in combination with other flowers to perfume coconut oil in Polynesia. An exquisite, uniquely Pacific perfume is made from the aromatic fruits of selected traditional cultivated varieties in the Cook Islands. In Southland Southeast Asia, the male flowers and preparations derived from them are used to scent clothes and incorporated into cosmetics, soaps, hair oils, and incense sticks. In Hawaii, the male flowers were used to scent tapa.

12.3. Pandan Edible Colouring and Flavouring Powder. A study on the production of spray-dried pandan (*P. amaryllifolius*) powder was conducted and optimized using response surface methodology (RSM). Parameters investigated include inlet temperature (170–200°C) and feed rate (6–12 rpm), with a preset outlet temperature of 90°C. The estimated regression coefficients (R^2) for the physicochemical characteristic and sensory responses of pandan powder were ≥0.800, except for overall acceptability. Some mathematical models could be developed with confidence based on the results from all responses. An optimum drying process for spray drying represents conditions that would yield acceptably high colour index (such as L value, a value, and b value), low moisture content, low water activity (a_w), high solubility and high colour, flavour, odour, and overall acceptability for sensory responses. Optimum conditions of 170°C inlet temperature and 6 rpm feed rate, with a constant outlet temperature of 90°C, were established for producing spray-dried pandan powder as an edible colouring and flavouring powder [47].

12.4. Separation of Divalent Metal Ions. Desorption by dead biomass has been studied on *P. amaryllifolius* Roxb (*Pandanus* leaves) by conducting batch experiments. The recovery of heavy metals such as lead and copper ions from biomass was examined using a variety of desorbing chemicals. This study aims to discover the best chemical which is able to leach the metal effectively with highest desorbing capacity. The results showed that HCl at pH 2 and 3.0 mM EDTA at pH 4.58 were effective in desorbing the copper and lead ions from the biomass. The recovery of copper is very feasible since over 90% of copper was removed from the biomass. The percentage of lead recovery is about 70%. In contrast, Na_2CO_3 and NaOH are not effective in desorbing both of the metals. The results indicated that low PH is preferable for desorbing the metal ions. The binding ability of HCl is explained using ion-exchanging principle. More concentrated protons are able to replace those ions thus regenerating the biomass. EDTA is functioning as polydentate ligands, which appear to grasp the metal between the six donor atoms. It was suggested that recovery of metal ions is mainly due to the strength of bonding between the fraction of functional group of biomass and metal ions. Recovery of the deposited metals can be accomplished because they can be released from the saturated biomass in a concentrated wash solution, which also regenerates the biomass for reuse. Desorbing chemicals such as HCl and EDTA have proved successful for desorbing the metal ions. Thus, biosorption of heavy metals by biomass will

be emerged as one of the alternative technologies in removing the heavy metals [48].

12.5. A Natural Cockroach Repellent Activity. Seven compounds and fractions prepared from pandan leaves (*P. amaryllifolius*) were evaluated for repellent activity against *Blattella germanica* Linn. using a modification of the linear tract olfactometer. 2-Acetyl-1-pyrroline, pandan essence, and the hexane-pandan extract were repellent (65–93% repellency) at all concentrations tested; the acetone-pandan extract was attractive at increasing concentrations (minimum of 62% attractancy); artificial pandan flavouring and the dichloromethane-pandan extract gave erratic results. Undiluted crude aqueous pandan extract displayed an attractancy of 62%. The potential of *P. amaryllifolius* as a natural and environmentally friendly pest management tool is discussed [49].

13. Analytical Evaluation

13.1. HPTLC Analysis for Polyphenols. A densitometry HPTLC analysis was performed for the development of characteristic finger printing profile. The *P. odoratissimus* methanolic extract of root was dissolved with HPLC grade methanol 100 mg/0.5 mL. The solution was centrifuged at contents which were centrifuged at 3000 rpm for 5 min and used for HPTLC analysis. Then 2 μL of the samples was loaded as 7 mm band length in the 10 × 10 Silica gel 60F254 TLC plate using Hamilton syringe and CAMAG LINOMAT 5 instrument. The samples loaded plate was kept in TLC twin through developing chamber (after saturation with solvent vapor) with respective mobile phase (polyphenolic compound) and the plate was developed in the respective mobile phase (toluene-acetone-formic acid 4.5 : 4.5 : 1) up to 90 mm. The developed plate was dried using hot air to evaporate solvents from the plate and sprayed with stannic chloride reagent. The plate was kept Photo-documentation chamber (CAMAG REPROSTAR 3) and captured the images at UV 366 nm. Finally, the plate was fixed in scanner stage and scanned at 254 nm. The upsurging interest in the health benefits of the Peak table, Peak display, and Peak densitogram was identified [50].

13.2. High Performance Liquid Chromatography. Fifteen (1–15) compounds including ten phenolic compounds and five flavonoids were isolated from the fruits of *Pandanus tectorius*. All of the compounds were isolated and purified by various column chromatographies especially by semipreparative high performance liquid chromatography (HPLC). Their structures were determined under the aid of spectral methods. All compounds were isolated from this medicinal plant for the first time. The biological activities of some compounds were discussed according to the results of related literature [51].

14. Conclusion

The scientific research on *P. odoratissimus* suggests a huge biological potential of this plant. It is strongly believed that detailed information as presented in this review on the phytochemical and various biological properties of the plant might provide detailed evidence for the use of this plant in different diseases.

Pandanus odoratissimus is said to be restorative, indolent, promoting a feeling of well-being and acting as a counter to tropical climates. It may be chewed as a breath sweetener or used as a preservative in foods. It is also believed to have health-related properties, including antiviral, antiallergy, antiplatelet, anti-inflammatory, antioxidant, and anticancer action. Ayurvedic science has found the medicinal action of essential oil yielded by the screw pine's highly scented flowers to be useful in headaches, earaches and as a liniment for rheumatic pains. The distilled water from flowers is used for inducing perspiration.

It is also prescribed as a stimulant aphrodisiac and an antispasmodic agent. The flowers are powdered and included in medicines, which are either sniffed like snuff or smoked for asthma and other bronchial infections [52]. The leaves are thought to be useful in leprosy, smallpox, scabies, and diseases of the heart and brain.

Preliminary qualitative chemical studies indicated the presence of lignan, isoflavones, phenolic contents, steroids, saponin, terpenoids, glycosides, tannins, flavonoids, and phenolic in the extract. And isoflavones, polyphenol, namely, lignan, are responsible for regulating the rat fertility [17]; maybe it is helpful for the regulating and enhancing the human fertility [17, 19, 53].

On the basis of biological activities of *P. odoratissimus*, crude extract and derived phytochemicals and their uses as pharmacological agents in traditional and modern research are possible but will first require more clinical trials and product development. The current evidence is largely limited to correlation between identified phytochemicals and mode of action for any pharmacological activity.

Mechanisms of action studies are expected to lead the way into the discovery of new agents with improved and intriguing pharmacological properties. This could be achieved by molecular modeling studies involving interaction of bioactive phytochemicals from *P. odoratissimus* with their respective molecular and therapeutic targets. The extract of *P. odoratissimus* could be further explored in the future as a source of useful phytochemicals for the pharmaceutical industry [17].

Conflict of Interests

The authors declare that there is no conflict of interests regarding the publication of this paper.

Acknowledgments

The authors are thankful to Professor T. J. Sawant Sir, founder secretary of Jayawant Shikshan Prasarak Mandal, Pune, and Dr. V. I. Hukkeri, Principal, for providing all necessary facilities to carry out the present review. Authors are also thankful to National Informatics Centre (NIC), Pune, India; Botanical Survey of India (BSI), Pune; and University of Pune, Pune, India, for contribution in this review. They thank Dr. S.D. Ambavade, Dr. Tushar Shelke, and Dr. Sneha Prafulla Adkar, Faculty of Pharmacology Department, for their kind help and suggestion during review and research.

References

[1] K. R. Kirtikar, B. D. Basu, and E. Blatter, *Indian Medicinal Plants*, vol. 4, Indian Book Center, New Delhi, India, 1991.

[2] A. Chatterjee and S. C. Pakrashi, *The Treatise of Indian Medicinal Plants*, vol. 6, National Institute of Science Communication, New Delhi, India, 2nd edition, 2001.

[3] Anonymous, *The Wealth of India: Raw Materials*, vol. 7, Publications and Information Directorate, Council for Scientific and Industrial Research, New Delhi, India, 1966.

[4] N. D. Prajapati, S. S. Purohit, A. Sharmak, and T. Kumar, *A Handbook of Medicinal Plants*, Agrobios, Jodhpur, India, 1st edition, 2003.

[5] C.-S. Wen and J.-Y. Hsiao, "Genetic differentiation of *Lilium longiflorum* Thunb. var. *Scabrum Masam.* (Liliaceae) in Taiwan using random amplified polymorphic DNA and morphological characters," *Botanical Bulletin of Academia Sinica*, vol. 40, no. 1, pp. 65–71, 1999.

[6] A. J. Thomson, L. Englberger, L. Guarino, R. R. Thaman, and C. R. Elevitch, *Pandanus tectorius (pandanus)*, Species Profiles for Pacific Island Agroforestry, 2006

[7] V. K. Raina, A. Kumar, S. K. Srivastava, K. V. Syamsundar, and A. P. Kahol, "Essential oil compostion of "kewda" (*Pandanus odoratissimus*) from India," *Flavour and Fragrance Journal*, vol. 19, no. 5, pp. 434–436, 2004.

[8] S. Rajuh, N. V. Subbaiah, K. S. Reddy, A. Das, and K. B. Murugan, "Potential of *Pandanus odoratissimus* as a CNS depressant in Swiss albino mice," *Brazilian Journal of Pharmaceutical Sciences*, vol. 47, no. 3, pp. 630–634, 2011.

[9] R. Kusuma, V. P. Reddy, B. N. Bhaskar, and S. Venkatesh, "Phytochemical and pharmacological studies of *Pandanus odoratissimus* Linn," *International Journal of Pharmacognosy and Phytochemical*, vol. 2, no. 4, pp. 171–174, 2012.

[10] N. R. Kumar, Sanjeeva, D. Padmalaxmi et al., "Antioxidant activity of methanol extract of *Pandanus fascicularis* Lam," *Journal of Pharmacy Research*, vol. 4, no. 4, pp. 1234–1236, 2011.

[11] L. Englberger, "Are Pacific islanders still enjoying the taste of pandanus?" in *Pacific Islands Nutrition*, vol. 58, pp. 10–11, 2003.

[12] L. Englberger, W. Aalbersberg, U. Dolodolotawake et al., "Carotenoid content of pandanus fruit cultivars and other foods of the Republic of Kiribati," *Public Health Nutrition*, vol. 9, no. 5, pp. 631–643, 2006.

[13] L. Englberger, W. Aalbersberg, J. Schierle et al., "Carotenoid content of different edible pandanus fruit cultivars of the Republic of the Marshall Islands," *Journal of Food Composition and Analysis*, vol. 19, no. 6-7, pp. 484–494, 2006.

[14] M. Murai, F. Pen, and C. D. Miller, *Some Tropical South Pacific Island Foods. Description, History, Use, Composition, and Nutritive Value*, University of Hawai'I Press, Honolulu, Hawaii, USA, 1958.

[15] C. D. Miller, M. Murai, and F. Pen, "The use of Pandanus fruit as food in Micronesia," *Pacific Science*, vol. 10, pp. 3–16, 1956.

[16] C. A. Dignan, B. A. Burlingame, J. M. Arthur, R. J. Quigley, and G. C. Milligan, *The Pacific Islands Food Composition Tables*, South Pacific Commission, Noumea, NC, USA, 1994.

[17] P. P. Adkar and V. H. Bhaskar, *Pharmacological evaluation of some medicinal plants for fertility [Ph.D. thesis]*, Vinayaka Missions University, Salem, India, 2014.

[18] S. K. Jain, *Dictionary of Indian Folk Medicine and Ethno Botany*, Deep Publications, New Delhi, India, 1991.

[19] P. P. Adkar, P. P. Jadhav, S. D. Ambavade, T. T. Shelke, and V. H. Bhaskar, "Protective effect of leaf extract of *Pandanus odoratissimus* Linn on experimental model of epilepsy," *International Journal of Nutrition, Pharmacology, Neurological Diseases*, vol. 4, no. 2, pp. 81–87, 2014.

[20] Sanjeeva, N. R. Kumar, D. Padmalaxmi et al., "Antioxidant activity of methanol extract of *Pandanus fascicularis* Lam," *Pharmacologyonline*, vol. 1, pp. 833–841, 2011.

[21] R. Londonkar and A. Kamble, "Evaluation of free radical scavenging activity of *Pandanus odoratissimus*," *International Journal of Pharmacology*, vol. 5, no. 6, pp. 377–380, 2009.

[22] R. Londonkar, A. Kamble, and V. C. Reddy, "Anti-inflammatory activity of *Pandanus odoratissimus* extract," *International Journal of Pharmacology*, vol. 6, pp. 311–314, 2010.

[23] A. L. Udupa, N. Ojeh, G. Gupta et al., "Analgesic activity of *Pandanus fascicularis* Lam.," *Pharmacologyonline*, vol. 2, pp. 837–840, 2011.

[24] S. Venkatesh, R. Kusuma, V. Sateesh, R. B. Madhava, and R. Mullangr, "Antidiabetic activity of pandanus odoratissimus root extract," *Indian Journal of Pharmaceutical Education and Research*, vol. 46, no. 4, pp. 340–345, 2012.

[25] J. Rajeswari, K. Kesavan, and B. Jayakar, "Antidiabetic activity and chemical characterization of aqueous/ethanol prop roots extracts of Pandanus fascicularis Lam in streptozotocin-induced diabetic rats," *Asian Pacific Journal of Tropical Biomedicine*, vol. 2, no. 1, pp. S170–S174, 2012.

[26] S. Sasidharan, V. Sumathi, N. R. Jegathambigai, and L. Y. Latha, "Antihyperglycaemic effects of ethanol extracts of *Carica papaya* and *Pandanus amaryfollius* leaf in streptozotocin-induced diabetic mice," *Natural Product Research*, vol. 25, no. 20, pp. 1982–1987, 2011.

[27] R. Londonkar and A. Kamble, "Hepatotoxic and in vivo antioxidant potential of *Pandanus odoratissimus* against carbon tetrachloride induced liver injury in rats," *Oriental Pharmacy and Experimental Medicine*, vol. 11, pp. 229–234, 2011.

[28] R. Ilanchezhian and R. Joseph, "Hepatoprotective and hepatocurative activity of the traditional medicine ketaki (*Pandanus odoratissimus* Roxb.)," *Asian Journal of Traditional Medicines*, vol. 5, no. 6, pp. 212–218, 2006.

[29] D. Kumar, S. Kumar, J. Singh, C. Sharma, and K. R. Aneja, "Antimicrobial and preliminary phytochemical screening of crude leaf extract of *Pandanus odoratissimus* L," *Pharmacologyonline*, vol. 2, pp. 600–610, 2010.

[30] M. E. Bungihan, M. G. Nonato, S. Draeger, and T. E. E. dela Cruz, "Antimicrobial and antioxidant activities of fungal leaf endophytes associated with *Pandanus amaryllifolius* roxb," *Philippine Science Letters*, vol. 6, no. 2, pp. 128–137, 2013.

[31] M. E. Bungihan, M. G. Nonato, S. Draeger, S. Franzblau, and T. E. E. dela Cruz, "Antimicrobial and antioxidant activities of fungal leaf endophytes associated with *Pandanus amaryllifolius* roxb," *Philippine Science Letters*, vol. 6, no. 2, pp. 129–137, 2013.

[32] P. Singh, R. Bundiwale, and L. K. Dwivedi, "*In-vitro* study of antifungal activity of various commercially available itra (Volatile plant oil) against the keratinophilic fungi isolated from soil," *International Journal of Pharma and Bio Sciences*, vol. 2, no. 3, pp. 178–184, 2011.

[33] S. L. Ooi, S. M. Sun, and V. E. Ooi, *Purification and Characterization of a New Antiviral Protein from the Leaves of Pandanu amaryllifolius (Pandanaceae)*, Department of Biology, The Chinese University of Hong Kong, Shatin, Hong Kong, 2000.

[34] N. B. Shankar and J. P. Kumar, "Phytochemical screening and evaluation of anthelmintic activity of pandanus odoratissimus leafy extract," *International Journal of Universal Pharmacy and Life Sciences*, vol. 1, no. 1, pp. 64–71, 2011.

[35] S. R. Chilakwad, K. P. Manjunath, K. S. Akki, R. V. Savadi, and N. Deshpande, "Pharmacognostic and Phytochemical investigation of leaves of *Pandanus odoratissimus* Linn. f.," *Ancient Science of Life*, vol. 28, no. 2, pp. 3–6, 2008.

[36] T. Jong and S. Chau, "Antioxidative activities of constituents isolated from *Pandanus odoratissimus*," *Phytochemistry*, vol. 49, no. 7, pp. 2145–2148, 1998.

[37] F. Busqué, P. de March, M. Figueredo, J. Font, and E. Sanfeliu, "Total synthesis of four *Pandanus* alkaloids: pandamarilactonine-A and -B and their chemical precursors norpandamarilactonine-A and -B," *Tetrahedron Letters*, vol. 43, no. 32, pp. 5583–5585, 2002.

[38] A. Kayser, *Nauru, One Hundred Years Ago. Pandanus. (trans : A. Blum)*, University of the South Pacific, Suva, Fiji, 2002.

[39] E. L. Little and R. G. Skolmen, *Common Forest Trees of Hawaii (Native and Introduced). Agricultural Handbook 679*, USDA, Washington, DC, USA, 1989.

[40] B. A. Meilleur, M. B. Maigret, and R. Manshardt, "Hala, Wauke in Hawai'i," *Bishop Museum Bulletin in Anthropology*, vol. 7, pp. 1–55, 1997.

[41] "Herbal Medicine: Pandan (*Pandanus tectorius*) Fragrant Screw Pine Fleurizon," Herbal Plant, http://www.philippineherbalmedicine.org/pandan.htm.

[42] F. B. Yahya, *Extraction of aroma compound from Pandan leaf and use of the compound to enhance rice flavor [Ph.D. thesis]*, The University of Birmingham, 2012.

[43] D. Rosario and N. M. Esguerra, *Medicinal Plants in Palau*, vol. 1 of *Publication 28/03 (3.0C)*, Palau Community College, Koror, Palau, 2003.

[44] I. E. Adam, M. J. Balick, and R. A. Lee, *Useful Plants of Pohnpei: A Literature Survey and Database*, Institute of Economic Botany, Bronx, NY, USA, 2003.

[45] V. Madhavan, J. C. Nagar, A. Murali, R. Mythreyi, and S. N. Yoganarasimhan, "Antihyperglycemic activity of alcohol and aqueous extracts of pandanus fascicularis lam. roots in alloxan induced diabetic rats," *Pharmacologyonline*, vol. 3, pp. 529–536, 2008.

[46] T. T. Mani, R. Senthil Kumar, M. Saravana, nayathulla, and B. Rajkapoor, "Antitumor activity of *Pandanus odoratissimus* Lam. on Daltons Ascitic Lymphoma (DAL) in mice," *Hamdard Medicus*, vol. 51, no. 3, pp. 27–31, 2008.

[47] K. L. Seng, Y. B. Che Man, C. P. Tan, A. Osman, and N. S. A. Hamid, "Process optimisation of encapsulated pandan (*Pandanus amaryllifolius*) powder using spray-drying method," *Journal of the Science of Food and Agriculture*, vol. 85, no. 12, pp. 1999–2004, 2005.

[48] M. Z. Abdullah and K. P. Loo, "Separation of divalent metal ions using *Pandanus amaryllifolius* Roxb (Pandanus) leaves: desorption study," in *Waste Management and the Environment III*, vol. 92, pp. 313–321, 2006.

[49] J. Li and S. H. Ho, *Pandan Leaves (Pandanus amaryllifolius Roxb) As A Natural Cockroach Repellent*, School of Biological Sciences, National University of Singapore, Singapore, 1926.

[50] J. M. Sasikumar, U. Jinu, and R. Shamna, "Antioxidant activity and HPTLC analysis of *Pandanus odoratissimus* L. root," *European Journal of Biological Sciences*, vol. 1, no 2, pp. 17–22, 2009.

[51] X. Zhang, P. Guo, G. Sun et al., "Phenolic compounds and flavonoids from the fruits of Pandanus tectorius Soland," *Journal of Medicinal Plants Research*, vol. 6, no. 13, pp. 2622–2626, 2012.

[52] K. R. Kirtikar and B. D. Basu, *Text Book of Indian Medicinal Plants, Volume 2*, pp. 3566–3569, 2000.

[53] P. P. Adkar, P. P. Jadhav, S. D. Ambavade, V. H. Bhaskar, and T. T. Shelke, "Adaptogenic activity of lyophilized hydroethanol extract of *Pandanus odoratissimus* in Swiss Albino mice," *International Scholarly Research Notices*, vol. 2014, Article ID 429828, 10 pages, 2014.

Effect of Hydroalcoholic Extract of *Cydonia oblonga* Miller (Quince) on Sexual Behaviour of Wistar Rats

Muhammad Aslam[1] and Ali Akbar Sial[2]

[1] *Department of Basic Medical Sciences, Faculty of Pharmacy, Ziauddin University, Karachi 75600, Pakistan*
[2] *Department of Pharmaceutics, Faculty of Pharmacy, Ziauddin University, Karachi 75600, Pakistan*

Correspondence should be addressed to Muhammad Aslam; pharmacologist1@yahoo.com

Academic Editor: Neal Davies

Cydonia oblonga Miller (quince) is regarded as a potent libido invigorator in Tib-e-Nabvi and Unani System of Medicine. This study was carried out to evaluate the aphrodisiac activity of the hydroalcoholic extract of the fruits of *Cydonia oblonga* Miller (quince) in Wistar rats. The extract was administered orally by gavage in the dose of 500 mg/kg and 800 mg/kg body weight per day as a single dose for 28 days. The observed parameters were mounting frequency, assessment of mating performance, and orientation activities towards females, towards the environment, and towards self. The results showed that after administration of the extract mounting frequency and the mating performance of the rats increased highly significantly ($P < 0.01$). The extract also influenced the behaviour of treated animals in comparison to nontreated rats in a remarkable manner, making them more attracted to females. These effects were observed in sexually active male Wistar rats.

1. Introduction

Male infertility is mostly caused by abnormalities in the male reproductive system. These abnormalities include impotence, erectile dysfunction, premature ejaculation, and decreased sexual desire. Sexual desire is an inescapable function of life. The principal role of sex and sexuality is the "continuation of progeny" and the survival of living organisms [1]. An aphrodisiac substance is a drug which enhances sexual desire. Etymologically, the term aphrodisiac had been derived from *Aphrodite*, the Greek goddess of sexuality and love [2]. There are a number of allopathic drugs used to enhance sexual desire in males and females, but these drugs have various adverse effects [3]. Today, most commonly used aphrodisiac drugs are phosphodiesterase type 5 inhibitors such as sildenafil (Viagra) and tadalafil. The adverse reactions produced by sildenafil and tadalafil include transient headache, dyspepsia, flushing, diarrhoea, dizziness, pulse irregularities, visual disturbance, and priapism.

Therefore, it is needed to explore the newer aphrodisiac drugs with a better safety profile. Traditional herbal drugs have proven to be a better choice when compared to modern synthetic drugs. These drugs have a few or no side effects and are claimed to be safer ones [4]. However, certain studies have shown that herbal drugs have the potential to interact with other drugs and food [5–10]. *Cydonia oblonga* Miller (quince) family Rosaceae also known as bahi (Urdu) and safarjal (Arabic) is official in Tib-e-Nabvi and is mentioned in the Holy Quran [11]. Traditionally, *Cydonia oblonga* had been used as an antidiarrhoeal, gastric tonic, ulcer-healing, anti-inflammatory, antiemetic and astringent agent. The fruit is suitable for uterine and hemorrhoid bleeding [12]. A number of pharmacological studies have also revealed antimicrobial activity [13], antiradical activity [14], antioxidant activity [15], the inhibitory effect on IgE immune reactions [16], antiulcerative activity [17], antiproliferative activity [18], antihemolytic activity [15], antiallergic activity [19], lipid-lowering activity [20], antidiabetic activity [21], and healing effects of *Cydonia oblonga* [22]. This study was carried out to evaluate the aphrodisiac activity of the hydroalcoholic extract of *Cydonia oblonga* Miller. To the best of our knowledge, this is the first study on the aphrodisiac effects of *Cydonia oblonga* Miller.

2. Materials and Methods

2.1. The Collection of Plant Material. Fresh fruits of *Cydonia oblonga* Miller, *at mature stage*, were purchased from local markets in Malir, Karachi 24°51N 67°02E, in November 2012. The sample was authenticated by an herbalist of the Department of Herbal Extracts, Avicenna Foundation, Pakistan. Voucher specimen (RP/PHARM/1103) was deposited in the institute for future reference.

2.2. Preparation of Hydroalcoholic Extract. The fruits of *Cydonia oblonga* along with their peels were cut into slices and shade-exsiccated at room temperature. Fine powder was made from 200 grams of the slices and soaked in sufficient volume of ethanol/water (70/30) for 1 hour. Further extraction was carried out using a percolator for 72 hours to complete the extracting process [23]. The extract was then subjected to filtration and made solvent-free using a rotary evaporator. To obtain a semisolid concentrated extract, the fluid extract obtained in the preceding step was further freeze-dried until a dry powder was produced [24].

2.3. Drugs and Chemicals. Sildenafil citrate (PZ0003 SIGMA), estradiol benzoate (46552 FLUKA), and progesterone (P0130 SIGMA) were purchased from Sigma-Aldrich.

2.4. The Selection of Animals. Male albino rats (Wistar strain) weighing between 150 and 200 g were used in this research. The specifications given in Helsinki Resolution 1964 were followed during animal handling. This research was approved by our institutional ethical committee vide Resol. number 12/PHA/89.

2.5. Determination of Acute Oral Toxicity. The extract in the dose range of 500–3000 mg/kg was given through oral route to different groups of rats. The control group received distilled water. Animals were kept in fasting condition before the administration of the doses. Following the period of fasting, the animals were weighed and properly marked and the extract was administered. After administration of the extract, food was withheld for two hours. Litchfield and Wilcoxon method was used to determine the acute toxicity. Acute toxicity study of the extract showed that the extract in the present investigation was nontoxic up to 3000 mg/kg body weight [25].

2.6. Dosing. The dose of the extract was calculated according to the body weight of the animals. The dosing of the drug was done daily in normal doses according to the body weight of the animals.

2.7. Methodology. Healthy adult albino rats (Wistar strain) weighing 150–200 g were procured from animal house of University of Karachi, Pakistan. Before administration of the drug, the animals were kept in the laboratory for one week for the conditioning period. They were kept individually in polypropylene cages under controlled conditions at room temperature (25–30°C) with 12/12 hours light-dark cycle. The rats were given a standard rat diet and water *ad libitum*.

2.7.1. Preparation of Male Rats. Male rats were given training, for sexual behaviour, twice a day for a period of 10 days. In case a rat showed a lack of sexual interest during the test period, it was considered as an inactive male and was replaced by another sexually active rat [26].

2.7.2. Preparation of Female Rats. The female rats were artificially brought into oestrus (heat) by the sequential administration of estradiol benzoate (10 μg/100 g body weight) and progesterone (0.5 mg/100 g body weight) through subcutaneous injections, 48 hours and 4 hours, respectively, before mating. After the confirmation of receptivity of the female rats, the experiment was started [26].

2.7.3. Experimental Details. The sexually active male rats were divided into four groups of six animals as follows.

> Group I: normal control, given vehicle (distilled water, 2 mL/kg) orally for 28 days;
>
> Group II: treated group, given hydroalcoholic extract at the dose of 500 mg/kg (orally, 2 mL/kg) for 28 days;
>
> Group III: treated group, given hydroalcoholic extract at the dose of 800 mg/kg (orally, 2 mL/kg) for 28 days;
>
> Group IV: standard drug group, given sildenafil citrate at the dose of 5 mg/kg (orally, 2 mL/kg) for 28 days.

To determine the aphrodisiac activity of the extract, several parameters were observed. These include measuring and observing the mounting frequency, assessment of mating performance, and orientation activities towards females, towards the environment, and towards self.

2.7.4. Mounting Behaviour Test. The mount is operationally defined as the male assuming the copulatory position, but failing to achieve intromission. To quantify mounting frequency, mounting behaviour test was used. Non-oestrus female rats were paired with males treated with the drug (500 mg/kg and 800 mg/kg; p.o.). Animals were observed for 3 hours and their behaviours were scored on the 14th and the 28th day of dosing. Males were placed individually in glass cages. After 15 minutes of acclimatization, a non-oestrus female was introduced into each cage. The number of mounts were noted during a 15-minute observation period at the start of 1st hour. Then the female was withdrawn from each cage for a period of 105 minutes. Again, the female was introduced and the number of mounts were observed for 15 minutes as before at 3rd hour. All the experiments were carried out between 9:00 a.m. to 12:00 p.m. during daytime at room temperature 26-27°C [27, 28].

2.7.5. Assessment of Mating Performance. Males were placed individually in glass cages. After 15 minutes of acclimatization, five oestrus females were admitted into each cage and they cohabited overnight. Microscopic examination of the vaginal smear of each female mouse was done to detect the presence of any sperms. The number of sperm positive females was recorded in each group [28].

TABLE 1: Effect of *Cydonia oblonga* on the mounting behaviour of male rats on the 14th day of the study.

Group	Number of mounts per 15 minutes	
	1st hour	3rd hour
Normal control	2.2 ± 0.61	1.3 ± 0.40
Treated group (500 mg/kg)	5.4 ± 0.20^a	6.9 ± 0.51^a
Treated group (800 mg/kg)	9.4 ± 0.27^a	10.3 ± 0.92^a
Standard group (5 mg/kg)	12.7 ± 0.73^a	13.9 ± 0.22^a

[a]$P < 0.01$: significant difference when compared with the control group.
Values are mean ± standard deviation.

TABLE 2: Effect of *Cydonia oblonga* on the mounting behaviour of male rats on the 28th day of the study.

Group	Number of mounts per 15 minutes	
	1st hour	3rd hour
Normal control	1.7 ± 0.54	1.9 ± 0.76
Treated group (500 mg/kg)	7.3 ± 0.49^a	7.9 ± 0.41^a
Treated group (800 mg/kg)	12.2 ± 0.46^a	11.9 ± 0.72^a
Standard group (5 mg/kg)	13.5 ± 0.35^a	15.4 ± 0.63^a

[a]$P < 0.01$: highly significant difference when compared with the control group.
Values are mean ± standard deviation.

2.7.6. Assessment of the Orientation Activities of Male Rats. The orientation activities of male rats towards females, towards the environment, and towards self were evaluated. After thirty minutes of the administration of the extract, the rats were observed for the next one hour and the number of lickings, anogenital sniffings, climbings, and genital groomings was counted for one hour [2].

2.7.7. Statistical Analysis. All values are mean ± standard deviation (SD). All values were compared with control and standard drug. The significance of difference in the mean was determined by Student's *t*-test. Values of $P < 0.05$ were considered as significant and $P < 0.01$ as highly significant. The data were analysed by using SPSS program Version 20.

3. Results

3.1. Effect of Cydonia oblonga on the Mounting Behaviour of Male Rats. Male rats treated with *Cydonia oblonga* (500 mg/kg and 800 mg/kg) showed a highly significant increase ($P < 0.01$) in the mounting behaviour after 1 hour and 3 hours of drug administration when compared to normal control group. The effect was observed on the 14th and the 28th day of the drug treatment. The increase in the number of mounts produced by *Cydonia oblonga* extract was comparable to the standard drug (Tables 1 and 2).

3.2. Effect of Cydonia oblonga on the Mating Performance of Male Rats. After administration of the extract of *Cydonia oblonga* (500 mg/kg; p.o.), *Cydonia oblonga* (800 mg/kg; p.o.), and sildenafil citrate (5 mg/kg; p.o.) there was observed an increase in the mating performance of the rats. On the 14th day of the study, out of six animals in Group I (normal

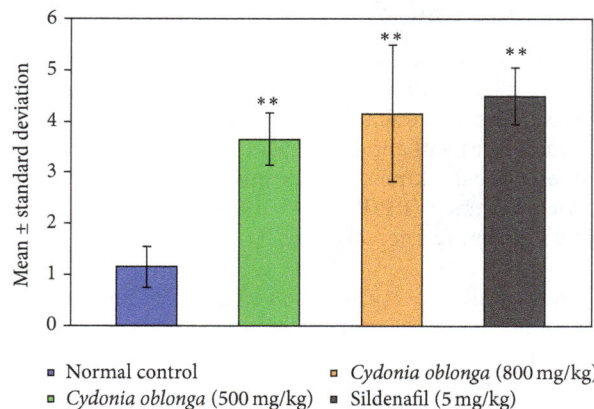

FIGURE 1: Effect of *Cydonia oblonga* on the mating performance of male rats on the 14th day of the study.

control), one male mated with (inseminated) two females and the remaining five males mated with one female each during the overnight experimental period. However, in Group II (*Cydonia oblonga* 500 mg/kg; p.o.), two males mated with three females and the remaining four rats mated with four females each. In Group III, (*Cydonia oblonga* 800 mg/kg; p.o.), one male mated with three females, one male mated with two females, and the remaining four rats mated with five females each. In Group IV (standard drug group), three males mated with five females each and three males mated with four females each. The mean number of females (mean ± SD) mated by one male in the control group was 1.16 ± 0.40 while it was 3.66 ± 0.51 ($P < 0.001$), 4.16 ± 1.33 ($P < 0.001$), and 4.50 ± 0.55 ($P < 0.001$) in the groups treated by *Cydonia oblonga* (500 mg/kg; p.o.), *Cydonia oblonga* (800 mg/kg; p.o), and sildenafil citrate, respectively (Figure 1).

On the 28th day of the study, out of six animals in Group I (normal control), only one male mated with (inseminated) three females and the remaining five males mated with one female each during the overnight experimental period. Whereas, in Group II (*Cydonia oblonga* 500 mg/kg; p.o.), two males mated with three females, one male mated with four females, and the remaining three males mated with five females each. In Group III, (*Cydonia oblonga* 800 mg/kg; p.o.), four males mated with five females each; two males mated with three females each. In Group IV (standard drug group), five males mated with five females each and one male mated with four females. The mean number of females (mean ± SD) mated by one male in the control group was 1.33 ± 0.81 while it was 4.16 ± 0.98 ($P < 0.001$), 4.66 ± 0.51 ($P < 0.001$), and 4.33 ± 1.03 ($P < 0.001$) in the groups treated by *Cydonia oblonga* (500 mg/kg; p.o.), *Cydonia oblonga* (800 mg/kg; p.o.), and sildenafil citrate, respectively, (Figure 2).

3.3. Effect of Cydonia oblonga on the Orientation Activities of Male Rats. The extract also influenced the behaviour of treated animals in a noteworthy manner, making them more attracted to females. The assessment of general parameters such as licking, anogenital sniffing, climbing, and genital grooming also proved the aphrodisiac activity of the plant.

TABLE 3: Effect of *Cydonia oblonga* extract on orientation activities of male rats towards females, towards environment, and towards self on the 14th day of the study.

Groups	Towards female (1 hour)		Towards environment (1 hour)	Towards self (1 hour)
	Licking	Anogenital sniffing	Climbing	Genital grooming
Normal control	3.12 ± 0.14	2.92 ± 0.59	9.85 ± 0.78	6.33 ± 0.29
Treated group (500 mg/kg)	3.66 ± 0.78^{IS}	3.51 ± 0.35^a	10.76 ± 0.49^a	6.74 ± 0.31^a
Treated group (800 mg/kg)	4.13 ± 0.23^a	3.71 ± 0.15^b	11.92 ± 0.33^b	8.18 ± 0.47^b
Standard group	5.82 ± 0.45^b	6.31 ± 0.74^b	14.56 ± 0.32^b	9.66 ± 0.27^b

Values are mean ± standard deviation.
[a] $P < 0.05$: significant difference when compared with the control group.
[b] $P < 0.01$: highly significant difference when compared with the control group.
IS: insignificant difference when compared with the control group.

TABLE 4: Effect of *Cydonia oblonga* extract on orientation activities of male rats towards females, towards environment, and towards self on the 28th day of the study.

Groups	Towards female (1 hour)		Towards environment (1 hour)	Towards self (1 hour)
	Licking	Anogenital sniffing	Climbing	Genital grooming
Normal control	3.23 ± 0.21	2.61 ± 0.13	8.69 ± 0.43	5.85 ± 0.71
Treated group (500 mg/kg)	3.98 ± 0.78^a	3.20 ± 0.41^a	9.41 ± 0.53^a	7.62 ± 0.58^b
Treated group (800 mg/kg)	4.73 ± 0.17^b	3.98 ± 0.54^b	12.29 ± 0.18^b	8.67 ± 0.53^b
Standard group	7.11 ± 0.45^b	8.73 ± 0.74^b	15.40 ± 0.93^b	10.34 ± 0.69^b

Values are mean ± standard deviation.
[a] $P < 0.05$: significant difference when compared with the control group.
[b] $P < 0.01$: highly significant difference when compared with the control group.
IS: insignificant difference when compared with the control group.

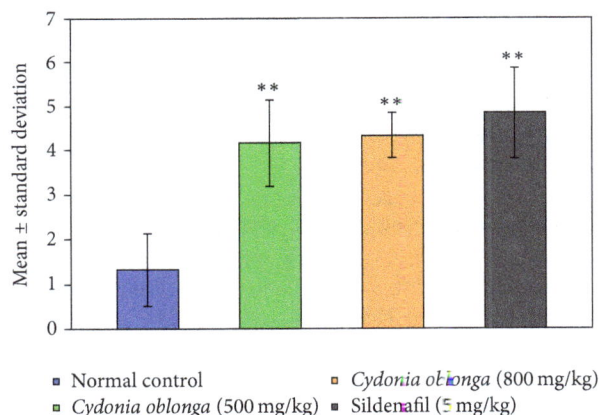

FIGURE 2: Effect of *Cydonia oblonga* on the mating performance of male rats on the 28th day of the study.

3.3.1. Licking. On the 14th day of the study, the results of licking showed a significant ($P < 0.05$) increase in the animals treated with hydroalcoholic extract at 800 mg/kg body weight. Whereas there was only an insignificant increase at 500 mg/kg body weight. However, on the 28th day a significant increase ($P < 0.05$) in the number of lickings was observed in the animals treated with hydroalcoholic extract 500 mg/kg body weight and a highly significant increase ($P < 0.01$) in the number of lickings was observed in the animals treated with hydroalcoholic extract at 800 mg/kg body weight (Tables 3 and 4).

3.3.2. Anogenital Sniffing. On the 14th and the 28th day of the study, the results of anogenital sniffing showed a highly significant ($P < 0.01$) increase in the animals treated with hydroalcoholic extract at 800 mg/kg body weight. Whereas a significant ($P < 0.05$) increase in the number of anogenital sniffings was observed in the animals treated with hydroalcoholic extract at 500 mg/kg body weight (Tables 3 and 4).

3.3.3. Climbing. On the 14th and the 28th day of the study, the results of climbing showed a highly significant ($P < 0.01$) increase in the animals treated with hydroalcoholic extract at 800 mg/kg body weight. Whereas a significant ($P < 0.05$) increase in the number of climbings was observed in the animals treated with hydroalcoholic extract at 500 mg/kg body weight (Tables 3 and 4).

3.3.4. Genital Grooming. On the 14th and the 28th day of the study, the results of genital grooming exhibited a highly significant ($P < 0.01$) increase in the animals treated with hydroalcoholic extract at 800 mg/kg body weight. Whereas a significant ($P < 0.05$) increase in the number of genital groomings was observed in the animals treated with hydroalcoholic extract at 500 mg/kg body weight (Tables 3 and 4).

4. Discussion

Cydonia oblonga Miller (quince) is regarded as a potent libido invigorator in Tib-e-Nabvi and Unani System of Medicine. The results of the current study demonstrated that after administration of the hydroalcoholic extract the sexual activity of male Wistar rats was increased highly significantly. The aphrodisiac potential of *Cydonia oblonga* may be due to its secondary metabolites such as flavonoids, glycosides, tannins, and phenolic compounds present in the extract. It has been observed that drug-induced alterations in the levels of neurotransmitters or their actions at the cellular level could also alter sexual behaviour [29]. Limbic system is the area of the human brain that has the main regulatory role in sexual behaviour. The literature shows a very close relationship between dopamine and 5-hydroxytryptamine and sexual behaviour [30]. The association of human sexual behaviour with dopamine is substantiated by reports of sexual behaviour induced by L-dopa in Parkinsonian patients. Stimulant drugs and antidepressant drugs have been well known to affect libido, erection, ejaculation, and orgasm. Dopamine is one of the most extensively studied central neurotransmitters involved in the control of sexual behaviour. As a matter of fact, while the nigrostriatal system is important for the control of the sensory-motor coordination needed for copulation, the mesolimbic-mesocortical system performs a key role in the preparatory phase of the behaviour, principally in sexual arousal, motivation, and possibly reward. The dopaminergic receptors, which are involved in the control of male sexual behaviour, belong to the D2 receptor subtype. Most studies have shown that drugs, which increase dopaminergic transmission, improve male sexual behaviour, and those drugs, which decrease dopaminergic transmission, worsen male sexual behaviour [31]. *Cydonia oblonga* is a good and cheap natural source of potent antioxidants such as phenolic acids and flavonoids [32, 33]. The fruits of *Cydonia oblonga* contain phenolic compounds, including chlorogenic acid, which is the principal phenolic compound of the fruits and has potent antioxidant [34] as well as anti-inflammatory [29] effects which can halt edema, inflammation, neutrophil migration, and TNF-α expression [35, 36]. Rutin, quercetin, and kaempferol are the well-known quince flavonoids with very potent antioxidant and immunomodulatory effects [37, 38]. Flavonoids react with free radicals and form more stable radicals with lower toxicity. Flavonoids also cause chelation of Fe^{2+} that results in the inhibition of the effects of free radicals [38]. These antioxidants act as cell saviours through their abilities as reducing agents, hydrogen donors, free radical scavengers, and singlet oxygen quenchers [13]. Therefore, it may be that the antioxidative potential of *Cydonia oblonga* might have protected the dopaminergic neurons, including serotenergic and adrenergic neurons against oxidative stress and their number has increased; correspondingly sexual behaviour has also been increased. The free radical scavenging potential of quince is associated with its antihemolytic activities [15] so it may be that the positive effects of the drug on blood are involved in its aphrodisiac activity.

5. Conclusion

Based on the results of our study, we conclude that the oral use of hydroalcoholic extract of *Cydonia oblonga* has sexual behaviour-enhancing effect in male Wistar rats. However, the mechanism of the sexual behaviour enhancing-effect of this miracle herb is yet to be elucidated.

Conflict of Interests

The authors declare that there is no conflict of interests regarding the publication of this paper.

References

[1] P. Kothari, *Common Sexual Problems*, UBS publishers, New Delhi, India, 3rd edition, 2001.

[2] P. Milind and P. Anupam, "Aphrodisiac activity of roots of *Mimosa pudica* Linn ethanolic extract in mice," *International Journal of Pharmaceutical Sciences and Nanotechnology*, vol. 2, pp. 477–486, 2009.

[3] S. K. Kulkarni and D. S. Reddy, "Pharmacotherapy of male erectile dysfunction with sildenafil," *Indian Journal of Pharmacology*, vol. 30, no. 6, pp. 367–378, 1998.

[4] B. N. Shah and A. K. Seth, "Pharmacognostic studies of the *Lagenaria siceraria* (MOLINA) standley," *International Journal of PharmTech Research*, vol. 2, no. 1, pp. 121–124, 2010.

[5] N. Minaz, "Herb-drug interactions," *International Journal of Pharmaceutical Research and Development*, vol. 3, pp. 97–98, 2011.

[6] A. A. Izzo, "Herb-drug interactions: an overview of the clinical evidence," *Fundamental and Clinical Pharmacology*, vol. 19, no. 1, pp. 1–16, 2005.

[7] L. Cranwell-Bruce, "Herb-drug interactions," *Medsurg Nursing*, vol. 17, no. 1, pp. 52–54, 2008.

[8] L. G. Miller, "Herbal medicinals: selected clinical considerations focusing on known or potential drug-herb interactions," *Archives of Internal Medicine*, vol. 158, no. 20, pp. 2200–2211, 1998.

[9] C. Haller, T. Kearney, S. Bent, R. Ko, N. Benowitz, and K. Olson, "Dietary supplement adverse events: report of a one-year poison center surveillance project," *Journal of Medical Toxicology*, vol. 4, no. 2, pp. 84–92, 2008.

[10] S. T. Anusha, V. Prakash, S. Annie, and S. Arun, "Herb-drug interactions: a review," *Hygeia*, vol. 4, pp. 33–40, 2012.

[11] K. M. Sarfaraz, A. K. Mir, A. K. Muhammad, A. Mushtaq, Z. Muhammad, and S. S. Fazal-ur-Rehman, "Fruit plant species mentioned in the Holy Qur'an and ahadith and their ethnomedicinal importance," *The American-Eurasian Journal of Agricultural and Environmental Sciences*, vol. 5, pp. 284–295, 2009.

[12] W. C. Evans, D. Evans, and G. E. Trease, *Trease and Evans Pharmacognosy*, WB Saunders, New York, NY, USA, 15th edition, 2002.

[13] S. Fattouch, P. Caboni, V. Coroneo et al., "Antimicrobial activity of tunisian quince (*Cydonia oblonga* Miller) pulp and peel polyphenols extracts," *Journal of Agricultural and Food Chemistry*, vol. 55, no. 3, pp. 963–969, 2007.

[14] A. S. Magalhães, B. M. Silva, J. A. Pereira, P. B. Andrade, P. Valentão, and M. Carvalho, "Protective effect of quince (*Cydonia oblonga* Miller) fruit against oxidative hemolysis of human erythrocytes," *Food and Chemical Toxicology*, vol. 47, no. 6, pp. 1372–1377, 2009.

[15] R. M. Costa, A. S. Magalhães, J. A. Pereira et al., "Evaluation of free radical-scavenging and antihemolytic activities of quince (*Cydonia oblonga*) leaf: a comparative study with green tea (*Camellia sinensis*)," *Food and Chemical Toxicology*, vol. 47, no. 4, pp. 860–865, 2009.

[16] T. Kawahara and T. Iizuka, "Inhibitory effect of hot-water extract of quince (*Cydonia oblonga*) on immunoglobulin E-dependent late-phase immune reactions of mast cells," *Cytotechnology*, vol. 63, no. 2, pp. 143–152, 2011.

[17] Y. Hamauzu, M. Irie, M. Kondo, and T. Fujita, "Antiulcerative properties of crude polyphenols and juice of apple, and Chinese quince extracts," *Food Chemistry*, vol. 108, no. 2, pp. 488–495, 2008.

[18] C. Márcia, B. M. Silva, S. Renata, V. Patrícia, and P. B. Andrade, "First report on *Cydonia oblonga* miller anticancer potential: differential antiproliferative effect against human kidney and colon cancer cells," *Journal of Agricultural and Food Chemistry*, vol. 58, no. 6, pp. 3366–3370, 2010.

[19] F. Shinomiya, Y. Hamauzu, and T. Kawahara, "Anti-allergic effect of a hot-water extract of quince (*Cydonia oblonga*)," *Bioscience, Biotechnology and Biochemistry*, vol. 73, no. 8, pp. 1773–1778, 2009.

[20] F. Khademi, *The efficay of quince leave extract on atherosclerotic plaques induced by atherogenic diet in coronary and aorta, hyperlipidemia and liver in rabbit [MSc dissertation]*, Tabriz University of Medical Sciences, Tabriz, Iran, 2009.

[21] M. Aslan, N. Orhan, D. D. Orhan, and F. Ergun, "Hypoglycemic activity and antioxidant potential of some medicinal plants traditionally used in Turkey for diabetes," *Journal of Ethnopharmacology*, vol. 128, no. 2, pp. 384–389, 2010.

[22] A. A. Hemmati, H. Kalantari, A. Jalali, S. Rezai, and H. H. Zadeh, "Healing effect of quince seed mucilage on T-2 toxin-induced dermal toxicity in rabbit," *Experimental and Toxicologic Pathology*, vol. 64, no. 3, pp. 181–186, 2012.

[23] *Ian Herbal Pharmacopeia*, Iranian Ministry of Health and Medical Education Publications, IranTehran, Iran, 1st edition, 2002.

[24] M. Minaiyan, A. Ghannadi, M. Etemad, and P. Mahzouni, "A study of the effects of *Cydonia oblonga* Miller (Quince) on TNBS-induced ulcerative colitis in rats" *Research in Pharmaceutical Sciences*, vol. 7, pp. 103–110, 2012.

[25] J. T. Litchfield and F. A. Wilcoxon, "A simplified method of evaluating dose-effect experiments," *Journal of Pharmacology and Experimental Therapeutics*, vol. 96, pp. 99–113, 1949.

[26] A. W. Javeed, N. Rajeshwara, and R. K. Nema, "Phytochemical screening and aphrodisiac property of *Asparagus racemosus*," *International Journal of Pharmaceutical Sciences and Drug Research*, vol. 3, pp. 112–115, 2011.

[27] L. J. Lawler, "Ethnobotany of the orchidaceace," in *Orchid Biology: Review and Perspectives*, A. Joseph, Ed., pp. 27–149, Cornell University Press, Ithaca, NY, USA, 3rd edition, 1984.

[28] A. Tajuddin, S. Ahmad, A. Latif, and I. A. Qasmi, "Aphrodisiac activity of 50% ethanolic extracts of *Myristica fragrans* Houtt. (nutmeg) and *Syzygium aromaticum* (L) Merr. & Perry. (clove) in male mice: a comparative study," *BMC Complementary and Alternative Medicine*, vol. 3, article 6, 2003.

[29] P. K. Suresh Kumar, A. Subramoniam, and P. Pushpangadan, "Aphrodisiac activity of *Vanda tessellata* (Roxb.) Hook. ex Don extract in male mice," *Indian Journal of Pharmacology*, vol. 32, no. 5, pp. 300–304, 2000.

[30] G. Singh and T. Mukerjee, "Herbal aphrodisiacs: a review," *Indian Drugs*, vol. 34, pp. 175–182, 1998.

[31] M. R. Melis and A. Argiolas, "Dopamine and sexual behaviour," *Neuroscience and Biobehavioral Reviews*, vol. 19, no. 1, pp. 19–38, 1995.

[32] B. M. Silva, P. B. Andrade, F. Ferreres, A. L. Domingues, R. M. Seabra, and M. A. Ferreira, "Phenolic profile of quince fruit (*Cydonia oblonga* Miller) (pulp and peel)," *Journal of Agricultural and Food Chemistry*, vol. 50, no. 16, pp. 4615–4618, 2002.

[33] A. P. Oliveira, J. A. Pereira, P. B. Andrade, P. Valentão, R. M. Seabra, and B. M. Silva, "Phenolic profile of *Cydonia oblonge* miller leaves," *Journal of Agricultural and Food Chemistry*, vol. 55, no. 19, pp. 7926–7930, 2007.

[34] Y. Sato, S. Itagaki, T. Kurokawa et al., "In vitro and in vivo antioxidant properties of chlorogenic acid and caffeic acid," *International Journal of Pharmaceutics*, vol. 403, no. 1-2, pp. 136–138, 2011.

[35] D. A. Chagas-Paula, R. B. D. Oliveira, V. C. da Silva et al., "Chlorogenic acids from *Tithonia diversifolia* demonstrate better anti-inflammatory effect than indomethacin and its sesquiterpene lactones," *Journal of Ethnopharmacology*, vol. 136, no. 2, pp. 355–362, 2011.

[36] P. S. Chauhan, N. K. Satti, V. K. Sharma, P. Dutt, K. A. Suri, and S. Bani, "Amelioration of inflammatory responses by chlorogenic acid via suppression of pro-inflammatory mediators," *Journal of Applied Pharmaceutical Science*, vol. 1, pp. 67–75, 2011.

[37] B. M. Silva, P. B. Andrade, P. Valentão, F. Ferreres, R. M. Seabra, and M. A. Ferreira, "Quince (*Cydonia oblonga* Miller) fruit (pulp, peel, and seed) and jam: antioxidant activity," *Journal of Agricultural and Food Chemistry*, vol. 52, no. 15, pp. 4705–4712, 2004.

[38] R. J. Nijveldt, E. Van Nood, D. E. C. Van Hoorn, P. G. Boelens, K. Van Norren, and P. A. M. Van Leeuwen, "Flavonoids: a review of probable mechanisms of action and potential applications," *The American Journal of Clinical Nutrition*, vol. 74, no. 4, pp. 418–425, 2001.

3

Evaluation of the Potential Nephroprotective and Antimicrobial Effect of *Camellia sinensis* Leaves versus *Hibiscus sabdariffa* (*In Vivo* and *In Vitro* Studies)

Doa'a Anwar Ibrahim[1] and Rowida Noman Albadani[2]

[1] *Department of Pharmacology, Faculty of Pharmacy, University of Science and Technology, Sana'a, Yemen*
[2] *Department of Pharmacognosy, Faculty of Pharmacy, University of Science and Technology, Sana'a, Yemen*

Correspondence should be addressed to Doa'a Anwar Ibrahim; dr_d_anwar@hotmail.com

Academic Editor: Robert Gogal

Green tea and hibiscus are widely consumed as traditional beverages in Yemen and some regional countries. They are relatively cheap and the belief is that they improve health state and cure many diseases. The aim of this study was to evaluate the potential protective and antibacterial activity of these two famous plants *in vitro* through measuring their antibacterial activity and *in vivo* through measuring nonenzymatic kidney markers dysfunction after induction of nephrotoxicity by gentamicin. Gram positive bacteria like MRSA (methicillin resistant *Staphylococcus aureus*) were isolated from hospitalized patients' different sources (pus and wound) and Gram negative bacteria including *E. coli* and *P. aeruginosa* were used *in vitro* study. In addition, the efficacy of these plants was assessed *in vivo* through measuring nonenzymatic kidney markers including S. creatinine and S. urea. Green tea was shown antimicrobial activity against MRSA with inhibition zone 19.67 ± 0.33 mm and MIC 1.25 ± 0.00 mg/mL compared with standard reference (vancomycin) 18.00 ± 0.00 mg/mL. Hibiscus did not exhibit a similar effect. Both Hibiscus- and green tea-treated groups had nephroprotective effects as they reduced the elevation in nonenzymatic kidney markers. We conclude that green tea has dual effects: antimicrobial and nephroprotective.

1. Introduction

In China, the usage of green tea was started for more than 4,000 years. The major species is originated from leaves of *Camellia sinensis*. Currently, this herb's use is widespread in Asia and West countries [1]. Many polyphenols are present in green tea leaves like catechins and epigallocatechin gallate. In addition, it contains tocopherols, carotenoids, ascorbic acid (vitamin C), minerals such as chromium, manganese, selenium, or zinc, and other minor phytochemical compounds [1, 2]. Consequently, animal and human studies showed that regular intake of green tea may have health benefits against cardiovascular diseases, cancer, and many types of infectious pathogens [3]. Green tea can support the immune system as well as improve the cognitive function [4]. *Hibiscus sabdariffa* calyces are a famous plant cultivated and used widely in

Africa, especially Egypt and Sudan as this region has a long history of the use of this drink. Hibiscus tea is known to be effective in lowering blood pressure [5] and cholesterol [6]. In addition, researchers propose that consuming hibiscus could aid in the prevention of human cancer [7]. *Hibiscus sabdariffa* calyces contain different components including mucilage, polysaccharides, pectins, polyphenols, organic acids, ascorbic acid, citric, malic and tartaric acids [8].

This study aimed firstly to assess and evaluate the antibacterial activity of two plants *Camellia sinensis* leaves and *Hibiscus sabdariffa* calyces through measuring the inhibition zone of tested plants compared with antibiotic references *in vitro* study. Secondly, the study aimed to compare the potential nephroprotective effect of two tested plants in *in vivo* study.

2. Materials and Methods

2.1. Materials

2.1.1. Drugs and Natural Products. Gentamicin sulfate was purchased from Alpha Aleppo pharmaceutical Ind.

Fresh green tea leaves and *Hibiscus sabdariffa* calyces were bought from special herbal stores in Sana'a city. The two plants were identified and authenticated at Pharmacognosy department, University of Science and Technology (UST).

2.1.2. Animals and Bacteria

(i) Different bacteria species Gram positive including methicillin resistant *Staphylococcus aureus* (MRSA) and Gram negative bacteria including *Escherichia coli* and *Pseudomonas aeruginosa* were supplied by the UST hospital laboratory where these were isolated freshly from infected patients.

(ii) Experimental animals being adult male New Zealand White Rabbits with weight range from 1–1.5 kg and age 7 months ±1 week were supplied by the Faculty animal house. They were fed with fresh green grass and housed in stainless steel cages (2500 cm^2 with a height of 35 cm) away from direct sunlight.

2.2. Preparation of Extracts. The dried plants subsequently were ground separately using a blender to fine powder.

Two kilograms (2 kg) of each dried plant material (green tea and hibiscus) were introduced separately into a Whatman paper thimble and then extracted by refluxing with water as solvent system in a Soxhlet apparatus for six hours. A second extraction was made using 80% methanol and concentrated using a rotary evaporator at 40°C and finally dried in a vacuum dissector at 40°C. The resulting residue which weighed 32.52 g (recovery 10.33%) was later stored under 4°C until required. A 10 mg/mL solution of the extract was prepared in distilled water before administration to the rabbits [9].

2.3. Determination of Antibacterial Activity. Disc diffusion assay [10] was used to determine the antimicrobial activity of the investigated extracts. Sterile filter paper discs of 6 mm diameter were impregnated with 35 µL of the extracted solution (equivalent to 7 mg of dried extract). The paper's discs were allowed to evaporate and then placed on the surface of agar plates that were previously inoculated with microbial cell. Plates were kept for 2 hours in refrigerator to enable prediffusion of extract into the agar. The plates then were incubated overnight (18 hours) at 37°C. Vancomycin, co-trimoxazole, and piperacillin were used as positive control for methicillin resistant *Staphylococcus aureus*, *Escherichia coli*, and *Pseudomonas aeruginosa*, respectively. At the end of incubation period, the antibacterial activity was evaluated by measuring the inhibition zones (diameter of inhibition zone plus diameter of the disc). An inhibition zone of 14 mm or greater is considered as high antibacterial activity [10].

2.4. Minimum Inhibitory Concentration. According the method of Olaleye and Mary Tolulope, 2007, serial dilution of plant extract was used: 20, 10, 5, 2.5, 1.25, 0.625, and 0.313 mg/mL. Each mL (innocula) was poured into petri dish and allowed to set after the agar was also poured. A 3 mm sterile cork borer was used to make wells. The serial freshly prepared dilutions were poured into these wells. The plates were incubated at 37°C for 24 h. Finally, the growth of tested microorganisms (m.o) was observed and compared with clear zone. The least concentration of plant extract that inhibits growth of tested m.o is considered as minimum inhibitory concentration (MIC) [11].

2.5. Animal Study Design. Twenty-four rabbits were divided into four groups randomly. Each group contained six animals. Before starting the experiment, all animals were kept for five days to be acclimatized.

Nephrotoxicity was induced in groups II, III, and IV intraperitoneally by gentamicin (80 mg/kg body weight) for seven consecutive days [12, 13]. Dose of 250 mg/kg body weight, of the *Hibiscus sabdariffa* calyx extract was administered to rabbits in group III, and 300 mg/kg body weight, of *Camellia sinensis* was given to rabbits in group IV, respectively. Rabbits in group I were given distilled water and kept as a control. All groups received tested agents via an oral route using a gavage needle once daily for seven days.

At the end of experiment, light anesthesia with halothane was used, and the animals were dissected. Blood samples were collected directly through the cardiac puncture and kept in container free from anticoagulant and allowed to clot for 20 minutes and centrifuged at 4000 rpm for 15 minutes.

Sera were collected using micropipettes and analyzed. Nonenzymatic markers of kidney dysfunction were measured including serum creatinine [14] and urea [15]. All the experimental procedures were in accordance with the guidelines for the care and use of laboratory animals, and approval from the Institutional Research and Ethics Committee, UST, was received prior to the experiments.

2.6. Statistical Analysis. Results of this work were expressed as mean ± standard error of the mean (S.E.M) by using the Statistical Analysis (SPSS) software package version 18.0. ANVOA was used to compare between groups. $P < 0.05$ was considered as significant.

3. Results

In *in vitro* study, water and methanolic extracts of both *Camellia sinensis* and *Hibiscus sabdariffa* were tested against MRSA (pus), MRSA (wound), *E. coli*, and *P. aeruginosa* and compared with the documented references. Only water and methanolic extracts of *Camellia sinensis* were shown 21, 22, 18, and 19 mm inhibiting zones, respectively. Extracts of *Hibiscus sabdariffa* did not produce antibacterial activity against tested bacterial species. This experiment was repeated three times to get the average inhibition zone of the tested extracts as shown in (Tables 1 and 2).

(a)

(b)

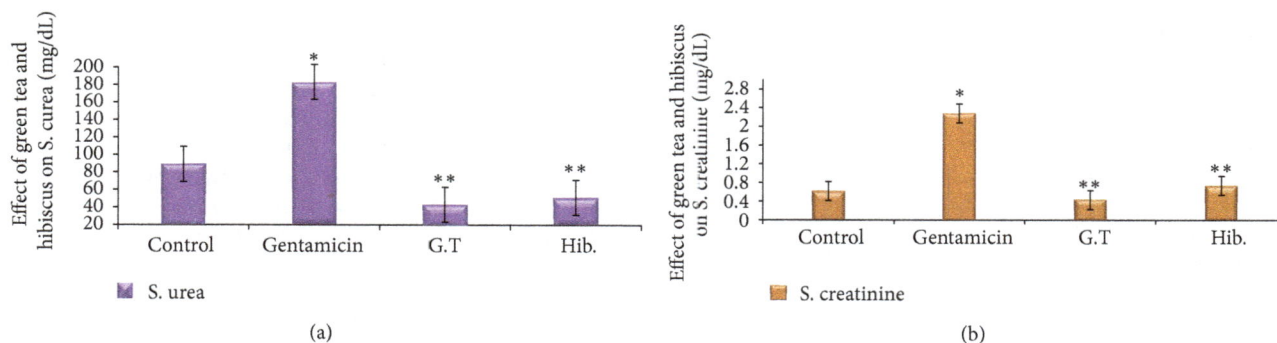

FIGURE 1: (a) Effect of green tea (300 mg/d) and hibiscus (250 mg/d) on the (mean ± SE) nonenzymatic markers of kidney dysfunction (serum urea mg/dL) for 7 days in adult rabbits ($n = 6$). *Significant as compared with control at P value < 0.05. **Significant as compared with gentamicin-induced nephrotoxicity at P value < 0.05. G.T: green tea, Hib: hibiscus. (b) Effect of green tea (300 mg/d) and hibiscus (250 mg/d) on the (mean ± SE) nonenzymatic markers of kidney dysfunction (serum creatinine mg/dL) for 7 days in adult rabbits ($n = 6$). *Significant as compared with control at P value < 0.05. **Significant as compared with gentamicin-induced nephrotoxicity at P value < 0.05. G.T: green tea, Hib: hibiscus.

TABLE 1: Antibacterial activity of water and methanolic extracts of *Camellia sinensis* and *Hibiscus sabdariffa* on tested Gram positive and Gram negative bacteria.

Bacteria species	Reference	T.w	T.m	H.w	H.m
MRSA (pus)	Van. [19]	21	22	R	10
MRSA (wound)	Van. [17]	18	19	R	R
E. coli	GT. [33]	R	R	R	R
P. aeruginosa	Pi. [30]	R	R	R	11

T.w: water extract of green tea; T.m: methanolic extract of green tea; H.w: water extract of hibiscus; H.m: methanolic extract of hibiscus; Van.: vancomycin; GT: gentamicin; Pi: piperacillin; R: resistance.

TABLE 2: Detection of MIC (mg/mL) of methanolic extract of *Camellia sinensis* by using MRSA (wound) species ($n = 3$).

Bacteria	Inhibition zone (mm)		MIC (mg/mL)
	10 mg/L	Van. 1 mg/L	G.T
Staph. aureus	19.67 ± 0.33	18.00 ± 0.00	1.25 ± 0.00
E. coli	0	0	0
P. aeruginosa	0	0	0

Results are expressed as mean ± SE; $n = 3$; MIC: minimum inhibitory concentration; G.T: green tea; Van.: vancomycin.

Regarding the *in vivo* study, levels of creatinine and urea in sera, gentamicin group displayed significant increase in urea (110.5 ± 17.52 mg/dL) and creatinine (1.62 ± 0.72 mg/dL) compared with control group. However, the green tea-treated group demonstrated significant reduction in urea (43.83 ± 3.45 mg/dL) and creatinine (0.617 ± 0.167 mg/dL) compared with gentamicin group. The hibiscus-treated group also revealed significant reduction in both nonenzymatic markers of kidney dysfunctions urea (43.30 ± 6.47 mg/dL) and creatinine (0.733 ± 0.114 mg/dL) compared with gentamicin group. There was insignificant difference between two tested plants as shown in (Figures 1(a) and 1(b)).

4. Discussion

Staphylococcus aureus is a contagious type of bacteria that can cause serious infection, especially nosocomial infections [16]. In the present study, both methanolic and water extracts of plant *Camellia sinensis* have been tested. The extracts displayed antimicrobial effect especially against Gram-positive bacteria as they inhibited the growth of methicillin resistant *Staph. aureus*. The antimicrobial effect of green tea extract is similar to that of the reference used (vancomycin), although it had no activity against gram negative bacteria like *E. coli* and *P. aeruginosa*. Hamilton-Miller, 1995, and Yamada et al., 2006, supported our findings. They found that green tea catechins possess strong antibacterial activity [17, 18].

The antimicrobial activity of green tea (*Camellia sinensis*) against MRSA may be related to the presence of epicatechin gallate (ECG) and epigallocatechin gallate (EGCG). These two polyphenols that are abundant in green tea (*Camellia sinensis*) were identified as candidates for treating *S. aureus*. Chromosomal factors, known as "fem factors", are links between branched-chain cell wall peptide formation and β-lactam rings that are necessary for *S. aureus*, to show resistance to methicillin. Scientists have identified ECG as a potential inhibitor of these fem factors. In addition, ECG also has been recognized as a selective growth inhibitor of MRSA because it damages the cell wall of the bacteria. It is only effective when ECG is present in high concentrations [19–22].

However, this study showed that methanolic and water extracts of hibiscus flowers were free from antimicrobial activity being neither against Gram-positive nor against Gram-negative bacteria. Our result disagreed with Mahadevan et al., 2009 and VimalinHena, 2010, who found that the organism *Staphylococcus aureus* is sensitive towards both the leaves and flowers hot aqueous extract of hibiscus. This effect is due to the polyphenolic nature of the flavonoid gossypetin [23, 24].

Antioxidant compounds are very important for inhibition of oxidative damage to biological target molecules.

They are used for prevention and treatment of many diseases such as cancer and cardiovascular, autoimmune, and neurodegenerative diseases as well as inflammatory effect [25]. Gentamicin was used in this study to induce kidney dysfunction as a model of nephrotoxicity. Silan et al. 2007 and Soliman et al. 2007 supported our findings. They showed that gentamicin produced an elevation in the concentrations of biochemical indicators of kidney function such as blood urea nitrogen (BUN) and serum creatinine [26]. Both green tea- and hibiscus-treated group had shown significant nephroprotective effects. They reduced biochemical indicators or nonenzymatic markers of the kidney dysfunction compared with gentamicin-induced nephrotoxicity. Okoko and Oruambo 2008 agree with our outcomes. They found that *Hibiscus sabdariffa* extract reduced the levels of serum creatinine, urea, and the elevation of the levels of kidney GSH and catalase in rats [27].

The exact mechanism of action is not clear. There are many suggestions; the extract of this plant may lower the level of lipid peroxidation that is elevated in response to some toxic materials like gentamicin. Another suggestion points toward the interaction between the phytochemicals and the toxic materials. In addition, calyces of *Hibiscus sabdariffa* contain potent antioxidant components including vitamin C and tocopherol. This explains the protective effect of this plant as it functions in the conversion of α-tocopheroxy radical to α-tocopherol or reduction of Ca^{+2} dependent permeabilization of renal cortex mitochondria [27–29]. On the other hand, antioxidant and radical scavenger of these calyces are related to the presence of flavonoids known as anthocyanins [27, 30, 31].

Koyner et al., 2008 and Ali et al., 2011, showed that several extracts of medicinal plants including green tea have been tested against gentamicin-induced nephrotoxicity in rats. The basis of the protective action of those plant extracts is not known with certainty, but it was thought to be directly related to their antioxidant properties [32, 33]. In addition, Kadkhodaee et al., 2005 and Kadkhodaee et al., 2007, found that the nephroprotective effect of green tea may be due to the presence of vitamins C and E in its composition [34, 35]. As previously noted, green catechins can act as scavengers of free radicals caused by reactive oxygen species and prevent free radical damage [36].

5. Conclusion

From this study, we conclude that green tea is a good and potent antimicrobial agent, mainly against MRSA, since it has a superior effect than hibiscus in this manner. According to their potential nephroprotective effect, both plants showed very close efficacy without any significant difference between them in their ability to ameliorate nephrotoxicity induced by gentamicin. This may due to the potent antioxidant activity of these two plants. Further studies are needed to elucidate the presence of other components in green tea and hibiscus that may have other health benefits such as anticancer or neuroprotective effects.

Conflict of Interests

There is no conflict of interests regarding the publication of this paper.

Acknowledgments

This study was funded by University of Science and Technology. The senior author would like to thank Faculty of Pharmacy and UST hospital lab team as well as the Aulaqi Specialized Med. Lab. that supported this work. Special thanks to Professor Lenny Rhine for his hard work to revise and edit this paper.

References

[1] E. Reich, A. Schibli, V. Widmer, R. Jorns, E. Wolfram, and A. DeBatt, "HPTLC methods for identification of green tea and green tea extract," *Journal of Liquid Chromatography and Related Technologies*, vol. 29, no. 14, pp. 2141–2151, 2006.

[2] C. Cabrera, R. Artacho, and R. Giménez, "Beneficial effects of green tea—a review," *Journal of the American College of Nutrition*, vol. 25, no. 2, pp. 79–99, 2006.

[3] H. Gradišar, P. Pristovšek, A. Plaper, and R. Jerala, "Green tea catechins inhibit bacterial DNA gyrase by interaction with its ATP binding site," *Journal of Medicinal Chemistry*, vol. 50, no. 2, pp. 264–271, 2007.

[4] X. Chen, W. Li, and H. Wang, "More tea for septic patients?—green tea may reduce endotoxin-induced release of high mobility group box 1 and other pro-inflammatory cytokines," *Medical Hypotheses*, vol. 66, no. 3, pp. 660–663, 2006.

[5] A. M. L. Seca, A. M. S. Silva, A. J. D. Silvestre, J. A. S. Cavaleiro, F. M. J. Domingues, and C. P. Neto, "Phenolic constituents from the core of kenaf (Hibiscus cannabinus)," *Phytochemistry*, vol. 56, no. 7, pp. 759–767, 2001.

[6] H. Mozaffari-Khosravi, B.-A. Jalali-Khanabadi, M. Afkhami-Ardekani, and F. Fatehi, "Effects of sour tea (*Hibiscus sabdariffa*) on lipid profile and lipoproteins in patients with type II diabetes," *Journal of Alternative and Complementary Medicine*, vol. 15, no. 8, pp. 899–903, 2009.

[7] M. M. Yajloo et al., "Inhibition of human breast cancer cells by aqueous extract of Hibiscus gossypifolius Mill (Sour tea)," *Journal of the Iranian Chemical Society*, vol. 6, pp. S115–S143, 2009.

[8] C.-J. Wang, J.-M. Wang, W.-L. Lin, C.-Y. Chu, F.-P. Chou, and T.-H. Tseng, "Protective effect of Hibiscus anthocyanins against tert-butyl hydroperoxide-induced hepatic toxicity in rats," *Food and Chemical Toxicology*, vol. 38, no. 5, pp. 411–416, 2000.

[9] D. Dahiru, O. J. Obi, and H. Umaru, "Effect of *Hibiscus sabdariffa* calyx extract on carbon tetrachloride induce liver damage," *Biokemistri*, vol. 15, no. 1, pp. 27–33, 2003.

[10] A. W. Bauer, W. M. Kirby, J. C. Sherris, and M. Turck, "Antibiotic susceptibility testing by a standardized single disk method," *American Journal of Clinical Pathology*, vol. 45, no. 4, pp. 493–496, 1966.

[11] M. T. Olaleye, "Cytotoxicity and antibacterial activity of Methanolic extract of *Hibiscus sabdariffa*," *Journal of Medicinal Plants Research August*, vol. 1, no. 1, pp. 9–13, 2007.

[12] P. V. A. Babu, K. E. Sabitha, and C. S. Shyamaladevi, "Green tea impedes dyslipidemia, lipid peroxidation, protein glycation and ameliorates Ca^{2+}-ATPase and Na^{+}/K^{+}-ATPase activity in

the heart of streptozotocin-diabetic rats," *Chemico-Biological Interactions*, vol. 162, no. 2, pp. 157–164, 2006.

[13] C. Silan, O. Uzun, N. U. Comunoglu, S. Gokcen, S. Bedirhan, and M. Cengiz, "Gentamicin-induced nephrotoxicityin rats ameliorated and healing effects of reveratrol," *Biological & Pharmaceutical Bulletin*, vol. 30, pp. 79–83, 2007.

[14] R. C. Rock, W. G. Walker, and C. D. Jennings, "Nitrogen metabolites and renalfunction," in *Fundamentals of Clinical Chemistry*, N. W. Tietz, Ed., pp. 669–704, WB Saunders, Philadelphia, Pa, USA, 3rd edition, 1987.

[15] C. A. Burtis and E. R. Edward, Eds., *Tietz Fundamentals of Clinical Chemistry*, W.B. Saunders Company, 5th edition, 2001.

[16] P. S. Mead, L. Slutsker, V. Dietz et al., "Food-related illness and death in the United States," *Emerging Infectious Diseases*, vol. 5, no. 5, pp. 607–625, 1999.

[17] J. M. T. Hamilton-Miller, "Antimicrobial properties of tea (*Camellia sinensis* L.)," *Antimicrobial Agents and Chemotherapy*, vol. 39, no. 11, pp. 2375–2377, 1995.

[18] H. Yamada, M. Tateishi, K. Harada et al., "A randomized clinical study of tea catechin inhalation effects on methicillin-resistant staphylococcus aureus in disabled elderly patients," *Journal of the American Medical Directors Association*, vol. 7, no. 2, pp. 79–83, 2006.

[19] T. S. Yam, J. M. T. Hamilton-Miller, and S. Shah, "The effect of a component of tea (*Camellia sinensis*) on methicillin resistance, PBP2' synthesis, and β-lactamase production in Staphylococcus aureus," *Journal of Antimicrobial Chemotherapy*, vol. 42, no. 2, pp. 211–216, 1998.

[20] A. S. Roccaro, A. R. Blanco, F. Giuliano, D. Rusciano, and V. Enea, "Epigallocatechin-gallate enhances the activity of tetracycline in staphylococci by inhibiting its efflux from bacterial cells," *Antimicrobial Agents and Chemotherapy*, vol. 48, no. 6, pp. 1968–1973, 2004.

[21] E. A. boulmagd, H. I. Al-Mohammed, and S. Al-Badry, "Synergism and postantibiotic effect of green tea extract and imipenem against methicillin-resistant staphylococcus aureus," *Microbiology Journal*, vol. 1, no. 3, pp. 89–96, 2011.

[22] S. Rohrer and B. Berger-Bächi, "FemABX peptidyl transferases: a link between branched-chain cell wall peptide formation and β-lactam resistance in gram-positive cocci," *Antimicrobial Agents and Chemotherapy*, vol. 47, no. 3, pp. 837–846, 2003.

[23] J. VimalinHena, "Antibacterial potentiality of *Hibiscus rosa-sinensis* solvent extract and aqueous extracts against some pathogenic bacteria," *Herbal Tech Industry*, vol. 6, no. 11, pp. 21–23, 2010.

[24] N. Mahadevan, S. Shivali, and P. Kamboj, "Hibiscus sabdariffa linn.—an overview," *Natural Product Radiance*, vol. 8, no. 1, pp. 77–83, 2009.

[25] N. Zamani, M. Mianabadi, and M. Younesabadi, "Evaluation of anti-oxidant properties and phenolic content of Thymus transcaspicus," *Journal of the Iranian Chemical Society*, vol. 6, pp. S115–S143, 2009.

[26] K. M. Soliman, M. Abdul-Hamid, and A. I. Othman, "Effect of carnosine on gentamicin-induced nephrotoxicity," *Medical Science Monitor*, vol. 13, no. 3, pp. BR73–BR83, 2007.

[27] T. Okoko and I. F. Oruambo, "The effect of *Hibiscus sabdariffa* calyx extract on cisplatin-induced tissue damage in rats," *Biokemistri*, vol. 20, no. 2, pp. 47–52, 2008.

[28] L. Packer and V. E. Kagan, *Vitamin E: the Antioxidant Harvesting Centre of Membranes and Lipoproteins*, Marcel Dekker, New York, NY, USA, 1993.

[29] P. I. Campbell and I. A. Al-Nasser, "Renal insufficiency induced by cisplatin in rats is ameliorated by cyclosporine-A," *Toxicology*, vol. 114, no. 1, pp. 11–17, 1996.

[30] Q. Zhou, H. Xie, L. Zhang, J. K. Stewart, X.-X. Gu, and J. J. Ryan, "*cis*-terpenones as an effective chemopreventive agent against aflatoxin B1-induced cytotoxicity and TCDD-induced P450 1A/B activity in HepG2 cells," *Chemical Research in Toxicology*, vol. 19, no. 11, pp. 1415–1419, 2006.

[31] J. M. Sini, I. A. Umar, and H. M. Inuwa, "The beneficial effects of extracts of *Hibiscus sabdariffa* calyces in alloxan-diabetic rats: reduction of free-radical load and enhancement of antioxidant status," *Journal of Pharmacognosy and Phytotherapy*, vol. 3, no. 10, pp. 141–149, 2011.

[32] B. H. Ali, M. Al Za'abi, G. Blunden, and A. Nemmar, "Experimental gentamicin nephrotoxicity and agents that modify it: a mini-review of recent research," *Basic and Clinical Pharmacology and Toxicology*, vol. 109, no. 4, pp. 225–232, 2011.

[33] J. L. Koyner, R. Sher Ali, and P. T. Murray, "Antioxidants: do they have a place in the prevention or therapy of acute kidney injury?" *Nephron Experimental Nephrology*, vol. 109, no. 4, pp. e109–e117, 2008.

[34] M. Kadkhodaee, H. Khastar, M. Faghihi, R. Ghaznavi, and M. Zahmatkesh, "Effects of co-supplementation of vitamins E and C on gentamicin-induced nephrotoxicity in rat," *Experimental Physiology*, vol. 90, no. 4, pp. 571–576, 2005.

[35] M. Kadkhodaee, H. Khastar, H. A. Arab, R. Ghaznavi, M. Zahmatkesh, and M. Mahdavi-Mazdeh, "Antioxidant vitamins preserve superoxide dismutase activities in gentamicin-induced nephrotoxicity," *Transplantation Proceedings*, vol. 39, no. 4, pp. 864–865, 2007.

[36] S. Liao, Y.-H. Kao, and R. A. Hiipakka, "Green tea: biochemical and biological basis for health benefits," *Vitamins and Hormones*, vol. 62, pp. 1–94, 2001.

4

Prophylactic Role of *Averrhoa carambola* (Star Fruit) Extract against Chemically Induced Hepatocellular Carcinoma in Swiss Albino Mice

Ritu Singh, Jyoti Sharma, and P. K. Goyal

Radiation & Cancer Biology Laboratory, Department of Zoology, University of Rajasthan, Jaipur 302 004, India

Correspondence should be addressed to P. K. Goyal; pkgoyal2002@gmail.com

Academic Editor: Mustafa F. Lokhandwala

Liver cancer remains one of the severe lethal malignancies worldwide and hepatocellular carcinoma (HCC) is the most common form. The current study was designed to evaluate the prophylactic role of the fruit of *Averrhoa carambola* (star fruit or Kamrak) on diethylnitrosamine- (DENA-) induced (15 mg/kg b.wt.; single i.p. injection) and CCl_4-promoted (1.6 g/kg b.wt. in corn oil thrice a week for 24 weeks) liver cancer in Swiss albino mice. Administration of ACE was made orally at a dose of 25 mg/kg b.wt/day for 5 consecutive days and it was withdrawn 48 hrs before the first administration of DENA (preinitiational stage). CCl_4 was given after 2 weeks of DENA administration. A cent percent tumor incidence was noted in carcinogen treated animals while ACE administration resulted in a considerable reduction in tumor incidence, tumor yield, and tumor burden. Further, ACE treatment brings out a significant reduction in lipid peroxidation ($P < 0.001$) along with an elevation in the activities of enzymatic antioxidants (superoxide dismutase, $P < 0.001$, and catalase, $P < 0.001$), nonenzymatic antioxidant (reduced glutathione, $P < 0.001$), and total proteins ($P < 0.001$) when compared to the carcinogen treated control. These results demonstrate that ACE prevents the DENA/CCl_4 induced adverse physical and biochemical alterations during hepatic carcinogenesis in mice. This study suggests the prophylactic role of *Averrhoa carambola* against hepatocellular carcinoma in mice; therefore, it could be employed for the further screening as a good chemopreventive natural supplement against cancer.

1. Introduction

Cancer is a global challenge as this disease remains the second largest cause of death around the world, with some predictions that it will move into the top rank in coming time. Cancer accounts for one out of every eight deaths annually. Increase in life expectancy and adoption of western diet and lifestyles, owing to tobacco abuse and widespread exposure to carcinogens, are some of the major key factors for increasing the burden of cancer in the developing countries like India.

Hepatocellular carcinoma (HCC) is one of the most frequent malignant tumors worldwide and a leading cause of cancer related death killing 5 lacs people annually [1]. HCC has been linked to diverse etiologies including chronic hepatitis B and C viral infection and alcohol exposure [2]. Due to the high tolerance of liver, HCC is seldom detected at the early stage and treatment has a poor prognosis in most of the cases, making it a significant global health problem [3–5].

The recurrence rates of HCC are also very high and long-term survival rate of the patients has not improved much from the past few decades. Surgery, including transplantation resection, is currently the most effective treatment for HCC.

Since the liver is the major site of metabolism of ingested materials, it is more susceptible to carcinogenic insult. DENA (diethylnitrosamine) is a potent carcinogen entering the environment through the food chain [6]. DENA is synthesized endogenously and found in work place, processed meats, tobacco smoke, whiskey, and wide variety of foods, and it is also produced from metabolism of some drugs [7]. In addition, DENA is extensively used as a solvent in fiber industry, softener for copolymer, additive for lubricants, in condensers to increase the dielectric constant, and for the synthesis of 1,1-diethylhydrazine [8]. It is a potent hepatocarcinogen known to cause perturbations in the nuclear enzymes involved in DNA repair or replication [9].

Free radicals and other reactive oxygen species (ROS) are constantly formed in the human body accumulation which causes oxidative damage. Normal cells have evolved defense mechanisms for protection against this oxidative damage by developing multiple antioxidative defenses [10]. If such delicate balance of free radical production and antioxidant defenses goes out of control, it results in the pathology of several human diseases, including cancer, atherosclerosis, malaria, rheumatoid arthritis, and neurodegenerative diseases [11, 12].

Chemoprevention is a pharmacological way of interference in order to arrest or reverse the process of carcinogenesis. Chemopreventive substances are identified on the basis of their antioxidant, antimutagenic, and anti-inflammatory activities capable of arresting proliferation and enhancing apoptosis which are the major criteria for their anticarcinogenic activity. Progress in the area of chemoprevention during the past two decades has been very impressive. Accumulating epidemiological and experimental evidences have revealed the chemopreventive influence of number of naturally occurring compounds and their role in prevention of the diseases [13–17].

Herbal products are gaining progressively attention these days for primary health care owing to less toxicity, better compatibility with the body, and high efficacy against free radical mediated diseases. Many studies have suggested that a healthy diet, especially fruits and vegetables that are rich in natural antioxidants, is efficacious to prevent oxidative stress and thus plays a vital role in cancer prevention [18].

Averrhoa carambola L. (Oxalidaceae) is also known as the star fruit tree. Studies have shown that the fruit of *A. carambola* has several medicinal properties and it is rich in antioxidants which act against reactive oxygen species. The ripe star fruit has digestive and biliousness properties. It is also a good source of vitamin C and used to treat headache, vomiting, coughing, hangovers, and eczemas [19, 20]. Furthermore, it is used as an appetite stimulant, diuretic, antidiarrheal, and febrifugal agent. In addition, the extract obtained through the leaves of such planthas been used in the treatment of diabetes [21].

Looking into the pharmacological and medicinal properties of this plant, the present study has been targeted to investigate the possible anticancer potential of *A. carambola* fruit extract against chemical induced hepatocellular carcinoma in mammals.

2. Materials and Methods

2.1. Chemicals. Diethylnitrosamine (DENA) and carbon tetrachloride (CCl_4) were purchased from Sigma Chemical Co. (St. Louis, MO, USA). DENA at a dose 15 mg/kg b.wt (single i.p. injection in normal saline) was injected to initiate hepatic carcinogenesis, while CCl_4 (1.6 g/kg b.wt.) in 1 : 1 dilution with corn oil was given orally to animals by gavage to stimulate liver cell proliferation and regeneration.

2.2. Preparation of Plant Extract. Carambola fruits were cleaned, air dried, and grinded into the form of fine powder. The powder was extracted with 90% ethyl alcohol using Soxhlet apparatus and concentrated by evaporating its liquid contents. The required dose for further treatment was prepared by dissolving the extract in DDW.

2.3. Animals. Swiss albino mice (3-week old) were taken for the experiment from an inbred colony, and they were provided feed and water *ad libitum*. All studies were carried out in accordance with the guidelines of the Institutional Animal Ethics Committee & INSA, New Delhi.

2.4. Dose Selection of ACE. For deciding the optimum dose, experiments were conducted in which Swiss albino mice were divided into different groups and were given orally *Averrhoa carambola* extract (ACE) at the dose of 05, 15, 25, 50, and 75 mg/kg b.wt./day mg/animal/day. Animals from each group were observed for 30 days for any sign of sickness, morbidity, mortality, gait, weight, behavioral alterations, and so forth, and were necropsied on 16th and 31st day. Various doses of ACE were selected (i.e., 15, 25, and 50 mg/kg/b.wt./animal), from the above doses, after evaluation of various biochemical parameters in the liver of mice. Out of these, 25 mg dose was found to be the optimum dose for this experiment.

2.5. Chemopreventive Activity of ACE. Animals for this experiment were divided into the following groups.

Group I: Negative Control (Vehicle Treated Normal Mice). In this group, animals were given single i.p. injection of normal saline and later administered with corn oil by oral gavage, three times in a week for the entire experimental period, that is, for 24 weeks.

Group II: Positive Control (Carcinogen Treated). The animals in this group were given DENA in normal saline. After 2 weeks of DENA administration, CCl_4 was given 3 times in a week until the end of the experiment.

Group III: Drug Treated Control. In this group, the animals were administered *Averrhoa carambola* extract (ACE) at a dose of 25 mg/kg/b.wt/animal/day for the entire experimental period.

Group IV: ACE Treated Experimental. The animals of this group were provided ACE at a dose of 25 mg/kg b.wt./day for 5 consecutive days. ACE source was withdrawn 48 hrs before the first administration of DENA. CCl_4 was given after 2 weeks as 3 times a week for 24 weeks.

The following parameters were taken into account for the study:

(1) Morphological:

   (i) *Body Weight.* The weights of the animals from each group were recorded at the beginning and at the termination of the experiments.

   (ii) *Tumor Incidence.* It is the number of mice carrying at least 1 tumor expressed as percentage incidence.

TABLE 1: Variations in body weight, liver weight, and morphometry of liver tumor after DENA/CCl₄ treatment with or without ACE treatment.

Group	Body weight (gm)		Liver weight (gm)	Tumor		
	Initial	Final		Incidence (%)	Burden	Yield
I	13.10 ± 1.48	31.60 ± 0.37	2.54 ± 0.92	0	0	0
II	12.60 ± 0.34	35.00 ± 0.44	3.90 ± 0.54	100	24	24
III	15.40 ± 1.83	33.83 ± 0.97	2.60 ± 0.28	0	0	0
IV	12.50 ± 1.19	30.93 ± 0.22	3.05 ± 0.33	80	8.1	10.12

(iii) *Tumor Yield.* It refers to the total number of tumors per group (number of tumors/total number of mice).

(iv) *Tumor Burden.* The average number of tumors per tumor bearing mouse (total number of tumors in all mice/total number of tumor bearing mice).

(2) Biochemical. All the animals were autopsied after the end of experiment, that is, 24 weeks, and the whole liver was taken out from each mice. Biochemical analysis for the following parameters was performed in the liver.

(i) *Lipid Peroxidation (LPO).* The level of LPO in liver was measured in terms of thiobarbituric acid reactive substances by the method of Ohkhawa et al. [22]. Briefly, thiobarbituric acid (0.8%), sodium dodecyl sulfate (0.1%), and acetic acid (20%) were added to 100 mL. of the tissue homogenate for 60 min. It was cooled and extracted with N-butanol-pyridine, and the optical density was recorded at 532 nm. The content of TBAS was expressed in nmol/mg.

(ii) *Glutathione (GSH).* The level of reduced GSH was estimated by the method of Moron et al. [23]. The GSH content in the liver was measured spectrophotometrically, using Ellman's reagent with 5,5'-dithiobis 2-nitrobenzoic acid (DTNB) as a coloring agent, according to the method of Beutler et al. [24]. The absorbance was recorded at 412 nm with levels expressed as nmol/mg of protein.

(iii) *Catalase (CAT).* The enzyme activity was assayed in the liver by the method of Aebi [25]. The content was estimated at 240 nm by monitoring the disappearance of H2O2.

(iv) *Superoxide Dismutase (SOD).* The activity of this enzyme was measured by utilizing the method of S. Marklund and G. Marklund [26].

(v) *Total Proteins.* The protein contents in liver were measured by the method of Lowry et al. [27]. The absorbance was recorded at 680 nm.

3. Results and Discussion

There was no considerable change in the average body weight of DENA (Group II), ACE (Group III), and DENA + ACE

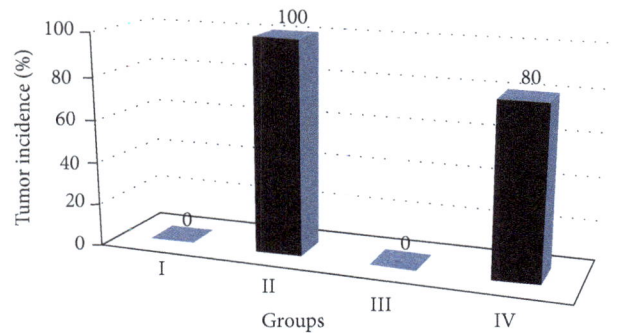

FIGURE 1: Variations in tumor incidence (%) after DENA/CCl₄ induced hepatic carcinogenesis with/without ACE administration.

(Group IV) treated animals when compared to vehicle treated control (Group I). However, the ACE treated mice (Group III) exhibited a spontaneous gain in body weight as similar to the control mice. The mice receiving DENA and CCl₄ (carcinogen control) exhibited a slight increase in mean body weight from that of the untreated (Group I) and ACE treated mice (Group III) till the end of experiment. On the contrary, liver weight was found to be significantly higher in DENA treated animals as compared to the ACE treated once. Further, no tumor appeared on the liver of the vehicle treated and ACE treated control animals while DENA treated mice had the appearance of the tumor incidence as 100%. On the other hand, such tumor appearance was reduced to 80% when DENA (Group III) treated mice were orally administered ACE (Group IV). Similarly, treatment with the carambola fruit extract leads to reduction in tumor burden and tumor yield to 33.75% and 42.16%, respectively, (Table 1, Figures 1, 2, and 3).

Morphologically several small white-grayish foci were detected on the liver of DENA treated mice at the end of the experimentation (i.e., 24 weeks). However, animals of vehicle treated control (Group I) as well as ACE treated control (Group III) did not show any such foci on the liver. On treatment of ACE with DENA (Group IV), the number of visible foci was found to be radically decreased and the liver surface was much smoother.

Induction of oxidative stress by DENA/CCl₄ was evidenced in the liver by the increase in LPO level and fall in the activities of GSH, SOD, CAT, and total proteins content. The levels of LPO in liver were measured to be significantly raised ($P < 0.001$) to 12.91 ± 1.38 n mole/mg tissue, while the activities of GSH, SOD, and catalase as well as the level of total proteins in the liver were obtained to be significantly

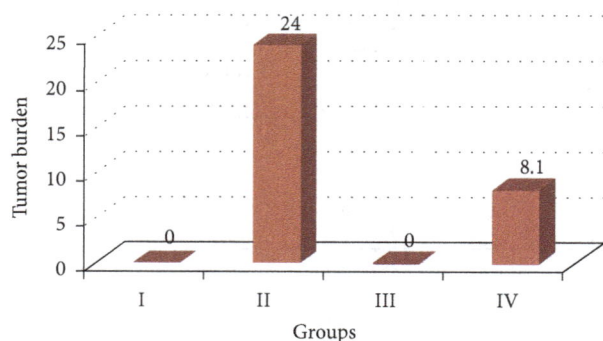

FIGURE 2: Variations in tumor burden in DENA/CCl$_4$ induced hepatic carcinogenesis with/without ACE administration.

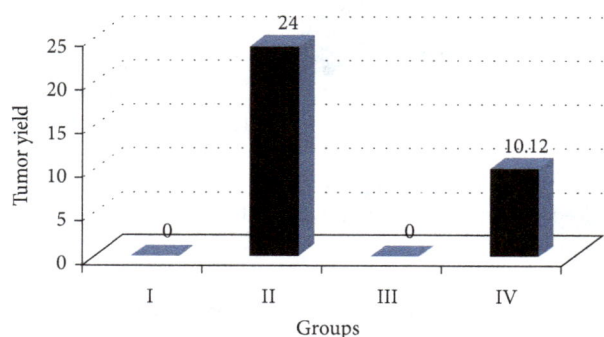

FIGURE 3: Variations in tumor yield after DENA/CCl$_4$ induced hepatic carcinogenesis with/without ACE administration.

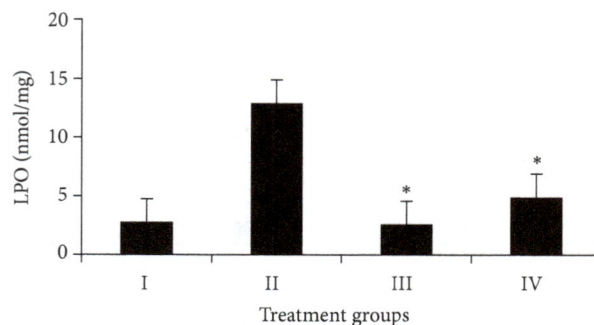

FIGURE 4: Variations in LPO levels after DENA/CCl$_4$ induced hepatic carcinogenesis with/without ACE administration. Significance level—normal versus carcinogen treated control; carcinogen treated control versus ACE treated experimental $^*P < 0.001$.

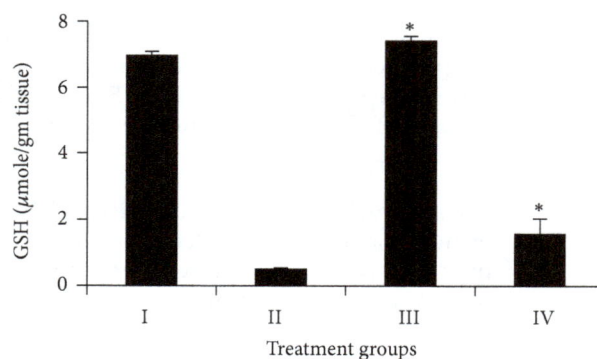

FIGURE 5: Variations in GSH level after DENA/CCl$_4$ induced hepatic carcinogenesis with/without ACE administration. Significance level—normal versus carcinogen treated control; carcinogen treated control versus ACE treated experimental $^*P < 0.001$.

lower ($P < 0.001$) to $0.51 \pm 0.02\,\mu$mole/gm tissue, 12.59 ± 2.08 U/mg tissue, 2.06 ± 0.42 U/mg tissue, 33.31 ± 5.95 mg/gm, respectively, than the vehicle treated control values.

Pretreatment of mice with the *A. carambola* fruit extract (25 mg/kg b.wt. for 5 consecutive days and was withdrawn 48 hrs before the first administration of DENA) significantly ($P < 0.001$) lowered down the activity of LPO to 4.92 ± 0.89 n mole/mg tissue, GSH to $1.58 \pm 0.45\,\mu$ mole/gm tissue, SOD to 13.05 ± 1.05 U/mg tissue, catalase to 3.95 ± 0.50 U/mg tissue, and the level of total proteins to 114.11 ± 11.55 mg/gm (Figures 4, 5, 6, 7, and 8).

Cancer continues to be a great challenge to scientists and practitioners interested in its biology, prevention, and therapy. Therefore, the search for new chemopreventive and antitumor agents, as more effective and less toxic than the existing ones, has kindled great interest in research for phytochemicals.

HCC is a complex disease with multiple underlying pathogenic mechanisms caused by a variety of risk factors. Hepatic carcinogenesis has been intensively studied in experimental animals, and numerous chemical compounds have been demonstrated to be carcinogenic to liver cells. DENA is used as hepatocarcinogen in this study, causing the tumor of the liver and not affecting any other organ. It has been used as an initiating agent in hepatocarcinogenic two-stage protocols, that is, initiation and promotion model.

There is a significant increase in the liver weight of mice receiving DENA and CCl$_4$ as compared to vehicle treated control. It may be because of the presence of tumors and the increased size of liver in such animals. The increase in the size of liver might be because hypertrophy took place in the liver to compensate the damage induced by the carcinogens. After 24 weeks of DENA treatment, hyperplastic nodules developed as a consequence of the appearance of renewed hepatocytes, degenerated hepatocytes, oval cells, and fibrotic changes.

Marked elevations in biochemical parameters like LPO and the fall in GSH, SOD, catalase, and total protein levels in the liver reflect the degree of hepatocellular dysfunctions which indicates that reactive oxygen species, induced by DENA, play an important role in DENA-induced hepatic carcinogenesis. Therefore, it is suggested that oxidative stress is one of the major causes of DENA-induced hepatic carcinogenesis.

Oxidative stress is the state of imbalance between the level of antioxidant defense system and production of reactive oxygen species (ROS). Increased generation of ROS and decreased antioxidant enzymes in liver tissue has been

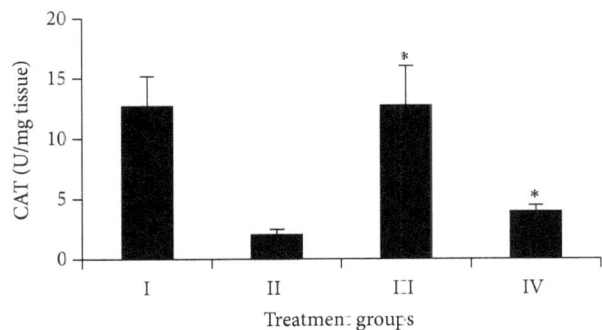

FIGURE 6: Variations in CAT level after DENA/CCl$_4$ induced hepatic carcinogenesis with/without ACE administration. Significance level—normal versus carcinogen treated control. carcinogen treated control versus ACE treated experimental $^*P < 0.001$.

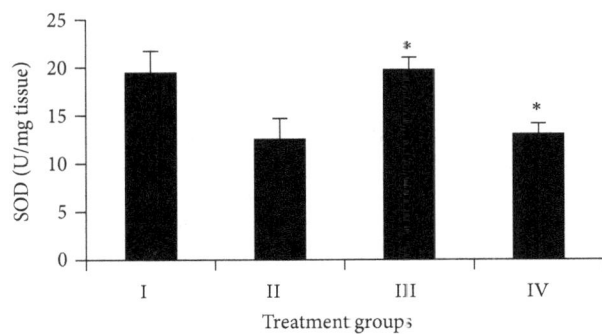

FIGURE 7: Variations in SOD level after DENA/CCl$_4$ induced hepatic carcinogenesis with/without ACE administration. Significance level—normal versus carcinogen treated control: carcinogen treated control versus ACE treated experimental $^*P < 0.001$.

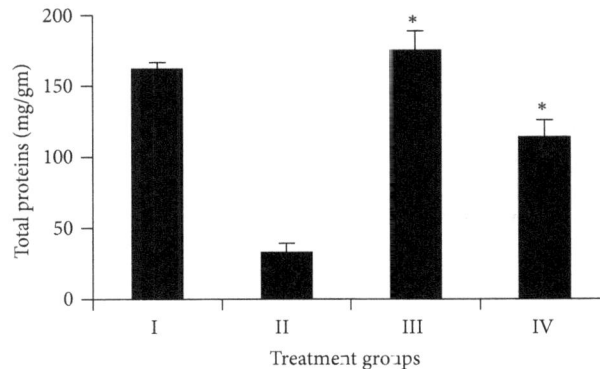

FIGURE 8: Variations in total proteins level after DENA/CCl$_4$ induced hepatic carcinogenesis with/without ACE administration. Significance level—normal versus carcinogen treated control; carcinogen treated control versus ACE treated experimental $^*P < 0.001$.

reported in many models of DENA-induced hepatocellular carcinoma [28–31].

The implication of reactive oxygen species (ROS) in carcinogenic nitrosamines, like DENA and CCl$_4$ toxic hepatic injury, is well documented [32]. It has been reported that ROS play a major role in tumor promotion through interaction with critical macromolecules including lipids, DNA, DNA repair systems, and other enzymes [33]. Increased O$_2$ concentration and production of ROS, such as superoxide radical (*O$_2$), hydroxyl radical (OH*), and hydrogen peroxide, cause oxidative stress in biological tissues. It may also act as tumor initiator by directly activating oncogenes through mutagenesis.

Herbal drugs play a role in the management of various liver disorders in addition to other natural healing processes of the liver [34]. There are studies which show that medicinal plants with hepatoprotective properties mediate their protection via antioxidant and free radical scavenging activities [35–37].

Further, the incidences of hepatic tumors were found to be significantly decreased in the experimental group (ACE treated) than the carcinogen treated control. The increase in the activities of the antioxidant enzymes in the experimental mice is attributed to the major antioxidative compounds

present in the *Averrhoa carambola* fruit. These include catechin, epicatechin, proanthocyanidins, and saponins [38, 39]. Polyphenols and flavonoids are known to have hepatoprotective role [40, 41].

In the present study fruit extract of *Averrhoa carambola* prevented the progression of DENA-induced hepatic carcinogenesis. Data presented here demonstrated that administration of ACE reversed the decrease in GSH, CAT, SOD, and total proteins induced by DENA in liver tissues. Significant reduction in the LPO levels elicited by carambola and enhanced GSH, SOD, catalase, and proteins levels suggest the protection of structural integrity of hepatocytes cell membrane or stimulatory effects on hepatic regeneration, also reflecting the recovery of liver from the toxic effects of DENA and CCl$_4$ towards the normal liver cell functions.

Lipid peroxidation plays an important role in the process of carcinogenesis [42] and may lead to the formation of several toxic products, such as malondialdehyde (MDE) and 4-hydroxynonenal. These products can attack cellular targets including DNA, thereby inducing mutagenicity and carcinogenicity [43]. Increase in lipid peroxidation has been reported during DENA-induced hepatocarcinogenesis [44]. An elevated level of lipid peroxidation during liver carcinogenesis was also observed in DENA treated control mice during the present study. Administration of carambola fruit extract resulted in a significant decrease in the levels of hepatic lipid peroxidation. The phytosterols present in the fruit of carambola showed to mediate the decrease in lipid peroxidation [45, 46].

Free radical scavenging enzymes such as superoxide dismutase (SOD) protect the biological systems from oxidative stress. SOD and CAT provide the first defense against oxygen toxicity by catalyzing the dismutation of superoxide anion to hydrogen peroxide and decomposition of hydrogen peroxide to water and molecular oxygen. Earlier reports showed the decreased activities of SOD and CAT in hepatoma [47]. The current study showed a significant decrease in SOD and CAT activity in mice treated with DENA. Decreased activities of SOD and CAT in DENA-treated mice could be due to overutilization of these nonenzymatic and enzymatic antioxidants to scavenge the products of lipid peroxidation. On the other hand, there was a significant increase in SOD and CAT activities in group treated with plant extract. It may be due to presence of the ascorbic acid which is known for its quenching abilities of the free radicals as well as for the conjugation with cytotoxic, genotoxic and lipid peroxidation products to ultimately lead their excretion [47, 48].

Glutathione is required to maintain the normal reduced state of cells and to counteract all the deleterious effects of oxidative stress. Thus, GSH is involved in many cellular processes including the detoxification of endogenous and exogenous compounds. The elevated level of GSH protects cellular proteins against oxidation through glutathione redox cycle and also directly detoxifies reactive species [49] while the increased level of glutathione reductase helps in maintaining the basal level of cellular GSH [50]. Administration of DENA depleted the level of glutathione (GSH) in this study. Such depletion is also reported in many studies [51–53]. It has been proposed that glutathione peroxidase is responsible for the detoxification of hydrogen peroxide in low concentration whereas catalase comes into play when glutathione peroxidase is saturated with the substrate [54]. GSH level was observed significantly higher in ACE treated mice than the carcinogen alone treated ones.

4. Conclusion

The exact mechanism of the chemopreventive action of ACE against DENA-induced hepatic tumor is not studied in the present experiment, but this investigation demonstrates that the *Averrhoa carambola* fruit extract has a prophylactic role against chemical induced hepatic carcinogenesis in the mammals.

Conflict of Interests

The authors declare that there is no conflict of interests regarding the publication of this paper.

Acknowledgment

The authors are thankful to Council of Scientific & Industrial Research, New Delhi, India, for providing the financial assistance in the form of Senior Research Fellowship to Ms. Ritu Singh under the supervision of Professor P. K. Goyal.

References

[1] T. Severi, H. van Malenstein, C. Verslype, and J. F. van Pelt, "Tumor initiation and progression in hepatocellular carcinoma: risk factors, classification, and therapeutic targets," *Acta Pharmacologica Sinica*, vol. 31, no. 11, pp. 1409–1420, 2010.

[2] S. Badvie, "Hepatocellular carcinoma," *Postgraduate Medical Journal*, vol. 76, no. 891, pp. 4–11, 2000.

[3] K. J. Jeena, K. L. Joy, and R. Kuttan, "Effect of Emblica officinalis, Phyllanthus amarus and Picrorrhiza kurroa on N-nitrosodiethylamine induced hepatocarcinogenesis," *Cancer Letters*, vol. 136, no. 1, pp. 11–16, 1999.

[4] F. X. Bosch, J. Ribes, R. Cléries, and M. Díaz, "Epidemiology of Hepatocellular carcinoma," *Clinics in Liver Disease*, vol. 9, pp. 191–211, 2005.

[5] H. B. El-Serag and K. L. Rudolph, "Hepatocellular carcinoma: epidemiology and molecular carcinogenesis," *Gastroenterology*, vol. 132, no. 7, pp. 2557–2576, 2007.

[6] G. Mittal, A. P. Brar, and G. Soni, "Impact of hypercholesterolemia on toxicity of N-nitrosodiethylamine: biochemical and histopathological effects," *Pharmacological Reports*, vol. 58, no. 3, pp. 413–419, 2006.

[7] L. Verna, J. Whysner, and G. M. Williams, "N-Nitrosodiethylamine mechanistic data and risk assessment: bioactivation, DNA-adduct formation, mutagenicity, and tumor initiation," *Pharmacology and Therapeutics*, vol. 71, no. 1-2, pp. 57–81, 1996.

[8] D. J. Liano, A. Blanck, P. Eneroth, J. Gustafsson, and I. P. Hällström, "Diethylnitrosamine causes pituitary damage, disturbs hormone levels, and reduces sexual dimorphism of certain liver functions in the rat," *Environmental Health Perspectives*, vol. 109, no. 9, pp. 943–947, 2001.

[9] K. Pashupathy and R. K. Bhattacharya, *Schriftenr. Forschungszent.Juliech, Bilateral Sem. Int. Bur*, vol. 29, pp. 159–161, 1998.

[10] B. Demple and L. Harrison, "Repair of oxidative damage to DNA: enzymology and biology," *Annual Review of Biochemistry*, vol. 63, pp. 915–948, 1994.

[11] O. Lux and D. Naidoo, "Biological variability of superoxide dismutase and glutathione peroxidase in blood," *Redox Report*, vol. 1, pp. 331–335, 1995.

[12] U. Bandyopadhyay, O. Das, and R. K. Banerjee, "Reactive oxygen species: oxidative damage and pathogenesis," *Current Science*, vol. 77, no. 5, pp. 658–666, 1999.

[13] G. Block, B. Patterson, and A. Subar, "Fruit, vegetables, and cancer prevention: a review of the epidemiological evidence," *Nutrition and Cancer*, vol. 18, no. 1, pp. 1–29, 1992.

[14] K. A. Steinmetz and J. D. Potter, "Vegetables, fruit, and cancer prevention: a review," *Journal of the American Dietetic Association*, vol. 96, no. 10, pp. 1027–1039, 1996.

[15] M. J. Wargovich, "Experimental evidence for cancer preventive elements in foods," *Cancer Letters*, vol. 114, no. 1-2, pp. 11–17, 1997.

[16] M. A. Eastwood, "Interaction of dietary antioxidants in vivo: how fruit and vegetables prevent disease?" *QJMed*, vol. 92, no. 9, pp. 527–530, 1999.

[17] E. J. Park and J. M. Pezzuto, "Botanicals in cancer chemoprevention," *Cancer and Metastasis Reviews*, vol. 21, no. 3-4, pp. 231–255, 2002.

[18] P. Vitaglione, F. Morisco, N. Caporaso, and V. Fogliano, "Dietary antioxidant compounds and liver health," *Critical Reviews in Food Science and Nutrition*, vol. 44, no. 7-8, pp. 575–586, 2004.

[19] A. D. Corrêa, *Plantas Medicinais: Do Cultivo à Terapêutica*, Editora Vozes, Petrópolis, Brazil, 1998.

[20] R. O. G. Carolino, R. O. Beleboni, A. B. Pizzo et al., "Convulsant activity and neurochemical alterations induced by a fraction obtained from fruit *Averrhoa carambola* (Oxalidaceae: Geraniales)," *Neurochemistry International*, vol. 46, no. 7, pp. 523–531, 2005.

[21] M. Provasi, C. E. Oliveira, M. C. Martino, L. G. Pessini, R. B. Bazotte, and D. A. G. Cortez, "Avaliacao da toxicidade e do potencial antihiperglicemiante da *Averrhoa carambola* L. Oxalidaceae," *Acta Scientiarum*, vol. 23, no. 3, pp. 665–669, 2001.

[22] H. Ohkhawa, N. Ohishi, and K. Yogi, "Assay for lipid peroxidation in animal tissue by thiobarbituric acid reaction," *Analytical Biochemistry*, vol. 95, pp. 351–358, 1979.

[23] M. A. Moron, J. W. Depierre, and B. Mannervik, "Levels of glutathione, glutathione reductase and glutathione S-transferase activities in rat lung and liver," *Biochimica et Biophysica Acta*, vol. 582, no. 1, pp. 67–78, 1979.

[24] E. Beutler, O. Duron, B. M. Kelly, and E. Butler, "Improved method for the determination of blood glutathione," *The Journal of laboratory and Clinical Medicine*, vol. 61, pp. 882–888, 1963.

[25] H. Aebi, "Catalase: in vitro," in *Method in Enzymology*, S. P. Colowick and N. O. Kaplan, Eds., vol 105, pp. 121–126, Academic Press, New York, NY, USA, 1984.

[26] S. Marklund and G. Marklund, "Involvement of the superoxide anion radical in the autoxidation of pyrogallol and a convenient assay for superoxide dismutase," *European Journal of Biochemistry*, vol. 47, no. 3, pp. 469–474, 1974.

[27] O. H. Lowry, N. J. Rosenbrough, A. L. Farr, and R. J. Landall, "Protein measurement with the Folin phenol reagent," *The Journal of Biological Chemistry*, vol. 193, no. 1, pp. 265–275, 1951.

[28] S. Kweon, K. A. Park, and H. Choi, "Chemopreventive effect of garlic powder diet in diethylnitrosamine-induced rat hepatocarcinogenesis," *Life Sciences*, vol. 73, no. 19, pp. 2515–2526, 2003.

[29] G. Ramakrishnan, H. R. Raghavendran, R. Vinodhkumar, and T. Devaki, "Suppression of N-nitrosodiethylamine induced hepatocarcinogenesis by silymarin in rats," *Chemico-Biological Interactions*, vol. 161, no. 2, pp. 104–114, 2006.

[30] A. S. Yadav and D. Bhatnagar, "Chemo-preventive effect of star anise in N-nitrosodiethylamine initiated and phenobarbital promoted hepato-carcinogenesis," *Chemico-Biological Interactions*, vol. 169, no. 3, pp. 207–214, 2007.

[31] V. Sivaramakrishnan, P. N. Shilpa, V. R. Praveen, and D. S. Niranjali, "Attenuation of N-nitrosodiethylamine-induced hepatocellular carcinogenesis by a novel flavonol-Morin," *Chemico-Biological Interactions*, vol. 171, no. 1, pp. 79–88, 2008.

[32] A. Ravid and R. Koren, "The role of reactive oxygen species in the anticancer activity of vitamin D," *Anticancer Research*, vol. 164, pp. 357–367, 2003.

[33] T. W. Kensler and M. A. Trush, "Role of oxygen radicals in tumor promotion," *Environmental Mutagenesis*, vol. 6, no. 4, pp. 593–616, 1984.

[34] A. Subramoniam, D. A. Evans, S. Rajasekharan, and P. Pushpangadan, "Hepatoprotective activity of *Trichopus zeylanicus* extract against paracetamol—induced hepatic damage in rats," *Indian Journal of Experimental Biology*, vol. 36, no. 4, pp. 385–389, 1998.

[35] A. A. Adeneye and A. S. Benebo, "Protective effect of the aqueous leaf and seed extract of Phyllanthus amarus on gentamicin and acetaminophen-induced nephrotoxic rats," *Journal of Ethnopharmacology*, vol. 118, no. 2, pp. 318–323, 2008.

[36] S. R. Parmar, P. H. Vashrambhai, and K. Kiran, "Hepatoprotective activity of some plants extract against paracetamol induced hepatotoxicity in rats," *Journal of Herbal Medicine and Toxicology*, vol. 4, no. 2, pp. 101–106, 2010.

[37] A. V. Rupal, D. M. Savalia, and A. V. R. L. Narasimhacharya, "Plant extracts as biotermiticides," *Electronic Journal of Environmental Sciences*, vol. 4, pp. 73–77, 2011.

[38] G. Shui and L. P. Leong, "Analysis of polyphenolic antioxidants in star fruit using liquid chromatography and mass spectrometry," *Journal of Chromatography A*, vol. 1022, no. 1-2, pp. 67–75, 2004.

[39] J. Ghosh, J. Das, P. Manna, and P. C. Sil, "Cytoprotective effect of arjunolic acid in response to sodium fluoride mediated oxidative stress and cell death via necrotic pathway," *Toxicology in Vitro*, vol. 22, no. 8, pp. 1918–1926, 2008.

[40] L. H. Yao, Y. M. Jiang, J. Shi et al., "Flavonoids in food and their health benefits," *Plant Foods for Human Nutrition*, vol. 59, no. 3, pp. 113–122, 2004.

[41] M. Meydani, "Effect of functional food ingredients: vitamin E modulation of cardiovascular diseases and immune status in the elderly," *The American Journal of Clinical Nutrition*, vol. 71, no. 6, pp. 1665–1668, 2000.

[42] M. C. Banakar, S. K. Paramasivan, M. B. Chattopadhyay et al., "1α, 25-dihydroxyvitamin D3 prevents DNA damage and restores antioxidant enzymes in rat hepatocarcinogenesis induced by diethylnitrosamine and promoted by phenobarbital," *World Journal of Gastroenterology*, vol. 10, no. 9, pp. 1268–1275, 2004.

[43] L. L. de Zwart, J. H. Meerman, J. N. Commandeur, and N. P. Vermeulen, "Biomarkers of free radical damage applications in experimental animals and in humans," *Free Radical Biology and Medicine*, vol. 26, no. 1-2, pp. 202–226, 1999.

[44] P. V. Jeyabal, M. B. Syed, M. Venkataraman, J. K. Sambandham, and D. Sakthisekaran, "Apigenin inhibits oxidative stress-induced macromolecular damage in N-nitrosodiethylamine (NDEA)-induced hepatocellular carcinogenesis in Wistar albino rats," *Molecular Carcinogenesis*, vol. 44, no. 1, pp. 11–20, 2005.

[45] Y. Yoshida and E. A. Niki, "Antioxidant effects of phytosterol and its components," *Journal of Nutritional Science and Vitaminology*, vol. 49, no. 4, pp. 277–280, 2003.

[46] G. Ferretti, T. Bacchetti, S. Masciangelo, and V. Bicchiega, "Effect of phytosterols on copper lipid peroxidation of human low-density lipoproteins," *Nutrition*, vol. 26, no. 3, pp. 296–304, 2010.

[47] R. Corrocher, M. Casaril, G. Bellisola et al., "Severe impairment of antioxidant system in human hepatoma," *Cancer*, vol. 58, no. 8, pp. 1658–1662, 1986.

[48] J. Sowell, B. Frei, and J. F. Stevens, "Vitamin C conjugates of genotoxic lipid peroxidation products: structural characterization and detection in human plasma," *Proceedings of the National Academy of Sciences of the United States of America*, vol. 101, pp. 17964–17969, 2004.

[49] B. Ketterer, "Glutathione S-transferases and prevention of cellular free radical damage," *Free Radical Research*, vol. 28, no. 6, pp. 647–658, 1998.

[50] J. Lopez-Baria, J. A. Barcena, and J. A. Bocanegra, "Structure, mechanism, functions and regulatory properties of glutathione reductase," in *Glutathione*, J. V. B. Raton, Ed., pp. 105–116, CRC Press, Boca Raton, Fla, USA, 1990.

[51] A. K. Bansal, M. Bansal, G. Soni, and D. Bhatnagar, "Protective role of Vitamin E pre-treatment on N-nitrosodiethylamine induced oxidative stress in rat liver," *Chemico-Biological Interactions*, vol. 156, no. 2-3, pp. 101–111, 2005.

[52] V. Sivaramakrishnan, P. N. Shilpa, V. R. Praveen Kumar, and S. Niranjali Devaraj, "Attenuation of N-nitrosodiethylamine-induced hepatocellular carcinogenesis by a novel flavonol-Morin," *Chemico-Biological Interactions*, vol. 171, no. 1, pp. 79–88, 2008.

[53] K. Pradeep, C. V. Mohan, K. Gobianand, and S. Karthikeyan, "Silymarin modulates the oxidant-antioxidant imbalance during diethylnitrosamine induced oxidative stress in rats," *European Journal of Pharmacology*, vol. 560, no. 2-3, pp. 110–116, 2007.

[54] G. F. Gaetani, S. Galiano, L. Canepa, A. M. Ferraris, and H. N. Kirkman, "Catalase and glutathione peroxidase are equally active in detoxification of hydrogen peroxide in human erythrocytes," *Blood*, vol. 73, no. 1, pp. 334–339, 1989.

5

Evaluation of Cytotoxicity and Antifertility Effect of *Artemisia kopetdaghensis*

Davood Oliaee,[1] Mohammad Taher Boroushaki,[2,3] Naiime Oliaee,[2] and Ahmad Ghorbani[2]

[1] Student Research Committee, Mashhad University of Medical Sciences, Mashhad 913750345, Iran
[2] Pharmacological Research Center of Medicinal Plants, School of Medicine, Mashhad University of Medical Sciences, Mashhad 9177948564, Iran
[3] Department of Pharmacology, School of Medicine, Mashhad University of Medical Sciences, Mashhad 9177948564, Iran

Correspondence should be addressed to Ahmad Ghorbani; ghorbania@mums.ac.ir

Academic Editor: Berend Olivier

To date, there is no report on safety of *Artemisia Kopetdaghensis*. This study aimed to determine the possible undesirable effects of *A. Kopetdaghensis* on reproduction of female rats. The pregnant rats were treated (i.p.) with vehicle or 200 and 400 mg/kg of *A. Kopetdaghensis* hydroalcoholic extract from the 2nd to 8th day of pregnancy. Then, number and weight of neonates, duration of pregnancy, and percent of dead fetuses were determined. Also, cytotoxicity of this plant was tested using fibroblast (L929) and ovary (Cho) cell lines. The *A. Kopetdaghensis* had no significant effect on duration of pregnancy, average number of neonates, and weight of neonates. However, administration of 200 and 400 mg/kg of the extract led to 30 and 44% abortion in animals, respectively. The extract at concentrations $\geq 200\,\mu g/mL$ significantly ($P < 0.001$) inhibited the proliferation of L929 fibroblast cells. Regarding the Cho cells, the extract induced toxicity only at concentration of $800\,\mu g/mL$ ($P < 0.01$). Our results showed that continuous consumption of *A. Kopetdaghensis* in pregnancy may increase the risk of abortion and also may have toxic effect on some cells.

1. Introduction

Today, medicinal plants are widely used around the world as an alternative to pharmaceutical drugs. Although herbal products are considered to have fewer adverse effects compared with synthetic drugs, they are not completely free from side effects or toxicity [1]. Adverse effects of medicinal plants may result from contamination of herbs with toxic metals, adulteration with active synthetic compounds, improperly prepared herbal products, misidentification of herbal ingredients, and inherent toxicity of certain herbs [2]. Therefore, the potential side effects of any medicinal plant need to be determined before its clinical applications. Special care should be taken when a herbal product is used by pregnant women, children, and geriatrics. Unfortunately, unlike those synthetic drugs not recommended for use in pregnancy because of known unwanted effects, there are insufficient data about undesirable maternal and perinatal consequences of use of herbal agents.

Artemisia kopetdaghensis, aromatic shrubs belonging to the Asteraceae family, is traditionally used in Iran for its anti-inflammatory, antimicrobial, antifungal, and sedative activities [3, 4]. However, to date, there is no report on safety or toxicity of this plant. Only Ebrahimi and coworkers reported that methanolic extract and essential oil of *A. kopetdaghensis* exhibited tumor growth induction at some concentrations and cytotoxicity at other concentrations [5]. The aim of the present study was to determine the possible undesirable effects of *A. kopetdaghensis* on reproduction of female rats. Also, the possible cytotoxicity of this plant was assessed using fibroblast and ovary cells *in vitro*.

2. Materials and Methods

2.1. Chemicals and Reagents. High glucose Dulbecco's Modified Eagles Medium (DMEM) and fetal bovine serum were purchased from Gibco. Penicillin, streptomycin, and

TABLE 1: Effect of *Artemisia kopetdaghensis* on reproduction of female rats. The pregnant rats were treated (i.p.) with vehicle or *A. kopetdaghensis* hydroalcoholic extract from the 2th to 8th day of pregnancy. Values are mean ± SEM ($n = 8$–10).

Animal groups	Duration of pregnancy (day)	Abortion (%)	Percent of dead fetuses (%)
Control	22 ± 0.3	0	6
A. kopetdaghensis (200 mg/kg)	23 ± 0.3	30	7
A. kopetdaghensis (400 mg/kg)	22 ± 0.4	44	0

3-(4,5-Dimethyl-2-thiazolyl)-2,5-Diphenyl-2H-tetrazolium bromide (MTT) were obtained from Sigma. Dimethyl sulfoxide (DMSO) was purchased from Fluka. Tween 80 was purchased from Merck.

2.2. Preparation of Plant Extract.
The fresh *A. kopetdaghensis* was collected from Gonabad (Eastern area of Iran) and identified by the herbarium of Ferdowsi University of Mashhad, Iran (voucher specimen number: 35205). The aerial parts of plant were cleaned and grounded to fine powder with a blender. Then, macerated extract was prepared as described previously [6, 7], briefly by suspension of 200 g of the powder in 500 mL of 50% ethanol and incubation for 72 h at 37°C. The hydroalcoholic extract was then dried on a water bath and the yield dissolved in distilled water containing 1% Tween 80.

2.3. Animals.
Male and female Wistar rats (200–250 g) and female mice (26–32 g) were obtained from Laboratory Animals Research Center, Mashhad University of Medical Sciences (Iran) and housed in a room with controlled lighting (12 h dark, 12 h light) and temperature ($22 \pm 2°C$). The animals were given standard pellets diet and water *ad libitum*. All animal procedures were in accordance with ethical guidelines approved by the Animal Care Use Committee of Shiraz University of Medical Sciences (Iran).

2.4. Evaluation of A. kopetdaghensis Effect on Reproduction.
Prior to the mating, the female rats were isolated for 30 days to rule out preexisting pregnancy. Then, they were caged overnight with a male rat of proven fertility in the ratio of 1:1. Rats exhibiting vaginal plug on the following morning were separated, and that day was considered as the first day of pregnancy. The pregnant rats were randomized into three groups: (1) control group receiving 1% Tween 80 as vehicle ($n = 8$), (2) experimental rats treated with 200 mg/kg of *A. kopetdaghensis* extract ($n = 10$), and (3) experimental rats receiving 400 mg/kg of the plant extract ($n = 9$). The extract was injected intraperitoneally from the 2nd to the 8th day of pregnancy (early period of organogenesis). The animals were kept individually in cages until parturition. Then, number and weight of neonates, duration of pregnancy, and percent of dead fetuses were determined.

2.5. Acute Toxicity Determination.
Acute toxicity of *A. kopetdaghensis* extract was evaluated by the method of Akhila et al. [8], as described in our previously published work [9]. Five groups of two mice received vehicle (1% Tween 80) or 400, 800, 1600, and 3200 mg/kg of the plant extract intraperitoneally. The treated animals were monitored for 24 h and also one week for mortality. The lowest dose which led to death of animals and the highest dose which did not kill any mice were recorded.

2.6. Cytotoxicity Assessment.
The L929 (mouse fibroblast) and Cho (Chinese hamster ovary) cells were seeded in 96-well plates and cultured for 24 h in DMEM supplemented with 10% FBS, penicillin (100 units/mL), and streptomycin (100 μg/mL) at 37°C and 5% CO_2. Then, the medium was changed to fresh one containing vehicle (1% DMSO) or 50–800 μg/mL of *A. kopetdaghensis* extract. The cells were further incubated for 24 h at 37°C and 5% CO_2. At the end of the treatment, the cell proliferation was measured using MTT assay as previously described [10–12]. The assay was carried out using 2 culture plates, 4 wells for each concentration ($n = 8$).

2.7. Statistical Analysis.
The values were compared using the one-way analysis of variance (ANOVA) followed by Tukey's post hoc test for multiple comparisons. The P values less than 0.05 were considered to be statistically significant. All results are presented as mean ± SEM.

3. Results

3.1. Effect of A. kopetdaghensis on Reproduction.
As shown in Table 1, the *A. kopetdaghensis* extract at concentrations of 200 and 400 mg/kg had no significant effect on duration of pregnancy. However, administration of 200 and 400 mg/kg of the extract led to 30 and 44% abortion in animals, respectively. The percent of dead neonates was 6% in control group and 7% and 0% in experimental groups treated with 200 and 400 mg/kg, respectively. The average number of the neonates in the animals receiving vehicle during pregnancy was 8.13 ± 1.5 (Figure 1(a)). None of the *A. kopetdaghensis* doses could cause a significant change in the neonate number. Likewise, the extract had virtually no significant effect on weight of neonates (Figure 1(b)).

3.2. Acute Toxicity of A. kopetdaghensis.
Different groups of mice ($n = 2$) were treated with 400, 800, 1600, and 3200 mg/kg of *A. kopetdaghensis* hydroalcoholic extract. After 24 h, it was found that 1600 and 3200 mg/kg are the highest dose which did not kill any mice and the lowest dose which led to death of both mice, respectively. The treated animals were further monitored until one week and no mortality or any sign of toxicity was observed at doses ≤1600 mg/kg.

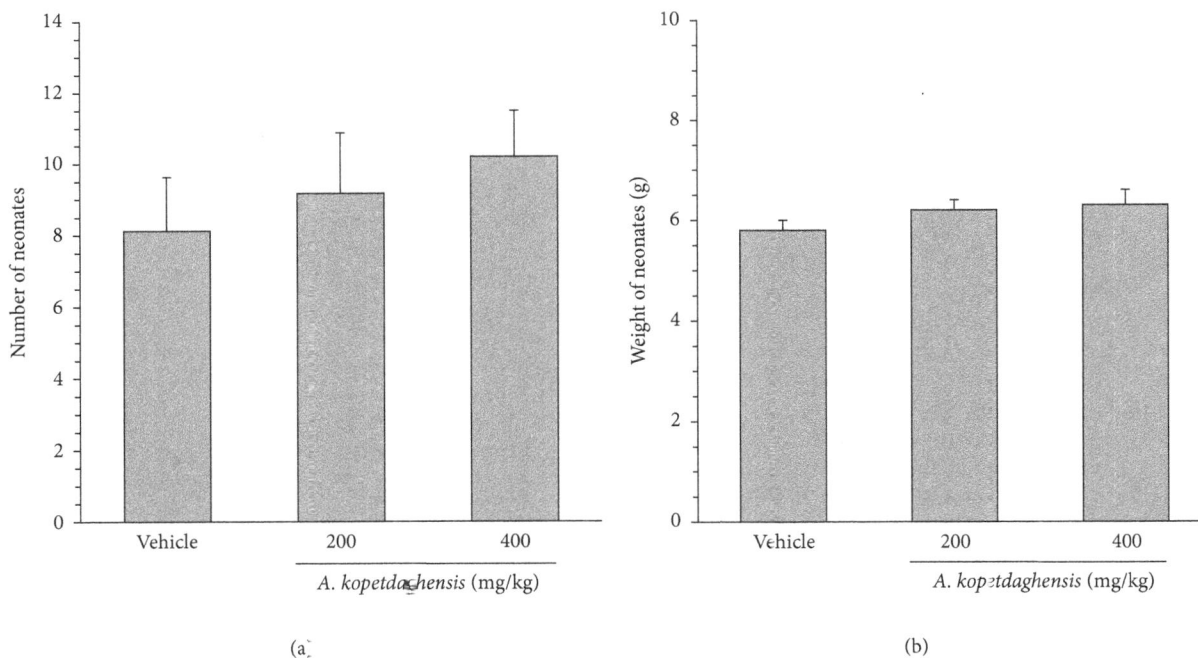

(a)

(b)

FIGURE 1: Effect of *Artemisia kopetdaghensis* hydroalcoholic extract on number (a) and weight (b) of neonates. The pregnant rats were treated (i.p.) with vehicle or 200 and 400 mg/kg of *A. kopetdaghensis* hydroalcoholic extract from the 2th to 8th day of pregnancy. Values are mean ± SEM (n = 8–10).

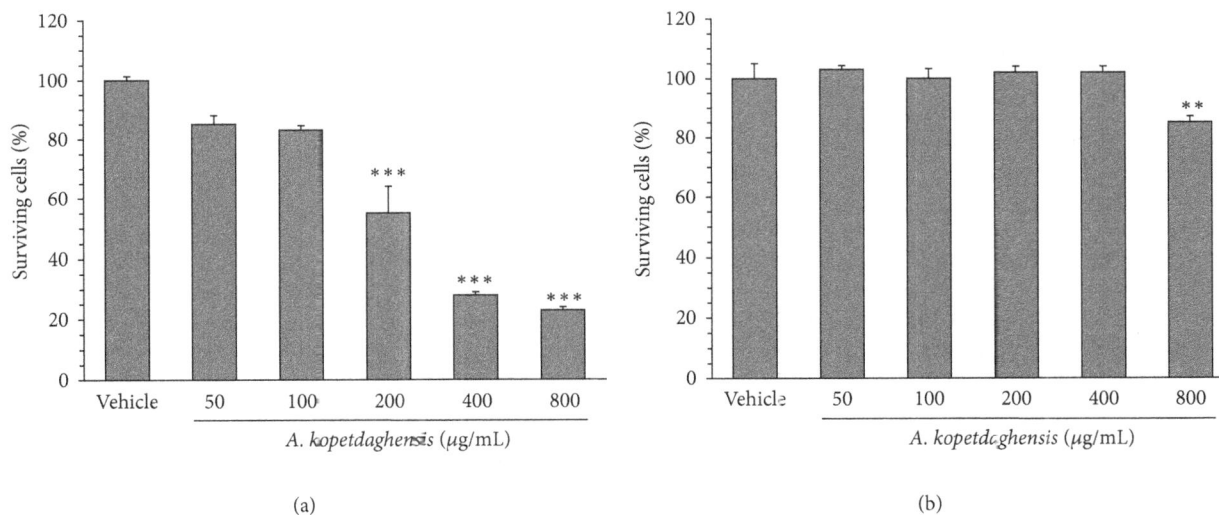

(a)

(b)

FIGURE 2: Effect of *Artemisia kopetdaghensis* hydroalcoholic extract on proliferation of fibroblast L929 (a) and Cho (b) cell lines. The cells were cultured for 24 h in the medium containing vehicle (1% DMSO) or 50–800 μg/mL of *A. kopetdaghensis* extract. Values are mean ± SEM (n = 8).

3.3. *Cytotoxicity of A. kopetdaghensis.* Figure 2 shows the effect of *A. kopetdaghensis* hydroalcoholic extract on proliferation of L929 and Cho cells. Following incubation of L929 fibroblast cells with 50, 100, 200, 400, and 800 μg/mL of the extract, approximately 15, 17, 45, 72, and 77% inhibition in cell growth, was observed, respectively, as compared with untreated cells. The cytotoxic effect of *A. kopetdaghensis* was statistically significant at concentrations ≥200 μg/mL ($P < 0.001$). On the other hand, the extract induced toxicity on Cho cells only at concentration of 800 μg/mL ($P < 0.01$).

In the presence of 50, 100, 200, 400 and 800 μg/mL of *A. kopetdaghensis*, surviving of Cho cells was 103 ± 1.3, 100 ± 3.2, 102 ± 2, 102 ± 2 and 85 ± 2%, respectively, as compared to untreated cells (100 ± 5).

4. Discussion

Many medicinal plants are used by pregnant women for their therapeutic effects. For example, it has been shown that about 36% of pregnant women in Norway use herbs [13]. However, these plants are consumed mostly based on personal experience or traditional knowledge and in most cases it is unclear how safe the use of them is during pregnancy. Previous studies highlighted that some of plants have different antifertility activities [14]. The present study was aimed to examine the possible toxic effects of *A. kopetdaghensis* on reproduction of female rats. Our data demonstrated that the plant extract has no effect on duration of pregnancy and number or weight of neonates. However, it can induce abortifacient effect when consumed at early period of pregnancy. This antifertility effect of *A. kopetdaghensis* has been also reported for some other plants of the Asteraceae family such as *Achillea millefolium* and *Aspilia africana* which showed antispermatogenic and antiovulatory activities, respectively [15, 16]. On the other hand, we observed that administration of *A. kopetdaghensis* extract (400 mg/kg) did not lead to stillbirth. The exact cause of this discrepancy should be explored in the future experiments. However, it may be attributed to high rate of abortion in animals receiving high concentration of the extract.

According to the previously published work, camphene, camphor, davanone, eucalyptol, eugenol, and geranial are of major components of *A. kopetdaghensis*. Camphor accounted for about 1.5 g/100 g of this plant [17]. Rabl and coworkers have reported that camphor crosses the placenta and may lead to abortion [18]. In another study, Linjawi reported that camphor induces significant structural changes on uterus of pregnant rats [19]. Therefore, it is rational to assume that camphor is involved in the abortifacient effect of *A. kopetdaghensis*.

Cytotoxicity evaluation of *A. kopetdaghensis* showed that its hydroalcoholic extract decreases proliferation of fibroblast cells. This finding may describe the camphor induced degeneration of luminal epithelium and decrease of endometrium thickness in uterus of pregnant animals [19].

In conclusion, our results showed that continuous consumption of *A. kopetdaghensis* in pregnancy may increase the risk of abortion and also may have toxic effect on some cells of body. Therefore, its continuous use is not recommended in pregnancy.

Conflict of Interests

The authors declare that there is no conflict of interests regarding the publication of this paper.

Acknowledgment

This work was supported by Vice Chancellor for Research, Mashhad University of Medical Sciences, Mashhad, Iran.

References

[1] P. A. G. M. De Smet, "Health risks of herbal remedies: an update," *Clinical Pharmacology and Therapeutics*, vol. 76, no. 1, pp. 1–17, 2004.

[2] S. A. Jordan, D. G. Cunningham, and R. J. Marles, "Assessment of herbal medicinal products: challenges, and opportunities to increase the knowledge base for safety assessment," *Toxicology and Applied Pharmacology*, vol. 243, no. 2, pp. 198–216, 2010.

[3] M. Ramezani, J. Behravan, and A. Yazdinezhad, "Composition and antimicrobial activity of the volatile oil of Artemisia kopetdaghensis Krasch., M.Pop. & Linecz ex Poljak from Iran," *Flavour and Fragrance Journal*, vol. 21, no. 6, pp. 869–871, 2006.

[4] S. Z. Mirdeilami, H. Barani, M. Mazandarani, and G. A. Heshmati, "Ethnopharmacological survery of medicinal plants in Marraveh Tappeh region, north of Iran," *Iranian Journal of Plant Physiology*, vol. 2, pp. 327–380, 2011.

[5] M. Ebrahimi, M. Ramezani, S. O. Tehrani, O. M. Malekshah, and J. Behravan, "Cytotoxic effects of methanolic extract and essential oil of Artemisia Kopetdaghensis," *Journal of Essential Oil-Bearing Plants*, vol. 13, no. 6, pp. 732–737, 2010.

[6] A. Ghorbani, M. R. Hadjzadeh, Z. Rajaei, and S. B. Zendehbad, "Effects of fenugreek seeds on adipogenesis and lipolysis in normal and diabetic rat," *Pakistan Journal of Biological Sciences*, vol. 17, no. 4, pp. 523–528, 2014.

[7] R. Shafiee-Nick, A. Ghorbani, F. Vafaee, and H. Rakhshandeh, "Chronic administration of a combination of six herbs inhibits the progression of hyperglycemia and decreases serum lipids and aspartate amino transferase activity in diabetic rats," *Advances in Pharmacological Sciences*, vol. 2012, Article ID 789796, 6 pages, 2012.

[8] A. Ghorbani, H. Rakhshandeh, and H. R. Sadeghnia, "Potentiating effects of *Lactuca sativa* on pentobarbital-induced sleep," *Iranian Journal of Pharmaceutical Research*, vol. 12, pp. 401–406, 2013.

[9] J. S. Akhila, S. Shyamjith, D. Deepa, and M. C. Alwar, "Acute toxicity studies and determination of median lethal dose," *Current Science*, vol. 93, no. 7, pp. 917–920, 2007.

[10] F. Forouzanfar, A. A. Goli, E. Assadpour, A. Ghorbani, and H. R. Sadeghnia, "Protective effect of *Punica granatum* L. against serum/glucose deprivation-induced PC12 cells injury," *Evidence-Based Complementary and Alternative Medicine*, vol. 2013, Article ID 7167730, 9 pages, 2013.

[11] S. M. Mortazavian and A. Ghorbani, "Antiproliferative effect of viola tricolor on neuroblastoma cells in vitro," *Australian Journal of Medical Herbalism*, vol. 24, pp. 93–96, 2010.

[12] S. M. Mortazavian, A. Ghorbani, and T. G. Hesari, "Effect of hydro-alcoholic extract of Viola tricolor and its fractions on proliferation of uterine cervix carcinoma cells," *The Iranian Journal of Obstetrics, Gynecology and Infertility*, vol. 15, pp. 9–16, 2012.

[13] H. Nordeng and G. C. Havnen, "Use of herbal drugs in pregnancy: a survey among 400 Norwegian women," *Pharmacoepidemiology and Drug Safety*, vol. 13, no. 6, pp. 371–380, 2004.

[14] G. Priya, K. Saravanan, and C. Renuka, "Medicinal plants with potential antifertility activity—a review of sixteen years of herbal medicine research (1994–2010)," *International Journal of PharmTech Research*, vol. 4, pp. 481–494.

[15] T. Montanari, J. E. De Carvalho, and H. Dolder, "Antispermatogenic effect of *Achillea millefolium* L. in mice," *Contraception*, vol. 58, no. 5, pp. 309–313, 1998.

[16] T. O. Oyesola, O. A. Oyesola, and C. S. Okoye, "Effects of aqueous extract of *Aspilia Africana* on reproductive functions of female wistar rats," *Pakistan Journal of Biological Sciences*, vol. 13, no. 3, pp. 126–131, 2010.

[17] R. Costa, M. R. De Fina, M. R. Valentino et al., "An investigation on the volatile composition of some *Artemisia* species from Iran," *Flavour and Fragrance Journal*, vol. 24, no. 2, pp. 75–82, 2009.

[18] W. Rabl, F. Katzgraber, and M. Steinlechner, "Camphor ingestion for abortion (case report)," *Forensic Science International*, vol. 89, no. 1-2, pp. 137–140, 1997.

[19] S. A. Linjawi, "Effect of camphor on uterus histology of pregnant rats," *Journal of King Abdulaziz University*, vol. 16, no. 2, pp. 77–90, 2009.

6

Effects of Resveratrol and Nebivolol on Isolated Vascular and Cardiac Tissues from Young Rats

Candice Pullen, Fiona R. Coulson, and Andrew Fenning

School of Medical and Applied Sciences, CQ University, Rockhampton, Australia

Correspondence should be addressed to Candice Pullen; c.bowen@cqu.edu.au

Academic Editor: Antonio Ferrer-Montiel

The mechanisms by which resveratrol and nebivolol induce vasodilation are not clearly understood. It has been postulated that both agents stimulate the production of nitric oxide; however, this remains to be conclusively established. The major aim of this study was to examine the vasodilatory and antiarrhythmic effects of both resveratrol and nebivolol and to provide further insight into possible mechanisms of action. Cardiac and vascular tissues were isolated from healthy male rodents. Results indicate that resveratrol and nebivolol decrease the action potential duration and induce mild vasorelaxation in aortic and mesenteric segments. Relaxation induced by resveratrol was prevented by the addition of verapamil, Nω-nitro-L-arginine-methyl ester, and 4-aminopyridine. This suggests that nebivolol and resveratrol act as putative antiarrhythmic and vasodilatory agents *in vitro* through possible indirect nitric oxide mechanisms.

1. Introduction

Currently it is estimated that 3.7 million Australians over the age of 25 have been diagnosed with hypertension [1], making it one of the most common health concerns in Australia. It has been well documented that hypertension has been commonly associated with endothelial dysfunction due, in part, to diminished circulation of nitric oxide [2, 3].

As nitric oxide plays such an important role in maintaining cardiovascular health, much research has been invested in studying various compounds, which may act on or improve the release of nitric oxide [3]. These include nutraceuticals that display novel antioxidant and anti-inflammatory action such as resveratrol and pharmacological agents such as nebivolol. Resveratrol and nebivolol have been demonstrated in both animal and human based studies to increase the bioavailability of nitric oxide [2, 4–6]. These two compounds have also been shown to exhibit beneficial effects on myocardial function by preventing hypertrophy [7, 8] as well as acting to decrease inflammation [9, 10] and oxidative stress [11, 12].

Epidemiological research has cited numerous health benefits related to the regular consumption of red wine. These

putative health improvements have been attributed in part to the presence of the antioxidant, resveratrol [2, 13, 14]. Resveratrol has been shown to have not only cardioprotective [8] but also anti-inflammatory [15] and antioxidant properties [2]. Resveratrol's cardioprotective effects, such as improved endothelium function, decreased left ventricular and vascular remodeling, and a decrease in ischemia-induced arryhthmias have been demonstrated in numerous chronic rodent models of diabetes and hypertension [8, 16–18], in patients with coronary artery disease [19] and overweight and/or obese patients [20]. Vasodilatory effects have been observed in isolated rodent mesenteric arteries [21] and in porcine coronary arteries [13]. It has been postulated that in animal models of diabetes and hypertension, resveratrol may be acting to improve nitric oxide release ultimately restoring endothelial function and thus preventing further damage.

Nebivolol is a novel, third generation β-blocker, which is administered as a racemic combination of both d- and l-nebivolol. What sets nebivolol apart from other β-blockers are its unique haemodynamic properties. Of the two different enantiomers, d-nebivolol has shown to be highly β_1 specific [22], whereas the l-enantiomer has been demonstrated to increase nitric oxide (NO) bioavailability [23]. Research carried out on aortic rings isolated from 10-week-old rats showed that nebivolol was able to induce both endothelial-dependent and NO-dependent relaxation [24]. In human patients, nebivolol may be beneficial in decreasing the risk of developing lethal ventricular arrhythmias, possibly due to modulation of sympathetic hyperactivity [25]. Patients treated with nebivolol had significantly decreased heart rates in comparison to untreated patients [25]. It is therefore possible that nebivolol's antiarrhythmic action may be due to blockade of the β_1-adrenoreceptors. This is further supported by research conducted in numerous animal models and has been associated with various mechanisms including the blockade of the myocardial β_1-adrenoreceptors, reduction of refractory period, and increased release of NO [26].

It remains unclear as to the mechanisms by which resveratrol and nebivolol may be acting to provide the reported protection to the cardiovascular system. Our aim was to investigate the antiarrhythmic and vasodilatory properties of resveratrol and nebivolol and their putative mechanisms of action using healthy cardiac and vascular tissues obtained from rodents.

2. Methods

Ethical clearance was granted through Central Queensland University Ethics Committee (AEC 099/11-251). All experimental protocols were carried out using guidelines set out by the committee. Experiments were conducted on male Wistar rats, approximately 9–11 weeks of age. Animals were purchased from the Animal Resources Centre (Perth, Australia) and housed in a 12 hr light/dark cycle under controlled environmental conditions. The animals were permitted a minimum of 1 week to acclimatise to the conditions before euthanasia via an overdose of sodium pentobarbital (375 mg/mL via i.p).

2.1. Assessment of Electrophysiological Function. Cardiac electrophysiological function was examined using a protocol similar to previously published studies [11, 27]. The papillary muscle was excised from the left ventricle and a stainless steel hook was inserted through the superior end. The muscle was then placed between two platinum electrodes in a 1.0 mL experimental chamber filled with Tyrode's physiological salt solution (37°C; aerated with 95% oxygen and 5% CO_2) and fixed into position with a stainless steel pin. The muscle was then slowly stretched to a maximum preload (5–10 mN). The field stimulation was then undertaken using a Grass SD-9 and contractions were induced at 1 Hz, with a pulse width of 0.5 msec and stimulus strength 20% above threshold. After a five-minute equilibration period, the muscle was then impaled by a glass electrode filled with potassium chloride (World Precision Instruments filamented borosilicate glass, outer diameter 1.5 mm, tip resistance of 5–15 mΩ when filled with 3 M potassium chloride). A silver/silver chloride was used as a reference electrode. The electrical activity of a cell was recorded with a Cyto 721 electrometer (World Precision Instruments) connected to an iMAC G5 computer through analogue digital converter (PowerLab 4/25).

After 20 minutes of baseline recordings, tissues were exposed to 30 μM resveratrol (dissolved in Tyrode's solution) followed by exposure to 120 μM resveratrol. Tissues were then rinsed with fresh Tyrode's solution for 10 min and then exposed to 10 μM nebivolol followed by 100 μM nebivolol.

2.2. Assessment of Vascular Function. Both thoracic aortic rings and mesenteric arteries were utilised. Aortic and mesenteric segments were freed from any connective or adipose tissue. Eight aortic segments from each animal were suspended in 25 mL organ baths containing Tyrode's solution (37°C; aerated with 95% oxygen and 5% CO_2). Mesenteric vessels (eight per animal) were suspended in 12 mL myograph chambers containing Tyrode's solution as in the aortic preparation. To ensure consistency, the secondary branch of the mesenteric vessels was utilised for each preparation. All vessels (mesenteric and aortic rings) were allowed to equilibrate for a minimum of 30 minutes, after which the mesenteric vessels were normalised using the standard DMT normalisation process [28].

Half of the tissues from each animal were precontracted with Tyrode's solution containing 10 mM potassium chloride. Once the contractile response had plateaued, relaxation response curves were generated to either resveratrol ($1e^{-8}$–$3e^{-4}$ M) or nebivolol ($1e^{-8}$–$3e^{-5}$ M). It is important to note that if a relaxation response was induced by one of the above-mentioned compounds, the response was allowed to plateau before the next dose of the compound was added. If no response was induced after approximately 3 minutes, the next dose was added to the baths. Following this, the remaining tissues were precontracted with noradrenaline ($3e^{-7}$ M) and relaxation response curves were generated to either resveratrol ($1e^{-8}$–$3e^{-4}$ M) or acetylcholine ($1e^{-8}$–$3e^{-4}$ M). Once completed, all tissues were rinsed repeatedly with fresh Tyrode's solution and were given 30 minutes to equilibrate back to baseline. The tissues were then precontracted a second time using Tyrode's solution containing 5 mM potassium chloride. The relaxation response curves to resveratrol and nebivolol were repeated but in the presence of one of the following antagonists: $3e^{-7}$ M verapamil, $1e^{-5}$ M Nω-nitro-L-arginine-methyl ester(L-NAME), or $1e^{-3}$ M 4-aminopyridine (resveratrol only).

2.3. Statistical Analysis. Data are expressed as mean ± standard error mean (SEM). Statistical analysis was performed using one-way analysis of variance (ANOVA) with a Bonferroni posttest and Student's t-test. Results were considered significant when $P < 0.05$. Analysis was carried out using Graphpad Prism v4 (GraphPad Software, CA, USA).

2.4. Drugs. All drugs used were purchased from Sigma Aldrich (St. Louis, MO, USA). Resveratrol and nebivolol were dissolved in dimethyl sulfoxide (DMSO) to a stock concentration of 10^{-1} M. The final concentration of DMSO in the organ baths was not sufficient to induce any physiological response in the tissues tested. Noradrenaline, acetylcholine, L-NAME, 4-aminopyridine, and verapamil were all dissolved in distilled water to a stock solution of 1 M.

3. Results

3.1. Electrophysiological Function. Resveratrol did not significantly alter the resting membrane potential, action potential amplitude, or the force of contraction recorded from the left ventricular papillary muscles (Table 1). Resveratrol did display a trend to dose dependently decrease the action potential duration at all three-time points analysed; however, this trend was more pronounced at 50% and 90% of repolarisation (Figure 1) but did not reach statistical significance.

Similar results were seen after the addition of nebivolol. There were no significant changes in the resting membrane potential, action potential amplitude, or force of contraction after exposure to nebivolol (Table 1). As with resveratrol, nebivolol displayed a nonsignificant trend to decrease action potential duration; however, these effects were not dose dependent (Figure 1).

3.2. Vascular Function

3.2.1. Thoracic Aorta. When precontracted with both potassium chloride and noradrenaline, resveratrol only induced relaxation at high doses (Figures 2(a) and 2(b)). It was not as effective as acetylcholine in relaxing the precontracted aortic tissues (Figure 2(b)). The addition of L-NAME, 4-aminopyridine, and verapamil abolished the response to resveratrol (Figure 2(c)). Nebivolol also acted as a moderate vasodilator in aortic tissue (Figure 2(a)). Neither L-NAME nor verapamil significantly altered the relaxation response due to nebivolol (Figure 2(d)).

3.2.2. Mesenteric Vessels. Resveratrol was more effective at inducing a relaxation response, in the mesenteric vessels, when precontracted with noradrenaline than with potassium chloride (Figures 3(a) and 3(b)). However, as with the aorta, resveratrol was not as effective as acetylcholine in producing a relaxation response (Figure 3(b)). The addition of L-NAME did not significantly inhibit the resveratrol-induced relaxation (Figure 3(c)). Nebivolol was only able to induce relaxation in potassium chloride precontracted tissues at relatively high doses (Figure 3(a)). The addition of the nitric oxide synthase inhibitor, L-NAME, did not affect the relaxation induced by nebivolol (Figure 3(d)).

4. Discussion

The major aim of this study was to investigate the possible antiarrhythmic and vasodilatory role of both resveratrol and nebivolol on isolated tissues. The electrophysiological studies demonstrated that both nebivolol and resveratrol have the potential to reduce action potential duration. This trend, though found not to be significant, was seen at both 50 and 90% of repolarisation. There was no significant effect on the force of the contraction, resting membrane potential, or the action potential amplitude after treatment with either compound.

Resveratrol and nebivolol acted as moderate vasodilators on both large conduit arteries (aorta) and small resistance vessels (mesenteric arteries). These effects were only noted at relatively high concentrations and appear to be more subtle in healthy tissues compared to those reported in diseased models. The addition of various antagonists inhibited resveratrol's effect in the aortic segments, but not in the mesenteric vessels. The relaxant effect of nebivolol was not hampered by the addition of either L-NAME or verapamil in both types of blood vessels studied.

4.1. Electrophysiological Function. Resveratrol's effect on cardiomyocytes remains unclear. Some studies report that exposure to resveratrol decreases the action potential duration (APD) in isolated cardiomyocytes [29, 30], whereas others report that resveratrol prolongs the APD [16]. Although the literature indicates conflicting results, the consensus is that resveratrol mediates its electrophysiological effects via alterations in ionic calcium and potassium channels [5, 16, 29, 30].

In our study, both resveratrol and nebivolol decreased the duration of the potentials recorded from the isolated papillary muscles at both 50% and 90% of repolarisation. In the case of resveratrol, these effects appear to be dose dependent. Although the results were not deemed to be significant after statistical analysis, the trends are noteworthy. There was no alteration in either the resting membrane potential, action potential amplitude, or the force of contraction after the muscles were exposed to either resveratrol or nebivolol indicating that there were minimal changes in basal cell function.

The decreases in action potential duration after exposure to resveratrol, seen in the current study, are similar to those observed in the guinea pig which concluded that resveratrol may inhibit calcium influx in myocytes [30]. As the duration of repolarisation is heavily dependent on potassium efflux and calcium influx, it would be expected that inhibition of calcium influx would result in a faster repolarisation of the cardiomyocytes. These findings are further supported by patch-clamp studies carried out in ventricular myocytes isolated from male Sprague-Dawley rats [31]. In the rodent myocytes it is found that resveratrol inhibited the activation of the L-type calcium channel, which may account, at least in part, for resveratrol's acute antiarrhythmic actions [31] and also contribute to its vascular function.

Similar alterations in the action potential were seen after the papillary muscles were exposed to nebivolol. At this stage, it is unclear as to the exact mechanism that may be at play behind the decrease in action potential duration after nebivolol exposure. A related study examining the negative inotropic effects of the β_1-selective adrenoceptor blocker esmolol found similar results [32]. The authors proposed that the mechanism behind esmolol's effects was through the inhibition of the calcium current [32]. The reduction in action potential duration by esmolol was also accompanied by a reduction in the force of the contraction [32]. This can be explained through the inhibition of the calcium current resulting in less calcium available intracellularly to initiate a contractile response. These findings are consistent with clinical studies investigating long QT syndrome. Long QT

TABLE 1: Effect of resveratrol and nebivolol on resting membrane potential (RMP), action potential amplitude (APA) and force of contraction (FOC) in isolated papillary muscle cells.

	Control	30 μM Res	120 μM Res	10 μM Neb	100 μM Neb
RMP	-62.2 ± 1.9 $n = 8$	-63.5 ± 2.5 $n = 5$	-65.5 ± 1.7 $n = 4$	-66.3 ± 2.4 $n = 4$	-65.5 ± 1.1 $n = 4$
APA	69.7 ± 6.1 $n = 8$	65.7 ± 4.3 $n = 5$	66.9 ± 4.3 $n = 4$	65.4 ± 8.7 $n = 4$	68.4 ± 9.3 $n = 4$
FOC	1.2 ± 0.4 $n = 8$	1.2 ± 0.3 $n = 5$	1.5 ± 0.6 $n = 4$	1.9 ± 0.5 $n = 4$	2.0 ± 0.6 $n = 4$

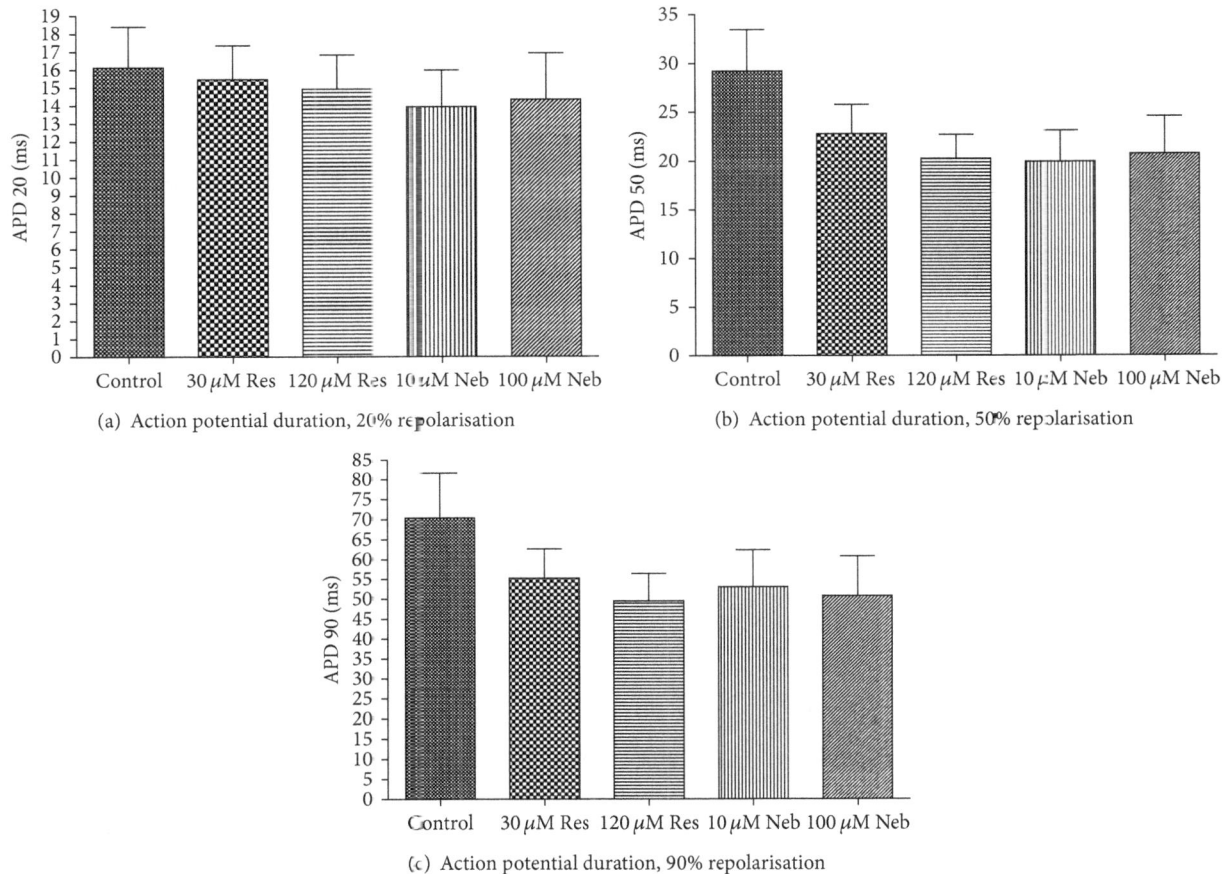

(a) Action potential duration, 20% repolarisation

(b) Action potential duration, 50% repolarisation

(c) Action potential duration, 90% repolarisation

FIGURE 1: Effects of various doses of resveratrol and nebivolol on the action potential duration in normal rat papillary muscles. Res: resveratrol; Neb: Nebivolol. (a) Action potential duration at 20% of repolarisation. (b) Action potential duration at 50% of repolarisation. (c) Action potential duration at 90% of repolarisation. Data presented as mean $\pm$ SEM; $n = 5$–8.

syndrome is considered a clinical marker for ventricular arrhythmia and end-organ damage in hypertensive patients. The reduction of QT dispersion induced by nebivolol treatment has been reported to be independent of a decrease in blood pressure [25].

4.2. Vascular Function. Our study suggests that the resveratrol has the ability to induce mild relaxation in vascular tissue; however, the effects were more pronounced in the small resistance vessels than in the large aortic vessels precontracted with noradrenaline. In aortic tissues precontracted with potassium chloride, 4-aminopyridine, L-NAME,

and verapamil completely abolished the relaxation induced by resveratrol, suggesting that the vasodilation induced by resveratrol in large conduit arteries, such as the aorta, may be both endothelium dependent and independent. However, L-NAME appeared to potentiate the vasorelaxation response induced in small resistance vessels.

There is much debate in the current literature regarding the exact mechanism by which resveratrol induces vasorelaxation. In retinal arterioles, resveratrol induced relaxation in a dose-dependent manner [14]. The authors found that the addition of L-NAME partially prevented the resveratrol-mediated relaxation [14], suggesting that the activation of

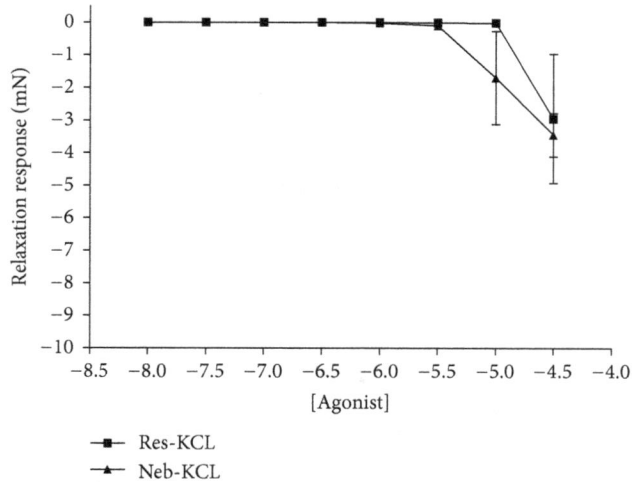

(a) Effect of resveratrol and nebivolol in thoracic aorta segments precontracted with potassium chloride

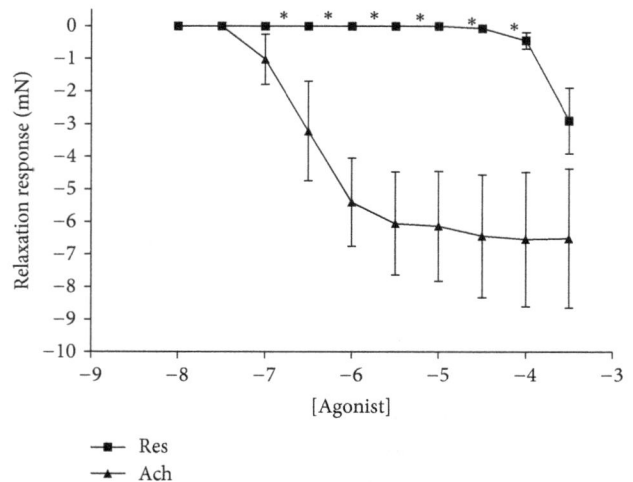

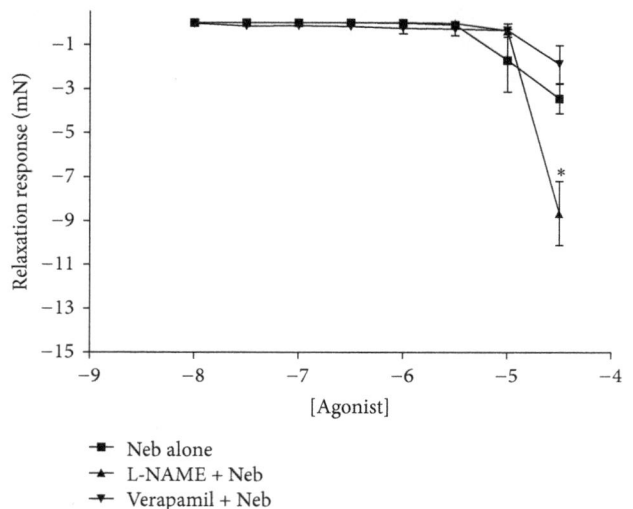

(b) Comparison of the effect of resveratrol and acetylcholine in thoracic aorta segments precontracted with noradrenaline

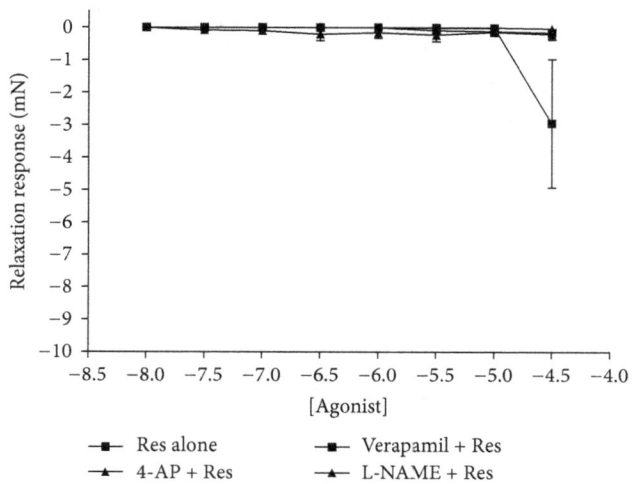

(c) Effect of various antagonists on relaxation induced by resveratrol in thoracic aorta segments precontracted with potassium chloride

(d) Effect of L-NAME and verapamil on relaxation induced by nebivolol in thoracic aorta segments precontracted with potassium chloride

FIGURE 2: Vasorelaxation induced by the addition of either resveratrol or nebivolol in isolated thoracic aortic segments. KCL: tydrodes solution containing potassium chloride; Res: resveratrol; Neb: nebivolol; Ach: acetylcholine; 4-AP: 4-aminopyridine; L-NAME: Nω-nitro-L-arginine-methyl ester. $^*P < 0.05$; data presented as mean $\pm$ SEM; $n = 9$ for all groups.

endothelial nitric oxide synthase may be partially responsible for the vasorelaxation. However, other published studies have speculated that potassium channels may play a role [21, 33]. In studies conducted in isolated rat aortic rings, the presence of 4-aminopyridine and magatoxin (a Kv1 channel inhibitor) completely abolished the resveratrol-induced vasorelaxation [33]. Similar results have been reported in mesenteric arteries collected from healthy rats [21]. The possibility exists that the discrepancies reported regarding resveratrol's mechanism of action may be due to the fact that responses may vary between healthy and diseased tissue, and in acute versus chronic administration.

Data gained in our study demonstrated that nebivolol induced mild relaxation in both the aortic and mesenteric

vessels that were precontracted with potassium chloride. The addition of either L-NAME or verapamil did not appear to hinder the relaxation produced by nebivolol. These results suggest that the response exhibited was not due to the release of nitric oxide or mediated through calcium channels. Adding nebivolol directly to the vascular tissue effectively bypassed metabolism; it is possible that it is the metabolites of nebivolol that are responsible for the reported effect on nitric oxide. This conclusion is supported by previously published studies [22]. A 50/50 mixture of both d- and l-nebivolol, once metabolised, was demonstrated to induce the release of nitric oxide in mouse aortas. These effects were not seen with nonmetabolised nebivolol or nebivolol bound to plasma [22]. The same study also found that even if nebivolol had been

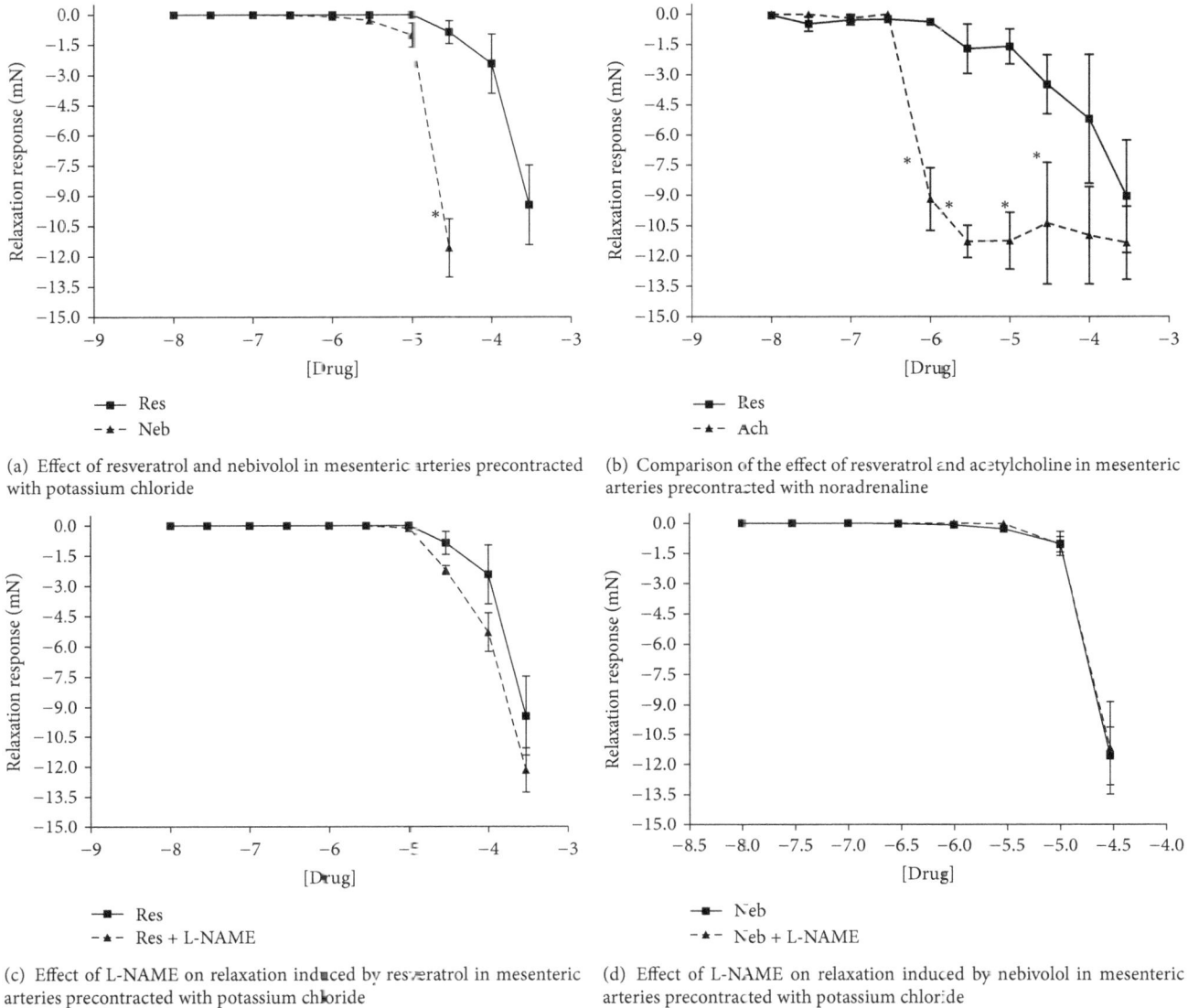

(a) Effect of resveratrol and nebivolol in mesenteric arteries precontracted with potassium chloride

(b) Comparison of the effect of resveratrol and acetylcholine in mesenteric arteries precontracted with noradrenaline

(c) Effect of L-NAME on relaxation induced by resveratrol in mesenteric arteries precontracted with potassium chloride

(d) Effect of L-NAME on relaxation induced by nebivolol in mesenteric arteries precontracted with potassium chloride

FIGURE 3: Relaxation responses induced by the addition of either resveratrol or nebivolol in isolated segments of mesenteric arteries. Res: resveratrol; Neb: nebivolol; Ach: acetylcholine; L-NAME: Nω-nitro-L-arginine-methyl-ester. $^*P < 0.05$, data presented as mean ± SEM; $n = 3$–6.

metabolised, it was still unable to induce an increase in NO if there was an insufficient amount of either intracellular or extracellular calcium.

The mechanisms by which nebivolol induces vasodilation are more established than resveratrol. Current literature places a heavy emphasis on the beneficial effect that nebivolol has not only on cardiovascular function but also on providing protection to the endothelium [4]. Patients with coronary artery disease treated with nebivolol for four weeks displayed an improvement in endothelium-dependent vasodilation in the brachial artery [34]. The authors suggest that these improvements were due to an increase in nitric oxide production and/or bioactivity [34].

One limitation of this study was the use of verapamil as a calcium channel antagonist in the vascular tissue. A more appropriate choice may have been a compound such

as nifedipine (vascular selective) or diltiazem (mixed cardiac and vascular effects). Verapamil has been shown to antagonise calcium channels in both cardiac and vascular tissues [35]. As this study examines various responses in both cardiac and vascular tissues, it was necessary to select a compound that would act on calcium channels in both experimental protocols. Verapamil was selected in order to explore any common effects.

5. Conclusion

Our results agree with the previously published data suggesting that both resveratrol and nebivolol display antiarrhythmic properties as demonstrated in their ability to decrease the duration of the cardiac action potential. Both compounds only elicit minor relaxation responses in both conduit and small resistance vessels at high concentrations. Drinking red wine alone would not provide a high enough concentration of resveratrol to benefit from its vasodilatory effects as red wine only contains 1.5–3.0 mg/L of resveratrol [36]; however, it can be achieved through supplementation.

In the aorta, resveratrol-induced relaxation was mediated mainly through independent mechanisms. The vasorelaxation response induced by nebivolol was not nitric oxide mediated. Both resveratrol and nebivolol displayed relatively mild effects when added acutely to healthy tissues. This effect may be more significant when examined in a chronic and/or diseased model as both compounds have been demonstrated to improve oxidative stress, decrease inflammation, and provide protection to the delicate endothelial lining of blood vessels.

Conflict of Interests

The authors declare that there is no conflict of interests regarding the publication of this paper.

References

[1] National Heart Foundation, *Data and Statistics*, 2012.

[2] S. R. Bhatt, M. F. Lokhandwala, and A. A. Banday, "Resveratrol prevents endothelial nitric oxide synthase uncoupling and attenuates development of hypertension in spontaneously hypertensive rats," *European Journal of Pharmacology*, vol. 667, no. 1–3, pp. 258–264, 2011.

[3] M. Mudau, A. Genis, A. Lochner, and H. Strijdom, "Endothelial dysfunction: the early predictor of atherosclerosis," *Cardiovascular Journal of Africa*, vol. 23, pp. 222–231, 2012.

[4] S. Chlopicki, V. I. Kozlovski, and R. J. Gryglewski, "No-dependent vasodilation induced by nebivolol in coronary circulation is not mediated by β-adrenoceptors or by 5 HT1A-receptors," *Journal of Physiology and Pharmacology*, vol. 53, no. 4, pp. 615–624, 2002.

[5] B. Turan, E. Tuncay, and G. Vassort, "Resveratrol and diabetic cardiac function: focus on recent in vitro and in vivo studies," *Journal of Bioenergetics and Biomembranes*, vol. 44, pp. 281–296, 2012.

[6] J. R. Cockcroft, P. J. Chowienczyk, S. E. Brett et al., "Nebivolol vasodilates human forearm vasculature: evidence for an L-arginine/NO-dependent mechanism," *Journal of Pharmacology and Experimental Therapeutics*, vol. 274, no. 3, pp. 1067–1071, 1995.

[7] G. Sacco, S. Evangelista, S. Manzini, M. Parlani, and M. Bigioni, "Combined antihypertensive and cardioprotective effects of nebivolol and hydrochlorothiazide in spontaneous hypertensive rats," *Future Cardiology*, vol. 7, no. 6, pp. 757–763, 2011.

[8] S. J. Thandapilly, P. Wojciechowski, J. Behbahani et al., "Resveratrol prevents the development of pathological cardiac hypertrophy and contractile dysfunction in the SHR without lowering blood pressure," *American Journal of Hypertension*, vol. 23, no. 2, pp. 192–196, 2010.

[9] N. Merchant, S. T. Rahman, K. C. Ferdinand, T. Haque, G. E. Umpierrez, and B. V. Khan, "Effects of nebivolol in obese African Americans with hypertension (NOAAH): markers of inflammation and obesity in response to exercise-induced stress," *Journal of Human Hypertension*, vol. 25, no. 3, pp. 196–202, 2011.

[10] S. J. Wang, Q. Y. Bo, X. H. Zhao, X. Yang, Z. F. Chi, and X. W. Liu, "Resveratrol pre-treatment reduces early inflammatory responses induced by status epilepticus via mtor signaling," *Brain Research*, vol. 1492, pp. 122–129, 2013.

[11] X. Zhou, L. Ma, J. Habibi et al., "Nebivolol improves diastolic dysfunction and myocardial remodeling through reductions in oxidative stress in the zucker obese rat," *Hypertension*, vol. 55, no. 4, pp. 880–888, 2010.

[12] C.-C. Chang, C.-Y. Chang, Y.-T. Wu, J.-P. Huang, T.-H. Yen, and L.-M. Hung, "Resveratrol retards progression of diabetic nephropathy through modulations of oxidative stress, proinflammatory cytokines, and AMP-activated protein kinase," *Journal of Biomedical Science*, vol. 18, no. 1, article 47, 2011.

[13] H.-F. Li, Z.-F. Tian, X.-Q. Qiu, J.-X. Wu, P. Zhang, and Z.-J. Jia, "A study of mechanisms involved in vasodilatation induced by resveratrol in isolated porcine coronary artery," *Physiological Research*, vol. 55, no. 4, pp. 365–372, 2006.

[14] T. Nagaoka, T. W. Hein, A. Yoshida, and L. Kuo, "Resveratrol, a component of red wine, elicits dilation of isolated porcine retinal arterioles: role of nitric oxide and potassium channels," *Investigative Ophthalmology and Visual Science*, vol. 48, no. 9, pp. 4232–4239, 2007.

[15] S. K. Manna, A. Mukhopadhyay, and B. B. Aggarwal, "Resveratrol suppresses TNF-induced activation of nuclear transcription factors NF-κB, activator protein-1, and apoptosis: potential role of reactive oxygen intermediates and lipid peroxidation," *Journal of Immunology*, vol. 164, no. 12, pp. 6509–6519, 2000.

[16] W.-P. Chen, M.-J. Su, and L.-M. Hung, "In vitro electrophysiological mechanisms for antiarrhythmic efficacy of resveratrol, a red wine antioxidant," *European Journal of Pharmacology*, vol. 554, no. 2-3, pp. 196–204, 2007.

[17] S. Rimbaud, M. Ruiz, J. Piquereau et al., "Resveratrol improves survival, hemodynamics and energetics in a rat model of hypertension leading to heart failure," *PLoS ONE*, vol. 6, no. 10, Article ID e26391, 2011.

[18] V. Chan, A. Fenning, A. Iyer, A. Hoey, and L. Brown, "Resveratrol improves cardiovascular function in DOCA-salt hypertensive rats," *Current Pharmaceutical Biotechnology*, vol. 12, no. 3, pp. 429–436, 2011.

[19] J. Lekakis, L. S. Rallidis, I. Andreadou et al., "Polyphenolic compounds from red grapes acutely improve endothelial function in patients with coronary heart disease," *European Journal of Cardiovascular Prevention and Rehabilitation*, vol. 12, no. 6, pp. 596–600, 2005.

[20] R. H. X. Wong, P. R. C. Howe, J. D. Buckley, A. M. Coates, I. Kunz, and N. M. Berry, "Acute resveratrol supplementation improves flow-mediated dilatation in overweight/obese individuals with mildly elevated blood pressure," *Nutrition, Metabolism and Cardiovascular Diseases*, vol. 21, no. 11, pp. 851–856, 2011.

[21] L. Gojkovic-Bukarica, A. Novakovic, V. Kanjuh, M. Bumbasirevic, A. Lesic, and H. Heinle, "A role of ion channels in the endothelium-independent relaxation of rat mesenteric artery induced by resveratrol," *Journal of Pharmacological Sciences*, vol. 108, no. 1, pp. 124–130, 2008.

[22] M. A. W. Broeders, P. A. Doevendans, B. C. A. M. Bekkers et al., "Nebivolol: a third-generation β-blocker that augments vascular nitric oxide release. Endothelial β2-adrenergic receptor-mediated nitric oxide production," *Circulation*, vol. 102, no. 6, pp. 677–684, 2000.

[23] L. J. Ignarro, "Different pharmacological properties of two enantiomers in a unique β-blocker, nebivolol," *Cardiovascular Therapeutics*, vol. 26, no. 2, pp. 115–134, 2008.

[24] T. Tran Quang, B. Rozec, L. Audigane, and C. Gauthier, "Investigation of the different adrenoceptor targets of nebivolol enantiomers in rat thoracic aorta," *British Journal of Pharmacology*, vol. 156, no. 4, pp. 601–608, 2009.

[25] F. Galetta, F. Franzoni, A. Magagna et al., "Effect of nebivolol on QT dispersion in hypertensive patients with left ventricular hypertrophy," *Biomedicine and Pharmacotherapy*, vol. 59, no. 1-2, pp. 15–19, 2005.

[26] H. R. Lu, P. Remeysen, and F. De Clerck, "Antiarrhythmic effects of nebivolol in experimental models in vivo," *Journal of Cardiovascular Pharmacology*, vol. 24, no. 6, pp. 986–993, 1994.

[27] A. Fenning, G. Harrison, R. Rose'meyer, A. Hoey, and L. Brown, "L-Arginine attenuates cardiovascular impairment in DOCA-salt hypertensive rats," *The American Journal of Physiology—Heart and Circulatory Physiology*, vol. 289, no. 4, pp. H1408–H1416, 2005.

[28] M. J. Mulvany, *Procedures For Investigation of Small Vessels Using Small Vessel Myograph*, Danish Myo Technology, 2004.

[29] R. Liew, M. A. Stagg, K. T. MacLeod, and P. Collins, "The red wine polyphenol, resveratrol, exerts acute direct actions on guinea-pig ventricular myocytes," *European Journal of Pharmacology*, vol. 519, no. 1-2, pp. 1–8, 2005.

[30] J. Zhao, H.-J. Ma, J.-H. Dong, L.-P. Zhang, E.-L. Liu, and Q.-S. Wang, "Electrophysiological effects of resveratrol on guinea pig papillary muscles," *Acta Physiologica Sinica*, vol. 56, no. 6, pp. 708–712, 2004.

[31] L.-P. Zhang, J.-X. Yin, Z. Liu, Y. Zhang, Q.-S. Wang, and J. Zhao, "Effect of resveratrol on L-type calcium current in rat ventricular myocytes," *Acta Pharmacologica Sinica*, vol. 27, no. 2, pp. 179–183, 2006.

[32] P. Arlock, B. Wohlfart, T. Sjöberg, and S. Steen, "The negative inotropic effect of esmolol on isolated cardiac muscle," *Scandinavian Cardiovascular Journal*, vol. 39, no. 4, pp. 250–254, 2005.

[33] A. Novakovic, L. G. Bukarica, V. Kanjuh, and H. Heinle, "Potassium channels-mediated vasorelaxation of rat aorta induced by resveratrol," *Basic and Clinical Pharmacology and Toxicology*, vol. 99, no. 5, pp. 360–364, 2006.

[34] J. P. Lekakis, A. Protogerou, C. Papamichael et al., "Effect of nebivolol and atenolol on brachial artery flow-mediated vasodilation in patients with coronary artery disease," *Cardiovascular Drugs and Therapy*, vol. 19, no. 4, pp. 277–281, 2005.

[35] S. Yesmine, K. Connolly, N. Hill, F. R. Coulson, and A. S. Fenning, "Electrophysiological, vasoactive, and gastromodulatory effects of stevia in healthy wistar rats," *Planta Medica*, vol. 79, no. 11, pp. 909–915, 2013.

[36] H. D. Hao and L. R. He, "Mechanisms of cardiovascular protection by resveratrol," *Journal of Medicinal Food*, vol. 7, no. 3, pp. 290–298, 2004.

7

Influence of Flunixin on the Disposition Kinetic of Cefepime in Goats

Mohamed El-Hewaity

Department of Pharmacology, Faculty of Veterinary Medicine, University of El-Sadat City, Minoufiya 32897, Egypt

Correspondence should be addressed to Mohamed El-Hewaity; melhewaty@yahoo.com

Academic Editor: Antonio Ferrer-Montiel

The pharmacokinetic profile of cefepime (10 mg/kg b.w.) was studied following intravenous and intramuscular administration of cefepime alone and coadministered with flunixin (2.2 mg/kg b.w.) in goats. Cefepime concentrations in serum were determined by microbiological assay technique using *Escherichia coli* (MTCC 443) as test organism. Following intravenous injection of cefepime alone and in combination with flunixin, there are no significant changes in the pharmacokinetic parameters. Following intramuscular injection of cefepime alone and in combination with flunixin, the maximum serum concentration was significantly increased in flunixin coadministered group compared with cefepime alone. However, no significant changes were reported in other pharmacokinetic parameters. The result of *in vitro* protein binding study indicated that 15.62% of cefepime was bound to goat's serum protein. The mean bioavailability was 92.66% and 95.27% in cefepime alone and coadministered with flunixin, respectively. The results generated from the present study suggest that cefepime may be coadministered with flunixin without change in dose regimen. Cefepime may be given intramuscularly at 12 h intervals to combat susceptible bacterial infections.

1. Introduction

It is well documented that concurrently administered drugs may alter pharmacokinetics of one or both drugs and in therapeutics antibiotic and nonsteroidal anti-inflammatory drugs (NSAIDs) are used most frequently in multiple drug prescriptions. Cefepime is a semisynthetic broad spectrum fourth generation cephalosporin antibiotic with a modified zwitterionic structure that allows more favorable penetration into the bacterial cells and reduced susceptibility to β-lactamases [1]. Cefepime shows broad spectrum of activity which includes Gram-positive cocci, enteric Gram-negative bacilli, and *Pseudomonas aeruginosa*. It lacks activity against methicillin-resistant *Staphylococcus aureus*, enterococci, *Bacteroides fragilis*, and *Listeria monocytogenes* [2]. Flunixin is nonsteroidal anti-inflammatory drug inhibiting cyclooxygenase enzymes in the arachidonic acid cascade, thus blocking the formation of cyclooxygenase derived eicosanoid inflammatory mediators [3]. Due to its anti-inflammatory, analgesic, and antipyretic effects [4], flunixin is widely used in veterinary medicine to treat the musculoskeletal conditions,

acute mastitis, endotoxemia, and calf pneumonia [5, 6]. The pharmacokinetics of cefepime administered as a single drug has been investigated in many animal species including goats [7, 8], calves [9–11], cow calves [12], and sheep [13]. However, there is no available information on the influence of flunixin on the disposition kinetic of cefepime in goats. But there is some literature available on the influence of other NSAIDs on pharmacokinetics of cefepime as the effect of ketoprofen on disposition kinetic of cefepime in cow calves [12] and sheep [14]. The aim of the study was to determine the disposition kinetic of cefepime in goats after a single intravenous and intramuscular administration. More to assess the effect of flunixin co-administration on the disposition kinetic of cefepime in goats.

2. Materials and Methods

2.1. Drugs and Chemicals. Cefepime hydrochloride powder (Onsime) was purchased from Sigmatec Pharmaceutical Industries Egypt. Flunixin meglumine (Megloxyine) was purchased from ADWIA Pharmaceuticals Company Egypt.

Mueller-Hinton agar was purchased from Mast Group Ltd., Merseyside, UK.

2.2. Animals. Twelve clinically normal goats were used in this investigation. The body weight ranged from 24 to 32 kg. Animals were housed in hygienic stable and fed on Berseem clover (*Trifolium alexandrinum*) dry concentrate. Water was provided *ad libitum*. None of the animals were treated with antibiotics for one month prior to the trial. The experiment was performed in accordance with the guidelines set by the Ethical Committee of El-Sadat City University, Egypt.

2.2.1. Experimental Design. Goats were randomly divided into two groups six goats each. The 1st group received cefepime 10 mg/kg b.w. as a single intravenous dose into the right jugular vein and single intramuscular dose into the deep gluteal muscle with 2-week washout period between each route. Those of the 2nd group were given a single dose of flunixin (2.2 mg/kg b.w. IM) followed immediately cefepime 10 mg/kg b.w. by intravenous and intramuscular routes with 2 weeks of washout period between each route. Blood samples were collected at 5, 10, 15, and 30 minutes and 1, 2, 4, 8, 12, 18, and 24 h after drug administration. Blood samples were left to clot for 1 hour at room temperature; the clear sera were separated by centrifugation at 3000 r.p.m for 15 minutes and stored at −20°C until assayed.

2.2.2. Drug Bioassay. The concentration of cefepime in serum samples was estimated by a standard microbiological assay method described by [15] using *Escherichia coli* (MTCC 443) as test organism [7]. This method estimated the level of drug having antibacterial activity, without differentiating between the parent drug and its active metabolites. The application of microbiological assay for measuring cefepime concentration is suitable [7]. Six wells were made at equal distances in standard Petri dishes containing 25 mL seeded agar. The wells were filled with 100 μL of either the test samples or the cefepime standard concentrations. The plates were kept at room temperature for 2 h before being incubated at 37°C for 18 h. Zones of inhibition were measured using micrometers, and the cefepime concentrations in the test samples were calculated from the standard curve. Cefepime standard solution of concentrations from 0.195 to 50 μg/mL. was prepared in antibiotic-free goat serum and phosphate buffer saline. Standard curves of cefepime were prepared in antibacterial-free goat serum by the appropriate serial dilution. The standard curve in goat serum was linear over the range of 0.195 to 50 μg/mL and the value of correlation coefficient (r) was 0.991. The limit of quantification was 0.195 μg/mL. Protein binding of cefepime was estimated according to [16].

2.3. Pharmacokinetic and Statistical Analysis. Following IV administration, the serum concentration versus time data of cefepime alone and coadministered with flunixin was fitted to a two-compartment open model system according to the following biexponential equation [17]:

$$C_p = Ae^{-at} + Be^{-\beta t}, \tag{1}$$

where C_p is the concentration of drug in the serum at time t, A and B are the zero-time drug intercepts of the distribution and elimination phase expressed as μg mL^{-1}, α and β are the distribution and elimination rate constants expressed in units of reciprocal time (h^{-1}), and e is the natural logarithm base.

A pharmacokinetic computer program (R-strip, Micromath, Scientific software, USA) was used to determine the least-squares best-fit curve for cefepime concentration versus time data. Following IV and IM administrations, the appropriate pharmacokinetic model was determined by visual examination of individual concentration-time curves and by application of Akaike's information criterion (AIC) [18]. The pharmacokinetic parameters were reported as mean ± SE. Mean pharmacokinetic parameters after IV and IM administrations were statistically compared in cefepime alone and coadministered with flunixin using Student's t-test [19].

3. Results

No clinical signs of adverse effects or intolerance were observed to cefepime after IV or IM injection. Mean serum concentrations of cefepime in goat following IV and IM injection of 10 mg/kg alone and coadministered with flunixin (2.2 mg/kg b.w.) are summarized in Figures 1 and 2. These data are best fitted to a two-compartment open model. The initial serum drug concentration following IV injection was 46.53 and 46.62 μg/mL in cefepime alone and coadministered with flunixin, respectively, and was detected above MIC up to 12 h of administration in cefepime alone and coadministered with flunixin. Following IM injection of cefepime alone or coadministered with flunixin, the mean peak serum concentrations (C_{max}) were 16.49 ± 0.53 and 19.03 ± 0.71 μg/mL achieved at time (T_{max}) 0.91 ± 0.08 and 1.01 ± 0.07 h, respectively. Cefepime could be detected in a therapeutic concentration for 12 h after IM injection in cefepime alone and coadministered with flunixin. The pharmacokinetic parameters of cefepime in goat following IV and IM injection of 10 mg/kg b.w. alone and coadministered with flunixin (2.2 mg/kg b.w.) are summarized in Tables 1 and 2. Following IV injection of cefepime alone and in combination with flunixin, there are no significant changes in the pharmacokinetic parameters. Following IM injection, the mean peak serum concentration (C_{max}) in goats was significantly increased in flunixin coadministered compared with cefepime alone. The result of *in vitro* protein binding study indicated that 15.62% of cefepime was bound to goat's serum protein. The mean bioavailability was 92.66% and 95.27% in cefepime alone and coadministered with flunixin, respectively.

4. Discussion

The pharmacokinetic of cefepime in goats is reported in the present study. The results revealed that serum cefepime concentration versus time decreased in a biexponential manner following IV injection either alone or when used concomitantly with flunixin, demonstrating the presence of distribution and elimination phases and justifying the use of

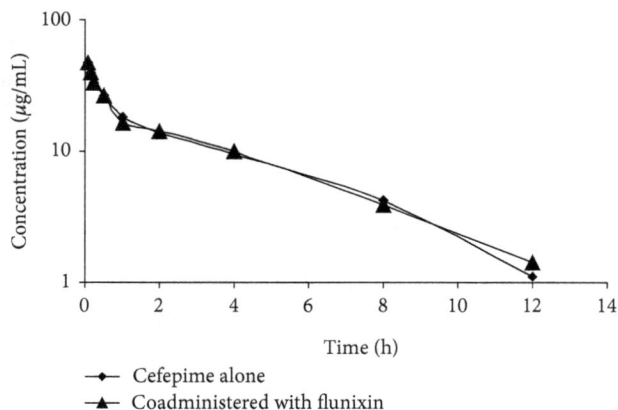

FIGURE 1: Serum concentrations of cefepime alone and in combination with flunixin following a single intravenous injection in goats.

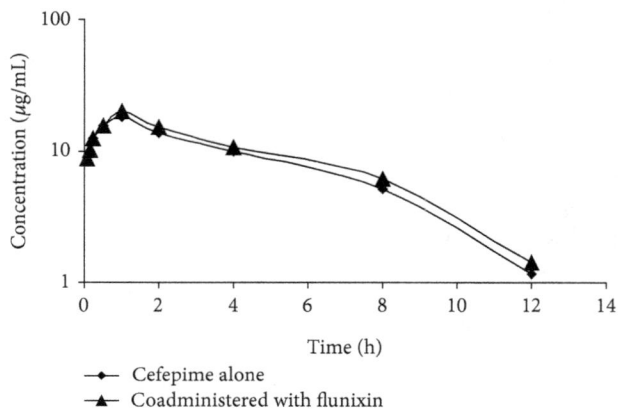

FIGURE 2: Serum concentrations of cefepime alone and in combination with flunixin following a single intramuscular injection in goats.

TABLE 1: Mean (±SE) kinetic parameters of cefepime (10 mg/kg b.w.) alone and in combination with flunixin (2.2 mg/kg b.w.) following a single intravenous injection in goats ($n = 6$).

Parameter	Units	Cefepime alone	Cefepime + flunixin
$T_{1/2(\alpha)}$	h	0.20 ± 0.004	0.20 ± 0.003
Vc	L kg^{-1}	0.18 ± 0.007	0.18 ± 0.006
Vd$_{(area)}$	L kg^{-1}	0.46 ± 0.02	0.48 ± 0.03
Vd$_{ss}$	L kg^{-1}	0.44 ± 0.01	0.47 ± 0.04
K_{12}	h^{-1}	2.17 ± 0.04	2.26 ± 0.09
K_{21}	h^{-1}	1.47 ± 0.09	1.40 ± 0.04
K_{el}	h^{-1}	0.49 ± 0.02	0.50 ± 0.03
$T_{1/2(\beta)}$	h	3.34 ± 0.12	3.50 ± 0.23
AUC$_{(0-inf)}$	μg mL^{-1} h^{-1}	102.38 ± 8.61	103.91 ± 10.08
MRT	h	3.35 ± 0.22	3.48 ± 0.24
Cl$_B$	L kg^{-1} h^{-1}	0.098 ± 0.0004	0.096 ± 0.0003

$T_{1/2(\alpha)}$: distribution half-life; Vc: apparent volume of central compartment; Vd$_{(area)}$: apparent volume of distribution calculated by area method; Vd$_{ss}$: volume of distribution at steady state; K_{12}: first-order constant for transfer from central to peripheral compartment; K_{21}: first-order constant for transfer from peripheral to central compartment; K_{el}: elimination rate constant; $T_{1/2(\beta)}$: elimination half-life; AUC$_{(0-inf)}$: area under serum concentration-time curve; MRT: mean residence time; Cl$_B$: total body clearance.

TABLE 2: Mean (±SE) kinetic parameters of cefepime (10 mg/kg b.w.) alone and in combination with flunixin (2.2 mg/kg b.w.) following a single intramuscular injection in goats ($n = 6$).

Parameter	Units	Cefepime alone	Cefepime + flunixin
$T_{1/2(ab)}$	h	0.25 ± 0.02	0.28 ± 0.03
$T_{1/2(el)}$	h	3.44 ± 0.31	3.50 ± 0.22
C_{max}	μg·mL^{-1}	16.49 ± 0.53	19.03 ± 0.71*
T_{max}	h	0.91 ± 0.08	1.01 ± 0.07
AUC$_{(0-inf)}$	μg·h·mL^{-1}	94.87 ± 3.89	98.99 ± 4.01
MRT	h	4.01 ± 0.33	4.08 ± 0.28

$^*P < 0.05$ significant difference.

$T_{1/2(ab)}$: absorption half-life; $T_{1/2(el)}$: elimination half-life; C_{max}: maximum serum concentration; T_{max}: time to peak serum concentration; AUC$_{(0-inf)}$: area under serum concentration-time curve; MRT: mean residence time.

two-compartment open model. This finding is in agreement with cefepime in goats [8]. Serum concentration showed a similar rapid distribution phase with elimination half-life of 3.34 and 3.50 h, respectively. This finding was similar to that recorded in calves 3.70 h [9] and cow calves 3.90 h [12]. Cefepime has moderate distribution in the body of goats with Vd$_{ss}$ of 0.44 and 0.47 L/kg in cefepime alone and coadministered with flunixin, respectively. This Vd$_{ss}$ was in agreement with that of the drug in cow calves 0.52 L/kg [12], in sheep 0.42 L/kg [13], and in calves 0.43 L/kg [9]. Mean value of the residence time (3.35 and 3.48 h) in cefepime alone and co-administered with flunixin, respectively. This finding was similar to that recorded in cow calves 3.38 h [10] and in calves 3.95 h [9], but longer than the value of 2.64 h recorded in goat [8]. Following intravenous injection of cefepime alone and in combination with flunixin, there are no significant changes in the pharmacokinetic parameters. These findings were similar to that recorded by [20] who found that there are no significant changes recorded in kinetic parameters of orbifloxacin (IV) when given with flunixin.

Following intramuscular administration of cefepime alone or coadministered with flunixin, no adverse effects

or toxic manifestations were observed. The drug was very rapidly absorbed with a short absorption half-life $T_{1/2(ab)}$ of 0.25 ± 0.02 h. The obtained result is consistent with those reported for cefepime in calves 0.21 ± 0.03 h [11]. The mean peak serum concentration (C_{max}) in goats was significantly increased in flunixin coadministered (19.03 ± 0.71 μg/mL) compared with cefepime alone (16.49 ± 0.53 μg/mL). A similar significant increase in peak serum level of cefepime following concomitant intramuscular administration of keto-profen with cefepime has been observed in sheep [14]. A significant increase in peak serum level of ceftizoxime following concomitant intramuscular administration of paracetamol with ceftizoxime has been observed in cross-bred calves [21]. However, no significant alteration in C_{max} was observed following coadministration of ketoprofen with cefepime in cow calves and coadministration of flunixin with orbifloxacin in buffalo calves [12, 20], respectively.

The $T_{1/2(el)}$ was 3.44 ± 0.31 h which was shorter than cefepime in goat 4.89 ± 0.24 h [8], in sheep 5.17 ± 0.44 h [13], and in cow calves 5.15 ± 0.09 h [12]. The MRT was 4.01 ± 0.33 h which was similar to cefepime in goats 4.89 h [8], while being shorter than cefepime in sheep 6.89 h [13]. These differences are relatively common and are frequently related to interspecies variation, assay methods used, the amount of time between blood samplings and/or the health status, and age of the animal [22].

Following intramuscular administration of cefepime with flunixin in goat, none of the pharmacokinetic parameters were altered significantly (except C_{max}) in comparison to cefepime alone. Similarly there was no significant alteration in pharmacokinetic parameters (except C_{max} and $T_{1/2(\alpha)}$) following coadministration of ketoprofen with cefepime in sheep [14], also the kinetic behavior of marbofloxacin in buffaloes was influenced by the coadministration with flunixin, and the affected parameters were C_{max} and MRT [23] which support the results of our study. However, there are no significant changes in all pharmacokinetic parameters recorded by [20] who found that there are no significant changes recorded in kinetic parameters of orbifloxacin when given with flunixin in buffalo calves. Also, there is no significant change have been recorded in kinetic parameters of cefepime when given with ketoprofen in cow calves [12]. Variations in the pharmacokinetics of cefepime and other cephalosporins when given with NSAIDs have been observed in many experiments that may be due to differences in the chemistry of drugs and species difference.

Average serum concentration of 0.004–1.0 μg/mL had been reported to be minimum inhibitory concentration (MIC_{90}) for cephalosporins with various pathogens [24]. An average MIC_{90} of 0.5 μg/mL of cefepime has been taken into consideration for calculation of efficacy predictors. Following intramuscular administration of cefepime alone or coadministered with flunixin in goats would result in a C_{max}/MIC_{90} ratio of 32.98- and 38.06-fold, respectively, which exceeds the recommended ratio of 10 and leads to potential clinical and bacteriological efficacy of cefepime [25, 26]. It is now accepted that high C_{max}/MIC_{90} values are necessary in order to avoid the emergence of bacterial resistance [27].

Based on this data, the intravenous and intramuscular injection of cefepime at dose of 10 mg/kg b.w. at 12 h interval in goat is sufficient to maintain serum concentration above MIC for most sensitive susceptible pathogens. The systemic bioavailability of cefepime in goats after IM administration alone and in combination with flunixin was 92.66 and 95.27%, respectively, which indicates excellent absorption of the drug. This finding was similar to that recorded in calves 98 ± 3% [11] and goats 86.45 ± 17.39% [7].

5. Conclusion

Cefepime can be used safely and effectively with flunixin for treating the infections and combating inflammatory conditions without alteration of the dose and dose intervals in goats. Further investigation should be done in the future to assess the effect of cefepime on the disposition kinetic of flunixin in goats.

Conflict of Interests

The author declares that there is no conflict of interests regarding the publication of this paper.

Acknowledgment

The author would like to thank Professor Dr. H. A. El-Banna, Pharmacology Department, Faculty of Veterinary Medicine, Cairo University, Giza, Egypt, for comments on the paper.

References

[1] P. Del Rio, M. Vellone, P. Fragapane et al., "Cefepime for prophylaxis of infections in the surgery of cholelithiasis. Results of a multicentric comparative trial," *Acta Biomedica de l'Ateneo Parmense*, vol. 79, no. 1, pp. 23–27, 2008.

[2] H. S. Sandhu and S. Rampal, *Essentials of Veterinary Pharmacology and Therapeutics*, Kalyani Publishers, New Delhi, India, 1st edition, 2006.

[3] Z. Cheng, A. M. Nolan, and Q. A. Mckellar, "Measurement of cyclooxygenase inhibition in vivo: a study of two non-steroidal anti-inflammatory drugs in sheep," *Inflammation*, vol. 22, no. 4, pp. 353–366, 1998.

[4] C. Beretta, G. Garavaglia, and M. Cavalli, "COX-1 and COX-2 inhibition in horse blood by phenylbutazone, flunixin, carprofen and meloxicam: an in vitro analysis," *Pharmacological Research*, vol. 52, no. 4, pp. 302–306, 2005.

[5] K. Odensvik and U. Magnusson, "Effect of oral administration of flunixin meglumine on the inflammatory response to endotoxin in heifers," *The American Journal of Veterinary Research*, vol. 57, no. 2, pp. 201–204, 1996.

[6] M. Rantala, L. Kaartinen, E. Välimäki et al., "Efficacy and pharmacokinetics of enrofloxacin and flunixin meglumine for treatment of cows with experimentally induced *Escherichia coli* mastitis," *Journal of Veterinary Pharmacology and Therapeutics*, vol. 25, no. 4, pp. 251–258, 2002.

[7] S. Prawez, R. Raina, D. Dimitrova, N. K. Pankaj, A. A. Ahanger, and P. K. Verma, "The pharmacokinetics of cefepime in goats following single-dose i.v. and i.m. administration," *Turkish Journal of Veterinary and Animal Sciences*, vol. 34, no. 5, pp. 427–431, 2010.

[8] K. Patani, U. Patel, S. Bhavsar, A. Thaker, and J. Sarvaiya, "Single dose pharmacokinetics of cefepime after intravenous and intramuscular administration in goats," *Turkish Journal of Veterinary and Animal Sciences*, vol. 32, no. 3, pp. 159–162, 2008.

[9] U. D. Patel, S. K. Bhavsar, and A. M. Thaker, "Pharmacokinetics and dosage regimen of cefepime following single dose intravenous administration in calves," *Iranian Journal of Pharmacology and Therapeutics*, vol. 5, no. 2, pp. 127–130, 2006.

[10] M. M. Ismail, "Disposition kinetics, bioavailability and renal clearance of cefepime in calves," *Veterinary Research Communications*, vol. 29, no. 1, pp. 69–79, 2005.

[11] U. Patel, K. Patani, S. Bhavsar, and A. Thaker, "Disposition kinetics of cefepime following single dose IM administration in calves," *International Journal of Cow Science*, vol. 2, no. 1, pp. 49–51, 2006.

[12] A. Patil, S. Bhavsar, H. Patel et al., "Effect of ketoprofen coadministration on pharmacokinetic of cefepime in cow calves," *International Journal of Veterinary Science*, vol. 1, no. 2, pp. 72–75, 2012.

[13] P. N. Patel, U. D. Patel, S. K. Bhavsar, and A. M. Thaker, "Pharmacokinetics of cefepime following intravenous and intramuscular administration in sheep," *Iranian Journal of Pharmacology and Therapeutics*, vol. 9, no. 1, pp. 7–10, 2010.

[14] N. Patel, H. Patel, S. Patel, J. Patel, S. Bhavsar, and A. Thaker, "Effect of ketoprofen co-administration or febrile state on pharmacokinetic of cefepime in sheep," *Veterinarski Arhiv*, vol. 82, no. 5, pp. 473–481, 2012.

[15] B. Arret, D. P. Johnson, and A. Kirshbaum, "Outline of details for microbiological assays of antibiotics: second revision," *Journal of Pharmaceutical Sciences*, vol. 60, no. 11, pp. 1689–1694, 1971.

[16] A. W. Craig and B. Suh, "Protein binding and the antibacterial effects: methods for determination of protein binding," in *Antibiotics in Laboratory Medicine*, V. Lorian, Ed., pp. 265–297, Williams and Wilkins, Baltimore, Md, USA, 1980.

[17] J. D. Baggot, "Some aspects of clinical pharmacokinetics in veterinary medicine," *Journal of Veterinary Pharmacology and Therapeutics*, vol. 1, no. 1, pp. 5–18, 1978.

[18] K. Yamaoka, T. Nakagawa, and T. Uno, "Statistical moments in pharmacokinetics," *Journal of Pharmacokinetics and Biopharmaceutics*, vol. 6, no. 6, pp. 547–558, 1978.

[19] G. W. Snedecor and T. Cochran, *Statistical Methods*, Ames, Iowa, USA, 6th edition, 1976.

[20] M. Tohamy, "Pharmacokinetic interaction of flunixin and orbifloxacin in buffalo calves," *Insight Pharmaceutical Sciences*, vol. 1, no. 3, pp. 29–33, 2011.

[21] R. Singh, R. K. Chaudhary, and V. K. Dumka, "Influence of paracetamol on the pharmacokinetics and dosage regimen of ceftizoxime in cross bred calves," *Israel Journal of Veterinary Medicine*, vol. 63, no. 3, pp. 72–76, 2008.

[22] N. S. Haddad, W. M. Pedersoli, W. R. Ravis, M. H. Fazel, and R. L. Carson, "Pharmacokinetics of gentamicin at steady-state in ponies: serum, urine, and endometrial concentrations," *The American Journal of Veterinary Research*, vol. 46, no. 6, pp. 1268–1271, 1985.

[23] E. Baroni, C. Rodriguez, M. D. San Andres et al., "Influence of the combination flunixin and marbofloxacin after its IM administration on the pharmacokinetics of marbofloxacin in buffaloes (preliminary study)," *Revista Veterinaria*, vol. 21, no. 1, pp. 317–319, 2010.

[24] J. Hardman and L. Limbird, *Goodman and Gilman's the Pharmacological Basis of Therapeutics*, McGraw-Hill, New York, NY, USA, 10th edition, 2001.

[25] M. N. Dudley, "Pharmacodynamics and pharmacokinetics of antibiotics with special reference to the fluoroquinolones," *The American Journal of Medicine*, vol. 91, no. 6, pp. 45–50, 1991.

[26] P. L. Toutain, J. R. E. Del Castillo, and A. Bousquet-Mélou, "The pharmacokinetic-pharmacodynamic approach to a rational dosage regimen for antibiotics," *Research in Veterinary Science*, vol. 73, no. 2, pp. 105–114, 2002.

[27] R. D. Walker, "The use of fluoroquinolones for companion animal antimicrobial therapy," *Australian Veterinary Journal*, vol. 78, no. 2, pp. 84–90, 2000.

8

Development of an Antioxidant Phytoextract of *Lantana grisebachii* with Lymphoprotective Activity against *In Vitro* Arsenic Toxicity

Elio A. Soria,[1] Patricia L. Quiroga,[1] Claudia Albrecht,[1] Sabina I. Ramos Elizagaray,[2] Juan J. Cantero,[3] and Guillermina A. Bongiovanni[4]

[1] *Facultad de Ciencias Médicas, Universidad Nacional de Córdoba, INICSA-CONICET/UNC, Enrique Barros S/N, 5014 Córdoba, Argentina*
[2] *Consejo Interuniversitario Nacional, Pacheco de Melo 2084, 1126 Ciudad Autónoma de Buenos Aires, Argentina*
[3] *Facultad de Agronomía y Veterinaria, Universidad Nacional de Río Cuarto, IMBIV-CONICET/UNC, Ruta 36 Km 601, 5804 Río Cuarto, Argentina*
[4] *Facultad de Ciencias Agrarias, Universidad Nacional del Comahue, PROBIEN-CONICET/UNCO, CP 8300, Neuquén, 1400 Buenos Aires, Argentina*

Correspondence should be addressed to Elio A. Soria; easoria@fcm.unc.edu.ar

Academic Editor: Robert Gogal

Phytochemicals have been presumed to possess prophylactic and curative properties in several pathologies, such as arsenic- (As-) induced immunosuppression. Our aim was to discover a lymphoprotective extract from *Lantana grisebachii* Stuck. (Verbenaceae) (LG). We assessed its bioactivity and chemical composition using cell-based assays. Fractions produced from a hexane extract acutely induced nitrite formation in T-activated cell cultures ($P < 0.0001$). Water extraction released a fraction lacking nitrite inducing activity in both lymphocyte types. Aqueous LG was found to be safe in proliferated and proliferating cells. The infusion-derived extract presented better antioxidant capacity in proportion to phenolic amount in lymphocytes (infusive LG-1i at 100 μg/mL), which protected them against *in vitro* As-induced lymphotoxicity ($P < 0.0001$). This infusive LG phytoextract contained 10.23 ± 0.43 mg/g of phenolics, with 58.46% being flavonoids. Among the phenolics, the only predominant compound was 0.723 mg of chlorogenic acid per gram of dry plant, in addition to 10 unknown minor compounds. A fatty acid profile was assessed. It contained one-third of saturated fatty acids, one-third of ω9, followed by ω6 (~24%) and ω3 (~4%), and scarce ω7. Summing up, *L. grisebachii* was a source of bioactive and lymphoprotective compounds, which could counteract As-toxicity. This supports its phytomedical use and research in order to reduce As-related dysfunctions.

1. Introduction

Many Argentinean plant species have been proposed as sources of bioactive compounds that might be used to prevent and treat several human health pathologies [1]. Among these compounds, phenolics are the main candidates for this biomedical potential, given their antioxidant and multitarget effects. These processes involve xenohormesis, which is an organic enhancement of cellular resistance against oxidative stress acquired by consuming plant-synthesized compounds [2]. Oxidative stress underlies numerous chronic dysfunctions by triggering a redox imbalance with free radical overproduction (reactive species of O, N, or S) and impairment of antioxidant defence [3]. Reactive species can be generated endogenously by cellular mechanisms or be induced exogenously by environmental agents, such as pollutants (e.g., arsenic, pesticides, etc.) [4].

The immune system involves a complex integration of biological defences intended to protect an organism against numerous pathogens, with B and T lymphocytes being the crucial cells involved [5]. Given that the immune system is one of the main targets affected by environmental oxidants (secondary immunosuppression), immune recovery might be achieved by implementing certain bioactive phytochemicals with immunoxenohormetic activity [6]. Accordingly, antioxidants could be used as chemopreventive immunoregulatory agents against chemically induced stress. A classic example is chronic hydroarsenicism or arsenicosis: a multisystem syndrome due to prolonged arsenic intake from drinking water. Worldwide, it presents high sanitary impact. Arsenic impairs the redox response of cells leading to oxidative damage by bottom-up cytotoxicity [7], with immunotoxic effects impairing cellular and antibody responses [8]. Furthermore, it exacerbates the inflammatory response [9].

In this area, phytopharmacological bioprospecting in Argentina is promising. Several potentially beneficial species inhabit in the mountainous region of central Argentina. *Lantana grisebachii* Stuck. ex Seckt. var. *grisebachii* (Verbenaceae) was selected after ethnopharmacological and experimental studies. Infusions of the aerial parts of this plant are traditional gastrointestinal stimulants, as they improve toxin clearance and possess antipyretic and antimicrobial activities [10]. All of this suggests an immunoactive potential. In addition, it exhibits antioxidant activity in food and prevents *in vitro* arsenic nephrotoxicity [11]. From these studies, this species has been proposed as sources of polyphenols [12]. Among these bioactive molecules, phenolic acids and flavonoids are the most extensive groups with antioxidant properties, whose acquisition depends on genetic, environmental, and technical variables [13].

The aim of this study was to develop an anti-As extract from *L. grisebachii* (LG), through establishing its bioactivity with cell-based assays and then its chemical composition. Specific objectives were to assess optimal extraction method, redox safety, and antioxidant and lymphoprotective effects.

2. Materials and Methods

2.1. Plant Processing.
Argentinean *Lantana grisebachii* (LG) of the Chaquenian phytogeographic region [14] was collected in summer (GPS coordinates: −31.28, −64.44), after obtaining government consent by MinCyT-Cba. Specimens were deposited in the RIOC Herbarium (UNRC, Argentina). One gram of pulverized, air-dried aerial parts was extracted in the dark at room temperature under constant shaking with 4 mL of hexane (LG-24h: hexanic extraction), water (LG-24m: 24 h aqueous maceration), or water initially at 95°C (LG-1i: 1 h aqueous infusion). Then, extracts were recovered from the supernatants by filtration (0.45 μm HAWG04756 filters, Millipore, Brazil) and 24 h lyophilisation to be later dissolved in 50% dimethylsulfoxide (Sigma, USA).

2.2. Animal Care and Cell Culture.
Wistar rats ($n \geq 6$) of both sexes were cared for according to US ethical guidelines and bred under standard laboratory conditions with *ad libitum* potable <0.01 mg As/L water (Aguas Cordobesas SA, Argentina) and commercial food (fatty acid profile: 14 : 0 (1.3%), 14 : 1 ω9 (1.8%), 16 : 0 (21%), 16 : 1 ω7 (0.6%), 18 : 0 (26%), 18 : 1 ω9 (11.5%), 18 : 2 ω6 (23.8%), 18 : 3 ω3 (2.1%), 20 : 1 ω9 (0.5%), 20 : 2 ω6 (1.3%), 20 : 4 ω6 (0.2%), 20 : 5 ω3

(6.7%), and 22 : 1 ω9 (0.2%)) (Cargill SACI, Argentina). After that, splenocytes were obtained by mechanical dispersion and chemical haemolysis of the spleens, and they were cultured at 37°C in a 5% CO_2 atmosphere in a RPMI-1640 medium with 10% foetal bovine serum, 100 μM ciprofloxacin, and 50 μM 2-mercaptoethanol (Sigma, USA). Then, *ex vivo* mitogen-induced activation (EVMIA) was achieved by treating 1000 cells/μL with 5 μg/mL of concanavalin A or lipopolysaccharide for 72 hours, to induce T-or B-activated splenocytes, respectively. All outcomes were standardized by results in unstimulated cell cultures, with a 72 h limit proliferation.

2.3. Experimental Design

2.3.1. Identification of Safe Fractions.
First, the effects of polar and nonpolar LG fractions (200 μg/mL, 2 h) were compared in already stimulated splenocytes (after EVMIA) to discard intrinsic extract toxicity. After the polar fraction was shown to be safe, aqueous extracts were studied in dividing cells (during all EVMIA; 100 μg/mL, 3 d). Also, given that *in vivo* insults could affect responses, two cell sources were used: C (control group) and As (2-month orally exposed rats to 5 mg/Kg/d of As from NaAsO$_2$, Anedra Lab, Argentina). These conditions were an accepted rat model of arsenicosis [15], with nitrites being oxidative (61% correlated to free radicals) and inflammatory biomarkers.

2.3.2. Identification of an Efficient Extract.
Redox efficiency (*see below*) of the safe aqueous fractions (100 μg/mL, 3 d) was tested during EVMIA.

2.3.3. Assessment of Direct In Vitro Protective Activity.
The most efficient and safe phytoextract was assayed during EVMIA in cells exposed to 0–7.5 μg/mL of As, with these conditions triggering high toxicity and allowing screening protective agents [16].

2.4. Biological Tests

2.4.1. Cellular Viability.
Since the Trypan blue exclusion test is not a sufficient determination of viability, a resazurin-based assay was employed. Viable cells were stained with resazurin (0.05 mg/mL in culture medium, 6–12 h; TOX-8 kit, Sigma-Aldrich, USA) [17]. Then, viability was calculated as the percentage of absorbance at 600 nm with respect to control (C = 100%). Absorbance readings were performed with a GloMax-Multi microplate multimode reader (Promega Corp., USA).

2.4.2. Cellular Nitrites.
Nitrites, used as nitrosative stress markers, were assayed by the Griess reaction [18], with reactants purchased by Wiener Lab (Argentina). Cell suspensions reacted with equal volumes of 0.1% naphthylethylenediamine dihydrochloride and 1% sulphanilamide in 0.1 N HCl (room temperature, 15 min). Percentages were calculated from a standard sodium nitrite curve (at 550 nm).

2.4.3. Free Radical Activity. Radicals oxidized an ethanolic 16 mM N,N,N′,N′-tetramethyl-p-phenylenediamine-1,4-dihydrochloride solution (Sigma, USA) to be read at 540 nm [3]. Equal volumes of cell sample and solution reacted for 30 min in an oxygen-free environment at room temperature. Percentages, with respect to control, were used to calculate redox efficiency as the quotient of radical activity (%) over the extract phenolic content (%).

2.5. Phytochemistry

2.5.1. Total Phenolics. A solution was created with 25 μL of extract, 25 μL of 2N Folin-Ciocalteau (Anedra, Argentina), and 150 μL of water, and then 50 μL of saturated sodium bicarbonate solution was added. After 30 min of incubation at 37°C in the dark, absorbance was recorded at 750 nm [19]. A standard curve was used to calculate mg equivalents of gallic acid per gram of dry extract (mg/g). Gallic acid was from Riedel-de-Haën (China).

2.5.2. Total Flavonoids. Flavones and flavonols were determined as follows [20]: 50 μL of extract was incubated for 30 min at room temperature with 150 μL of ethanol (96%) (Cicarelli, Argentina), 10 μL of aluminium chloride (10%), 10 μL of potassium acetate (1 M) (Anedra, Argentina), and 150 μL of water. Results were calculated at 415 nm as mg equivalents of quercetin dihydrate per gram of dry extract (mg/g) using a standard curve (Fluka, UK).

2.5.3. Phenolic Analysis. Phenolics were analyzed by high performance liquid chromatography with diode array detection with a HPLC-DAD Agilent Technologies 1200 Series system equipped with Agilent G1312B SL Binary gradient pump, Agilent G1379 B solvent degasser, Agilent G1367 D SL + WP autosampler, and Agilent G1315 C Starlight DAD (ISIDSA, UNC). Separation was achieved on a LUNA reversed-phase C18 column (5 μm, 250 mm × 4.60 mm i.d.; Phenomenex, USA), set at 35°C using an Agilent G1316 B column heater module. The mobile phase was 0.5% formic acid (Fluka, Germany) in ultrapure water (<5 μgL-1 TOC; Sartorius, Germany) (vv-1, solvent A) and 0.5% formic acid in methanol (Baker, Mex.) (vv-1, solvent B). It began at 20%, rising to 50% B in a period of 3 min, maintained for 5 min, followed by a second increase to 70% B in the course of 7 min, maintained for 5 min, and a third increase to 80% B in 1 min, maintained for 9 min, remaining at this last concentration for 10 min before being run. The flow rate was 0.4 mL/min, injecting 40 μL into the column. DAD was set at 280, 320, and 350 nm as preferred wavelengths and the UV-Vis spectra were 200–600 nm. Standards were ferulic acid and caffeic acids (Extrasynthese, France), naringin, kaempferol, and p-coumaric acid (Fluka, UK), and chlorogenic acid, naringenin, myricetin, trans-resveratrol, and rutin (Sigma-Aldrich, Germany).

2.5.4. Fatty Acid Profile. Lipids were taken from the lower phase of a Fölch extraction, which was dried under a nitrogen flow and methylated with toluene and sodium methoxide

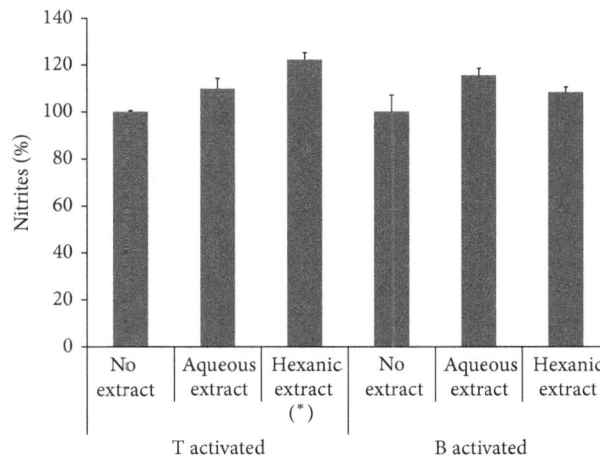

FIGURE 1: Nitrite % in T- and B-activated cultures treated for 2 h with 200 μg/mL of *L. grisebachii* extracts. Results were averaged from three separate experiments ($^*P < 0.01$).

(Sigma, USA) at room temperature for 24 hours. Then, fatty acid methyl esters were dissolved in 50% hexane and recovered from the hexane phase to be dried in nitrogen and suspended in hexane. Separation was achieved in a Supelco fused silica capillary column (30 m × 0.25 mm × 0.25 μm), with a 20 cm/s nitrogen flow rate (mobile phase) and 2°C/min gradient. A Perkin Elmer 500 CLARUS GLC chromatograph with flame ionization detection (Waltham, USA) was used for analysis (oven program: 180°C–240°C). The standard was from NU-Chek-Prep Inc. (USA) and results were expressed as percentages of total fatty acid content.

2.6. Statistical Analysis. Data were expressed as mean ± standard error (SE) from at least three separate experiments performed in triplicate, unless otherwise noted. ANOVA models were used to evaluate differences between treatments, followed by Tukey's test for mean comparisons. Then, GLM were suited to regress the effects of experimental conditions ($P < 0.05$). Analyses were performed with the InfoStat 2012 software (InfoStat Group, Argentina).

3. Results

3.1. Bioguided Extract Selection

3.1.1. Extraction. Given that solvent polarity determines the type of extracted compounds, hexane and water were compared. Hexanic *L. grisebachii* extraction produced an organic fraction that induced nitrite formation in T-activated cultures during the acute assay ($P < 0.0001$). On the other hand, water extraction released an aqueous fraction without nitrite inducing activity in either lymphocyte type. Thus, these polar derivatives were also safe for B- and T-activated cells, which came from *in vivo* As-exposed animals; that is, their safety was an exposure-independent effect and found in proliferated and proliferating cells (Figures 1 and 2). Therefore, aqueous extracts were selected for the next stage.

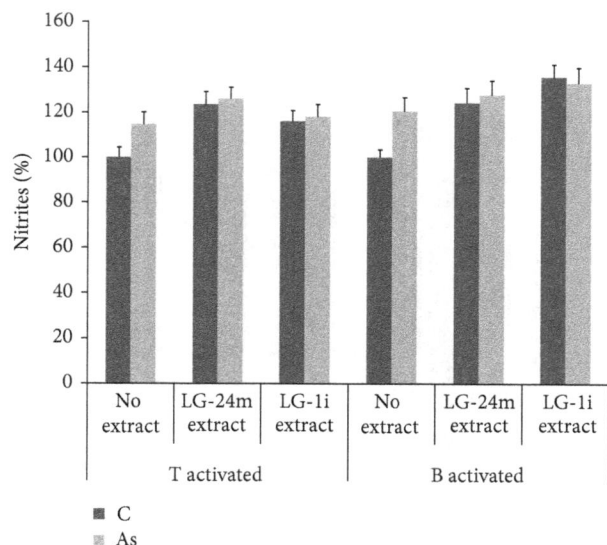

FIGURE 2: Nitrite % in T- and B-activated cultures from control (C) and arsenic-exposed rats (As), treated for 72 h with 100 μg/mL of aqueous *L. grisebachii* extracts (LG-24m: cold 24 h maceration versus LG-1i: hot 1 h infusion) or without them. Results were averaged from three separate experiments (*$P < 0.01$).

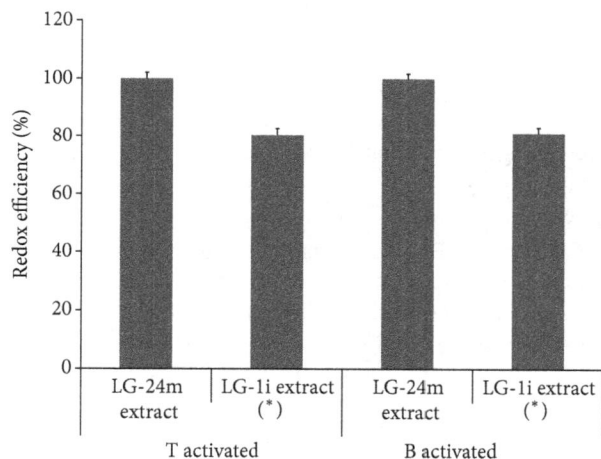

FIGURE 3: Redox efficiency (cell free radical level/extract phenolic content) of 100 μg/mL aqueous *L. grisebachii* extracts (LG-24m: cold 24 h maceration versus LG-1i: hot 1 h infusion) in T- and B-activated cultures treated for 72 h. Results were averaged from three separate experiments (*$P < 0.01$).

3.1.2. Redox Efficiency. Given that higher temperature promotes molecular mobility, caloric changes of water could modify the extraction profile. The 24 h water-macerated extract demonstrated higher quotients than the infusive extract ($P < 0.01$), without arsenic-related differences; that is, the last extract showed a better antioxidant capacity per phenolic amount in all cell cultures (Figure 3). Thus, the infusive fraction was selected.

3.1.3. Protection against Arsenotoxicity. Given that *in vivo* As exposure has been related to a decrease in splenocyte viability, an *in vitro* assaying of *L. grisebachii* to explore its potential to combat this toxin was encouraged. First, arsenic dose-dependent toxicity was confirmed (concentrations as low as 0.075 μg/mL) ($P < 0.05$). In this case, the infusive extract counteracted such toxicity in a dose-dependent manner (Figure 4) with 100 μg/mL reducing cell death at all As concentrations (including 7.5 μg/mL) ($P < 0.0001$). The dose of 10 μg/mL was protective up to 0.075 μg/mL of As in both cell types. On the other hand, B-activated splenocytes were protected up to 0.75 μg/mL of As, indicating increased resistance. Lower extract concentrations were not sufficient to prevent As-induced damage related to oxidant induction ($P < 0.05$). T-activated cells were more liable than B-activated ones (111.24 ± 0.40% versus 100.00 ± 0.73%, resp.) ($P < 0.005$), whereas the infusive extract was antioxidant in both ($P < 0.01$).

3.2. Phytochemistry of the Selected Infusive Lantana grisebachii Extract

3.2.1. Phenolics. It is known that solvent polarity and temperature determine extraction outcome. The employment of water yielded 1.67 times more phenolic extraction from LG than hexane (distinct polarities) after 24 h maceration at room temperature ($P < 0.05$). Also, water extraction could be reduced to 1 hour by increasing its temperature. This method increased phenolic extraction 1.55 times over the classic 24 h water maceration, with extraction being temperature dependent ($P < 0.02$). This infusive phytoextract contained 10.23 ± 0.43 mg/g of phenolics, with 58.46% of flavonoids (05.98 ± 0.12 mg/g). Among phenolics, chlorogenic acid was the predominant compound (0.723 mg/g), among 10 unknown minor compounds (Figure 5).

3.2.2. Lipids. Increased water temperature allows some organic compounds to be extracted; thus, a fatty acid fingerprint could be assessed. The result showed one-third of saturated fatty acids, one-third of ω9, ω6 (~24%), and ω3 (~4%), and scarce ω7 (Figure 5).

4. Discussion

This study pursued the bioguided identification of a plant extract of *L. grisebachii* (LG) that could combat As lymphotoxicity by comparing different extraction methods and lymphocyte responses (nitrites, free radicals, and cellular viability).

The phenolic increase found in aqueous LG extracts was caused by the presence of principal bioactive molecules, such as flavonoids and phenolic acids (chlorogenic). This was enhanced by the use of heated water, thus improving extraction [21]. Although hydrophilic organic solvents (e.g., ethanol) are usually utilized to obtain these kinds of compounds [22], a pharmacological equivalency has been demonstrated between alcoholic extracts and those derived from infusions [23]. Therefore, flavonoids become

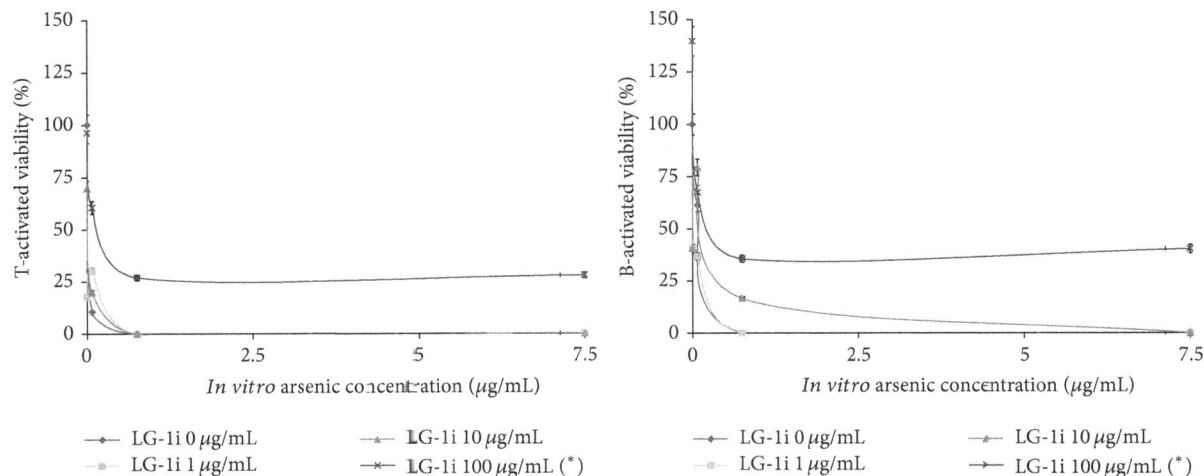

FIGURE 4: Viability of T- and B-activated cells treated for 72 h with 0–100 μg/mL of the 1h infusion *L. grisebachii* extract (LG-1i) and 0–7.5 μg/mL of arsenic. Percentages with respect to control (0 μg/mL LG-1i, 0 μg/mL As) were average from four separate experiments (*$P < 0.0001$).

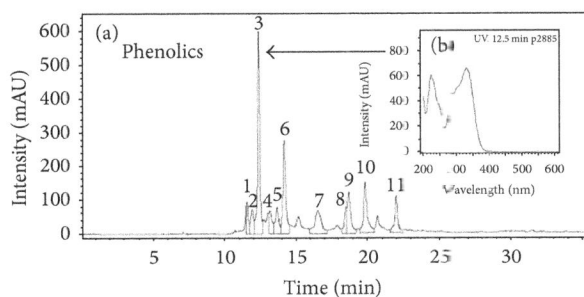

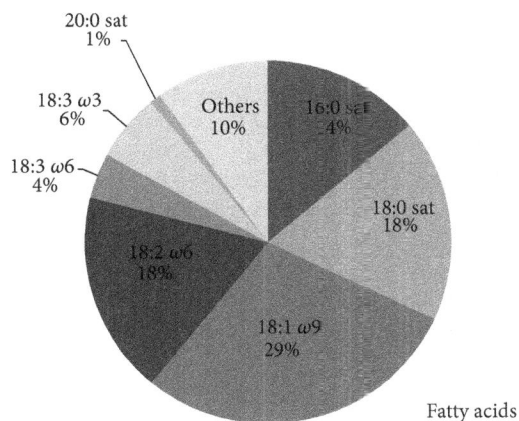

FIGURE 5: Chromatographic analysis of the infusive *Lantana grisebachii* extract: phenolics with a 0.723 mg/g chlorogenic (*arrow*) and fatty acids (%; others-each one <1%—: 14 : 0, 14 : 1 ω9, 16 : 1 ω7, 20 : 1 ω9, 20 : 3 ω3, 20 : 4 ω6, 22 : 1 ω9, 22 : 5 ω3, 24 : 0, and 24 : 1 ω9) (*$P < 0.05$).

bioavailable in humans due to the presence of functional chemical groups (e.g., hydrophilic hydroxyl and carbonyl) in their polycyclic structures [24]. Moreover, the better redox efficiency of infusions with respect to the other cold water-macerated extracts indicated qualitative differences with greater bioactivity per weight. This might be related to extraction of hydrosoluble thermostable antioxidants from plants [25]. Furthermore, organic extracts of other plants have been reported as antioxidants and cytoprotectors but in a lesser extent than their aqueous counterparts [26]. In this study, an elevation of nitrites was seen in cell cultures treated with the hexanic extract, which correlated with phenolic decrease. Concerning this, LG metabolome might present apolar oxidants (e.g., nitrosative inducers, oxygenated fatty acids) [27, 28].

Given that lymphocyte response can be affected by different factors (e.g., cell cycle progression, environmental exposure, etc.), the safety of aqueous extracts was reevaluated. Proliferating lymphocytes were more susceptible to oxidative stress induced by As, as was expected [29]. Nevertheless, aqueous extracts were safe in all lymphocyte cultures. Also, the infusive antioxidant phytoextract of *Lantana grisebachii* triggered a xenohormetic defence against arsenic lymphotoxicity. Some of the pathways involved in such protection have been established [30]. Also, differences between T- and B-activated splenocytes have shown higher B resistance to chemical/environmental stress related to their reduced biologically conditioned susceptibility [31, 32]. Furthermore, the extract may contain B lymphoproliferative compounds such as other plant phenolic derivatives [33]. On other hand, the involvement of apoptosis as the primary lymphotoxic effect has been demonstrated *in extenso* under the assayed conditions [34]; thus, lethal phenotype was not searched (in fact, late determinations in cell culture end could lead to confusions about the initial type). Therefore, a cell-based method for high throughput screenings of phytodrugs was selected [35] due to its representativeness of immune cell response and apoptosis [36].

These multiple effects (antioxidation, cytoprotection, and functional induction) have been seen in other *in vitro* systems. For example, 100 μg/mL LG-1i promoted kidney cells of *Cercopithecus aethiops* (viability with respect to control: $104.67 \pm 0.05\%$) with decreased γ-glutamyl transpeptidase activity after being treated for 2 h (control: 27.95 ± 1.55 versus LG-1i: 22.50 ± 0.51 nIU/cell, $P < 0.05$) and 4 h (control: 31.60 ± 0.64 versus LG-1i: 23.15 ± 0.64 nIU/cell, $P < 0.05$) (*unpublished data*). This cell type was the first one where cytoprotective LG was discovered to prevent As-induced oxidative stress [11], with the enzyme being a cell response to augment redox resistance [37]. This supported that phytodrugs (e.g., flavonoid-related compounds, flavolignanes) can stimulate molecular protective pathways [38]. Also, the beneficial effects of *Lantana grisebachii* infusion in both murine lymphocytes and monkey renocytes indicated that they were independent of species and cell types; that is, a general antioxidant bioactivity was found for this plant.

Given that temperature favours lipid kinetics in aqueous biological samples [39], solvent heating was mandatory to extract them from plant material during water extraction, with fatty acid assessment in a plant infusion being innovative. In fact, the extraction enhancement achieved by heating water was manifested by the presence of lipids in an aqueous infusion. This methodological approach favoured unsaturated fatty acids obtaining, including some essential ones for immunological responses, which are highly sensitive to arsenic-induced dysfunctions and disturbances [30].

5. Conclusion

Although further studies are required in order to establish other functional implications for lymphocytes, this study provides, for the first time, the basis to develop *Lantana grisebachii*-derived phytodrugs to reduce dysfunctions induced by arsenic, a well-known oxidative immunotoxic. In this regard, arsenicosis is a public health concern worldwide, despite efforts to remedy contaminated soil and water, with immune cells being major targets. Accordingly, sequential bioguided bioprospecting of antioxidant plants, such as *Lantana grisebachii*, is a valuable approach. Moreover, the mentioned plant is immunoactive and common in Argentine flora, which might represent an abundant source of compounds for phytopharmaceutical development by easy extraction using a water-based photoprotected thermoassisted method.

Conflict of Interests

The authors declare that there is no conflict of interests.

Acknowledgments

The authors would like to thank Marta Goleniowski, Ph.D. degree holder, and Ana Figueroa, B.S. degree holder, for their valuable contribution, and Garrett Gardner, M.D. degree student, a native English speaker, for the paper revision. This work was supported by the National Agency of Scientific and Technological Promotion (Grant no. 171/08); the Science Agency of Cordoba (Grant no. 969/05); and the National University of Cordoba (Grant no. 162/12).

References

[1] M. E. Goleniowski, G. A. Bongiovanni, L. Palacio, C. O. Nuñez, and J. J. Cantero, "Medicinal plants from the "Sierra de Comechingones", Argentina," *Journal of Ethnopharmacology*, vol. 107, no. 3, pp. 324–341, 2006.

[2] Y.-J. Surh, "Xenohormesis mechanisms underlying chemopreventive effects of some dietary phytochemicals," *Annals of the New York Academy of Sciences*, vol. 1229, no. 1, pp. 1–6, 2011.

[3] G. A. Bongiovanni, E. A. Soria, and A. R. Eynard, "Effects of the plant flavonoids silymarin and quercetin on arsenite-induced oxidative stress in CHO-K1 cells," *Food and Chemical Toxicology*, vol. 45, no. 6, pp. 971–976, 2007.

[4] L. Nasreddine and D. Parent-Massin, "Food contamination by metals and pesticides in the European Union. Should we worry?" *Toxicology Letters*, vol. 127, no. 1–3, pp. 29–41, 2002.

[5] C. A. Janeway Jr., P. Travers, M. Walport, and M. J. Shlomchik, *Immunobiology: The Immune System in Health and Disease*, Garland Science, New York, NY, USA, 5th edition, 2001.

[6] M. K. Singh, S. S. Yadav, V. Gupta, and S. Khattri, "Immunomodulatory role of *Emblica officinalis* in arsenic induced oxidative damage and apoptosis in thymocytes of mice," *BMC Complementary and Alternative Medicine*, vol. 13, article 193, 2013.

[7] E. A. Soria, A. R. Eynard, and G. A. Bongiovanni, "Cytoprotective effects of silymarin on epithelial cells against arsenic-induced apoptosis in contrast with quercetin cytotoxicity," *Life Sciences*, vol. 87, no. 9-10, pp. 309–315, 2010.

[8] R. Colognato, F. Coppedè, J. Ponti, E. Sabbioni, and L. Migliore, "Genotoxicity induced by arsenic compounds in peripheral human lymphocytes analysed by cytokinesis-block micronucleus assay," *Mutagenesis*, vol. 22, no. 4, pp. 255–261, 2007.

[9] K. A. Ramsey, R. E. Foong, P. D. Sly, A. N. Larcombe, and G. R. Zosky, "Early life arsenic exposure and acute and long-term responses to influenza a infection in mice," *Environmental Health Perspectives*, vol. 121, no. 10, pp. 1187–1193, 2013.

[10] G. E. Barboza, J. J. Cantero, C. Núñez, A. Pacciaroni, and L. Ariza Espinar, "Medicinal plants: a general review and a phytochemical and ethnopharmacological screening of the native Argentine Flora," *Kurtziana*, vol. 34, no. 1-2, pp. 7–365, 2009.

[11] E. A. Soria, M. E. Goleniowski, J. J. Cantero, and G. A. Bongiovanni, "Antioxidant activity of different extracts of Argentinian medicinal plants against arsenic-induced toxicity in renal cells," *Human and Experimental Toxicology*, vol. 27, no. 4, pp. 341–346, 2008.

[12] R. Borneo, A. E. León, A. Aguirre, P. Ribotta, and J. J. Cantero, "Antioxidant capacity of medicinal plants from the Province of Córdoba (Argentina) and their in vitro testing in a model food system," *Food Chemistry*, vol. 112, no. 3, pp. 664–670, 2009.

[13] R. Tsao, "Chemistry and biochemistry of dietary polyphenols," *Nutrients*, vol. 2, no. 12, pp. 1231–1246, 2010.

[14] A. L. Cabrera, "Regiones fitogeográficas argentinas," in *Enciclopedia Argentina de Agricultura Y Jardinería*, p. 85, ACME SA, Buenos Aires, Argentina, 1976.

[15] P. N. Rubatto Birri, R. D. Pérez, D. Cremonezzi, C. A. Pérez, M. Rubio, and G. A. Bongiovanni, "Association between As and Cu renal cortex accumulation and physiological and histological alterations after chronic arsenic intake," *Environmental Research*, vol. 110, no. 5, pp. 417–423, 2010.

[16] D. Sinha, S. Dey, R. K. Bhattacharya, and M. Roy, "In vitro mitigation of arsenic toxicity by tea polyphenols in human

lymphocytes," *Journal of Environmental Pathology, Toxicology and Oncology*, vol. 26, no. 3, pp. 207–220, 2007.

[17] U. J. Strotmann, B. Butz, and W.-R. Bias, "The dehydrogenase assay with resazurin: practical performance as a monitoring system and Ph-dependent toxicity of phenolic compounds," *Ecotoxicology and Environmental Safety*, vol. 25, no. 1, pp. 79–89, 1993.

[18] L. C. Green, D. A. Wagner, J. Glogowski, P. L. Skipper, J. S. Wishnok, and S. R. Tannenbaum, "Analysis of nitrate, nitrite, and [15N]nitrate in biological fluids," *Analytical Biochemistry*, vol. 126, no. 1, pp. 131–138, 1982.

[19] G. Ait Baddi, J. Cegarra, G. Merlina, J. C. Revel, and M. Hafidi, "Qualitative and quantitative evolution of polyphenolic compounds during composting of an olive-mill waste-wheat straw mixture," *Journal of Hazardous Materials*, vol. 165, no. 1–3, pp. 1119–1123, 2009.

[20] G. S. Grosso, I. V. C. Carvajal, and J. Principal, "Perfil de flavonoides e índices de oxidación de algunos propóleos colombianos," *Zootecnia Tropical*, vol. 25, no. 2, pp. 95–102, 2007.

[21] Q. V. Vuong, J. B. Golding, C. E. Stathopoulos, M. H. Nguyen, and P. D. Roach, "Optimizing conditions for the extraction of catechins from green tea using hot water," *Journal of Separation Science*, vol. 34, no. 21, pp. 3099–3106, 2011.

[22] M. A. Abbasi, K. Rubab, T. Riaz, T. Shahzadi, M. Khalid, and M. Ajaib, "In vitro assessment of relief to oxidative stress by different fractions of Boerhavia procumbens," *Pakistan Journal of Pharmaceutical Sciences*, vol. 25, no. 2, pp. 357–364, 2012.

[23] T. Ito, M. Kakino, S. Tazawa et al., "Quantification of polyphenols and pharmacological analysis of water and ethanol-based extracts of cultivated agarwood leaves," *Journal of Nutritional Science and Vitaminology*, vol. 58, no. 2, pp. 136–142, 2012.

[24] S. S. Beevi, L. N. Mangamoori, and B. B. Gowda, "Polyphenolics profile and antioxidant properties of Raphanus sativus L.," *Natural Product Research*, vol. 26, no. 6, pp. 557–563, 2012.

[25] S. Jäger, M. Beffert, K. Hoppe, D. Nadberezny, B. Frank, and A. Scheffler, "Preparation of herbal tea as infusion or by maceration at room temperature using mistletoe tea as an example," *Scientia Pharmaceutica*, vol. 79, no. 1, pp. 145–155, 2011.

[26] Y. B. Tripathi, A. P. Chaturvedi, and N. Pandey, "Effect of nigella sativa seeds extracts on inos through antioxidant potential only: crude/total extract as molecular therapy drug," *Indian Journal of Experimental Biology*, vol. 50, no. 6, pp. 413–418, 2012.

[27] N. Morihara, I. Sumioka, N. Ide, T. Moriguchi, N. Uda, and E. Kyo, "Aged garlic extract maintains cardiovascular homeostasis in mice and rats," *Journal of Nutrition*, vol. 136, no. 3, pp. 777S–781S, 2006.

[28] D. C. Doehlert, P. Rayas-Duarte, and M. S. McMullen, "Inhibition of fusarium graminearum growth in flour gel cultures by hexane-soluble compounds from oat (Avena sativa L.) flour," *Journal of Food Protection*, vol. 74, no. 12, pp. 2188–2191, 2011.

[29] A. Thomas-Schoemann, F. Batteux, C. Mongaret et al., "Arsenic trioxide exerts antitumor activity through regulatory T cell depletion mediated by oxidative stress in a murine model of colon cancer," *Journal of Immunology*, vol. 189, no. 11, pp. 5171–5177, 2012.

[30] S. I. Ramos Elizagaray, *Actividad quimiopreventiva e inmunoprotectora del extracto acuoso de Lantana grisebachii var. grisebachii en hidroarsenicismo experimental [M.S. thesis]*, National University of Cordoba, Cordoba, Spain, 2013.

[31] J. E. Turner, J. A. Bosch, and S. Aldred, "Measurement of exercise-induced oxidative stress in lymphocytes," *Biochemical Society Transactions*, vol. 39, no. 5, pp. 1299–1304, 2011.

[32] C.-C. Shen, H.-J. Liang, C.-C. Wang, M.-H. Liao, and T.-R. Jan, "A role of cellular glutathione in the differential effects of iron oxide nanoparticles on antigen-specific T cell cytokine expression," *International Journal of Nanomedicine*, vol. 6, pp. 2791–2798, 2011.

[33] T. Francus, "Plant polyphenolic-protein conjugates activate murine spleen cells and bind to multiple cell surface components," *Proceedings of the Society for Experimental Biology and Medicine*, vol. 207, no. 1, pp. 117–126, 1994.

[34] H.-S. Yu, W.-T. Liao, K.-L. Chang, C.-L. Yu, and G.-S. Chen, "Arsenic induces tumor necrosis factor α release and tumor necrosis factor receptor 1 signaling in T helper cell apoptosis," *Journal of Investigative Dermatology*, vol. 119, no. 4, pp. 812–819, 2002.

[35] T. E. O'Neill, H. Li, C. D. Colquhoun, J. A. Johnson, D. Webster, and C. A. Gray, "Optimisation of the microplate resazurin assay for screening and bioassay-guided fractionation of phytochemical extracts against mycobacterium tuberculosis," *Phytochemical Analysis*, 2014.

[36] Y. Zhi-Jun, N. Sriranganathan, T. Vaught, S. K. Arastu, and S. A. Ahmed, "A dye-based lymphocyte proliferation assay that permits multiple immunological analyses: mRNA, cytogenetic, apoptosis, and immunophenotyping studies," *Journal of Immunological Methods*, vol. 210, no. 1, pp. 25–39, 1997.

[37] A. Quiroga, P. L. Quiroga, E. Martínez, E. A. Soria, and M. A. Valentich, "Anti-breast cancer activity of curcumin on the human oxidation-resistant cells ZR-75-1 with γ-glutamyltranspeptidase inhibition," *Journal of Experimental Therapeutics and Oncology*, vol. 8, no. 3, pp. 261–266, 2010.

[38] J. Sonnenbichler, F. Scalera, I. Sonnenbichler, and R. Weyhenmeyer, "Stimulatory effects of silibinin and silicristin from the milk thistle Silybum marianum on kidney cells," *Journal of Pharmacology and Experimental Therapeutics*, vol. 290, no. 3, pp. 1375–1383, 1999.

[39] J. Milhaud, "New insights into water-phospholipid model membrane interactions," *Biochimica et Biophysica Acta—Biomembranes*, vol. 1663, no. 1-2, pp. 19–51, 2004.

9

Antihyperglycemic Activity of *Houttuynia cordata* Thunb. in Streptozotocin-Induced Diabetic Rats

Manish Kumar, Satyendra K. Prasad, Sairam Krishnamurthy, and Siva Hemalatha

Pharmacognosy Research Laboratory, Department of Pharmaceutics, Indian Institute of Technology, Banaras Hindu University, Varanasi 221005, India

Correspondence should be addressed to Siva Hemalatha; shemalatha.phe@itbhu.ac.in

Academic Editor: Todd C. Skaar

Present study is an attempt to investigate plausible mechanism involved behind antidiabetic activity of standardized *Houttuynia cordata* Thunb. extract in streptozotocin-induced diabetic rats. The plant is used as a medicinal salad for lowering blood sugar level in North-Eastern parts of India. Oral administration of extract at 200 and 400 mg/kg dose level daily for 21 days showed a significant ($P < 0.05$) decrease in fasting plasma glucose and also elevated insulin level in streptozotocin-induced diabetic rats. It also significantly reversed all the alterations in biochemical parameters, that is, total lipid profile, blood urea, creatinine, protein, and antioxidant enzymes in liver, pancreas, and adipose tissue of diabetic rats. Furthermore, we have demonstrated that the extract significantly reversed the expression patterns of various glucose homeostatic enzyme genes like GLUT-2, GLUT-4, and caspase-3 levels but did not show any significant effect on PPAR-γ protein expressions. Additionally, the extract positively regulated mitochondrial membrane potential and succinate dehydrogenase (SDH) activity in diabetic rats. The findings justified the antidiabetic effect of *H. cordata* which is attributed to an upregulation of GLUT-4 and potential antioxidant activity, which may play beneficial role in resolving complication associated with diabetes.

1. Introduction

Diabetes mellitus (DM) is a disease that results in chronic inflammation and apoptosis in pancreatic islets in patients with either type 1 or 2 DM and is characterized by abnormal insulin secretion [1]. Insulin-resistant glucose use in peripheral tissues such as muscle and adipose tissues is a universal feature of both insulin-dependent DM and non-insulin-dependent DM. In this process, glucose transporters (GLUTs) play crucial role [2]. Glucose transporter 4 is mainly expressed in skeletal muscle, heart, and adipose tissues which plays critical role in insulin stimulated glucose transport in these tissues, with glucose uptake occurring when insulin stimulates the translocation of GLUT-4 from the intracellular pool to the plasma membrane [3]. Glucose transporter 2, being the primary GLUT isoform in the liver, plays a pivotal role in glucose homeostasis by mediating bidirectional transport of glucose [4]. It is reported that oxidative stress plays a major role in the development of diabetes associated disorders, possibly due to overproduction of reactive oxygen species (ROS) [5]. Glucose and lipid metabolism are largely dependent on the mitochondrial functional state and physiology which, on excessive ROS formation, leads to mitochondrial oxidative damage and reduced mitochondria biogenesis that contributes to insulin resistance and associated diabetic complications [6, 7].

Medicinal plants continue to be an important source in search of a suitable active principle(s), wherein they are currently being investigated for their potential pharmacological properties in the regulation of conditions such as elevated blood glucose level in diabetes [8]. *Houttuynia cordata* Thunb. (HC) is a single species of its genus and is native to Japan, South-East Asia, and Himalayas. Ethnomedically, whole plant of *H. cordata* is being used for the treatment of diabetes. In the Ri-Bhoi district of Meghalaya, India, whole plant of *H. cordata* is eaten raw as a medicinal salad for lowering the blood sugar level and is commonly known by the name Jamyrdoh [9, 10]. The plant is also used as an ingredient in insulin secretion promoter compositions [11]. In southern China, green leaves and young roots are used as vegetable while dry leaves are used to prepare drink by boiling decoction [12, 13]. Reported pharmacological activities of plant including hypoglycaemic [14], antileukemic [15], anticancer [16], adjuvanticity [14], antioxidant [17] and inhibitory effects on anaphylactic reaction and mast cell activation [16].

A recent study has shown that the volatile oil from *H. cordata* restored the alterations in blood glucose, insulin, adiponectin, and connective tissue growth factor levels in diabetic rats, induced by the combination of a high-carbohydrate and high-fat diet, and STZ injection which may be attributed to the reduced insulin resistance, adiponectin, and connective tissue growth factor levels [18]. Jang et al. [19] reported the potential advanced glycation end products formation and rat lens aldose reductase inhibitory activity of two flavonol rhamnosides 4 and 5 isolated from the whole plant of *H. cordata*. On the basis of the above reports, the present study was undertaken for the first time to assess the mechanism involved in protective role of *H. cordata* against STZ-induced glucose toxicity using rat liver, pancreas, and adipose tissue as the working model. In addition, a mechanistic approach of *H. cordata* against STZ-induced inflammation, apoptosis, and mitochondrial dysfunction was proposed for evaluation. Moreover, GLUT-2 in liver and pancreas and GLUT-4 in adipose tissue were expressed to explain the probable mechanism of *H. cordata* against STZ-induced impaired glucose utilization.

2. Material and Methods

2.1. Chemicals Used. Streptozotocin, tetra methyl rhodamine methyl ester (TMRM), glutamate, and *o*-phthalaldehyde (OPA) were procured from Sigma-Aldrich (St. Louis, MO, USA). Glibenclamide (standard drug) was obtained as a gift sample from Accent pharma (QC. Ref. No. GLB/B129/10/11) Pvt. Ltd. Thiobarbituric acid (TBA), ethylene glycol tetra-acetic acid (EGTA), and 2-[4-(2-hydroxyethyl)1-piperazinyl]ethanesulfonic acid (HEPES buffer, acid free) were purchased from Hi-media (Mumbai) and sodium succinate, sodium azide, phenazine methanesulphonate (PMS), and nitro blue tetrazolium were purchased from Merck (Darmstadt, Germany). All other chemicals and reagents were procured from local suppliers and were of analytical grade. Plasma insulin was assayed by using commercial enzyme-linked immunosorbent assay kit (ELISA, Boerhringer Mannheim, Germany).

Total cholesterol (TC), high density lipoprotein (HDL) cholesterol, triglyceride (TG), blood urea nitrogen (BUN), creatinine (CRTN), and total protein (TPR) were estimated using kits from Span Diagnostics Ltd., India.

2.2. Animals. Albino rats of Charles foster strain with body weights of (160–200 g) were obtained from the Central Animal House (Registration number: 542/02/ab/CPCSEA), Institute of Medical Science (IMS), Banaras Hindu University (BHU), Varanasi, India. Before and during the experiment, rats were fed with normal laboratory pellet diet (Hindustan lever Ltd., India) and water *ad libitum*. After randomization into various groups, the rats were allowed to acclimatize for

a period of 2-3 days in the new environment before initiation of experiment. The experimental protocol has been approved by the institutional animal ethics committee (Reference number Dean/10-11/58 dated 07.03.2011).

2.3. Plant Material and Preparation of Extract. Houttuynia cordata Thunb. herb was collected from Jaintia Hills of Meghalaya, India. The plant was identified by Dr. B. K. Sinha, Botanical Survey of India. A voucher specimen number (COG/HC/011) was deposited in the Department of Pharmaceutics, Indian Institute of Technology, Banaras Hindu University, Varanasi (U.P), India. Whole plants of *H. cordata* were washed with water and after being shade dried, the plant material was ground in a mill, passed through sieve number 40 to obtain a coarse plant powder. Dried powdered material (1 kg) of whole plant of *H. cordata* was extracted with 3 liter ethanol by soxhlation for 6 h. The resulting extract was concentrated under reduced pressure to obtain a dark crude residue (yield: 13.2% w/w).

2.4. Phytochemical Analysis. The extract was subjected to various phytochemicals tests to determine the active constituents present in the crude ethanolic of *H. cordata* [20]. Total phenolic and tannin content in *H. cordata* was estimated according to the method of Makkar, [21] using Folin ciocalteu reagent, whereas the method proposed by Kumaran and Joel Karunakaran [22] was followed to estimate total flavonoid and flavonol contents in *H. cordata*.

Further, *H. cordata* was standardized with quercetin using high performance thin layer chromatography (HPTLC). A stock solution of both *H. cordata* and standard quercetin in methanol was prepared in concentration of 5 mg/mL and 0.2 mg/mL respectively. Mobile phase for developing the chromatogram was composed of chloroform: methanol and formic acid mixture in the ratio 7.5 : 1.5 : 1 (v/v/v). The study was carried out using Camag-HPTLC instrumentation equipped with Linomat V sample applicator, Camag TLC scanner 3, Camag TLC visualizer, and WINCATS 4 software for data interpretation. The R_f values were recorded and the developed plate was screened and photo-documented at ultraviolet range with wavelength (λ_{max}) of 254 nm.

2.5. Oral Toxicity Studies. Acute oral toxicity study of ethanolic extract from *H. cordata* was done according to "Organization for Environmental Control Development" guidelines (OECD: Guidelines 425; Up and Down Procedure). The study was performed on 24 h fasted rats by single dose administration each of 2000 and 5000 mg/kg, (p.o.). The toxicity sign and symptoms or any abnormalities associated with the ethanolic extract of *H. cordata* were observed at 0, 30, 60, 180, and 240 min and then once a day for the next 14 days. The number of rats that survived was recorded at the end of the study period.

2.6. Induction of Experimental Diabetes. The animals were fasted overnight and diabetes was induced by a single intraperitoneal injection of a freshly prepared solution of streptozotocin (65 mg/kg, b.w.) in 0.1 M citrate buffer (pH 4.5) [23]. The animals were allowed free access to 5% glucose solution to overcome the drug induced hypoglycemia. Diabetes was confirmed after 48 h and then on the 7th day of streptozotocin injection, the blood samples were collected through retroorbital venous plexus under light anesthesia and plasma glucose levels were estimated by enzymatic GOD-PAP (glucose oxidase peroxidase) diagnostic kit method. The rats having fasting plasma glucose (FPG) levels more than 200 mg/dL were selected and used for the present study [24].

2.7. Experimental Design.

The diabetic animals were divided into six groups ($n = 6$). Group-I, normal control (untreated) rats; group-II, diabetic control rats; group-III, diabetic rats given glibenclamide 10 mg/kg orally for 21 days; group-IV, group-V, and group-VI, diabetic rats that received *H. cordata* extract at 100, 200, and 400 mg/kg, p.o. body weight, respectively, once daily for 21 days. At the 0th, 7th, 14th, and 21st days blood from each rat was collected through retroorbital venous plexus under light anesthesia. Plasma was separated and the FPG level was estimated. Plasma lipid profile (TC, TG, LDL, HDL, and VLDL), insulin, and other biochemical parameters, that is, creatinine (CRT), blood urea nitrogen (BUN), and total protein (TPR), were also estimated on the 21st day of the experiment.

2.8. Evaluation of Mitochondrial Function and Oxidative Stress

2.8.1. Mitochondria Isolation Procedure.

Mitochondria were isolated by standard differential centrifugation [25]. The liver, pancreas, and adipose tissue were homogenized in (1:10, w/v) ice cold isolation buffer (250 mM sucrose, 1 mM EGTA, and 10 mM HEPES-KOH, pH 7.2). Homogenates were centrifuged at 600 ×g/5 min and the resulting supernatant was centrifuged at 10,000 ×g/15 min and supernatant discarded. Pellets were next suspended in medium (1 mL) consisting of 250 mM sucrose, 0.3 mM EGTA, and 10 mM HEPES-KOH, pH 7.2 and again centrifuged at 14,000 ×g/10 min. All centrifugation procedures were performed at 4°C. The final mitochondrial pellet was resuspended in medium (1 mL) containing 250 mM sucrose and 10 mM HEPES-KOH, pH 7.2, and used within 3 h. Mitochondrial protein content was estimated using the method of Lowry et al. [26].

2.8.2. Estimation of Mitochondrial Antioxidant Enzymes.

Mitochondrial malondialdehyde (MDA) content was measured based on the TBA reaction test [27]. The activity of superoxide dismutase (SOD) was assayed by the method of Kakkar et al. based on the formation of NADH-phenazine methosulphate-nitro blue tetrazolium formazan measured at 560 nm against butanol as blank [28]. Decomposition of hydrogen peroxide in presence of catalase (CAT) was followed at 240 nm [29]. The results were expressed as units (U) of CAT activity/min/mg of protein.

2.8.3. Estimation of Mitochondrial Succinate Dehydrogenase Activity (SDH).

The mitochondrial succinate: acceptor oxidoreductase (EC 1.3.99.1) was determined by standard protocol based on the progressive reduction of NBT to an insoluble colored compound [a diformazan (dfz)] used as a reaction indicator [30]. The reaction of NBT was mediated by H^+ released in the conversion of succinate to fumarate. The concentration of NBT-dfz produced was measured at 570 nm. The mean SDH activity of each region was expressed as micromole formazan produced per min per microgram of protein.

2.8.4. Estimation of Mitochondrial Membrane Potential (MMP).

The Rhodamine dye taken up by healthy mitochondria was measured by fluorometric methods [31]. The mitochondrial suspension was mixed with TMRM solution. The mixture was then incubated for 5 min at 25°C temperature and any unbound TMRM was removed by frequent washings (four times). Then the buffer was added to make up the final volume and florescence emission was read at an excitation λ 535 ± 10 nm and emission λ of 580 ± 10 nm using slit number 10. The peak fluorescence intensity recorded was around λ 570 ± 5 nm. The results are expressed as fluorescence intensity value per milligram of protein.

2.9. Evaluation of Caspase-3, PPAR-γ, GLUT-2, and 4 by Western Blotting.

Caspase-3, PPAR-γ, GLUT-4, and 2 antibodies were purchased from Santa Cruz Biotechnology Inc (Santa Cruz, CA, USA). The liver and pancreatic tissues were homogenized in lysis buffer and centrifuged. Lysates (80 μg proteins) were electrophoresed on 10% sodium dodecyl sulfate (SDS)-PAGE gels and then transferred to polyvinyl difluoride (PVDF) membranes (Bio-Rad, USA). The membranes were incubated with rabbit polyclonal anti-caspase-3 antibody (1:1000), rabbit polyclonal anti-GLUT-4, and anti-GLUT-2 antibody (1:2000 and 1:1500) or mouse monoclonal anti-PPAR-γ antibody (1:1000) overnight at 4°C, and then with horseradish peroxidise-conjugated goat anti-rabbit IgG (1:3000) or horseradish peroxidise-conjugated goat anti-mouse IgG (1:3000) for 60 min at room temperature. Western blotting luminescent reagent was used to visualize peroxidase activity. Normalization was carried out by stripping films and reprobing with a mouse monoclonal antibody to the β-isoform of actin (1:10000, Sigma). Films were scanned and subsequently analyzed by measuring optical densities of immunostained bands using an image processing and analysis system (Image J 1.37 software, NIH, USA).

2.10. Pancreatic Histology.

For histopathological studies the pancreas was blotted, dried, and fixed in 10% formalin for 48 h. Thereafter, the tissues were dehydrated in acetone for 1 h and embedded in paraffin wax. Section of pancreatic tissues was then taken through microtome and stained with Haematoxylin-Eosin for photomicroscopic observation [32], which was carried out on Nikon Trinocular Microscope, Model E-200, Japan.

2.11. Statistical Analysis.

The data were analyzed with GraphPad Prism version 5 (San Diego, CA). Statistical analysis was done by two-way ANOVA, followed by Bonferroni posttest for FPG, whereas other biochemical parameters were

Track 4, ID: H cordata

Peak	Start R_f	Start height	Max R_f	Max height	Max (%)	End R_f	End height	Area	Area (%)
1	0.48	0.1	0.51	103.7	100.00	0.54	0.9	2143.0	100.00

(a)

Track 8, ID: quercetin

Peak	Start R_f	Start height	Max R_f	Max height	Max (%)	End R_f	End hight	Area	Area (%)
1	0.47	3.5	0.52	186.5	100.00	0.54	14.1	4952.5	100.00

(b)

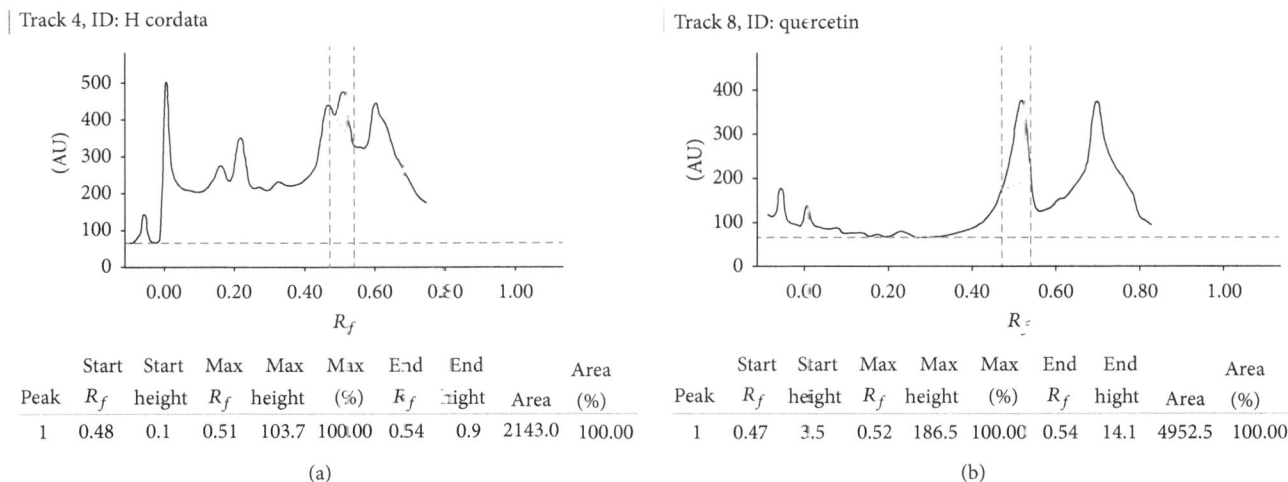

FIGURE 1: HPTLC densitogram of quercetin in ethanolic extract of *H. cordata* (HC). (a) Peak of quercetin present in HC and (b) standard peak of quercetin.

analysed by one-way ANOVA, followed by Tukey's multiple comparison test. Data are expressed as mean ± SEM. A level of $P < 0.05$ was accepted as statistically significant.

3. Results

3.1. Phytochemical Analysis. Preliminary phytochemical analysis of the extract revealed the presence of phenols, flavonoids, tannins, alkaloids, steroids, and carbohydrates as a major component. Total phenolic content of *H. cordata* was reported to be 45.74 mg/g gallic acid equivalent while total tannin content was estimated to be 33.29 mg/g tannic acid equivalent. Total flavonoid and flavonol contents were found to be 104.55 and 17.16 mg/g rutin equivalents. HPTLC studies revealed well-resolved peaks of *H. cordata* containing quercetin. The spots of the entire chromatogram were visualized under UV 254 nm and the percentage of quercetin (R_f 0.51) in *H. cordata* extract was found to be 4.39% (w/w) (Figure 1).

3.2. Effects of H. cordata on FPG Levels in STZ-Induced Diabetic Rats. Table 1 demonstrates a time-dependent effect on the level of FPG in STZ-induced diabetic rats showing significant interaction between groups ([$F(5, 15) = 10.16$, $P < 0.05$] and days [$F(3, 15) = 1.92$, $P < 0.05$]. Statistical analysis by two-way ANOVA revealed that there was no significant difference among the groups at the 0th and 7th days except glibenclamide (10 mg/kg, p.o.) treated rats. However, statistical analysis at the 14th and 21st days revealed a significant reduction in the plasma sugar level of glibenclamide and *H. cordata* (200 and 400 mg/kg, p.o.) treated groups compared to diabetic control groups.

3.3. Effect on Plasma Lipid Profile and Other Biochemical Parameters. The effect of *H. cordata* on TC, TG, LDL, HDL, and VLDL is represented in Table 2. The results demonstrated a significant decrease in TC [$F(5, 30) = 29.24$, $P < 0.05$],

TG [$F(5, 30) = 25.75$, $P < 0.05$], LDL [$F(5, 30) = 37.98$, $P < 0.05$] and VLDL [$F(5, 30) = 25.75$, $P < 0.05$] levels in glibenclamide and *H. cordata* (200 and 400 mg/kg, p.o.) treated groups. Moreover, glibenclamide and *H. cordata* also showed significant increase in HDL level [$F(5, 30) = 33.29$, $P < 0.05$]. The results also depicted a significant reduction in total creatinine [$F(5, 30) = 7.1$, $P < 0.05$] and blood urea nitrogen [$F(5, 30) = 21.46$, $P < 0.05$], content at 200 and 400 mg/kg, p.o. of *H. cordata*; however, a significant increase in total protein [$F(5, 30) = 21.53$, $P < 0.05$] was observed only at 400 mg/kg, p.o. of *H. cordata* (Table 3).

3.4. Effect on Body Weight. Table 4 represents the effect of *H. cordata* on body weight of treated rats. Although the mean body weight of treated groups (100 and 200 mg/kg; p.o.) was higher than diabetic control group, it was not statistically significant. However, the rats treated with glibenclamide (10 mg/kg; p.o.) and *H. cordata* (400 mg/kg, p.o.) showed significant increase in body weight compared to diabetic control.

3.5. Effect on Insulin Levels. The effect of *H. cordata* (100, 200 and 400 mg/kg, p.o.) on plasma insulin is depicted in Figure 2. Post hoc test revealed a significant reduction in plasma insulin level in diabetic rats compared to normal control. However, glibenclamide and *H. cordata* at 200 and 400 mg/kg, p.o. showed significant [$F(5, 30) = 23.94$, $P < 0.05$] increase in plasma insulin levels compared to diabetic control.

3.6. Effect of H. cordata on Mitochondrial Antioxidant Level. One-way ANOVA showed that, in liver [$F(5, 30) = 21.58$, $P < 0.05$], pancreas [$F(5, 30) = 53.6$, $P < 0.05$], and adipose tissue [$F(5, 30) = 47.39$, $P < 0.05$], there were significant differences in MDA levels among groups (Table 5). Post hoc analysis revealed that hyperglycaemia significantly increased MDA levels compared to normal control. However,

TABLE 1: Effect of HC on FPG in streptozotocin-induced diabetic rats.

| Group ($n = 3$) | Treatment (dose in mg/kg) | Fasting plasma glucose concentration (mg/dL) | | | |
		1st day	7th day	14th day	21st day
I	NC	85.62 ± 3.8	83.01 ± 3.05	85.40 ± 3.63	80.10 ± 2.92
II	DC	294.72 ± 11.07^a	319.72 ± 12.41^a	362.99 ± 13.63^a	365.15 ± 13.29^a
III	Glib (10)	327.67 ± 10.7^a	$184.91 \pm 6.72^{a,b}$	$152.63 \pm 4.67^{a,b}$	122.62 ± 3.87^b
IV	HC (100)	271.48 ± 18.87^a	$293.77 \pm 16.11^{a,c}$	$320.52 \pm 20.89^{a,c}$	$324.64 \pm 15.33^{a,c}$
V	HC (200)	275.07 ± 14.42^a	$322.25 \pm 12.68^{a,c}$	$260.82 \pm 12.95^{a,b,c,d}$	$190.50 \pm 11.36^{a,b,c,d}$
VI	HC (400)	316.20 ± 15.87^a	$299.68 \pm 14.57^{a,c}$	$208.56 \pm 11.56^{a,b,c,d,}$	$146.86 \pm 8.26^{a,b,d,e}$

Results are expressed as mean ± SEM, $n = 6$, $^aP < 0.05$ compared to normal control; $^bP < 0.05$ compared to diabetic control; $^cP < 0.05$ compared to glibenclamide; $^dP < 0.05$ compared to HC 100; $^eP < 0.05$ compared to HC 200 (two-way ANOVA followed by Bonferroni posttest).

TABLE 2: Effect of HC on lipid profile of streptozotocin-induced diabetic rats on the 21st day.

Group ($n=3$)	Treatment (dose in mg/kg)	TC (mg/dL)	TG (mg/dL)	VLDL (mg/dL)	HDL-C (mg/dL)	LDL (mg/dL)
I	NC	89.73 ± 3.91	82.67 ± 4.08	16.53 ± 0.81	38.06 ± 1.23	35.13 ± 2.70
II	DC	173.13 ± 6.99^a	177.41 ± 8.61^a	35.48 ± 1.72^a	21.01 ± 0.98^a	116.63 ± 7.4^a
III	Glib (10)	96.19 ± 4.26^b	$140.13 \pm 8.08^{a,b}$	$28.02 \pm 1.61^{a,b}$	40.96 ± 1.31^b	27.20 ± 3.60^b
IV	HC (100)	$161.09 \pm 7.68^{a,c}$	161.84 ± 8.70^a	32.36 ± 1.74^a	$24.13 \pm 1.09^{a,c}$	$104.58 \pm 8.33^{a,c}$
V	HC (200)	$132.95 \pm 7.59^{a,b,c,d}$	$138.15 \pm 5.55^{a,b}$	$27.63 \pm 1.11^{a,b}$	$31.02 \pm 1.6^{a,b,c,d}$	$74.29 \pm 6.34^{a,b,c,d}$
VI	HC (400)	$116.09 \pm 6.14^{b,d}$	$106.57 \pm 4.63^{b,c,d,e}$	$21.31 \pm 0.92^{b,c,d,e}$	$35.01 \pm 1.76^{b,c,d}$	$59.76 \pm 4.51^{b,c,d}$

Values are expressed as mean ± SEM of 6 animals in each group. One-way ANOVA showed a significant difference in drug treatment between the groups for HC for total cholesterol, triglyceride, very low density lipoprotein (VLDL), HDL-cholesterol (HDL-C), and low density lipoprotein (LDL). $^aP < 0.05$ compared to normal control; $^bP < 0.05$ compared to diabetic control; $^cP < 0.05$ compared to glibenclamide; $^dP < 0.05$ compared to HC 100; $^eP < 0.05$ compared to HC 200 (one-way ANOVA followed by Tukey's multiple comparison test).

TABLE 3: Effect of HC on other biochemical parameters.

Group ($n = 6$)	Treatment (dose in mg/kg)	CRTN (mg/dL) 21 day	BUN (mg/dL) 21 day	TPR (g/dL) 21 day
I	NC	0.641 ± 0.055	21.908 ± 1.392	0.717 ± 0.012
II	DC	1.165 ± 0.135^a	57.906 ± 4.831^a	0.615 ± 0.011^a
III	Glib (10)	0.59 ± 0.019^b	$35.241 \pm 2.654^{a,b}$	0.723 ± 0.012^b
IV	HC (100)	$1.039 \pm 0.087^{a,c}$	$52.573 \pm 2.474^{a,c}$	$0.614 \pm 1.028^{a,c}$
V	HC (200)	0.792 ± 0.095^b	$44.862 \pm 2.143^{a,b}$	$0.646 \pm 1.017^{a,c}$
VI	HC (400)	0.724 ± 0.074^b	$39.745 \pm 1.793^{a,b,d}$	$0.697 \pm 0.0.02^{b,d}$

Values are mean ± SEM of 6 animals in each group. One-way ANOVA showed a significant difference in drug treatment between the groups for HC for total creatinine (CRTN), blood urea nitrogen (BUN), and total protein (TPR); $^aP < 0.05$ compared to normal control; $^bP < 0.05$ compared to diabetic control; $^cP < 0.05$ compared to glibenclamide; $^dP < 0.05$ compared to HC 100; $^eP < 0.05$ compared to HC 200 (one-way ANOVA followed by Tukey's multiple comparison test).

TABLE 4: Effect of HC on body weight in streptozotocin-induced diabetic rats.

| Group ($n = 6$) | Treatment (dose in mg/kg) | Body weight (g) | |
		1st day	21st day
I	NC	147.83 ± 3.42	154.66 ± 4.18
II	DC	149.33 ± 4.15	110.66 ± 5.33^a
III	Glib (10)	154.83 ± 4.20	145.66 ± 3.89^b
IV	HC (100)	153.16 ± 5.32	$118.5 \pm 4.76^{a,c}$
V	HC (200)	155.33 ± 4.49	$124.5 \pm 4.02^{a,c}$
VI	HC (400)	151.83 ± 4.96	136.5 ± 4.48^b

Values are mean ± SEM of 6 animals in each group. One-way ANOVA reveals that there were significant differences among the experimental groups [$F(5, 30) = 14.12$, $P < 0.05$]. $^aP < 0.05$ compared to normal control; $^bP < 0.05$ compared to diabetic control; $^cP < 0.05$ compared to glibenclamide. (One-way ANOVA followed by Tukey's multiple comparison test.)

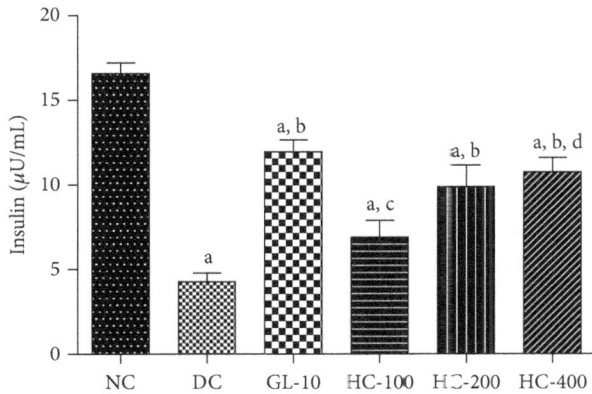

FIGURE 2: Effect of HC on plasma Insulin levels in control and experimental rats. Values are given as mean ± SD, $n = 6$, [a]$P < 0.05$ compared to normal control; [b]$P < 0.05$ compared to diabetic control; [c]$P < 0.05$ compared to glibenclamide; [d]$P < 0.05$ compared to HC 100 (one-way ANOVA followed by Tukey's multiple comparison test).

treatment with *H. cordata* (200 and 400 mg/kg, p.o.) reversed diabetes-induced MDA levels significantly in all the regions. The changes in mitochondrial SOD activity as a measure of mitochondrial antioxidant function are represented in Table 5. Analysis by one-way ANOVA showed that there was significant difference in the SOD activity in liver [$F(5, 30) = 7.31$, $P < 0.05$], pancreas [$F(5, 30) = 9.19$, $P < 0.05$], and adipose tissue [$F(5, 30) = 8.04$, $P < 0.05$] among groups. However, administration of *H. cordata* (200 and 400 mg/kg, p.o.) significantly increased the SOD activity in all the three tissues. Statistical analysis by one-way ANOVA showed that there was significant difference in the CAT activity in liver [$F(5, 30) = 11.13$, $P < 0.05$], pancreas [$F(5, 30) = 5.84$, $P < 0.05$], and adipose tissue [$F(5, 30) = 18.83$, $P < 0.05$] among groups. Nevertheless, treatment with *H. cordata* (200 and 400 mg/kg, p.o.) significantly increased the CAT activity in all three regions compared to diabetic control groups.

3.7. Effect of H. cordata Extract on Mitochondrial Function.
The mitochondrial function in terms of mitochondrial SDH activity was determined in STZ-induced diabetic animals (Table 5). One-way ANOVA showed that there were significant differences in mitochondrial function among groups in pancreas [$F(5, 30) = 34.81$, $P < 0.05$], liver [$F(5, 30) = 46.93$, $P < 0.05$], and adipose tissue [$F(5, 30) = 23.38$, $P < 0.05$]. Post hoc analysis revealed that the mitochondrial function was decreased in terms of decrease in the mitochondrial SDH activity in all the tissues of STZ-induced rats compared to control animals. *H. cordata* (200 and 400 mg/kg, p.o.) significantly reversed STZ-induced decrease in mitochondrial function in pancreatic tissues.

3.8. Effect of H. cordata Extract on Mitochondrial Membrane Potential $(\Delta\Psi_m)$.
The changes in $\Delta\Psi_m$ as a marker of mitochondrial integrity during the hyperglycaemic condition are represented in Figure 3. One-way ANOVA showed that there

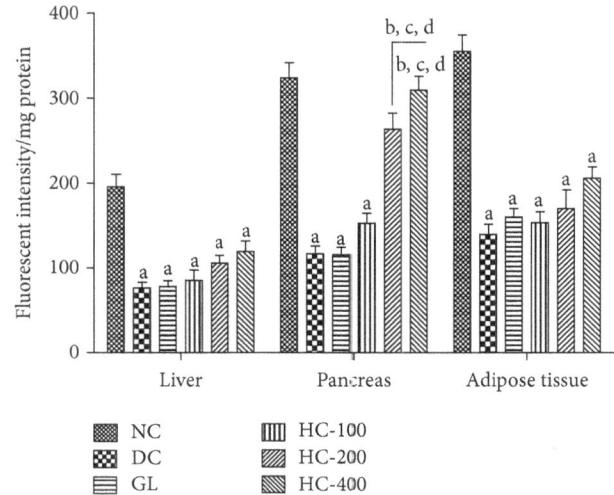

FIGURE 3: Effect of HC on MMP levels in liver, pancreas and adipose tissue in STZ-induced diabetic rats. Bars represent data as mean ± SEM, $n = 6$, [a]$P < 0.05$ compared to normal control; [b]$P < 0.05$ compared to diabetic control; [c]$P < 0.05$ compared to glibenclamide; [d]$P < 0.05$ compared to HC 100 (one-way ANOVA followed by Tukey's multiple comparison test).

were significant differences in mitochondrial integrity among groups in pancreas [$F(5, 30) = 41.95$, $P < 0.05$], adipose tissue [$F(5, 30) = 25.26$, $P < 0.05$], and liver [$F(5, 30) = 18.41$, $P < 0.05$]. Post hoc analysis showed that STZ caused loss in the mitochondrial integrity in all the tissues compared to control rats. *H. cordata* (200 and 400 mg/kg, p.o.) significantly mitigated mitochondrial integrity in pancreas compared to diabetic control. Glibenclamide treatment also showed no significant effect on diabetes-induced decline in $\Delta\Psi_m$ in all the regions under the investigation.

3.9. Effect on Apoptosis.
Figure 4 illustrates the effect of *H. cordata* on STZ-induced changes in the level of caspase-3 as a marker of apoptosis in liver, pancreas, and adipose tissues. One-way ANOVA revealed that there were significant differences in the level of expression of caspase-3 among groups in pancreas [$F(5, 12) = 50.19$, $P < 0.005$], liver [$F(5, 12) = 27.37$, $P < 0.005$] and adipose tissues [$F(5, 12) = 11.32$, $P < 0.005$]. Post hoc analysis showed that *H. cordata* (200 and 400 mg/kg, p.o.) significantly reversed the STZ-induced apoptosis in pancreas only.

3.10. PPAR-γ Expressions in Liver, Pancreas, and Adipose Tissue.
Figure 5 shows PPAR-γ expressions as a marker of inflammation in all three regions of normal control, diabetic control, and diabetic rats subjected to glibenclamide and *H. cordata* treatment after 21 days. The level of PPAR-γ expression was significantly increased among the groups in the pancreas [$F(5, 12) = 6.51$, $P < 0.005$]; however, there was no significant change observed in liver [$F(5, 12) = 1.93$, $P < 0.005$] and adipose tissue [$F(5, 12) = 0.79$, $P < 0.005$] compared to normal control rats. Further, post hoc analyses

TABLE 5: Effect of HC on mitochondrial MDA, SOD, CAT, and SDH levels in liver, pancreas, and adipose tissue of diabetic rats.

	Control	Diabetic	GL-10	HC-100	HC-200	HC-400
	MDA level (nmol MDA/mg protein)					
Liver	6.31 ± 0.322	10.625 ± 0.411[a]	7.436 ± 0.331[b]	9.95 ± 0.348[a,c]	8.253 ± 0.4[a,b,d]	7.23 ± 0.335[b,d]
Pancreas	3.66 ± 0.29	10.389 ± 0.381[a]	5.071 ± 0.327[b]	8.965 ± 0.396[a,c]	6.082 ± 0.376[a,b,d]	4.71 ± 0.373[b,d]
Adipose tissue	7.092 ± 0.334	13.19 ± 0.356[a]	8.336 ± 0.321[b]	11.93 ± 0.383[a,c]	10.14 ± 0.287[a,b,c,d]	8.218 ± 0.375[b,d,e]
	SOD activity (units/min/mg protein)					
Liver	0.152 ± 0.012	0.04 ± 0.007[a]	0.147 ± 0.009[b]	0.076 ± 0.021[a]	0.114 ± 0.015[b]	0.141 ± 0.022[b]
Pancreas	0.384 ± 0.024	0.134 ± 0.019[a]	0.331 ± 0.04[b]	0.17 ± 0.023[a,c]	0.276 ± 0.04[b]	0.319 ± 0.037[b,d]
Adipose tissue	0.512 ± 0.053	0.232 ± 0.018[a]	0.482 ± 0.042[b]	0.272 ± 0.032[a,c]	0.426 ± 0.029[b]	0.46 ± 0.057[b,d]
	CAT (units/min/mg protein)					
Liver	21.94 ± 1.415	8.864 ± 1.203[a]	18.733 ± 1.326[b]	11.611 ± 1.523[a,c]	16.631 ± 1.708[b]	20.938 ± 2.674[b,d]
Pancreas	9.605 ± 0.553	3.828 ± 0.505[a]	8.108 ± 1.472[b]	4.505 ± 1.026[a]	5.738 ± 0.644	7.875 ± 1.041[b]
Adipose tissue	13.672 ± 0.896	4.544 ± 0.711[a]	10.91 ± 0.857[b]	7.172 ± 0.784[a,c]	8.325 ± 0.733[a,b]	11.841 ± 0.618[b,d,e]
	SDH activity formazan produced (mM/min/mg/protein)					
Liver	1.701 ± 0.066	0.801 ± 0.078[a]	1.581 ± 0.064[b]	0.829 ± 0.35[a,c]	0.883 ± 0.056[a,c]	0.930 ± 0.045[a,c]
Pancreas	2.071 ± 0.058	0.589 ± 0.046[a]	1.882 ± 0.069[b]	0.836 ± 0.033[a,c]	1.591 ± 0.069[a,b,c,d]	1.832 ± 0.067[b,d]
Adipose tissue	2.307 ± 0.187	0.73 ± 0.083[a]	1.814 ± 0.185[b]	0.816 ± 0.056[a,c]	1.151 ± 0.103[a,c]	1.27 ± 0.064[a,c]

All results are expressed as mean ± SEM, $n = 6$, MDA: malondialdehyde, SOD: succinate dehydrogenase, CAT: catalase. [a]$P < 0.05$ compared to normal control; [b]$P < 0.05$ compared to diabetic control; [c]$P < 0.05$ compared to glibenclamide; [d]$P < 0.05$ compared to HC 100 and [e]$P < 0.05$ compared to HC 200 (one-way ANOVA followed by Tukey's multiple comparison test).

revealed that glibenclamide and *H. cordata* had no significant effect on PPAR-γ expression.

3.11. Effect of H. cordata on GLUT-2 in Liver and Pancreas and GLUT-4 in Adipose Tissue. As there was an increase in plasma insulin levels in *H. cordata*-treated diabetic rats and because of the physiologic importance of insulin-dependent GLUT-2 and GLUT-4 translocation to the cell membrane, attempts have been made to see the effect of *H. cordata* treatment on GLUT-4 level in adipose tissue membrane and GLUT-2 levels in liver and pancreas. In the liver and adipose tissue membrane fractions of diabetic rats, the translocation of GLUT-2 and GLUT-4 was very much reduced when compared with the band density of normal controls. This is quite rational because the deficiency of insulin in the diabetic state would decrease the translocation of GLUT-2 and GLUT-4 from the vesicles to cell membranes. Treatment with *H. cordata* resulted in the significant increase in membrane GLUT-2 and GLUT-4 levels at the dose of 400 mg/kg. However, there was no significant effect on GLUT-2 level in pancreatic cells. The modulation of GLUT-4 and GLUT-2 protein could thus be one of the mechanisms of antidiabetic properties of *H. cordata* (Figures 6 and 7).

3.12. Histopathological Studies. The effects of *H. cordata* on pancreatic cells are represented in Figure 8. The pancreas of the normal rats showed normal islets with intact β-cells, whereas, in case of diabetic control rats, atrophy of β-cells with vascular degeneration in islets was observed. The rats treated with glibenclamide (10 mg/kg; p.o.) and *H. cordata* (400 mg/kg; p.o.) depicted regeneration of β-cells which were found to be intact and also preserved islets justifying its protective effect.

4. Discussion

Regular administration of ethanolic extract of *H. cordata* for 3 weeks resulted in a significant diminution of FPG level with respect to diabetic rat, which clearly explains its antidiabetic activity. The results demonstrated a dose-dependent effect of *H. cordata* treatment in decreasing FPG. Treatment with *H. cordata* (200 and 400 mg/kg, p.o.) not only lowered the TC, TG, and LDL level, but also enhanced the HDL-cholesterol which is known to play an important role in the transport of cholesterol from peripheral cells to the liver by a pathway termed "reverse cholesterol transport," and is considered to be a cardioprotective lipid [33]. Decreased levels of BUN, creatinine and elevation in total protein again indicated that *H. cordata* can improve renal and liver function [34].

Dysfunctional mitochondria produce excessive amounts of ROS such as superoxide (O_2^-), hydrogen peroxide (H_2O_2), and peroxynitrite ($ONOO^-$). This, over production of ROS accumulated in the mitochondrial matrix, leads to collapse of mitochondrial membrane potential ($\Delta\Psi_m$), decrease in ATP production, and subsequent mitochondrial dysfunction [35]. In line with earlier studies, we also observed that STZ administration produced an increase in the oxidative damage and decreased the antioxidant enzyme activity [36]. Further, there was a significant decrease in mitochondrial function and integrity with the administration of STZ. This effect has been observed in other studies also [37]. *H. cordata* extract attenuated the STZ-induced mitochondrial oxidative stress and stabilized the mitochondrial function and integrity in the pancreatic tissues. It is well accepted that PPAR-γ plays a significant role in the pathogenesis of inflammation in several tissues [38]. Moderate amounts of PPAR-γ are expressed in pancreatic β-cells, which increases in the diabetic state [39], leading to accumulation of intracellular triglyceride. In

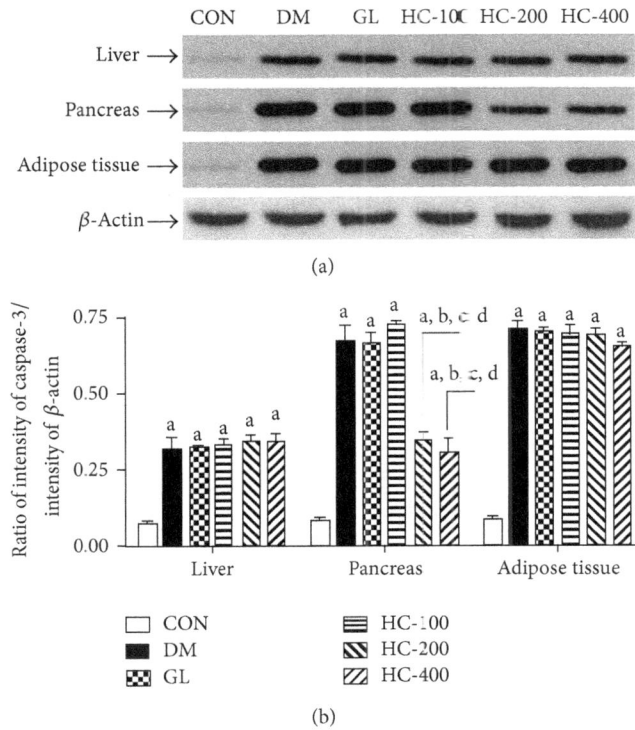

FIGURE 4: Effect of HC (100, 200 and 400 mg/kg) on STZ-induced changes in the levels of expression of caspase-3 in liver, pancreas, and adipose tissues. The blots (a) are representative of caspase-3 in liver, pancreas, and adipose tissues. The results in the histogram (b) are expressed as ratio of relative intensity of levels of protein expression of caspase-3 to β-Actin. All values are mean ± SEM of three separate sets of independent experiments. [a]$P < 0.05$ compared to normal control; [b]$P < 0.05$ compared to diabetic control; [c]$P < 0.05$ compared to glibenclamide; [d]$P < 0.05$ compared to HC 100; [e]$P < 0.05$ compared to HC 200 (One-way ANOVA followed by Tukey's multiple comparison test).

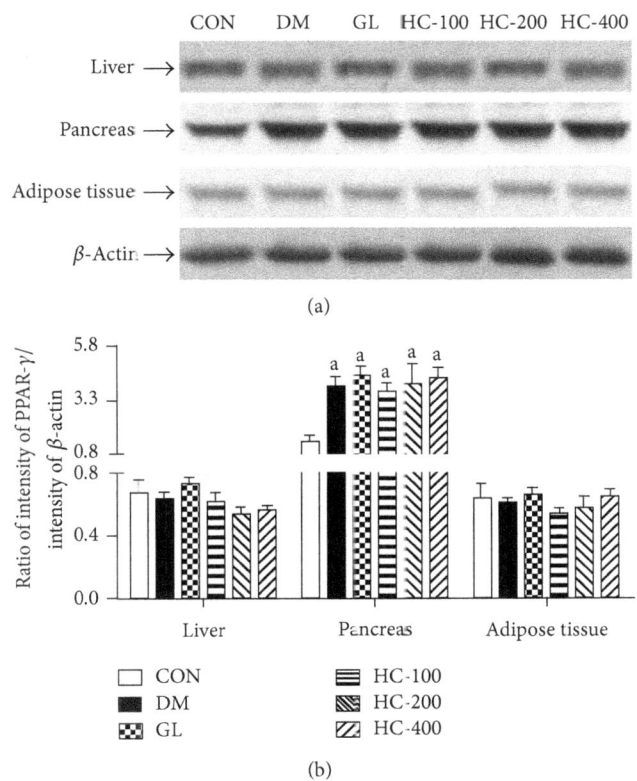

FIGURE 5: Effect of HC (100, 200 and 400 mg/kg) on STZ-induced changes in the levels of expression of PPAR-γ in liver, pancreas, and adipose tissues. The blots (a) are representative of PPAR-γ in liver, pancreas, and adipose tissues. The results in the histogram (b) are expressed as ratio of relative intensity of levels of protein expression PPAR-γ to β-Actin. All values are mean ± SEM of three separate sets of independent experiments. [a]$P < 0.05$ compared to normal control (one-way ANOVA followed by Tukey's multiple comparison test).

the present study, the level of expression of PPAR-γ was elevated in STZ-induced rats similar to earlier reports. *H. cordata* extract did not cause any change in the STZ-induced inflammation indicating that the extract was probably ineffective against STZ-induced inflammation.

It is reported that STZ injection causes apoptosis in several tissues such as liver, pancreas, and adipose tissues [37]. As a marker of apoptosis, the level of caspase-3 was increased with the STZ injection in all the tissues under the investigation. *H. cordata* extract showed significant lowering of caspase-3 level in pancreatic tissues of STZ-injected rats, indicating its promising effect on STZ-induced apoptosis. It is well documented that caspase-3 is a common product of both extrinsic and intrinsic mediated apoptotic pathways [40]. The effect was also well supported by the histopathological studies showing a considerable regeneration in the β-cells of pancreas in rats treated with *H. cordata* 400 mg/kg; p.o. In this context, it is quite impossible to explain the mechanism of *H. cordata* extract in the STZ-induced apoptosis; however further studies may elaborate the plausible antiapoptotic mechanism of *H. cordata* extract in STZ-induced model.

Several tissues are involved in maintaining glucose homeostasis. Among them, liver, pancreatic β-cells, and adipose tissue are the most important because they can sense and respond to changing blood glucose levels. Glucose is taken up into the cell through GLUT-2 and GLUT-4 in the plasma membrane of the cells. In pancreatic β-cells, glucose is the primary physiological stimulus for insulin secretion [41]. GLUT-2 is known to play more permissive roles, allowing rapid equilibration of glucose across the plasma membrane. However, it is also essential in glucose stimulating insulin signal (GSIS) because normal glucose uptake and subsequent metabolic signaling for GSIS cannot be achieved without GLUT-2. In diabetic subjects, GLUT-2 and GLUT-4 expression is decreased before the loss of GSIS [42]. Our study suggests that the modulation of GLUT-2 and GLUT-4 protein could thus be one of the mechanisms of antidiabetic potential of *H. cordata*.

The study revealed a significant increase in serum insulin level in rats treated with *H. cordata* (especially at 400 mg/kg, p.o.) and glibenclamide as a result of regeneration of pancreatic β-cells which were destroyed by streptozotocin

(a)

(b)

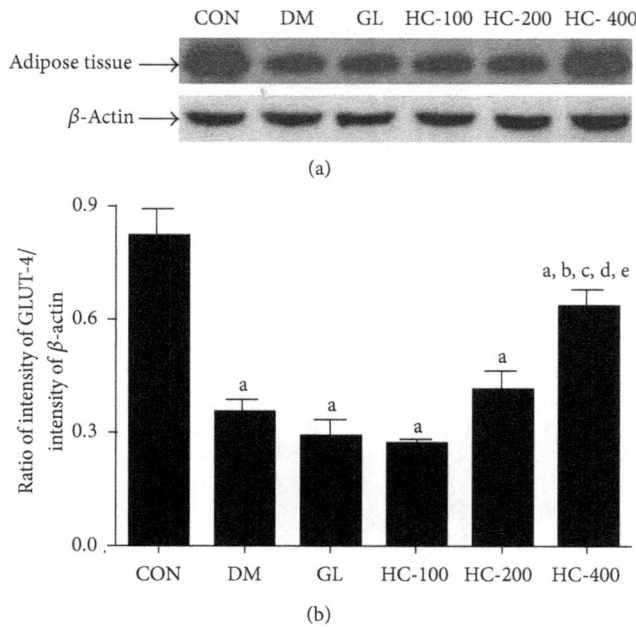

FIGURE 6: Effect of HC (100, 200 and 400 mg/kg) on STZ-induced changes in the levels of expression of GLUT-4 in adipose tissues. The blots (a) are representative of GLUT-4 in adipose tissues. The results in the histogram (b) are expressed as ratio of relative intensity of levels of protein expression of GLUT-4 to β-Actin. All values are mean $\pm$ SEM of three separate sets of experiments. [a]$P < 0.05$ compared to normal control; [b]$P < 0.05$ compared to diabetic control; [c]$P < 0.05$ compared to glibenclamide; [d]$P < 0.05$ compared to HC 100; [e]$P < 0.05$ compared to HC 200 (one-way ANOVA followed by Tukey's multiple comparison test).

(a)

(b)

FIGURE 7: Effect of HC (100, 200 and 400 mg/kg) on STZ-induced changes in the levels of expression of GLUT-2 in liver and pancreas. The blots (a) are representative of GLUT-2 in liver and pancreas. The results in the histogram (b) are expressed as ratio of relative intensity of levels of protein expression of GLUT-2 to β-Actin. All values are mean $\pm$ SEM of three separate sets of independent experiments. [a]$P < 0.05$ compared to normal control; [b]$P < 0.05$ compared to diabetic control; [c]$P < 0.05$ compared to glibenclamide; [d]$P < 0.05$ compared to HC 100; [e]$P < 0.05$ compared to HC 200 (one-way ANOVA followed by Tukey's multiple comparison test).

[43]. Thus, the antidiabetic effect of _H. cordata_ could be attributed to upregulation of GLUT-2 and GLUT-4 protein expressions resulting in potentiation of pancreatic secretion of insulin from existing β-cells of islets. Moreover, the study also demonstrated the beneficial role of _H. cordata_ in attenuating oxidative stress responsible for mitochondrial dysfunction.

Many works in the literature have shown the antioxidative, anticarcinogenic, antimicrobial, antidiabetic, and anti-inflammatory activities of phenols, flavonoids, and polysaccharides [44]. Among the polyphenols, gallic acid, resveratrol, and quercetin are widely distributed in the plant kingdom and are reported to possess antioxidant and antidiabetic properties [45]. In contrast to our results, _H. cordata_ shows anti-inflammatory activity in diabetic condition by improving the level of adiponectins [46]. This discrepancy in the results could be due to the different sets of diabetic condition. The above experiment was performed in the cell lines; however the present study was investigated as an _in vivo_ model of diabetes. Moreover, in both studies _H. cordata_ showed antiapoptotic effect in pancreatic tissues [46]. Studies on diabetic animal models have shown that quercetin significantly decreases the blood glucose level, plasma cholesterol, and TG in diabetic rats, in dose-dependent manner [47]. Beneficial effects of quercetin in increasing the number of

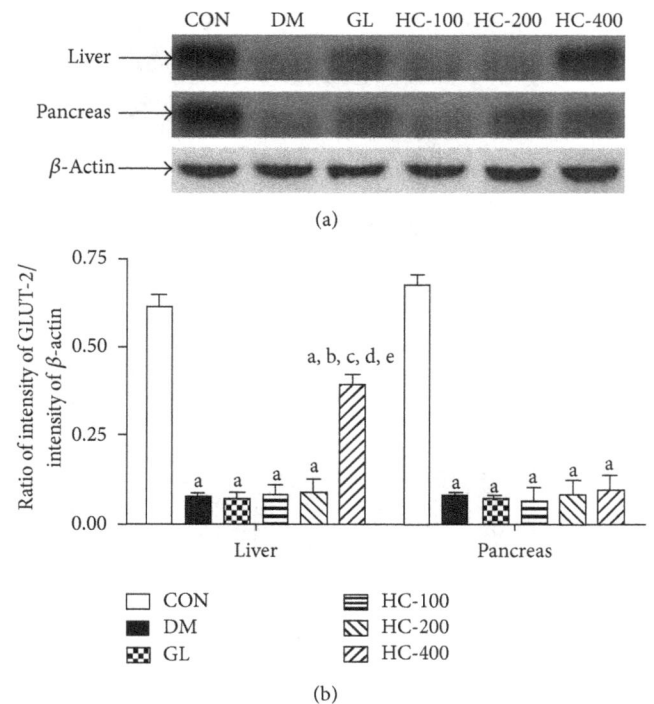

pancreatic islets and protective effect on degeneration of β-cells along with facilitation in translocation of GLUT-4 have also been reported in the literature [48, 49]. Thus, the presence of quercetin quantified in _H. cordata_ may play a contributing factor to the observed antidiabetic activity via the above mentioned pathways.

5. Conclusion

In conclusion, the present study justified the protective role of _H. cordata_ on pancreatic β-cells under high glucose toxic condition by reducing ROS-induced oxidative stress and apoptosis. These findings demonstrated that _H. cordata_ can be employed as a potential pharmaceutical agent against glucotoxicity induced by hyperglycaemia and in oxidative stress associated with diabetes.

Disclaimer

The authors alone are responsible for the content and writing of the paper.

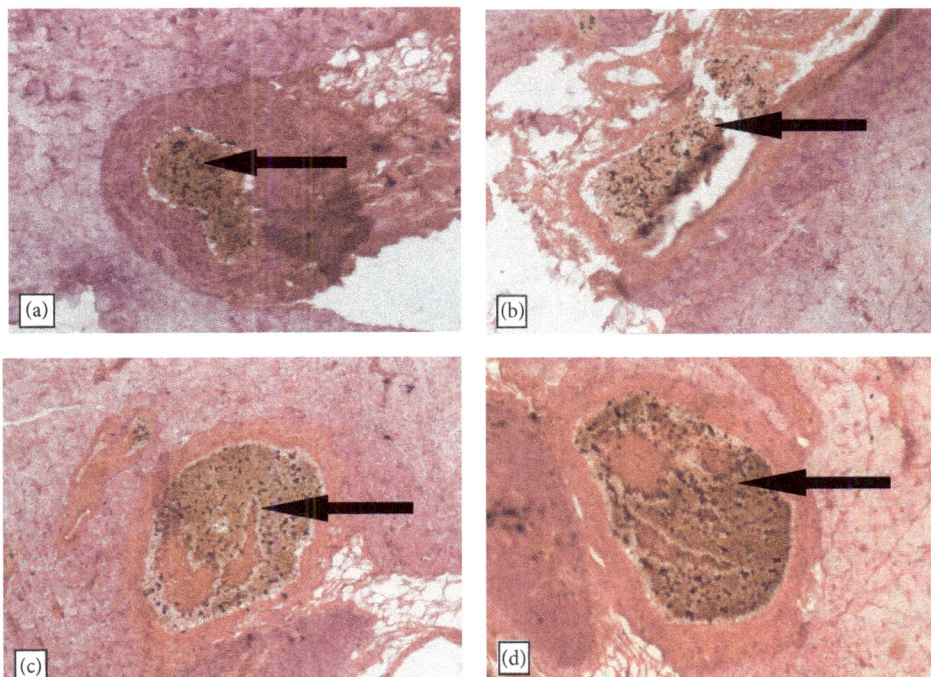

FIGURE 8: Histopathological view of rat pancreas on treatment with *H. cordata* at 400 mg/kg; p.o.; arrow indicates the location of β-cells of pancreas. (a) Normal control. (b) Diabetic control. (c) Diabetic treated with glibenclamide (10 mg/kg; p.o.) and (d) diabetic treated with *H. cordata* (400 mg/kg; p.o.).

Conflict of Interests

The authors report no conflict of interests.

Acknowledgments

Financial assistance provided by Rajiv Gandhi National Fellowship Scheme (RGNFS) to Mr. Manish Kumar is greatly acknowledged. Authors also would like to acknowledge Dr. B. K. Sinha, Botanical Survey of India, Shillong, Meghalaya, India, for identification and authentication of the plant. They are also thankful to Mr. H. Carehome Pakyntein (President and Herbal practitioner: Jaintia Indigenous Medicine Association) for providing information regarding the medicinal uses of the plant in lowering blood glucose level.

References

[1] J. F. Ndsing, "Role of hemeoxygenase in inflammation insulin signaling diabetes and obesity," *Mediators of Inflammation*, vol. 359, pp. 732–738, 2010.

[2] M. J. Charron, F. C. Brosius III, S. L. Alper, and H. F. Lodish, "A glucose transport protein expressed predominately in insulin-responsive tissues," *Proceedings of the National Academy of Sciences of the United States of America*, vol. 86, no. 8, pp. 2535–2539, 1989.

[3] P. R. Shepherd and B. B. Kahn, "Glucose transporters and insulin action: implications for insulin resistance and diabetes mellitus," *The New England Journal of Medicine*, vol. 341, no. 4, pp. 248–257, 1999.

[4] G. I. Bell, T. Kayano, J. B. Buse et al., "Molecular biology of mammalian glucose transporters," *Diabetes Care*, vol. 13, no. 3, pp. 198–208, 1990.

[5] J. W. Baynes, "Role of oxidative stress in development of complications in diabetes," *Diabetes*, vol. 40, no. 4, pp. 405–412, 1991.

[6] K. Green, M. D. Brand, and M. P. Murphy, "Prevention of mitochondrial oxidative damage as a therapeutic strategy in diabetes," *Diabetes*, vol. 53, supplement 1, pp. S110–S118, 2004.

[7] J.-A. Kim, Y. Wei, and J. R. Sowers, "Role of mitochondrial dysfunction in insulin resistance," *Circulation Research*, vol. 102, no. 4, pp. 401–414, 2008.

[8] K. Kamiya, W. Hamabe, S. Harada, R. Murakami, S. Tokuyama, and T. Satake, "Chemical constituents of *Morinda citrifolia* roots exhibit hypoglycemic effects in streptozotocin-induced diabetic mice," *Biological and Pharmaceutical Bulletin*, vol. 31, no. 5, pp. 935–938, 2008.

[9] R. J. Marles and N. R. Farnsworth, "Antidiabetic plants and their active constituents," *Phytomedicine*, vol. 2, no. 2, pp. 137–189, 1995.

[10] "Medicinal plants conservation and sustainable utilisation-Meghalaya (MPCSU)," in *Medicinal Plants Used in Ri-Bhoi District, Meghalaya, India*, pp. 72–75, 2003.

[11] T. Miho, K. Toshikazu, E. Tetsuo, and K. Santoshi, "Insulin secretion promoter," US Patent no. 6946451_B2, 2005.

[12] State Pharmacopoeia Commission of People's Republic of China, *Pharmacopoeia of the People'S Republic of China*, Chemical Industry Press, Beijing, China, 2005.

[13] H. M. Lu, Y. Z. Liang, L. Z. Yi, and X. J. Wu, "Anti-inflammatory effect of *Houttuynia cordata* injection," *Journal of Ethnopharmacology*, vol. 104, no. 1-2, pp. 245–249, 2006.

[14] World Health Organization, Regional Office for the Western Pacific, *Medicinal Plants in the Republic of Korea*, Western Pacific Series no. 21, WHO Regional Publications, Manila, Philippines, 1998.

[15] J.-S. Chang, L.-C. Chiang, C.-C. Chen, L.-T. Liu, K.-C. Wang, and C.-C. Lin, "Atileukemic activity of *Bidens pilosa* L. var. minor (blume) sherff and *Houttuynia cordata* thunb," *The American Journal of Chinese Medicine*, vol. 29, no. 2, pp. 303–312, 2001.

[16] S.-K. Kim, S. Y. Ryu, J. No, S. U. Choi, and Y. S. Kim, "Cytotoxic alkaloids from *Houttuynia cordata*," *Archives of Pharmacal Research*, vol. 24, no. 6, pp. 518–521, 2001.

[17] E. J. Cho, T. Yokozawa, D. Y. Rhyu et al., "Study on the inhibitory effects of Korean medicinal plants and their main compounds on the 1,1-diphenyl-2-picrylhydrazyl radical," *Phytomedicine*, vol. 10, pp. 554–551, 2003.

[18] W. Hai-Ying and B. Jun-Lu, "Effect of *Houttuynia cordata* aetherolea on adiponectin and connective tissue growth factor in a rat model of diabetes mellitus," *Journal of Traditional Chinese Medicine*, vol. 32, pp. 58–62, 2012.

[19] D. S. Jang, J. M. Kim, Y. M. Lee et al., "Flavonols from *Houttuynia cordata* with protein glycation and aldose reductase inhibitory activity," *Natural Product Sciences*, vol. 12, no. 4, pp. 210–213, 2006.

[20] K. R. Khandelwal, *Practical Pharmacognosy Techniques and Experiments*, Pune, India, 17th edition, 2007.

[21] H. P. S. Makkar, *Quantification of Tannins in Tree Foliage: A LaboraTory Manual for the FAO/IAEA Co-Ordinated Research Project on Use of Nuclear and Related Techniques to Develop Simple Tannin Assays for Predicting and Improving the Safety and Efficiency of Feeding Ruminants of Tanniniferous Tree Foliage. Working Document*, FAO/IAEA, Vienna, Austria, 2000.

[22] A. Kumaran and R. Joel Karunakaran, "*In vitro* antioxidant activities of methanol extracts of five Phyllanthus species from India," *LWT—Food Science and Technology*, vol. 40, no. 2, pp. 344–352, 2007.

[23] S. Hemalatha, A. K. Wahi, P. N. Singh, and J. P. N. Chansouria, "Hypoglycemic activity of *Withania coagulans* Dunal in strep-tozotocin induced diabetic rats," *Journal of Ethnopharmacology*, vol. 93, no. 2-3, pp. 261–264, 2004.

[24] H. Liu, X. Liu, J. Lee et al., "Insulin therapy restores impaired function and expression of P-glycoprotein in blood-brain bar-rier of experimental diabetes," *Biochemical Pharmacology*, vol. 75, pp. 1649–1658, 2008.

[25] P. L. Pedersen, J. W. Greenawalt, and B. Reynafarje, "Preparation and characterization of mitochondria and submitochondrial particles of rat liver and liver-derived tissues," *Methods in Cell Biology*, vol. 20, pp. 411–481, 1978.

[26] O. H. Lowry, N. J. Rosebrough, A. L. Farr, and R. J. Randall, "Protein measurement with the Folin phenol reagent," *The Journal of Biological Chemistry*, vol. 193, no. 1, pp. 265–275, 1951.

[27] F. W. Sunderman Jr., A. Marzouk, and S. M. Hopfer, "Increased lipid peroxidation in tissues of nickel chloride-treated rats," *Annals of Clinical and Laboratory Science*, vol. 15, no. 3, pp. 229–236, 1985.

[28] P. Kakkar, B. Das, and P. N. Viswanathan, "A modified spec-trophotometric assay of superoxide dismutase," *Indian Journal of Biochemistry and Biophysics*, vol. 21, no. 2, pp. 130–132, 1984.

[29] R. F. Beers Jr. and I. W. Sizer, "A spectrophotometric method for measuring the breakdown of hydrogen peroxide by catalase," *The Journal of Biological Chemistry*, vol. 195, no. 1, pp. 133–140, 1952.

[30] L. O. Sally and A. J. Margaret, "Methods of micro photometric assay of succinate dehydrogenase and cytochrome-C oxidase activities for use on human skeletal muscle," *Histochemical Journal*, vol. 21, pp. 545–555, 1989.

[31] S.-G. Huang, "Development of a high throughput screening assay for mitochondrial membrane potential in living cells," *Journal of Biomolecular Screening*, vol. 7, no. 4, pp. 383–389, 2002.

[32] C. Sunil, P. G. Latha, S. R. Suja et al., "Effect of ethanolic extract of *Pisonia alba* Span. Leaves on blood glucose levels and histological changes in tissues of alloxan-induced diabetic rats," *International Journal of Applied Research in Natural Products*, vol. 2, pp. 4–11, 2009.

[33] R. I. Levy, "High-density lipoproteins, an overview," *Lipids*, vol. 13, pp. 911–913, 1978.

[34] G. Mary and C. Charles, *Clinical Laboratory Parameters for Crl: CD, (SD) Rats*, Charles River Laboratories, Wilmington, NC, USA, 2006.

[35] D. G. Nicolls, "Mitochondrial function and dysfunction in the cell: its relevance to aging and aging-related disease," *International Journal of Biochemistry and Cell Biology*, vol. 34, pp. 1372–1381, 2002.

[36] T. Szkudelski, "The mechanism of alloxan and streptozotocin action in B cells of the rat pancreas," *Physiological Research*, vol. 50, no. 6, pp. 537–546, 2001.

[37] P. Manna, M. Sinha, and P. C. Sil, "Protective role of arjunolic acid in response to streptozotocin-induced type-I diabetes via the mitochondrial dependent and independent pathways," *Toxicology*, vol. 257, no. 1-2, pp. 53–63, 2009.

[38] P. Xu, X. L. Lou, C. Chen, and Z. W. Yang, "Effects of peroxisome proliferator-activated receptor-γ activation on apoptosis in rats with acute pancreatitis," *Digestive Diseases and Sciences*, vol. 58, no. 12, pp. 3516–3523, 2013.

[39] M. Dubois, F. Pattou, J. Kerr-Conte et al., "Expression of peroxisome proliferator-activated receptor gamma (PPAR-γ) in normal human pancreatic islet cells," *Diabetologia*, vol. 43, pp. 1165–1169, 2000.

[40] N. Liadis, K. Murakami, M. Eweida et al., "Caspase-3-dependent β-cell apoptosis in the initiation of autoimmune diabetes mellitus," *Molecular and Cellular Biology*, vol. 25, pp. 3620–3629, 2005.

[41] F. C. Schuit, P. Huypens, H. Heimberg, and D. G. Pipeleers, "Glucose sensing in pancreatic β-cells: a model for the study of other glucose-regulated cells in gut, pancreas, and hypotha-lamus," *Diabetes*, vol. 50, no. 1, pp. 1–11, 2001.

[42] B. Thorens, M.-T. Guillam, F. Beermann, R. Burcelin, and M. Jaquet, "Transgenic reexpression of GLUT1 or GLUT2 in pancreatic β cells rescues GLUT2-null mice from early death and restores normal glucose-stimulated insulin secretion," *The Journal of Biological Chemistry*, vol. 275, no. 31, pp. 23751–23758, 2000.

[43] A. Eidi, M. Eidi, and E. Esmaeili, "Antidiabetic effect of garlic (*Allium sativum* L.) in normal and streptozotocin-induced diabetic rats," *Phytomedicine*, vol. 13, no. 9-10, pp. 624–629, 2006.

[44] H. Y. Huang, M. Korivi, Y. Y. Chaing, T. Y. Chien, and Y. C. Tsai, "*Pleurotus tuber-regium* polysaccharides attenuate hyperglycemia and oxidative stress in experimental diabetic rats," *Evidence-Based Complementary and Alternative Medicine*, vol. 2012, Article ID 856381, 8 pages, 2012.

[45] M. López-Vélez, F. Martínez-Martínez, and C. Del Valle-Ribes, "The study of phenolic compounds as natural antioxidants in

wine," *Critical Reviews in Food Science and Nutrition*, vol. 43, no. 3, pp. 233–244, 2003.

[46] I. Rakatzi, H. Mueller, O. Ritzeler, N. Tennagels, and J. Eckel, "Adiponectin counteracts cytokine- and fatty acid-induced apoptosis in the pancreatic beta-cell line INS-1," *Diabetologia*, vol. 47, no. 2, pp. 249–258, 2004.

[47] M. Vessal, M. Hemmati, and M. Vasei, "Antidiabetic effects of quercetin in streptozocin-induced diabetic rats," *Comparative Biochemistry and Physiology C*, vol. 135, no. 3, pp. 357–364, 2003.

[48] O. Coskun, M. Kanter, A. Korkmaz, and S. Oter, "Quercetin, a flavonoid antioxidant, prevents and protects streptozotocin-induced oxidative stress and β-cell damage in rat pancreas," *Pharmacological Research*, vol. 51, no. 2, pp 117–123, 2005.

[49] J. M. Santos, S. B. Ribeiro, A. R. Gaya, H.-J. Appell, and J. A. Duarte, "Skeletal muscle pathways of contraction-enhanced glucose uptake," *International Journal of Sports Medicine*, vol. 29, no. 10, pp. 785–794, 2008.

10

Inhibitory Potential of Five Traditionally Used Native Antidiabetic Medicinal Plants on α-Amylase, α-Glucosidase, Glucose Entrapment, and Amylolysis Kinetics *In Vitro*

Carene M. N. Picot, A. Hussein Subratty, and M. Fawzi Mahomoodally

Department of Health Sciences, Faculty of Science, University of Mauritius, 230 Réduit, Mauritius

Correspondence should be addressed to M. Fawzi Mahomoodally; f.mahomoodally@uom.ac.mu

Academic Editor: Mustafa F. Lokhandwala

Five traditionally used antidiabetic native medicinal plants of Mauritius, namely, *Stillingia lineata* (SL), *Faujasiopsis flexuosa* (FF), *Erythroxylum laurifolium* (EL), *Elaeodendron orientale* (EO), and *Antidesma madagascariensis* (AM), were studied for possible α-amylase and α-glucosidase inhibitory property, glucose entrapment, and amylolysis kinetics *in vitro*. Only methanolic extracts of EL, EO, and AM (7472.92 ± 5.99, 1745.58 ± 31.66, and $2222.96 \pm 13.69 \, \mu g/mL$, resp.) were found to significantly ($P < 0.05$) inhibit α-amylase and were comparable to acarbose. EL, EO, AM, and SL extracts ($5000 \, \mu g/mL$) were found to significantly ($P < 0.05$) inhibit α-glucosidase (between 87.41 ± 3.31 and $96.87 \pm 1.37\%$ inhibition). Enzyme kinetic studies showed an uncompetitive and mixed type of inhibition. Extracts showed significant ($P < 0.05$) glucose entrapment capacities (8 to 29% glucose diffusion retardation index (GDRI)), with SL being more active (29% GDRI) and showing concentration-dependent activity (29, 26, 21, 14, and 5%, resp.). Amylolysis kinetic studies showed that methanolic extracts were more potent inhibitors of α-amylase compared to aqueous extracts and possessed glucose entrapment properties. Our findings tend to provide justification for the hypoglycaemic action of these medicinal plants which has opened novel avenues for the development of new phytopharmaceuticals geared towards diabetes management.

1. Introduction

Phytomedicine also known as herbal medicine has become a mainstream phenomenon worldwide. Recently, it has been reported that more than 80% of the world population is dependent on herbal medicine [1]. The utilisation of plants and their derivatives for the treatment and/or management of various diseases, including diabetes mellitus (DM), is becoming more and more prominent in pharmaceutical markets as an alternative and/or complementary therapy. DM is a growing epidemic and is highly prevalent in Mauritius with at least one out of two adults aged between 25 and 74 years being prediabetic or diabetic [2, 3].

The fundamental defect in DM is the lack of insulin which results in the impairment in glucose uptake, storage, and utilisation [4]. Type 2 DM is the most common form of diabetes and is usually caused by life-style factors and also related to

insufficient insulin production and resistance of target tissues to insulin. Several research works have been undertaken to elucidate the possible biochemical mechanisms involved in the pathogenesis of type 2 DM, but the exact mechanism is still unclear. However, hyperglycaemia, the hallmark of type 2 DM, has been considered as the principal cause of diabetes complications. Indeed, it was observed that strict glycaemic control lowered the incidence of retinopathy, nephropathy and neuropathy [5, 6].

Recently, there have been a growing number of scientific publications on the potential antidiabetic action of medicinal plants [7]. Indeed, advances in understanding the activity of key carbohydrate metabolising enzymes such as α-amylase and the role of dietary fibers have led to the development of new pharmacologic agents. Existing hypoglycemic agents such as metformin, voglibose, acarbose and miglitol effectively control glycemic level but carry prominent gastrointestinal side effects. The search for inhibitors devoid of side effects has been geared towards natural resources, namely, medicinal plants [8, 9]. Polyphenolic agents in plants have been shown to inhibit digestive enzymes due to their ability to bind to enzyme protein [10]. Moreover, the role of dietary fibres and viscous polysaccharides in the reduction of postprandial plasma glucose level in diabetic patients is highly documented [11].

The local population has a deep-rooted interest in the use of medicinal plants. Although a free advanced health care system exists, many Mauritians still rely on the use of folk medicine for the management of diabetes and related complications [7, 12]. Nonetheless, the majority of traditional antidiabetic medicinal plants await proper scientific and medical evaluation. In the present study selected medicinal plants of Mauritius were evaluated for their possible α-amylase and α-glucosidase inhibitory property, glucose movement entrapment and amylolysis kinetics effects using a battery of *in vitro* bioassays.

2. Materials and Method

2.1. Plant Materials and Extraction. Native traditionally used antidiabetic medicinal plants of Mauritius, namely, *Stillingia lineata* Lam. (Euphorbiaceae) (SL), *Faujasiopsis flexuosa* Lam. (Asteraceae) (FF), *Erythroxylum laurifolium* Lam. (Erythroxylaceae) (EL), *Elaeodendron orientale* Jacq. (Celastraceae) (EO), and *Antidesma madagascariensis* Lam. (Euphorbiaceae) (AM), were collected from a natural reserve situated on the upper humid regions of the island. The identity of the plants was confirmed by the natural reserve curator. The harvested plant materials were thoroughly washed under running tap water and air-dried until a constant weight was obtained. Subsequently, the dried samples were ground (Pacific mixer grinder, India) and stored in a cool-dry place prior to extraction. Crude methanolic extracts were obtained by soaking the dry powdered material into 70% methanol (1 : 10, sample : solvent w/v) for 72 h. Aqueous extracts, were prepared following traditional decoction method. Briefly, dried powdered material (50 g) was boiled into distilled water (200 mL) for 30 min. The filtrates were concentrated *in vacuo* using a rotary evaporator (Rotavap Stuart Scientific Ltd, Staffordshire, UK). The resulting paste-like material was stored at −20°C or dissolved in appropriate solvents.

2.2. α-Amylase Inhibition Assay. α-Amylase activity was assessed using the modified starch-iodine colour change method described previously by Mahomoodally et al. [9] and Kotowaroo et al. [13]. Briefly, 100 μL α-amylase solution from porcine origin (13 U/mL in 0.1 M sodium acetate buffer pH 7.2) was added to 3 mL soluble starch solution (1 g soluble starch was suspended into 10 mL distilled water and boiled for 2 min. The volume was then made up to 100 mL with distilled water. The starch solution was used within 2-3 days) and 2 mL sodium acetate buffer (0.1 M, pH 7.2). The reaction mixture was incubated for 37°C for 1 h. At timed interval ($t = 0$ min and $t = 60$ min) aliquot (0.1 mL) from the reaction mixture was discharged into 10 mL iodine solution. After mixing, the absorbance of the starch-iodine solution

was measured at 565 nm. As previously described [9] one unit of enzyme inhibitor was defined as that which reduced amylase activity by one unit and defined as $[(A_0 - A_t)/A_0] \times 100$; A_0 and A_t being absorbance of starch-iodine solution at $t = 0$ min and $t = 60$ min, respectively. For assessing the potential inhibitory activity of graded concentrations of plant extracts (5000–312.5 μg/mL) 100 μL extract was preincubated with 100 μL enzyme solution at 37°C for 15 min. The assay was then conducted as described above. Substrate and amylase blanks were carried out under similar assay conditions. The specific activity of amylase was described as U/mg protein/h.

2.3. Kinetics of α-Amylase Inhibition. A calibration curve using graded glucose concentration (10–0.156 mg/mL) was set up. Glucose solution (3 mL) was added to 3 mL dinitrosalicylic acid (DNS) reagent solution at 1% (10 g DNS, 0.5 g sodium disulphite, and 10 g sodium hydroxide) to capped tubes. The tubes were then placed in boiling water for 5–15 min until a reddish brown colour developed. Sodium potassium tartrate (1 mL, 40%) was then added to the mixture. After cooling, the absorbance was measured at 575 nm. The mode of inhibition of plant extracts on α-amylase action was determined by increasing the substrate (starch) concentration. The amount of glucose released after exactly 3 min was quantified using DNS reagent solution. 0.5 mL graded starch solution (4–0.25%), plant extract (0.25 mL; 5000 μg/mL) and α-amylase solution (0.25 mL; 13 U/mL) were allowed to react for 3 min at 37°C. DNS solution (2 mL) was then added to stop the reaction and the mixture was placed in a boiling water bath for 5–15 min. Sodium potassium tartrate (1 mL, 40%) was then added and absorbance was measured at 575 nm using a spectrophotometer [13]. Kinetic parameters namely, the Michaelis-Menten constant affinity (K_m) and maximum velocity ($V_{\max}$), were derived from appropriate Lineweaver-Burk plots.

2.4. α-Glucosidase Inhibition Assay. α-Glucosidase inhibition was assessed using modified methods previously described by Bachhawat et al. [14] and Mayur et al. [5]. Briefly, 10 μL α-glucosidase (1 U/mL), 50 μL sodium phosphate buffer (0.1 M, pH 6.9), and 20 μL p-nitrophenol-α-D-glucopyranoside (PNPG) substrate (1 mM) were incubated at 37°C for 30 min. After the incubation period, 50 μL sodium carbonate (0.1 M) was added to the reaction mixture to terminate the reaction. The hydrolysis of PNPG to p-nitrophenol was monitored using an ELISA microplate reader at 405 nm. The IC_{50} value and % inhibition of glucosidase were calculated as % inhibition = $[(Abs_{blank} - Abs_{sample})/Abs_{blank}] \times 100$; Abs_{blank} is absorbance of the blank and Abs_{sample} is absorbance of the sample.

2.5. α-Glucosidase Kinetic Studies. The type of inhibition of plant extracts on α-glucosidase action was determined by increasing PNPG concentration following the modified method of Gurudeeban et al. [8]. Graded concentrations of p-nitrophenol (0.6–0.019 mM) were allowed to react with sodium carbonate and the absorbance was measured at 405 nm. Plant extract (20 μL; 5000 μg/mL) was incubated with 10 μL α-glucosidase solution (1 U/mL), 50 μL sodium phosphate buffer (0.1 M, pH 6.9), and 20 μL graded concentrations of PNPG (1.25–0.039 mM) for 10 min at 37°C. The reaction was terminated by adding 50 μL sodium carbonate (0.1 M). Kinetic parameters, namely, the Michaelis-Menten constants affinity (K_m) and maximum velocity (V_{max}), were derived from appropriate Lineweaver-Burk plots.

2.6. Glucose Movement.

A simple model system was used to evaluate the effect of the plant extracts on glucose movement *in vitro*. This model was adapted from a method described by Shaukat et al. [15]. Briefly, the model used in the present experiment consisted of a one-sided sealed dialysis tube (15 cm × 25 mm, dialysis tubing membrane Sigma-Aldrich MW12173) into which 2 mL of 22 mM D-glucose in 0.15 M NaCl and 1 mL extract (160 mg/mL)/control (water) were incorporated. The other end was then sealed and the membrane was placed into a conical flask containing 45 mL 0.15 M NaCl. The conical flask was placed into an orbital shaking incubator (SI50, UK) at 37°C and speed of 100 rotations per minute. Aliquot (10 μL) of the external solution was withdrawn at timed intervals and tested for the presence of glucose using a glucose oxidase kit (Biosystems, Spain). As described by Gallagher et al. [16] concentration-dependent effect of plant extracts (160, 80, 40, 20, and 10 mg crude extract/mL) that exhibited the highest glucose diffusion retardation index was also evaluated. A standard curve was drawn using different glucose concentrations. Experiments were conducted in triplicate. The glucose diffusion retardation index (GDRI) was calculated using the following formula.

GDRI = (100 − glucose content (mg/mL) in external solution in the presence of plant extract/glucose content (mg/mL) in external solution in the absence of plant extract) * 100.

2.7. Amylolysis Kinetics.

This assay was adapted from Ahmed et al. [17]. Briefly, 8 g of soluble starch was dissolved in approximately 20 mL 0.1 M phosphate buffer (pH 6.5). The solution was boiled for 3 min and was made up to a final volume 100 mL to give an 8% (w/v) starch solution. The sample-α-amylase-starch system comprised extract (1 mL, 160 mg/mL), freshly prepared starch solution (3 mL, 8%), and enzyme solution (0.1% in 0.1 M phosphate buffer pH 6.5). The test system was dialysed against 45 mL distilled water at 37°C. The glucose concentration of the dialysate was monitored every hour for 4 h using a glucose oxidase kit (Biosystems, Spain). A control test was carried out with and without acarbose, a standard α-amylase inhibitor. After 4 h, the amount of starch remaining inside the dialysis tubing was quantified. To 5 mL iodine solution (0.254 g iodine and 4 g potassium iodide were dissolved in 1 L distilled water), 0.1 mL test mixture was added. The solution was vortexed and the absorbance was read at 565 nm. Then, using a calibration curve (4–0.125% starch solution) the amount of starch was quantified.

2.8. Statistical Analysis.

Results were expressed as mean ± standard deviation of three independent determinations. Difference between the samples and controls was determined using one-way analysis of variance (ANOVA) with statistical significance considered as $P < 0.05$ using SPSS 16.0.

3. Results

3.1. α-Amylase Inhibition Assay.

Data from the present study showed the variable inhibitory effect of tested plant extracts on α-amylase activity *in vitro*. Methanolic extracts of EL, EO, and AM were found to significantly ($P < 0.05$) inhibit α-amylase at different doses. IC_{50} values of extracts (methanolic EL, EO, and AM) are summarised in Table 1. As illustrated in Table 1, extracts activity (IC_{50} 1745.58–7472.92 μg/mL) was found to be significantly lower compared to positive standard acarbose (1100 μg/mL). In contrast, no dose-dependent response was observed for the other tested extracts (data not shown).

3.2. α-Amylase Kinetic Studies.

Since activity was observed for EL, EO, and AM methanolic extracts, kinetic studies were performed on these extracts. Methanolic EO and AM extracts showed an uncompetitive type of inhibition, whereby there was a reduction in both K_m and V_{max}. As presented in Table 2, in the presence of EO K_m was reduced from 3.73×10^{-1} mg to 3.05×10^{-1} mg and V_{max} from 0.03×10^{-1} mg mL^{-1} sec^{-1} to 0.01×10^{-1} mg mL^{-1} sec^{-1}. Similarly, K_m was reduced from 4.98×10^{-1} mg to 3.63×10^{-1} mg and V_{max} from 0.04×10^{-1} mg mL^{-1} sec^{-1} to 0.03×10^{-1} mg mL^{-1} sec^{-1} in the presence of methanolic AM. In contrast, in the presence of EL, K_m was raised from 3.73×10^{-1} mg to 4.37×10^{-1} mg while V_{max} was reduced to 0.02×10^{-1} mg mL^{-1} sec^{-1}.

3.3. α-Glucosidase Inhibition In Vitro.

α-Glucosidase activity was assessed by the release of *p*-nitrophenol from PNPG *in vitro*. IC_{50} (μg/mL) values of active extracts are presented in Table 3. Tested extracts exhibited various levels of effectiveness in inhibiting α-glucosidase. It was observed that both methanolic and aqueous extracts of EL, EO, AM, and SL were potent inhibitors (1.02–185.92 μg/mL) of α-glucosidase compared to acarbose (5115.73 μg/mL).

3.4. α-Glucosidase Kinetic Studies.

Table 4 presents the V_{max} and K_m values of active plants extracts against α-glucosidase. A decrease in both K_m and V_{max} as compared to the uninhibited reaction (61.40×10^{-2} mM (K_m), 2.50×10^{-2} mg mL^{-1} sec^{-1} (V_{max})) was noted for all tested extracts.

3.5. Glucose Movement.

Glucose movement for the control experiment (without plant extract) showed a mean glucose concentration of 0.906 mM. From Figures 1 and 2, it was observed that there was no apparent difference in glucose diffusion inhibition between the different types of extracts. As shown in Table 5, studied extracts exhibited glucose diffusion retardation index (GDRI) between 8 and 29%. Furthermore, it was observed that methanolic extracts were more potent inhibitors of glucose movement.

Dose-dependent studies on the effect of extracts on glucose retarding activity revealed a concentration-dependent inhibitory action (Figure 3). GDRI (%) decreased with

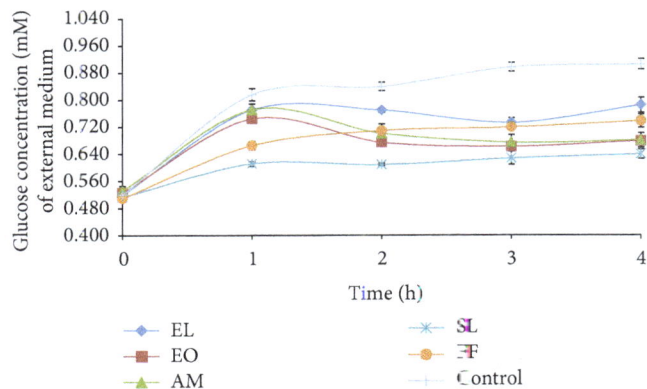

FIGURE 1: Effect of methanolic plant extracts (160 mg crude extract/mL) on glucose diffusion.

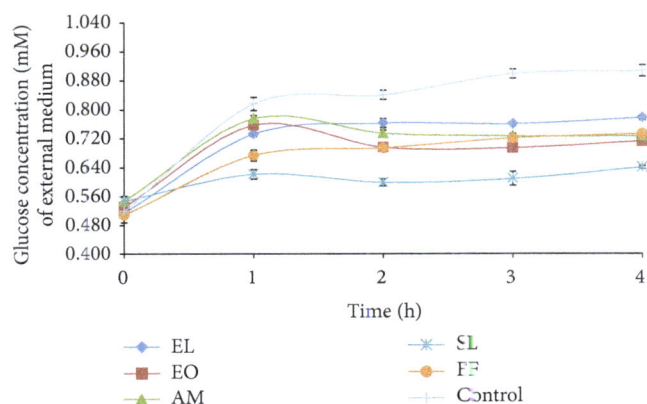

FIGURE 2: Effect of aqueous plant extracts (160 mg crude extract/mL) on glucose diffusion.

TABLE 1: IC$_{50}$ values of methanolic plants against α-amylase.

Plant extracts	IC$_{50}$ value (μg/mL)
EL	7472.92 ± 5.99[a]
EO	1745.58 ± 31.66[a]
AM	2222.96 ± 13.69[a]
Control	1100.06 ± 0.03

Data represents the mean ± standard deviation of triplicate values. [a]Values significantly lower ($P < 0.05$) than positive control (acarbose).

decreasing plant extract concentration. SL was found to exhibit greater GDRI at all concentrations tested.

3.6. Amylolysis Kinetics. Figures 4 and 5 summarise the starch concentration (%) of the reaction mixture inside the dialysis bag and the glucose concentration (mM) of the surrounding solution after 4 h. Methanolic extracts were found to be potent inhibitors compared to their corresponding aqueous extracts. As observed by the α-amylase inhibition assay, methanolic EL, EO, and AM gave the best inhibitory activity since starch concentration was the highest in the presence of these extracts (Figure 5). Glucose dialysis was the least in the presence of methanolic SL extract.

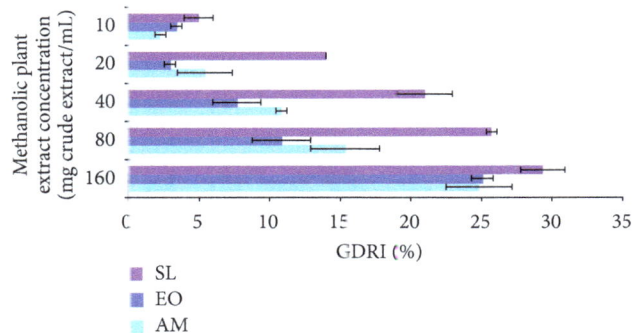

FIGURE 3: Dose-dependent effect of SL, EO, and AM extracts on glucose diffusion.

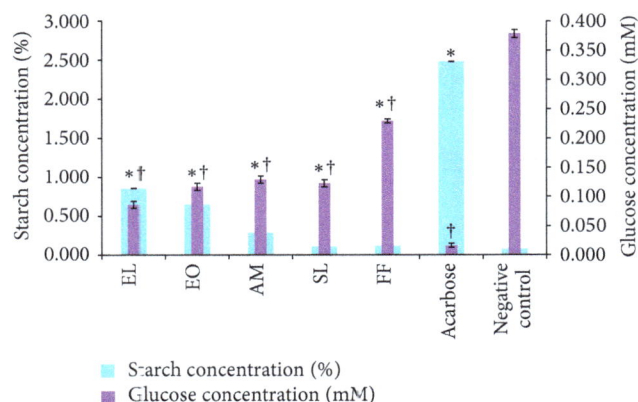

FIGURE 4: Percentage starch of reaction mixture and glucose concentration of dialysate in the presence of aqueous extracts. *Values [starch (%) concentration] significantly ($P < 0.05$) higher than negative control. †Values [glucose (mM) concentration] significantly ($P < 0.05$) lower than negative control.

TABLE 2: Kinetic parameters of active plant extracts on α-amylase activity *in vitro.*

Plants extracts (5000 μg/mL)	K_m (mg ×10^{-})	V_{max} (mgmL^{-1}sec^{-1} ×10^{-1})
EL	4.37	0.02
EO	3.05	0.01
AM	3.63	0.03

4. Discussion

The present study was geared towards investigating the potential effects of selected medicinal plants of Mauritius to inhibit key carbohydrate hydrolysing enzymes, namely, α-amylase and α-glucosidase. Furthermore, the ability of the extracts to entrap glucose and amylolysis kinetics were also evaluated. α-Amylase and α-glucosidase are key carbohydrate hydrolysing enzymes responsible for breaking α,1-4 bonds in disaccharides and polysaccharides, liberating glucose [18, 19]. The glucose surge observed a few minutes after ingestion contributes to hyperglycaemia, the hallmark of DM. Several scientific studies have shed light on the inhibition of these key

TABLE 3: IC$_{50}$ values (μg/mL) of methanolic and aqueous plants extracts that actively inhibit α-glucosidase.

Plant extracts	IC$_{50}$ value (μg/mL)
EL	[1.02 ± 0.02^b]
	(12.00 ± 1.57^b)
EO	[1.75 ± 0.26^b]
	(16.72 ± 2.81^b)
AM	[10.40 ± 0.26^b]
	(1.22 ± 0.05^b)
SL	[19.30 ± 3.59^b]
	(185.92 ± 9.00^b)
Control	5115.73 ± 3.91

^{b}Values significantly ($P < 0.05$) lower than control (acarbose); [] methanolic extracts; ( ) aqueous extracts.

TABLE 4: Kinetic parameters of methanolic and aqueous plant extracts on α-glucosidase activity *in vitro*.

Plant extracts (5000 μg/mL)	K_m (mM $\times 10^{-2}$)	V_{max} (mMmin^{-1} $\times 10^{-2}$)
EL	[0.60]	[0.90]
	(0.50)	(1.20)
EO	[0.70]	[0.70]
	(0.80)	(0.70)
AM	[0.80]	[0.90]
	(2.40)	(0.50)
SL	[2.60]	[0.50]
	(1.00)	(2.00)

[] methanolic extracts; ( ) aqueous extracts.

TABLE 5: Glucose concentration in external solution and glucose diffusion retardation index of methanolic plant extracts after 4 h.

Plant extracts	Glucose concentration in external solution^1 (mM)	GDRI^2 (%)
EL	[0.785 ± 0.022^c]	[13 ± 2.44]
	(0.777 ± 0.007^c)	(14 ± 0.78)
EO	[0.679 ± 0.007^c]	[25 ± 0.78]
	(0.712 ± 0.011^c)	(21 ± 1.17)
AM	[0.681 ± 0.021^c]	[25 ± 2.35]
	(0.726 ± 0.007^c)	(20 ± 0.78)
SL	[0.640 ± 0.014^c]	[29 ± 1.56]
	(0.640 ± 0.004^c)	(29 ± 0.39)
FF	[0.738 ± 0.020^c]	[19 ± 2.18]
	(0.732 ± 0.009^c)	(19 ± 0.78)
Control	0.906 ± 0.015	—

^{1}Values are mean ± SD of triplicate determinations; ^{c}values significantly ($P < 0.05$) different from negative control; ^{2}GDRI expressed as percentage; GDRI ± SD was calculated from triplicate determinations; [] methanolic extracts; ( ) aqueous extracts.

glycoside hydrolases to slow down carbohydrate digestion, reducing glucose absorption rate, consequently preventing postprandial glucose surge [20, 21]. The ability of plant

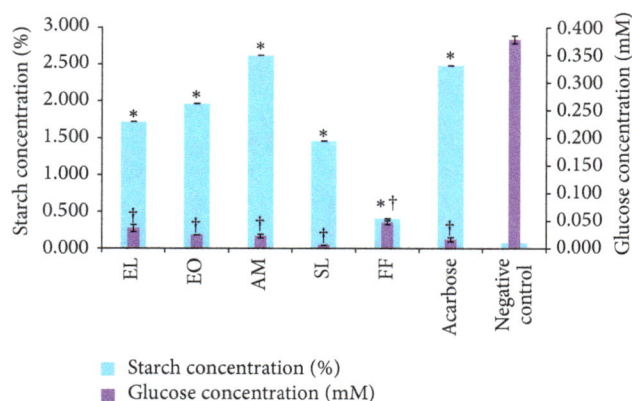

FIGURE 5: Percentage starch of reaction mixture and glucose concentration of dialysate in the presence of methanolic extracts. *Values [starch (%) concentration] significantly ($P < 0.05$) higher than negative control. †Values [glucose (mM) concentration] significantly ($P < 0.05$) lower than negative control.

extracts to modulate glucose liberation from starch and its absorption [10] has proved to be an attractive therapeutic modality in the management of DM. Polyphenolic compounds found in extracts have also been reported to interact with proteins and hence inhibit enzymatic activity [10, 22].

Results from this study tend to show that extracts of selected medicinal plants showed variable inhibitory effect on α-amylase and α-glucosidase *in vitro*. It was observed that three methanolic extracts (EL, EO, and AM) possessed dose-dependent α-amylase inhibitory activity. From data amassed, it was obvious that methanolic fractions carried higher concentration of inhibitory phytochemicals as previously reported [9, 23]. Furthermore, several scientific reports highlight the inhibitory action of plant phytochemicals on α-amylase [23, 24]. Additionally, the kinetic model of these extracts on α-amylase was studied and it was found that in the presence of methanolic extracts of EO and AM, a decrease in both K_m (the affinity of the enzymes for the substrate) and V_{max} (the velocity of reaction) were observed. This tends to suggest an uncompetitive mode of inhibition. Uncompetitive inhibitors bind to enzyme-substrate complex forming an enzyme-substrate-inhibitor complex [25, 26]. This complex reduces affinity for the enzyme active site for the substrate decreasing the affinity and delays rate of reaction [14, 27]. It was also noted that active extracts uncompetitively inhibited α-glucosidase. Furthermore, α-glucosidase inhibitory assay tends to show that extracts of medicinal plants were potent inhibitors of α-glucosidase as compared to acarbose. This finding was consistent with Shai et al. [28] who reported the little inhibitory action of acarbose on α-glucosidase. In contrast, methanolic extract of EL was found to follow mixed type of inhibition. Mixed inhibitor bind to free and to substrate bound enzyme and interfere with binding and catalysis of substrate [25, 26], increasing affinity and decreasing reaction rate [27]. Retarding glucose production and/or absorption might be important strategies in the management of diabetes.

We also investigated the effect of selected medicinal plants on glucose entrapment *in vitro*. A number of studies have unravelled the value of plants complex polysaccharides such as guar gum, oats, and psyllium husk in lowering blood glucose level [28]. The retardation in glucose diffusion *in vivo* might be attributed to the physical obstacles, insoluble fibre particles, which entrap glucose molecules within the fibre network preventing postprandial glucose rise [17, 29]. They form a viscous matrix which delay gastric emptying and slow glucose uptake [17, 30]. The viscous gel also impedes the access of glucose to the small intestines' epithelium, blunting postprandial glucose peaks. GDRI, a useful *in vitro* index to predict the effect of fibres present in the extracts on the delay in glucose absorption, was calculated in this study [24, 31]. SL was found to have the highest GDRI value. Similarly, Wood et al. [32] reported that plants showing between 6 and 48% inhibitory action on glucose diffusion across a semipermeable membrane possessed moderate inhibitory activity. Furthermore, widely studied sources of soluble fibres such as wheat bran, oats, and psyllium husk were found to inhibit between 10 and 23% glucose diffusion after 180 min *in vitro* [31]. However, in the present study we observed that SL was a poor α-amylase inhibitor. It could be argued that the antidiabetic action of SL might be due to this glucose movement retardation properties rather than α-amylase inhibition. Further studies demonstrated that glucose movement retardation properties were dose dependent. Published literature highlight the effect of soluble fibre's molecular weight and concentration along with viscosity on modulating glucose dialysis [11, 33]. Another possible mechanism is the sequestration of enzymatic activity on carbohydrates. As reported from previous study amylolysis assay showed that the retardation of glucose diffusion is also due to the inhibition of α-amylase, thus limiting the release of glucose from starch [31]. The inhibition of α-amylase might be due to the concerted action of encapsulation of the enzyme and/or starch in the fiber matrix and/or the action of inhibitors. Eventually, this leads to reduced glucose absorption and blunting of postprandial glucose rise [27].

5. Conclusion

The present study demonstrated the ability of native antidiabetic medicinal plants of Mauritius to inhibit key carbohydrate hydrolysing enzymes and unravelled their mode of inhibition. Furthermore, to date no such study has been conducted to evaluate the glucose entrapment properties and amylolysis kinetic effects of these extracts. Data gathered suggest that methanolic fractions of EO, EL, and AM were active enzyme inhibitors. Pertaining to the role of these enzymes in the control of post-prandial increase of blood glucose level, their inhibition could be useful in the development of new drug strategies. Further scientific validation is essential to understand the therapeutic potential of these medicinal plants for improving glycaemic control in diabetic subjects and confirm their antidiabetic mode of action.

Conflict of Interests

The authors declare that there is no conflict of interests.

Acknowledgments

The authors acknowledge the University of Mauritius and the Tertiary Education Commission for financial support.

References

[1] V. K. Prabhakar, A. Jaidka, and R. Singh, "*In vitro* study on α-amylase inhibitory activity and phytochemical screening of few Indian medicinal plant having anti-diabetic properties," *International Journal of Scientific and Research Publications*, vol. 3, no. 8, pp. 1–6, 2013.

[2] Ministry of Health and Quality of life (MOH), "The trends in diabetes and cardiovascular disease risk in Mauritius," The Mauritius Non Communicable Disease Survey 2009, 2009, http://health.gov.mu/English/Documents/ncd-2009.pdf.

[3] International Diabetes Federation, *IDF Diabetes Atlas*, 5th edition, 2013, http://www.idf.org/diabetesatlas/5e/the-global-burden.

[4] P. Pasupathi, V. Chandrasekar, and U. S. Kumar, "Evaluation of oxidative stress, enzymatic and non-enzymatic antioxidants and metabolic thyroid hormone status in patients with diabetes mellitus," *Diabetes and Metabolic Syndrome: Clinical Research & Reviews*, vol. 3, no. 3, pp. 160–165, 2009.

[5] B. Mayur, S. Sandesh, S. Shruti, and S. Sung-Yum, "Antioxidant and α-glucosidase inhibitory properties of *Carpesium abrotanoides* L.," *Journal of Medicinal Plants Research*, vol. 4, pp. 1547–1553, 2010.

[6] S. Pennathur and J. W. Heinecke, "Mechanisms of oxidative stress in diabetes: implications for the pathogenesis of vascular disease and antioxidant therapy," *Frontiers in Bioscience*, vol. 9, pp. 565–574, 2004.

[7] A. Mootoosamy and M. F. Mahomoodally, "Ethnomedicinal application of native remedies used against diabetes and related complications in Mauritius," *Journal of Ethnopharmacology*, vol. 10, pp. 413–444, 2014.

[8] S. Gurudeeban, K. Satyavani, and T. Ramanathan, "Alpha glucosidase inhibitory effect and enzyme kinetics of coastal medicinal plants," *Bangladesh Journal of Pharmacology*, vol. 7, pp. 186–191, 2012.

[9] M. F. Mahomoodally, A. H. Subratty, A. Gurib-Fakim, M. I. Choudary, and S. N. Khan, "Traditional medicinal herbs and food plants have the potential to inhibit key carbohydrates hydrolyzing enzymes *in vitro* and reduce postprandial blood glucose peaks *in vivo*," *The Scientific World Journal*, vol. 2012, Article ID 285284, 9 pages, 2012.

[10] E. Thilagam, B. Parimaladevi, C. Kumarappan, and S. C. Mandal, "α-glucosidase and α-amylase inhibitory activity of *Senna surattensis*," *Journal of Acupuncture and Meridian Studies*, vol. 6, pp. 24–30, 2013.

[11] C. A. Edwards, N. A. Blackburn, and L. Craigen, "Viscosity of food gums determined *in vitro* related to their hypoglycemic actions," *American Journal of Clinical Nutrition*, vol. 46, no. 1, pp. 72–77, 1987.

[12] A. Gurib-Fakim, J. Gueho, and M. D. Sewraj, *Plantes Medicinales de Maurice*, vol. 1, Editions de L'ocean Indien, Stanley, Rose Hill, Mauritius, 1996.

[13] M. I. Kotowaroo, M. F. Mahomoodally, A. Gurib-Fakim, and A. H. Subratty, "Screening of traditional antidiabetic medicinal plants of Mauritius for possible α-amylase inhibitory effects *in vitro*," *Phytotherapy Research*, vol. 20, no. 3, pp. 228–231, 2006.

[14] J. A. Bachhawat, M. S. Shihabudeen, and K. Thirumurugan, "Screening of Fifteen Indian ayurvedic plants for alpha-glucosidase inhibitory activity and enzyme kinetics," *International Journal of Pharmacy and Pharmaceutical Sciences*, vol. 3, no. 4, pp. 267–274, 2011.

[15] S. Shaukat, A. Waqar, and M. A. Waqar, "Investigating the influence of folk anti-diabetic plants on glucose diffusion," *Journal of the Chemical Society of Pakistan*, vol. 31, no. 3, pp. 480–484, 2009.

[16] A. M. Gallagher, P. R. Flatt, G. Duffy, and Y. H. A. Abdel-Wahab, "The effects of traditional antidiabetic plants on *in vitro* glucose diffusion," *Nutrition Research*, vol. 23, no. 3, pp. 413–424, 2003.

[17] F. Ahmed, S. Sairam, and A. Urooj, "*In vitro* hypoglycemic effects of selected dietary fiber sources," *Journal of Food Science and Technology*, vol. 48, no. 3, pp. 285–289, 2011.

[18] S. S. Gropper and J. L. Smith, *Advanced Nutrition and Human Metabolism*, Cengage Learning, Hampshire, UK, 2012.

[19] S. R. Rolfes, K. Pinna, and E. Whitney, *Understanding Normal and Clinical Nutrition*, Cengage Learning Inc., Belmont, Calif, USA, 2008.

[20] R. Rhabasa-Lhoret and J. L. Chiasson, "Alpha-glucosidase inhibition," in *International Textbook of Diabetes Mellitus*, R. A. Defronzo, E. Ferrannini, H. Keen, and P. Zimmet, Eds., pp. 901–914, John Wiley & Sons, London, UK, 2004.

[21] G. Oboh, A. O. Ademosun, O. V. Odubanjo, and I. A. Akinbola, "Antioxidative properties and inhibition of key enzymes relevant to type-2 diabetes and hypertension by essential oils from black pepper," *Advances in Pharmacological Sciences*, pp. 1–6, 2013.

[22] R. Sharma, *Enzyme Inhibition and Bio Applications*, In Tech, Beijing, China, 2012.

[23] K. Sama, K. Murugesan, and R. Sivaraj, "*In vitro* alpha amylase and alpha glucosidase inhibition activity of crude ethanol extract of *Cissus arnottiana*," *Asian Journal of Plant Science and Research*, vol. 2, no. 4, pp. 550–553, 2012.

[24] R. McEwan, R. P. Madivha, T. Djarova, O. A. Oyedeji, and A. R. Opoku, "Alpha-amylase inhibitor of amadumbe (*Colocasia esculenta*): isolation, purification and selectivity toward α-amylases from various sources," *African Journal of Biochemistry Research*, vol. 4, no. 9, pp. 220–224, 2010.

[25] A. Cornish-Bowden, *Fundamentals of Enzyme Kinetics*, John Wiley & Sons, London, UK, 2013.

[26] H. Bisswanger, *Enzyme Kinetics*, John Wiley & Sons, 2008.

[27] A. Cornish-Bowden, "A simple graphical method for determining the inhibition constants of mixed, uncompetitive and non competitive inhibitors," *Biochemical Journal*, vol. 137, no. 1, pp. 143–144, 1974.

[28] L. J. Shai, P. Masoko, M. P. Mokgotho et al., "Yeast alpha glucosidase inhibitory and antioxidant activities of six medicinal plants collected in Phalaborwa, South Africa," *South African Journal of Botany*, vol. 76, no. 3, pp. 465–470, 2010.

[29] S. K. Basha and V. S. Kumari, "*In vitro* antidiabetic activity of psidium guajava leaves extracts," *Asian Pacific Journal of Tropical Diseases*, pp. 98–100, 2012.

[30] C. Palanuvej, S. Hokputsa, T. Tunsaringkarn, and N. Ruangrungsi, "*In vitro* glucose entrapment and alpha-glucosidase inhibition of mucilaginous substances from selected Thai medicinal plants," *Scientia Pharmaceutica*, vol. 77, no. 4, pp. 837–849, 2009.

[31] F. Ahmed, N. S. Siddaraju, and A. Urooj, "*In vitro* hypoglycemic effects of *Gymnema sylvestre*, *Tinospora cordifolia*, *Eugenia jambolana* and *Aegle marmelos*," *Journal of Natural Pharmaceuticals*, vol. 2, no. 2, pp. 52–55, 2011.

[32] P. J. Wood, M. U. Beer, and G. Butler, "Evaluation of role of concentration and molecular weight of oat β-glucan in determining effect of viscosity on plasma glucose and insulin following an oral glucose load," *British Journal of Nutrition*, vol. 84, no. 1, pp. 19–23, 2000.

[33] A. Srichamroen and V. Chavasit, "*In vitro* retardation of glucose diffusion with gum extracted from malva nut seeds produced in Thailand," *Food Chemistry*, vol. 127, no. 2, pp. 455–460, 2011.

11

Susceptibility of *Porphyromonas gingivalis* and *Streptococcus mutans* to Antibacterial Effect from *Mammea americana*

Alejandra Herrera Herrera,[1] **Luis Franco Ospina,**[2] **Luis Fang,**[1] and **Antonio Díaz Caballero**[1]

[1] *Grupo de Investigaciones GITOUC, Facultad de Odontología, Universidad de Cartagena, Campus de la Salud, Cartagena, Colombia*
[2] *Grupo de Evaluación Biológica de Sustancias Promisorias, Facultad de Ciencias Farmacéuticas, Universidad de Cartagena, Campus de la Salud, Cartagena, Colombia*

Correspondence should be addressed to Alejandra Herrera Herrera; alejandrah03@gmail.com

Academic Editor: Abdelwahab Omri

The development of periodontal disease and dental caries is influenced by several factors, such as microorganisms of bacterial biofilm or commensal bacteria in the mouth. These microorganisms trigger inflammatory and immune responses in the host. Currently, medicinal plants are treatment options for these oral diseases. *Mammea americana* extracts have reported antimicrobial effects against several microorganisms. Nevertheless, this effect is unknown against oral bacteria. Therefore, the aim of this study was to evaluate the antibacterial effect of *M. americana* extract against *Porphyromonas gingivalis* and *Streptococcus mutans*. For this, an experimental study was conducted Ethanolic extract was obtained from seeds of *M. americana* (one oil phase and one ethanolic phase). The strains of *Porphyromonas gingivalis* ATCC 33277 and *Streptococcus mutans* ATCC 25175 were exposed to this extract to evaluate its antibacterial effect. Antibacterial activity was observed with the two phases of *M. americana* extract on *P. gingivalis* and *S. mutans* with lower MICs (minimum inhibitory concentration). Also, bactericidal and bacteriostatic activity was detected against *S. mutans*, depending on the concentration of the extract, while on *M. americana* extract presented only bacteriostatic activity against *P. gingivalis*. These findings provide important and promising information allowing for further exploration in the future.

1. Introduction

Oral diseases are a worldwide public health problem. Many epidemiological studies report that diseases such as dental caries and periodontal disease are the most prevalent oral disorders of humanity [1–3]. These conditions are caused by poor oral hygiene and biofilm forming bacteria residing in the mouth, able to communicate with each other through mechanisms of Quorum sensing [4]. Biofilms are complex structures, where different bacterial species are arranged to form a superorganism with advanced properties unlike planktonic bacteria. Dental or bacterial plaque is a type of biofilm on the tooth surface that plays an important role in the development of these oral conditions [5, 6]. *Streptococcus mutans* colonize the tooth surface and initiate biofilm formation by their ability to synthesize extracellular polysaccharides from sucrose [7]. The further accumulation of biofilm around the supra- and subgingival region leads to a shift in its microbial composition from *Streptococcus* spp.,

Actinomyces spp., and *Porphyromonas gingivalis* [8, 9]. Therefore, these microorganisms are considered to be the major etiological agents involved in dental caries and periodontal disease [3].

Clinical practice seeks to prevent the occurrences of these oral conditions or apply minimally invasive treatments, avoiding in most cases surgical interventions [10, 11]. Therefore, antimicrobial or antibacterial agents against these oral pathogens could play an important role in the prevention and treatment of dental caries and periodontal disease, principally those that can inhibit or reduce the growth of these microorganisms, inhibit biofilm formation, influence the adhesion of bacteria to surfaces, and reduce the clinic symptoms [12, 13]. Many of the currently available oral antimicrobials can change oral microbiota and have adverse side effects such as diarrhea, vomiting, and teeth staining. Therefore, it is necessary to find safe and effective therapeutic agents for everyone. Traditional herbal medicines are considered as a good source of therapeutic alternatives, depending on their properties [14, 15]. Antimicrobial agents isolated from plants represent a huge and poorly exploited source of drugs with great therapeutic potential. Some of these compounds are effective in the treatment of infectious diseases, while having the advantage of causing few side effects which are often associated with synthetic antimicrobials [16].

Mammea americana is an evergreen tree of the family Calophyllaceae, native of the Antilles, and introduced into central and northern South America, although it is currently cultivated in other tropical and humid areas. It is commonly known as mammee, mammee apple, mamey, mamey apple, Santo Domingo apricot, South American apricot, mamey de cartagena de indias, or mamey de santo domingo. Its fleshy fruit is edible and frequently consumed; they have a yellow-reddish and aromatic pulp and are round or slightly irregular, with a thick brown rind. Their diameter ranges from 10 to 20 cm. Small fruit contain a single seed, while larger ones might have up to four. The seeds are brown, rough, oval, and around 6 cm long [17].

Oral lore has referred the use of *M. americana* as a natural therapeutic alternative. However, the medicinal properties of the leaves, fruits, and seeds have not been widely elucidated. Several studies have reported some medicinal properties, such as anticonvulsant, antipyretic, antimalarial, anthelmintic, and digestive tonic, as well as a remedy for parasitic skin diseases [18]. It also provides inhibitory activity against *Mycobacterium tuberculosis* [19] and molluscicidal properties against *Biomphalaria glabrata* [20]. Furthermore, antitumor activity has been reported, as well as some coumarin, phloroglucinol derivatives [21, 22], xanthones, and benzophenones [23]. Currently, there are few studies reporting the *M. americana* antimicrobial activity, specifically for oral bacteria. Therefore, the aim of this study was to identify the mamey's antibacterial activity against pathogenic bacteria involved in dental caries and periodontal disease.

2. Materials and Methods

2.1. Plant Material. Mammea americana fruit was collected from rural areas in the Department of Bolivar on the Caribbean coast of Colombia. Geographical and environmental conditions in this tropical zone promote the wild growth of *M. americana*. Voucher specimens were prepared and identified at the Universidad de Antioquia Herbarium (*HUA 183928*).

2.2. Extract Preparation. From the ripe fruit of *M. americana*, we extracted the seeds. These were air dried at 25°C for 3 weeks and ground in a seed grinder into a fine powder. The powdered materials (1313 g) were soaked in ethanol (50% w/v) at room temperature for 72 h in dark conditions and then were filtered. The total extract was dried, and solvent was evaporated in a rotary evaporator (*Laborota 4001, Heidolph*) under reduced pressure at 50°C. We obtained two phases from the total extract: one hydroalcoholic phase called "ethanolic phase" and one "oily phase," 90 g and 109 g, respectively. Both phases were further dried at room

temperature; before evaluating the antibacterial activity, each phase was subjected to a solubility test in 2% ethanol, 2% methanol, 1% DMSO (dimethyl sulfoxide), and combinations from these solvents. We observed that 1% DMSO was the best solvent for both phases. In addition, 1% DMSO did not exert any damage on the bacterial strains.

2.3. Preliminary Phytochemical Screening. Several chemical tests were carried out on two phases of the *M. americana* extract using procedures to identify the following groups of metabolites: flavonoids and xanthone (Shinoda test and Action front of álcalis), leucoanthocyanidins (Rosenheim test, NaOH 10% test, and hydrochloric acid test), phenolic compounds ($FeCl_3$ test), quinones (RX with sulfuric acid), cardiotonic glycoside (Kedde test), steroid nucleus (Salkowski test), alkaloids (Dragendorff test, Mayer test, Wagner test, and $FeCl_3$ test), tannins ($FeCl_3$ test), saponins (Foam test), and coumarins (coumarins volatile test, ammonium hydroxide Rx) [24].

2.4. Microorganisms and Growth Conditions. This study only included *Porphyromonas gingivalis* (ATCC 33277) and *Streptococcus mutans* (ATCC 25175), both acquired from the American Type Culture Collection. *P. gingivalis* was grown in Brucella agar (BD, *Becton Dickinson*), supplemented with vitamin kl (1 mg/mL) - hemin (5 μg/mL) solution (BD, *Becton Dickinson*) and 5% human anticoagulated whole blood, and incubated at 37°C under anaerobic conditions in an anaerobic jar with AnaeroGen (90% N_2, 5% CO_2, and 5% H_2) (Oxoid Ltd.) for 5 days, while *S. mutans* was cultured in TYS20B agar. This culture medium contains 30 g trypticase soy (BD, *Becton Dickinson*), 10 g yeast extract (Oxoid Ltd.), 20% w/v sucrose (Merck), 0.2 U/mL bacitracin (Sigma-Aldrich), 11 g granulated agar, and distilled water and incubated at 37°C under anaerobiosis by AnaeroGen (Oxoid Ltd.) for 48 h.

From a few microbial colonies of *P. gingivalis* and *S. mutans* bacterial cultures, inocula and bacterial growth curves were performed for each strain. Isolated colonies were suspended in their corresponding culture media and turbidity of the inoculum was adjusted to reach 0.5 on the McFarland scale (optical density between 0.08 and 0.10) using a microplate reader (*Multiscan EX, Thermo Scientific*) at 620 nm, which is equivalent to $1–2 \times 10^8$ CFU/mL. *S. mutans* reached its stationary phase for approximately 13 h, whereas *P. gingivalis* required 22 h of incubation. These preliminary tests allowed establishing ideal experimental conditions.

2.5. Antibacterial Activity Assay. Antibacterial activity was determined by the microdilution technique with 96-well microplates. Using this technique, minimum inhibitory concentration (MIC) and minimum bactericidal concentration (MBC) values were obtained for the ethanolic phase and oily phase against the microorganisms under study. All assays were performed in triplicate.

2.5.1. Determination of the Minimum Inhibitory Concentration (MIC). The ethanolic and oily phases were serially diluted, ranging from 500 μg/mL to 0.06 μg/mL in the 96-well plate

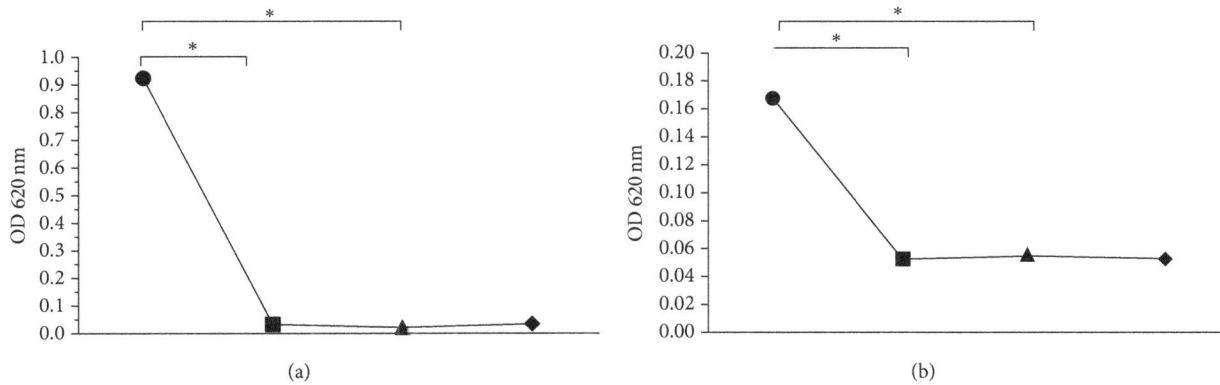

FIGURE 1: Bacterial sensitivity assays of *Mammea americana* extract. (a) Sensitivity of *Porphyromonas gingivalis* (ATCC 33277) to oily and ethanolic phases; exposure of *P. gingivalis* to mamey extract inhibited bacterial growth by approximately 96%. (b) Sensitivity of *Streptococcus mutans* (ATCC 25175) to mamey extract; the two phases inhibited bacterial growth by approximately 31.5%. Each symbol represents the mean for the group ($n = 6$ per group); inoculum: (●), oily phase (500 μg/mL): (■), ethanolic phase (500 μg/mL): (▲), control (gentamicin (16 μg/mL)): (◆), and P value < 0.05: (∗); Kruskal-Wallis test and Dunnett's posttest.

with bacterial suspension (5×10^5 CFU/mL); gentamicin (16 μg/mL) was used as negative control for bacterial growth, and a broth solution was used as control sterility. Elsewhere, microbial growth was indicated as changes in optical density from bacterial inoculum (positive control). The 96-well plates were incubated at 37°C under anaerobic conditions, for 13 h (*S. mutans*) and 22 h (*P. gingivalis*). The MIC was defined as the lowest concentration that inhibited microbial growth.

2.5.2. Determination of the Minimum Bactericidal Concentration (MBC).
The MBC was determined by adding 10 μL of the suspensions from the wells, which did not show any growth during MIC assays in petri dishes with corresponding agar to each bacterium. These petri dishes were incubated at 37°C under anaerobic conditions for 5 days (*P. gingivalis*) and for 48 h (*S. mutans*). After this incubation period, bacterial colonies were observed. The ethanolic and oily phases were designated as bacteriostatic (those in which bacterial colonies grew in petri dishes) or bactericide (those in which bacterial colonies did not grow in petri dishes).

2.6. Statistical Analysis.
The data were analyzed using Graph-Pad Prism v5 and compared by nonparametric Kruskal-Wallis and multiple-comparison tests as the Dunnett's test; this was applied for comparison between each treatment concentration and the respective control. The chosen level of significance for all statistical tests was $P < 0.05$.

3. Results

3.1. Antibacterial Activity.
The two phases of *M. americana* extract proved antibacterial activity against *S. mutans* and *P. gingivalis* strains. These bacteria were significantly sensitive to the extract from 500 μg/mL, from a mean optical density (OD) of 0.93 for the inoculums of *P. gigivalis* to 0.033 ($P = 0.005$) and 0.022 ($P = 0.005$) for wells with bacteria exposed to the oily and ethanolic phases, respectively. These results

are similar and do not differ from those of gentamicin OD: 0.034, ($P = 0.32$); therefore, mamey extract inhibits bacterial growth by 96% (Figure 1(a)). *S. mutans* was susceptible to mamey and inhibits bacterial growth by approximately 31.5%, from a mean OD of 0.170 for the inoculums of *S. mutans* to 0.053 ($P = 0.013$) for oily phase and 0.055 ($P = 0.013$) for ethanolic phase (Figure 1(b)).

This antibacterial activity was interpreted as minimum inhibitory concentration (MIC) and minimum bactericidal concentration (MBC). The oily and ethanolic phases showed very promising data on Gram-positive bacteria, which was reflected by their MICs against *S. mutans* (MIC: 15.62 μg/mL and 62.5 μg/mL, resp.), comparing broth solution at all tested concentrations (Figures 2(a) and 2(b)). While the two phases did not show prominent results against *P. gingivalis*, their MICs showed antibacterial activity; the MIC of the oily phase was 250 μg/mL and 500 μg/mL for the ethanolic phase (Figures 3(a) and 3(b)).

MBC was determined from 500 μg/mL of each phase. The oily phase showed bactericidal property against *S. mutans* from 500 μg/mL to 125 μg/mL, and concentrations <125 μg/mL behaved as bacteriostatic. While the ethanolic phase showed bactericidal activity from 500 μg/mL to 250 μg/mL, lower concentrations were bacteriostatic. *M. americana* extract did not show bactericidal activity against *P. gingivalis*. Both oily and ethanolic phases only showed bacteriostatic behavior even at 500 μg/mL (Table 1).

3.2. Phytochemical Screening.
The phytochemical screening of the oily and ethanolic phases showed the presence of phenolic compounds, tannins, and coumarins (Table 2). These metabolites possibly contribute to the antibacterial activity of *M. americana* extract.

4. Discussion

Oral bacteria have been amply tested for antimicrobial susceptibility to various plant extracts and natural substances.

(a)

(b)

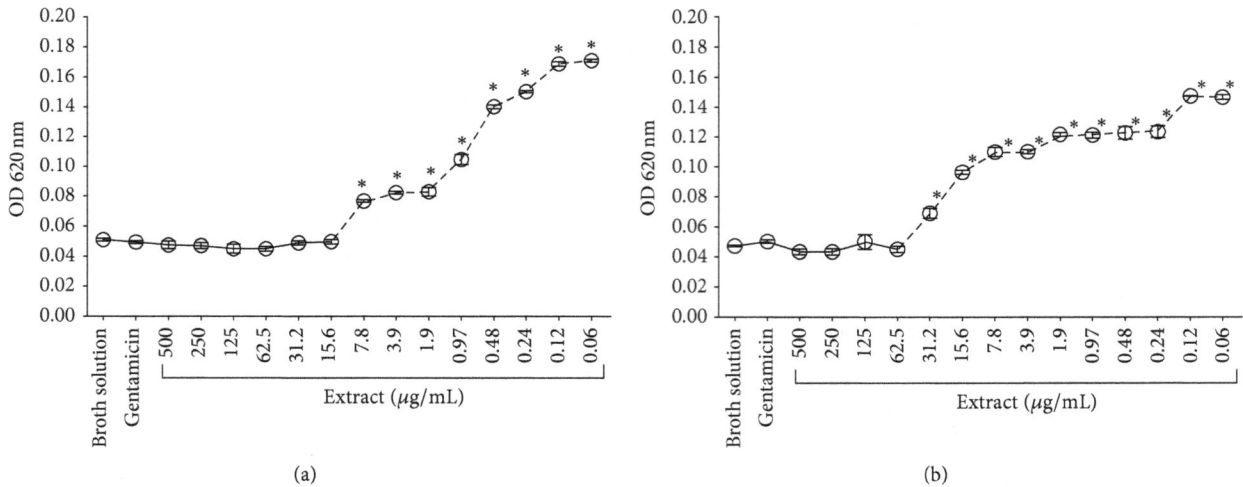

FIGURE 2: MIC of the oily and ethanolic phases from *Mammea americana* extract against *Streptococcus mutans*. (a) The minimum concentration of the oily phase which inhibited bacterial growth was 15.6 μg/mL, (b) whereas the MIC of ethanolic phase was 62.5 μg/mL. Each symbol represents the mean $\pm$ SEM for each concentration tested ($n = 4$ per (μg/mL)). P value < 0.05: ($*$); Kruskal-Wallis test and Dunnett's posttest.

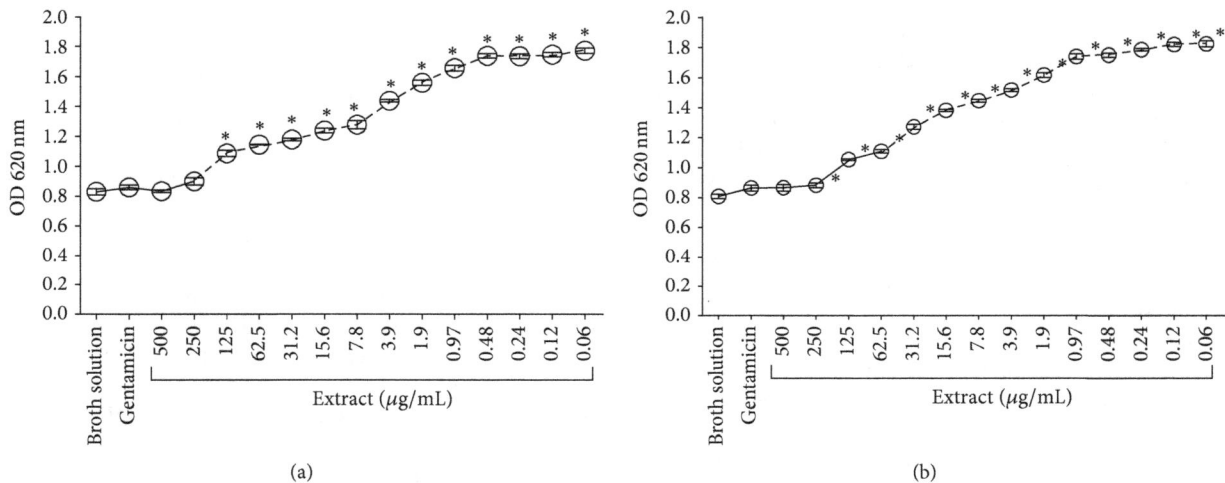

(a)

(b)

FIGURE 3: MIC of the oily and ethanolic phases from *Mammea americana* extract against *Porphyromonas gingivalis*. (a) The MIC of the oily phase was 250 μg/mL, (b) while the MIC of the ethanolic phase was 500 μg/mL. Each symbol represents the mean $\pm$ SEM for each concentration tested ($n = 4$ per (μg/mL)). P value < 0.05: ($*$); Kruskal-Wallis test and Dunnett's post-test.

According to our knowledge, this is the first report on the antibacterial effect of *M. americana* extract against bacteria representative of oral diseases such as dental caries and periodontal disease such as *S. mutans* and *P. gingivalis* [8, 9].

M. americana, commonly known as "mamey," is a tree widely used for its medicinal properties and its fruit is sought in communities of the Antilles and central and northern South America. Morris and Pagán. were the first to report some properties of mamey, including antimicrobial and toxic properties of fruit seeds of this tree [25]; other parts of mamey, such as leaves, stems, and fruit, have also shown medicinal properties. Frame et al. evaluated the antituberculous effect against *Mycobacterium smegmatis* from 50 extracts of plants belonging to tropical flora in Puerto Rico. The *Mammea americana* extract showed the

best antituberculous effect with low concentration (50 μg) unlike 49 remaining extracts whose concentrations are close at 500 μg, this showed promising properties for *M. americana* [19]. We also observe similar promising results of fruit seeds of mamey against oral bacteria.

For a better knowledge, there are no papers reporting antimicrobial activity of *Mammea americana* extract tested on bacteria such as *Streptococcus mutans* and *Porphyromonas gingivalis*. However, other plant extracts were tested on the same bacteria; for instance, Fani and Kohanteb, in 2012 [26], assessed Aloe Vera against *Streptococcus mutans* and they founded a MIC with 25 ppm against that bacterium. Iauk et al., in 2003 [27], reported that extract of *Hamamelis virginiana* had a MIC of 512 ppm against *Porphyromonas gingivalis*. Regarding the MBC Moreno et al. in 2007 [28] reported that

TABLE 1: Minimum bactericidal concentration MBC from the oily and ethanolic phases against *Streptococcus mutans* and *Porphyromonas gingivalis* strains.

Bacterial strain	Phase	Results
Streptococcus mutans	Oily	Bactericidal activity from 500–125 μg/mL; lower concentrations were bacteriostatic.
	Ethanolic	Bactericidal activity from 500–250 μg/mL; lower concentrations were bacteriostatic.
Porphyromonas gingivalis	Oily	It showed bacteriostatic activity at all concentrations.
	Ethanolic	It showed bacteriostatic activity at all concentrations.

TABLE 2: Phytochemical screening of the oily and ethanolic phases.

Chemical components	Oily phase	Ethanolic phase
Flavonoides (xanthone and flavone)	–	+
Leucoanthocyanidins	–	–
Phenolic compounds	+++	+++
Quinones	–	–
Cardiac glycosides	–	–
Steroid nucleus	–	+
Alkaloids	–	–
Coumarins	+++	+++
Tannins	++	+++
Saponins	–	–

Absent: –; present: + (mild), ++ (moderate), and +++ (severe).

460 ppm of *propolis* was a MBC against *Streptococcus mutans*. Bakri and Douglas in 2005 [29] observed a MBC of *Allium sativum* (garlic) against *Porphyromonas gingivalis* 7.9 mg/mL. Comparing these results with the activity of the extract of *Mammea americana* proposed in this paper, it can be noted that present results of *Mammea americana* have a higher potential or more promising behavior such as medicament for the observed outcome of inhibitory activity against these oral bacteria.

Due to the fatty nature of the mamey fruit seeds, a total extract composed of two phases was obtained, which evaluated their antibacterial activity. Few studies have reported this property; Yasunaka et al. evaluate the antibacterial activity on *Escherichia coli* and *Staphylococcus aureus* of 32 crude extracts from 22 Mexican medicinal plants. Some extracts evaluated showed antibacterial activity in one of two bacterial strains, but only the leaves extract of *M. americana* inhibited bacterial growth of the two strains tested [30]. We also obtained similar results, considering that this property was assessed on *S. mutans* and *P. gingivalis*.

It remains to elucidate the active compounds and cytotoxic effect of *M. americana* seeds extract. However, some metabolites present in mamey have reported antimicrobial activity for other medicinal plants. The major metabolite of mamey reported in other studies is coumarin [31], including *Mammea africana*, another species of the Guttiferae family; coumarins of this species exhibit significant antimicrobial activity against *S. aureus* [32]. Other metabolites found in mamey are the phenolic compounds, the antimicrobial capacity of these, acting by the alteration of the permeability of the cell membrane that could result in the uncoupling of oxidative phosphorylation, inhibition of active transport, and

loss of pool metabolites due to cytoplasmic membrane from bacteria [33, 34]. These could be two possible explanations for the antibacterial activity of the *M. americana* seeds extract reported in our study.

In conclusion, we may point out that the *Mammea americana* extract showed antibacterial activity against *Porphyromonas gingivalis* ATCC 33277 and *Streptococcus mutans* ATCC 25175, and the MIC-MBC obtained in this work allows us to hypothesize that *M. americana* presents promising effects against oral bacteria which need to be further studied.

Ethical Approval

This study was approved by the Institutional Ethics Committee of the Universidad de Cartagena, according to resolution no. 62 of 28-02-2013.

Conflict of Interests

The authors declare that there is not any direct or indirect conflict of financial, academic, or personal interests, which may call into question the validity of this study.

Acknowledgments

The authors thank COLCIENCIAS for its Young-Researcher program, which granted scholarships to Alejandra Herrera Herrera, and Luis Fang. Also, the authors thank Professor Joseph Dunn and the Writing Center of the Faculty of Human Sciences of the Universidad de Cartagena for English revision of the paper. This research was financially supported by the Universidad de Cartagena, according to resolution no. 4681 of 2011.

References

[1] G. I. Lafaurie, A. Contreras, A. Barón et al., "Demographic, clinical, and microbial aspects of chronic and aggressive periodontitis in Colombia: a multicenter study," *Journal of Periodontology*, vol. 78, no. 4, pp. 629–639, 2007.

[2] K. M. Arrieta Vergara, A. Díaz Caballero, and F. González Martínez, "Prevalencia de caries y enfermedad periodontal en estudiantes de odontología," *Revista Cubana de Estomatología*, vol. 48, pp. 6–13, 2011.

[3] A. T. Merchant, "Periodontitis and dental caries occur together," *The Journal of Evidence-Based Dental Practice*, vol. 12, pp. 18–19, 2012.

[4] A. Díaz Caballero, R. Vivas Reyes, L. Puerta et al., "Biopelículas como expresión del mecanismo de quorum sensing: una

revisión," *Avances en Periodoncia e Implantología Oral*, vol. 23, pp. 195–201, 2011.

[5] A. D. Caballero, R. V. Reyes, L. P. Llerena et al., "Periodontitis, *Porphyromonas gingivalis* and its relation to quorum sensing expression," *Revista Cubana de Estomatologia*, vol. 47, no. 4, pp. 404–416, 2010.

[6] A. J. Díaz Caballero, R. Vivas Reyes, L. Puerta et al., "Papel de la Biopelícula dental en la Enfermedad Periodontal," *Acta Odontológica Venezolana*, vol. 50, p. 22, 2012.

[7] X. Li, M. A. Hoogenkamp, J. Ling, W. Crielaard, and D. M. Deng, "Diversity of *Streptococcus mutans* strains in bacterial interspecies interactions," *Journal of Basic Microbiology*, vol. 54, no. 2, pp. 97–103, 2014.

[8] A. Mannaa, A. Carlen, G. Campus, and P. Lingstrom, "Supragingival plaque microbial analysis in reflection to caries experience," *BMC Oral Health*, vol. 13, article 5, 2013.

[9] M. Kishi, Y. Hasegawa, K. Nagano, H. Nakamura, Y. Murakami, and F. Yoshimura, "Identification and characterization of novel glycoproteins involved in growth and biofilm formation by *Porphyromonas gingivalis*," *Molecular Oral Microbiology*, vol. 27, pp. 458–470, 2012.

[10] J. E. Frencken, M. C. Peters, D. J. Manton, S. C. Leal, V. V. Gordan, and E. Eden, "Minimal intervention dentistry for managing dental caries—a review: report of a FDI task group," *International Dental Journal*, vol. 62, pp. 223–243, 2012.

[11] N. Sugano, "Biological plaque control: novel therapeutic approach to periodontal disease," *Journal of Oral Science*, vol. 54, pp. 1–5, 2012.

[12] D. A. Apatzidou, "Modern approaches to non-surgical biofilm management," *Frontiers of oral biology*, vol. 15, pp. 99–116, 2012.

[13] A. Leszczyńska, P. Buczko, W. Buczko, and M. Pietruska, "Periodontal pharmacotherapy-an updated review," *Advances in Medical Sciences*, vol. 56, no. 2, pp. 123–131, 2011.

[14] E. A. Palombo, "Traditional medicinal plant extracts and natural products with activity against oral bacteria: potential application in the prevention and treatment of oral diseases," *Evidence-based Complementary and Alternative Medicine*, vol. 2011, Article ID 680354, 15 pages, 2011.

[15] Y. Ramakrishna, H. Goda, M. S. Baliga, and A. K. Munshi, "Decreasing cariogenic bacteria with a natural, alternative prevention therapy utilizing phytochemistry (plant extracts)," *Journal of Clinical Pediatric Dentistry*, vol. 36, no. 1, pp. 55–63, 2011.

[16] M. Lahlou, "Methods to study the phytochemistry and bioactivity of essential oils," *Phytotherapy Research*, vol. 18, no. 6, pp. 435–448, 2004.

[17] K. S. Mourão and C. M. Beltrati, "Morphology and anatomy of developing fruits and seeds of *Mammea americana* L. (Clusiaceae)," *Revista Brasileira De Biologia*, vol. 60, no. 4, pp. 701–711, 2000.

[18] H. Lorenzi and F. J. de Abreu Matos, *Plantas Medicinais no Brasil: Nativas e Exóticas*, Instituto Plantarum de Estudos da Flora, Sao Paulo, Brazil, 2nd edition, 2002.

[19] A. D. Frame, E. Ríos-Olivares, L. De Jesús, D. Ortiz, J. Pagán, and S. Méndez, "Plants from Puerto Rico with anti-Mycobacterium tuberculosis properties," *Puerto Rico Health Sciences Journal*, vol. 17, no. 3, pp. 243–252, 1998.

[20] P. A. Meléndez and V. A. Capriles, "Molluscicidal activity of plants from Puerto Rico," *Annals of Tropical Medicine and Parasitology*, vol. 96, no. 2, pp. 209–218, 2002.

[21] R. A. Finnegan, K. E. Merkel, and N. Back, "Constituents of *Mammea americana* L. 8. Novel structural variations on the mammein theme and antitumor activity of mammein and related coumarin and phloroglucinol derivatives," *Journal of Pharmaceutical Sciences*, vol. 61, no. 10, pp. 1599–1603, 1972.

[22] R. A. Finnegan and K. E. Merkel, "Constituents of *Mammea americana* L. IX. Oxidation of mammein and mammeisin," *Journal of Pharmaceutical Sciences*, vol. 61, no. 10, pp. 1603–1608, 1972.

[23] R. A. Finnegan, K. E. Merkel, and J. K. Patel, "Constituents of *Mammea americana* L. XII. Biological data for xanthones and benzophenones," *Journal of Pharmaceutical Sciences*, vol. 62, no. 3, pp. 483–485, 1973.

[24] O. A. Aiyegoro and A. I. Okoh, "Preliminary phytochemical screening and In vitro antioxidant activities of the aqueous extract of Helichrysum longifolium DC," *BMC Complementary and Alternative Medicine*, vol. 10, article 21, 2010.

[25] M. P. Morris and C. Pagán, "The isolation of the toxic principles of mamey," *Journal of the American Chemical Society*, vol. 75, no. 6, p. 1489, 1953.

[26] M. Fani and J. Kohanteb, "Inhibitory activity of Aloe vera gel on some clinically isolated cariogenic and periodontopathic bacteria," *Journal of Oral Science*, vol. 54, no. 1, pp. 15–21, 2012.

[27] L. Iauk, A. M. lo Bue, I. Milazzo, A. Rapisarda, and G. Blandino, "Antibacterial activity of medicinal plant extracts against periodontopathic bacteria," *Phytotherapy Research*, vol. 17, no. 6, pp. 599–604, 2003.

[28] H. Z. Moreno, A. P. Martinez, and J. Figueroa, "Efecto antimicrobiano in vitro de propóleos argentinos, colombianos y cubano sobre *Streptococcus mutans* ATCC, 25175," *NOVA*, vol. 5, pp. 70–75, 2007.

[29] I. M. Bakri and C. W. I. Douglas, "Inhibitory effect of garlic extract on oral bacteria," *Archives of Oral Biology*, vol. 50, no. 7, pp. 645–651, 2005.

[30] K. Yasunaka, F. Abe, A. Nagayama et al., "Antibacterial activity of crude extracts from Mexican medicinal plants and purified coumarins and xanthones," *Journal of Ethnopharmacology*, vol. 97, no. 2, pp. 293–299, 2005.

[31] H. Yang, B. Jiang, K. A. Reynertson, M. J. Basile, and E. J. Kennelly, "Comparative analyses of bioactive mammea coumarins from seven parts of *Mammea americana* by HPLC-PDA with LC-MS," *Journal of Agricultural and Food Chemistry*, vol. 54, no. 12, pp. 4114–4120, 2006.

[32] B. M. W. Ouahouo, A. G. B. Azebaze, M. Meyer, B. Bodo, Z. T. Fomum, and A. E. Nkengfack, "Cytotoxic and antimicrobial coumarins from *Mammea africana*," *Annals of Tropical Medicine and Parasitology*, vol. 98, no. 7, pp. 733–739, 2004.

[33] A. P. Pereira, I. C. F. R. Ferreira, F. Marcelino et al., "Phenolic compounds and antimicrobial activity of olive (*Olea europaea* L. Cv. Cobrançosa) leaves," *Molecules*, vol. 12, no. 5, pp. 1153–1162, 2007.

[34] S. O. Salawu, A. O. Ogundare, B. B. Ola-Salawu, and A. A. Akindahunsi, "Antimicrobial activities of phenolic containing extracts of some tropical vegetables," *African Journal of Pharmacy and Pharmacology*, vol. 5, no. 4, pp. 486–492, 2011.

12

Comparative Evaluation of Cytotoxic and Apoptogenic Effects of Several Coumarins on Human Cancer Cell Lines: Osthole Induces Apoptosis in p53-Deficient H1299 Cells

Yalda Shokoohinia,[1,2] **Leila Hosseinzadeh,**[1] **Maryam Alipour,**[3] **Ali Mostafaie,**[4] **and Hamid-Reza Mohammadi-Motlagh**[4]

[1] *Novel Drug Delivery Research Center, School of Pharmacy, Kermanshah University of Medical Sciences, Kermanshah 6734667149, Iran*

[2] *Department of Pharmacognosy and Biotechnology, School of Pharmacy, Kermanshah University of Medical Sciences, Kermanshah 6734667149, Iran*

[3] *Students Research Committee, School of Pharmacy, Kermanshah University of Medical Sciences, Kermanshah 6734667149, Iran*

[4] *Medical Biology Research Center, Kermanshah University of Medical Sciences, Kermanshah 6734667149, Iran*

Correspondence should be addressed to Leila Hosseinzadeh; lhosseinzadeh90@yahoo.com

Academic Editor: Ismail Laher

Natural products are excellent resources for finding lead structures for the development of chemotherapeutic agents. Coumarins are a class of natural compounds found in a variety of plants. In this study, we evaluated the cytotoxic potential of coumarins isolated from *Prangos ferulacea* (L.) Lindl. in PC3, SKNMC, and H1299 (p53 null) human carcinoma cell lines. Osthole proved to be an outstanding potent cytotoxic agent especially against PC3 cells. Isoimperatorin exhibited moderate inhibitory effect against SKNMC and PC3 cell lines. Oxypeucedanin and braylin did not display any cytotoxic activity. In the next set of experiments, the apoptotic potentials of osthole and isoimperatorin were investigated. Induction of apoptosis by isoimperatorin was accompanied by an increase in activation of caspase-3, -8, and -9 in SKNMC cells and caspase-3 and -9 in PC3 cells. Moreover, isoimperatorin induced apoptosis by upregulating Bax and Smac/DIABLO genes in PC3 and SKNMC cells. Osthole induced apoptosis by downregulating antiapoptotic Bcl-2 in only PC3 cells and upregulating the proapoptotic genes Bax and Smac/DIABLO in PC3, SKNMC, and H1299 cells. The effects of osthole on H1299 cells are important because the loss of p53 has been associated with poor clinical prognosis in cancer treatment.

1. Introduction

New anticancer therapeutics are necessary to minimize various complications endured by cancer patients. The most common tumors frequently resist treatment with a significant number of commercially available anticancer drugs; therefore, the growing demand for developing more effective anticancer agents continues to exist. Higher plants provide a good source of clinically relevant compounds with anticancer properties. These classes of compounds include terpenoids, alkaloids, and various phenolic compounds such as coumarins [1].

Coumarins (2*H*-1-benzopyran-2-one) represent a class of phenolic compounds isolated from plants; the structural characteristic of coumarins depicts a framework consisting of fused benzene and α-pyrone ring systems [2]. Coumarins are well-known for their potential pharmacological activities: anti-inflammatory, antioxidant [3], antiviral [4], antimicrobial [5], and anticancer [6].

Moreover, scientists have reported potent cytotoxic activity of a number of coumarin compounds in various cancer cell lines including A549 (lung), A375 (skin), MCF-7 (breast), HSCs (liver), and HL-60 (leukemia) [7–11].

In this study, we have used *Prangos ferulacea* (L.) Lindl. as a source for coumarin isolation because Apiaceous plants provide an attractive resource for obtaining furanocoumarins [12, 13]. The plant, *P. ferulacea* commonly grows in the Mediterranean and Middle-East regions including Iran [14]; the antioxidant, antibacterial [15], and antispasmodic effects [16, 17] of this plant have been reported, and also it is widely used as provender for mutton [12]. *P. ferulacea* provides a major source of coumarins compounds such as osthole, isoimperatorin, and oxypeucedanin and coumarins such as gosferol, pranferol, oxypeucedanin methnolate, oxypeucedanin hydrate, and psoralen [18, 19] occur in minor amounts. This is the first report describing the cytotoxicity of braylin (6-methoxyseselin) isolated from this plant. This compound belongs to the group of angular furanocoumarins, which are rare in nature. Braylin has shown to exhibit vasorelaxant [20] and moderate anti-HIV effect [21].

Further research is essential to gain better understanding of the anticancer activity of coumarins. The present study compares the cytotoxic and apoptotic inducing effects of four coumarin compounds, namely, osthole, isoimperatorin, oxypeucedanin, and braylin (isolated from *P. ferulacea*) on H1299 (human non-small cell lung carcinoma), SKNMC (human neuroblastoma), and PC3 (human prostate cancer) cell lines. The findings presented herein constitute the first report to demonstrate the proapoptotic activity of the coumarins osthole and isoimperatorin in SKNMC and PC3 cells. We have also demonstrated that osthole induced apoptosis in H1299 cells through a mechanism independent of tumor suppressing action of p53 protein because H1299 cell line is devoid of genes encoding p53 protein.

2. Materials and Methods

2.1. Plant Material and Coumarins Isolation. Plant material gathering, identification and extraction, and isolation of osthole, isoimperatorin, and oxypeucedanin (Figure 1) were performed as previously reported [22]. Braylin was purified by using HPLC (petroleum ether (P) : ethyl acetate (E), 6 : 94) separation from a fraction obtained from an open column chromatography (P : E, 10 : 90) of defatted acetone extract. Structures of all compounds were elucidated by using ^{1}H-NMR, ^{13}C-NMR, and Mass spectra, comparing to literature [12, 22–24].

2.2. Cell Culture Conditions. H1299 (human nonsmall cell lung carcinoma) cell line was a kind gift from Prof. G. Storm. The cells have a homozygous partial deletion of the p53 protein and lack p53 protein expression. SKNMC, human neuroblastoma cell line, and PC3, human prostate cancer cell line, were obtained from Pasteur Institute (Tehran, Iran). PC3 was established in 1979 from bone metastasis of grade IV of prostate cancer in a 62-year-old Caucasian male. This cell line is useful to assess prostatic cancer cells response

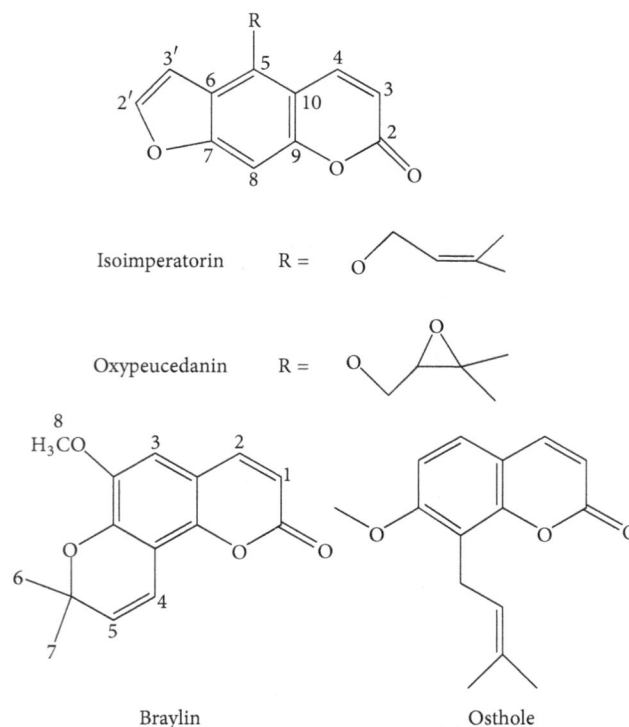

FIGURE 1: Chemical structures of isolated coumarins.

to chemotherapeutic agents [25]. SKMNC, is a neuroepithelioma cell line derived from a metastatic supraorbital human brain tumor [26]. The cells were cultured in Dulbecco's modified Eagle's medium (DMEM-F12) with 5% (v/v) fetal bovine serum, 100 Uml^{-1} penicillin, and 100 mgml^{-1} streptomycin. The medium was changed every 2-3 days and subcultured when the cell population density reached to 70–80% confluence.

2.3. Viability Assay. The cytotoxic effects of isolated coumarins were determined against cell lines by a colorimetric assay using 3-(4,5-dimethylthiazol-2-yl)-2, 5-diphenyltetrazolium bromide (MTT) and were compared with the untreated control. Cells were plated onto 96-well plates at a density of 2.0×10^4 cells/well and in a volume of $200\,\mu$L. Stock solutions of isolated coumarins were prepared in dimethyl sulfoxide (DMSO). The final concentration of the vehicle in the medium was always 0.5%. One day after seeding, $2\,\mu$L of the DMSO containing coumarins at different concentrations was added to each well. At appropriate time intervals, the medium was removed and replaced by $100\,\mu$L of 0.5 mg/mL of MTT in growth medium and then the plates were transferred to a 37°C incubator for 3-4 h. Supernatants were removed and the reduced MTT dye was solubilized with DMSO ($100\,\mu$L/well). Absorbance was determined on an ELISA plate reader (Biotek, H1M) with a test wavelength of 570 nm and a reference wavelength of 630 nm to obtain sample signal (OD570–OD630). Percentage of proliferation was calculated using the following formula: percent of control proliferation = (OD test/OD control) × 100. IC${}_{50}$ values were calculated by

TABLE 1: Cytotoxic activity of coumarins isolated from *Prangos ferulacea* against human cancer cell lines.

	SKNMC		PC3		H1299	
	IC$_{50}$ (μM)	MAE (%)	IC$_{50}$ (μM)	MAE (%)	IC$_{50}$ (μM)	MAE (%)
Osthole	28.81 ± 0.79	69.65 (5.93)	20.1 ± 2.1	70.38 ± 2.6	58.43 ± 2.15	52.18 ± 10.94
Isoimperatorin	182 ± 10.91	63.38 ± (10.94)	119.4 ± 8.65	55.14 ± 1.74	>300	13.89 ± 3.01
Oxypeucedanin	>300	<10	>300	<10	>300	<10
Braylin	>300	<10	>300	<10	>300	<10

MAE: maximum antiprolifrative effect.

plotting the log 10 of the percentage of proliferation versus drug concentration.

2.4. Detection of Caspase-3, -8, and -9 Activation.
Caspase 3, 8, and 9 assays were carried out using the sigma colorimetric caspase kit. This assay was based on the ability of the active enzyme to cleave the chromophore from the enzyme substrates, Ac-DEVD-pNA (for caspase-3), Ac-IETD-pNA (for caspase-8), and Ac-LEHD-pNA (for caspase-9), in equal amount of cells protein. The cells (5×10^5) were harvested and lysed in 70 μL of the cell lysis buffer included with the kit, and protein concentrations were equalized for each condition. Subsequently, 10 μL of cell lysate was combined with an equal amount of substrate reaction buffer containing caspase-3, -8, and -9 colorimetric substrates. This mixture was incubated for 2 h at 37°C, and then absorbance was measured with a plate reader (BioTek, H1M).

2.5. Real Time RT-PCR Analysis of Apoptosis-Related Gene Expression.
Total RNA from SKNMC, PC3 and H1299 cells pretreated with IC$_{50}$ concentration of coumarins were extracted using high pure isolation kit (Roche, Mannheim, Germany) according to the manufacture instructions. Quality and quantity of total RNA were assessed by spectrophotometer (NanoDrop 2000, USA) and samples were stored at −80°C until use. The primer sequences used for PCR were β-actin: 5′-TCATGAAGTGTGTGACGTGGACATC-3 (forward) and 5′-CAGGAGGAGCAATGATCTTGATCT-3′ (reverse); Bcl-2: 5′-ATCGCCCTGTGGATGACTGAG-3′ (forward) and 5′-GACCCAGGAGAAATCAAACAGAGG-3′ (reverse); Bax: 5′-GGACGAACTGGACAGTAACATCG-3′ (forward) and 5′-GCAAAGTAGAAAAGGGCGACAAC-3′ (reverse); and Smac/DIABLO: 5′-AGCTGGAAACCA-CTTGGATG-3′ (forward) and 5′-CCAGCTTGGTTTCTG-CTTT-3′ (reverse) [27, 28]. The performances of all primer pairs were tested by primer concentration to determine the optimal reaction conditions. Thermal cycler conditions were 15 min at 50°C for cDNA synthesis, 10 min at 95°C followed by 40 cycles of 15 s at 95°C to denature the DNA and 45 s at 60°C to anneal and extend the template. Melting curve analysis was performed to ascertain specificity by continuous acquisition from 65°C to 95°C with a temperature transient rate of 0.1°C/S. All reactions were performed in triplicate in a Corbett system (Australia). The value obtained for the target gene expression was normalized to β-actin and analyzed by the relative gene expression −ΔΔCT method, where −ΔΔCT =

(CT target − CT β-actin) unknown − (CT target − CT β-actin) calibrator.

2.6. Statistical Analysis.
Each experiment was performed at least three times, and the results were presented as mean ± S.E.M. One-way analysis of variance (ANOVA) followed by Turkey's test was used to compare the difference between means. A probability value of $P < 0.05$ was considered to be statistically significant.

3. Results

3.1. Inhibition of Cell Viability.
The potency of isolated coumarins to induce cell death was determined on SKNMC, PC3, and H1299 cell lines under MTT method. The results indicated that the cell proliferation was inhibited in the order of osthole > isoimperatorin > oxypeucedanin ≥ braylin in three cell lines. As shown in Figures 2(a)–2(c), exposure to osthole for 24 h resulted in a concentration dependent decrease in cell viability, with approximate IC$_{50}$ of 28.81 ± 0.79 μM, 20.08 ± 2.1 μM, and 58.43 ± 4.08 in SKNMC, PC3, and H1299 cells, respectively. Isoimperatorin possessed a moderate inhibitory effect against SKNMC (IC$_{50}$ = 182 ± 10.91 μM) and PC3 (IC$_{50}$ = 119.4 ± 8.65 μM) cell lines and had no effect against H1299 cell line. On the contrary, toxicity was not observed after exposure to oxypeucedanin and braylin at the concentrations up to 300 μM in the above mentioned cell lines (Table 1). The results indicated that osthole and isoimperatorin have the highest antiproliferative effect towards PC3, SKNMC, and H1299 cell lines, respectively. Therefore, they were selected and used for further studies.

3.2. Effects of Osthole and Isoimperatorin on Caspase-3, -8, and -9 Activity.
Activation of caspase cascade is critical in the initiation of apoptosis in various biological systems [29]. Therefore, for improvement of MTT results and also characterizing the type of cell death involved in our experiments, the activity of caspases was examined. A member of this family, caspase-3, has been identified as being a key mediator of apoptosis [30]. The obtained results showed that 24 h treatment with IC$_{50}$ concentration of osthole and isoimperatorin increased caspase-3 activation in human carcinoma cell lines. To determine which apoptotic pathway is activated by osthole and isoimperatorin, we evaluated the activation of caspase-8 and -9, the apical proteases in extrinsic and intrinsic pathways, respectively [31]. Osthole was able

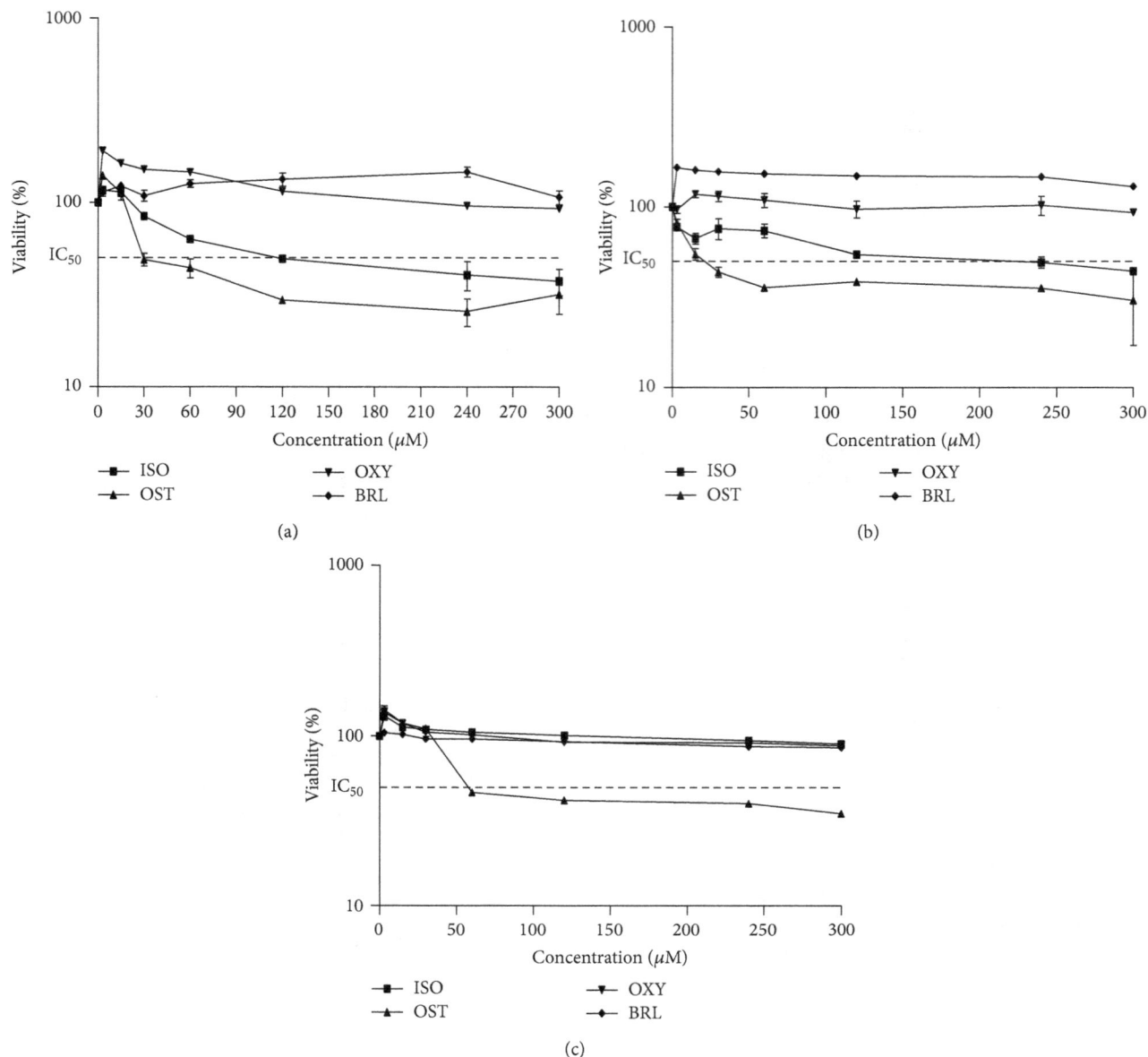

FIGURE 2: Cytotoxic effects of four isolated coumarins in (a) SKNMC, (b) PC3, and (c) H1299 cancer cells. The cells were incubated with at different concentrations of coumarins for 24 h. The cell proliferation inhibition was determined by MTT assay as described under materials and methods. Data are presented as mean ± S.E.M (n = 3).

to increase caspase-8 and -9 in H1299, PC3, and SKNMC cells, thus implying that osthole induces apoptosis in these cell lines through both intrinsic and extrinsic pathways. Like osthole, isoimperatorin increased both caspases activities in SKNMC cells. While in the PC-3 cells, isoimperatorin could only increase caspase-9 activity (Figure 3).

3.3. Effect of Osthole and Isoimperatorin on Some Critical Genes Involved in Apoptosis. The mitochondria are an integral part of the apoptotic machinery; therefore, we analyzed the most important proteins involved in mitochondrial pathway of apoptosis (Bax and Bcl-2) [32]. We found that osthole was able to decrease significantly Bcl-2 mRNA expression

in only PC-3 cell line. However, the Bax mRNA expression decreased significantly upon treatment with osthole in three cell lines. Next, the mRNA expression of Smac/DIABLO was measured. It is a protein released from mitochondria in response to apoptotic stimuli. Smac/DIABLO antagonizes inhibitor of apoptosis proteins (IAPs) to relieve their inhibitory effects on caspases [27]. The obtained results demonstrated that 24 h treatment with osthole increased significantly Smac/DIABLO in the level of mRNA expression in all cell lines. Furthermore, real time RT-PCR analysis clearly shows a significant reduction in the expression level of Bcl-2 after 24 h treatment with isoimperatorin in SKNMC cells. Moreover, induction of apoptosis by isoimperatorin was

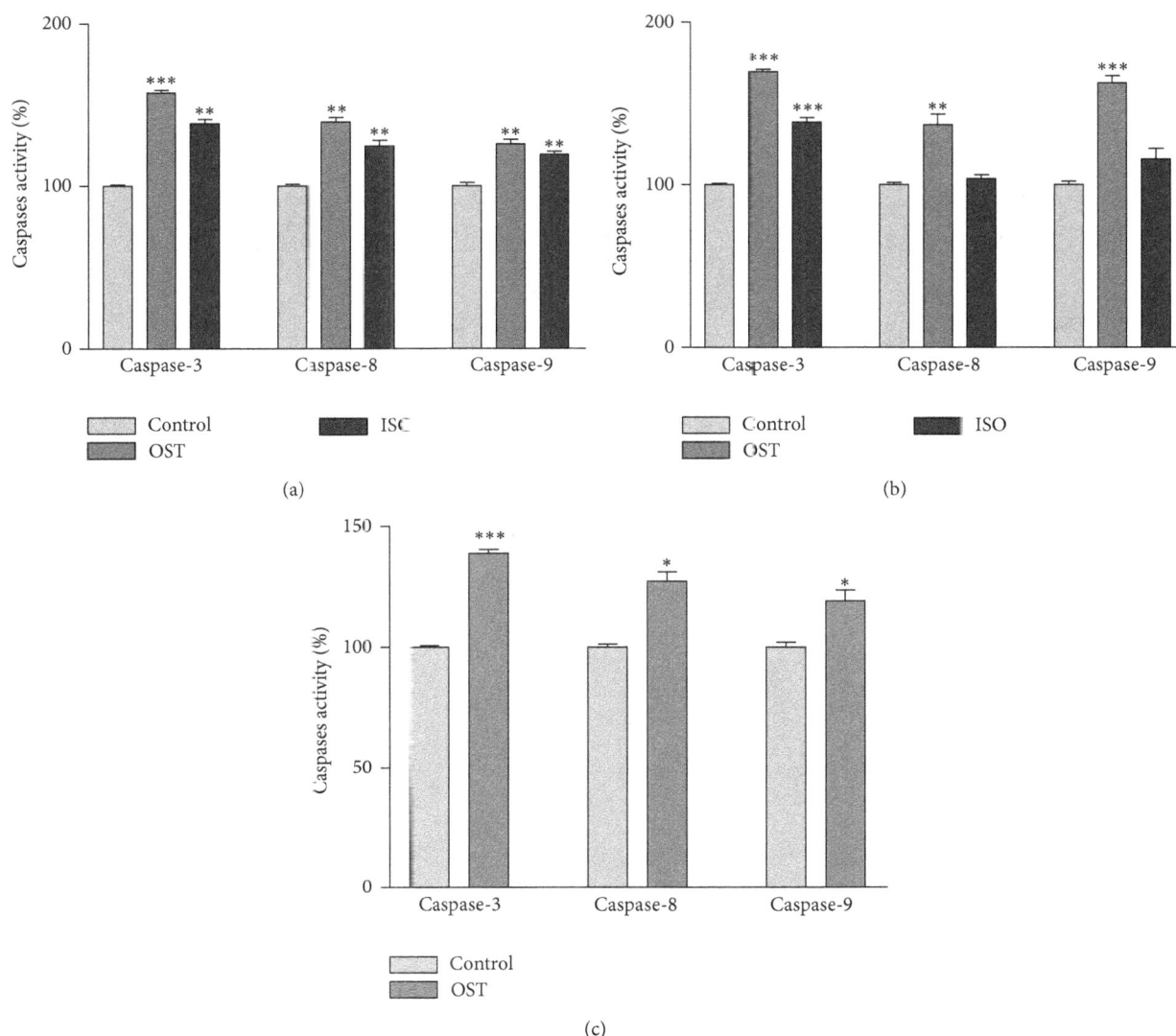

FIGURE 3: Involvement of activation of caspases in the induction of apoptosis on (a) SKNMC, (b) PC3, and (c) H1299 human cancer cells. Cells were incubated with IC_{50} concentration of the indicated compounds and harvested at 24 h and cell lysates were assayed using microplate reader for activation caspases. Significant differences were compared with the control. Data are presented as mean ± S.E.M. $^{*}P < 0.05$, $^{**}P < 0.01$, and $^{***}P < 0.001$ versus control.

accompanied by increase in mRNA levels of proapoptotic Bax and Smac/DIABLO genes in PC3 and SKNMC cells (Figure 4).

4. Discussion

Herbs and herbal extracts offer a wide variety of phytochemicals with diverse biological functions. Among these phytochemicals, coumarins play a significant role in plant biochemistry and physiology including antioxidants, enzyme inhibitors, and precursors of toxic substances in biochemical reactions involving different cellular systems [6]. Among their diverse biological properties, the antitumor activities and antiproliferative effects have been extensively studied and reported [33].

In the current study, the following four coumarins were isolated from *P. ferulacea*: osthole, isoimperatorin, oxypeucedanin, and braylin. Among the isolates, osthole and isoimperatorin showed the highest inhibitory potency against the growth of human carcinoma cell lines whereas oxypeucedanin and braylin failed to exhibit any cytotoxic effects. The present findings corroborate the findings reported by Yang et al., who evaluated cytotoxicity of coumarins isolated from fruits of *Cnidium monnieri* on leukemia cell lines. Their results revealed that, among osthole, imperatorin, bergapten, isopimpinellin, and xanthotoxin, osthole showed the strongest cytotoxic activity in tumor cell lines [34]. In our study, PC3 cells showed the highest sensitivity toward osthole and isoimperatorin. This result supports previous literature reports, which indicated that

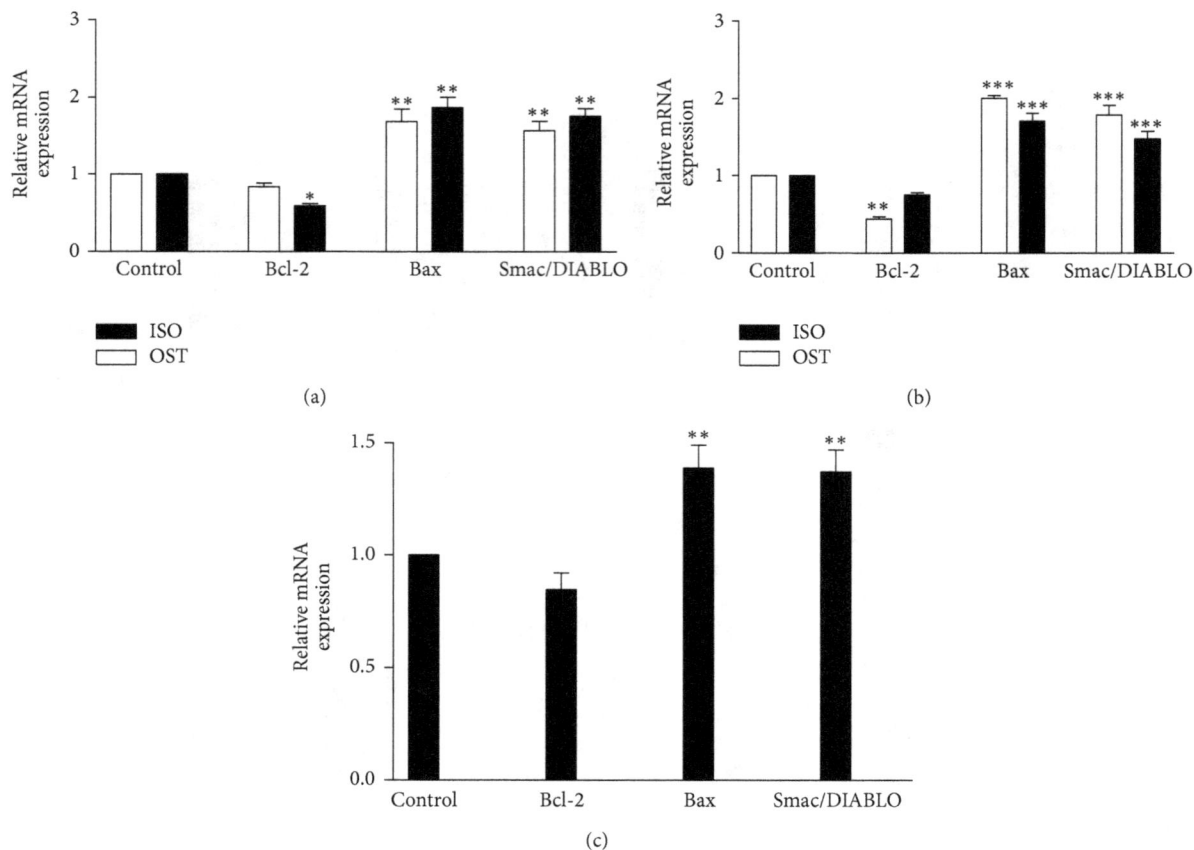

FIGURE 4: The effect of coumarins on expression of apoptotic-related genes on (a) SKNMC, (b) PC3, and (c) H1299 human cancer cells. Normalization relative to b-actin was performed. Levels of mRNA are expressed relative to control in the mean ± S.E.M values derived from three independent experiments. $^*P < 0.05$, $^{**}P < 0.01$, and $^{***}P < 0.001$ versus control.

osthole (100 μM) had a weak but significant antiproliferative activity against hormone independent PC3 and DU145 human prostate cancer cell lines [35]. In addition, there is a report showing antiproliferative effects of isoimperatorin on DU145 cell line [36]. We also found that H1299 cells were more susceptible to treatment with osthole but isoimperatorin had no antiproliferative effect on this cell line.

The apoptosis-inducing capacity rather than necrosis induction is preferably considered as a key feature of a potential antitumour drug. Accordingly, in the next set of experiments we investigated the apoptosis-inducing potentials of the cytotoxic agents. The Bcl-2 family proteins have emerged as a key component in regulating apoptosis; they either inhibit or promote cell death [28]. Bax and Bcl-2, the two important members of this family, influence the permeability of mitochondrial membrane. Cell survival in the early phases of apoptotic signaling cascade depends mostly on the balance between proapoptotic and antiapoptotic proteins of the Bcl-2 family [31]. Permeability of mitochondrial membrane allows the release of soluble molecules from the outer space of the mitochondria to the cytosol. One of these representative molecules which is called Smac/DIABLO activates a cascade of caspases in the cytosol [27]. The activation of caspases triggers the release of cytochrome C leading to

the deactivation of apoptosis inhibitory proteins belonging to the (IAP) family [29]. Our results showed that osthole was able to increase caspase-3, -8, and -9 activities in H1299, PC3, and SKNMC cells. Moreover, osthole induced apoptosis by downregulating antiapoptotic Bcl-2 in PC3 cells and upregulating proapoptotic genes Bax and Smac/DIABLO in PC3, SKNMC, and H1299 cells thereby, implying that osthole induces apoptosis in these cells via both mitochondrial and extrinsic pathways. As mentioned before, H1299 cells lack the expression of p53 protein. The p53 tumor suppressor proteins play a pivotal role in initiating apoptosis by sensing different intrinsic and extrinsic stresses. Defect in p53 function alone leads to phenotypic resistance resulting in chemotherapeutic failure of cancer treatment. The lack of p53 expression in H1299 may account for its higher resistance to cell death in comparison with other carcinoma cells [37].

Our results indicated that osthole caused an increase in expression of proapoptotic protein Bax via a p53 independent pathway and the increase in Bax expression induced the initiation of apoptotic cell death. The potential effect of osthole on H1299 cells is very promising as this compound can be applied to treat different types of tumors that display deregulated tumor suppression pathways under p53 control. However, further studies are needed to determine the exact molecular mechanisms induced by osthole in human non-small cell lung cancer carcinoma. In accordance with this finding, it has been previously reported that 7,8-dihydroxy-4-methylcoumarin (DHMC) mediates apoptosis in human leukemic HL-60 and U-937 cells via mechanisms independent of p53 activity [38]. Additionally, another study has described the p53 independent cytotoxic effects of coumarin and hydroxyl coumarins on squamous carcinoma cell lines [37]. We also found that isoimperatorin induces apoptosis by upregulating proapoptotic Bax and Smac/DIABLCO in PC3 and SKNMC cells. Moreover, isoimperatorin mediated apoptosis was accompanied by an increase in activation of caspase-3, -8, and -9 in SKNMC cells and caspase-3 and -9 in PC3 cells. Therefore, it appears that apoptosis induced by isoimperatorin occurred via an intrinsic pathway in PC3 cells.

It is difficult to render a structure activity relationship among the coumarin analogues tested from *P. ferulacea* because they come from different class types. For example, osthole is a prenylated coumarin, isoimperatorin and oxypeucedanin are linear furanocoumarins and braylin is an angular pyranocoumarin. However, Riveiro et al. proved that alkoxy residue could potentiate the antiproliferative effects of coumarins [39]. Although the tested coumarins were devoid of catechol moiety, which could have contributed to the growth inhibitory activity [40], it is highly likely that the presence of isoprenoid residue in osthole and isoimperatorin has contributed to various pharmacological interactions, which gave rise to the proapoptotic activity [41]. Important coumarin apoptotic features such as free catechol and isoprenoid moieties are absent in braylin and oxypeucedanin. Oxidation or cyclization of isoprenoid in isoimperatorin and osthole, respectively, resulted in inactive oxypeucedanin and braylin.

In conclusion, osthole showed the best cytotoxic activity among the four coumarin compounds tested. Osthole can induce apoptosis in PC3, H1299, and SKNMC cells at low micromolar concentrations. Therefore, osthole can be considered as a promising lead in cancer drug discovery and development.

Conflict of Interests

The authors declare there is no conflict of interests.

Acknowledgments

The results presented here are extracted from the Pharm.D. thesis of M. Alipour. This study was financially supported by the Research Council of Kermanshah University of Medical Sciences. The authors also appreciate the support of Professor Dr. G. Storm (University of Utrecht, Netherland).

References

[1] H. Itokawa, S. L. Morris-Natschke, T. Akiyama, and K.-H. Lee, "Plant-derived natural product research aimed at new drug discovery," *Journal of Natural Medicines*, vol. 62, no. 3, pp. 263–280, 2008.

[2] K. N. Venugopala, V. Rashmi, and B. Odhav, "Review on natural coumarin lead compounds for their pharmacological activity," *BioMed Research International*, vol. 2013, Article ID 963248, 14 pages, 2013.

[3] K. C. Fylaktakidou, D. J. Hadjipavlou-Litina, K. E. Litinas, and D. N. Nicolaides, "Natural and synthetic coumarin derivatives with anti-inflammatory/antioxidant activities," *Current Pharmaceutical Design*, vol. 10, no. 30, pp. 3813–3833, 2004.

[4] A. Ghannadi, K. Fattahian, Y. Shokoohinia, M. Behbahani, and A. Shahnoush, "Anti-viral evaluation of sesquiterpene coumarins from *Ferula assa-foetida* against HSV-1," *Iranian Journal of Pharmaceutical Research*, vol. 13, pp. 523–530, 2014.

[5] T. Ojala, S. Remes, P. Haansuu et al., "Antimicrobial activity of some coumarin containing herbal plants growing in Finland," *Journal of Ethnopharmacology*, vol. 73, no. 1-2, pp. 299–305, 2000.

[6] I. Kostova, "Synthetic and natural coumarins as cytotoxic agents," *Current Medicinal Chemistry—Anti-Cancer Agents*, vol. 5, no. 1, pp. 29–46, 2005.

[7] S. W. Yoo, J. S. Kim, S. S. Kang et al., "Constituents of the fruits and leaves of *Euodia daniellii*," *Archives of Pharmacal Research*, vol. 25, pp. 824–830, 2002.

[8] S. S. Bhattacharyya, S. Paul, A. de et al., "Poly (lactide-co-glycolide) acid nanoencapsulation of a synthetic coumarin: cytotoxicity and bio-distribution in mice, in cancer cell line and interaction with calf thymus DNA as target," *Toxicology and Applied Pharmacology*, vol. 253, no. 3, pp. 270–281, 2011.

[9] P.-C. Liao, S.-C. Chien, C.-L. Ho et al., "Osthole regulates inflammatory mediator expression through modulating NF-κB, mitogen-activated protein kinases, protein kinase C, and reactive oxygen species," *Journal of Agricultural and Food Chemistry*, vol. 58, no. 19, pp. 10445–10451, 2010.

[10] E. Shin, C. Lee, S. H. Sung, Y. C. Kim, B. Y. Hwang, and M. K. Lee, "Antifibrotic activity of coumarins from *Cnidium monnieri* fruits in HSC-T6 hepatic stellate cells," *Journal of Natural Medicines*, vol. 65, no. 2, pp. 370–374, 2011.

[11] T. Murata, M. Itoigawa, C. Ito et al., "Induction of apoptosis in human leukaemia HL-60 cells by furanone-coumarins from *Murraya siamensis*," *Journal of Pharmacy and Pharmacology*, vol. 60, no. 3, pp. 385–389, 2008.

[12] S. E. Sajjadi, H. Zeinvand, and Y. Shokoohinia, "Isolation and identification of osthol from the fruits and essential oil composition of the leaves of *Prangos asperula* Boiss," *Research in Pharmaceutical Sciences*, vol. 4, no. 1, pp. 19–23, 2009.

[13] S. E. Sajjadi, Y. Shokoohinia, and S. Hemmati, "Isolation and identification of furanocoumarins and a phenylpropanoid from the acetone extract and identification of volatile constituents from the essential oil of *Peucedanum pastinacifolium*," *Chemistry of Natural Compounds*, pp. 1–4, 2012.

[14] A. Ghahreman, *Flora of Iran*, Research Institute of Forests and Rangelands Publication, Tehran, Iran, 1986.

[15] N. Kafash-Farkhad, M. Asadi-Samani, and M. Rafieian-Kopaei, "A review on phytochemistry and pharmacological effects of *Prangos ferulacea* (L.) Lindl," *Life Science Journal*, vol. 10, no. 8, pp. 360–367, 2013.

[16] H. Sadraei, Y. Shokoohinia, S. E. Sajjadi, and B. Ghadirian, "Antispasmodic effect of osthole and prangos ferulacea extract on rat uterus smooth muscle motility," *Research in Pharmaceutical Sciences*, vol. 7, no. 3, pp. 141–149, 2012.

[17] H. Sadraei, Y. Shokoohinia, S. E. Sajjadi, and M. Mozafari, "Antispasmodic effects of *Prangos ferulacea* acetone extract and

its main component osthole on ileum contraction," *Research in Pharmaceutical Sciences*, vol. 8, no. 2, pp. 137–144, 2013.

[18] Y. Shokoohinia, S. E. Sajjadi, S. Gholamzadeh, A. Fattahi, and M. Behbahani, "Antiviral and cytotoxic evaluation of coumarins from *Prangos ferulacea* (L.) Lindl," *Pharmaceutical Biology*, 2014.

[19] A. Z. Abyshev, "Coumarin composition of the roots, stems, and fruit of *Prangos lophoptera*," *Chemistry of Natural Compounds*, vol. 10, no. 6, pp. 731–733, 1976.

[20] O. Rakotoarison, I. Rabenau, A. Lobstein et al., "Vasorelaxing properties and bio-guided fractionation of *Cedrelopsis grevei*," *Planta Medica*, vol. 69, no. 2, pp. 179–181, 2003.

[21] L. Xie, Y. Takeuchi, L. M. Cosentino, and K.-H. Lee, "Anti-AIDS agents. 37. Synthesis and structure-activity relationships of (3'R,4'R)-(+)-cis-khellactone derivatives as novel potent anti-HIV agents," *Journal of Medicinal Chemistry*, vol. 42, no. 14, pp. 2662–2672, 1999.

[22] L. Xie, Y. Takeuchi, L. M. Cosentino, and K.-H. Lee, "Anti-AIDS agents. 37. Synthesis and structure-activity relationships of (3'R,4'R)-(+)-cis-khellactone derivatives as novel potent anti-HIV agents," *Journal of Medicinal Chemistry*, vol. 42, no. 14, pp. 2662–2672, 1999.

[23] G. W. Ivie, "Linear furocoumarins (psoralens) from the seed of Texas *Ammi majus* L. (Bishop's weed)," *Journal of Agricultural and Food Chemistry*, vol. 26, no. 6, pp. 1394–1403, 1978.

[24] R. Liu, A. Li, and A. Sun, "Preparative isolation and purification of coumarins from *Angelica dahurica* (Fisch. ex Hoffm) Benth, et Hook. f (Chinese traditional medicinal herb) by high-speed counter-current chromatography," *Journal of Chromatography A*, vol. 1052, no. 1-2, pp. 223–227, 2004.

[25] M. E. Kaighn, K. S. Narayan, Y. Ohnuki, J. F. Lechner, and L. W. Jones, "Establishment and characterization of a human prostatic carcinoma cell line (PC-3)," *Investigative Urology*, vol. 17, no. 1, pp. 16–23, 1979.

[26] R. C. Seeger, S. A. Rayner, A. Banerjee et al., "Morphology, growth, chromosomal pattern, and fibrinolytic activity of two new human neuroblastoma cell lines," *Cancer Research*, vol. 37, no. 5, pp. 1364–1371, 1977.

[27] H. L. Mao, P. S. Liu, J. F. Zheng et al., "Transfection of Smac/DIABLO sensitizes drug-resistant tumor cells to TRAIL or paclitaxel-induced apoptosis in vitro," *Pharmacological Research*, vol. 56, no. 6, pp. 483–492, 2007.

[28] O. Porichi, M.-E. Nikolaidou, A. Apostolaki et al., "BCL-2, BAX and P53 expression profiles in endometrial carcinoma as studied by real-time PCR and immunohistochemistry," *Anticancer Research*, vol. 29, no. 10, pp. 3977–3982, 2009.

[29] L. Hosseinzadeh, J. Behravan, F. Mosaffa, G. Bahrami, A. R. Bahrami, and G. Karimi, "Effect of curcumin on doxorubicin-induced cytotoxicity in h9c2 cardiomyoblast cells," *Iranian Journal of Basic Medical Sciences*, vol. 14, no. 1, pp. 49–56, 2011.

[30] L. Hosseinzadeh, A. Khorand, and A. Aliabadi, "Discovery of 2-phenyl-N-(5-(trifluoromethyl)-1,3,4-thiadiazol-2-yl)acetamide derivatives as apoptosis inducers via the caspase pathway with potential anticancer activity," *Archiv der Pharmazie*, vol. 346, no. 11, pp. 812–818, 2013.

[31] W. Chen, Z. Zhao, L. Li et al., "Hispolon induces apoptosis in human gastric cancer cells through a ROS-mediated mitochondrial pathway," *Free Radical Biology and Medicine*, vol. 45, no. 1, pp. 60–72, 2008.

[32] L. Hosseinzadeh, J. Behravan, F. Mosaffa, G. Bahrami, A. Bahrami, and G. Karimi, "Curcumin potentiates doxorubicin-induced apoptosis in H9c2 cardiac muscle cells through generation of reactive oxygen species," *Food and Chemical Toxicology*, vol. 49, no. 5, pp. 1102–1109, 2011.

[33] M. Kawase, H. Sakagami, N. Motohashi et al., "Coumarin derivatives with tumor-specific cytotoxicity and multidrug resistance reversal activity," *In Vivo*, vol. 19, no. 4, pp. 705–712, 2005.

[34] L.-L. Yang, M.-C. Wang, L.-G. Chen, and C.-C. Wang, "Cytotoxic activity of coumarins from the fruits of *Cnidium monnieri* on leukemia cell lines," *Planta Medica*, vol. 69, no. 12, pp. 1091–1095, 2003.

[35] L. Wu, X. Huang, J. Li, and R. Zhang, "Haibo Hu Recent advances in the multifunction of a natural occurring coumarin: osthole," *Journal of Intercultural Ethnopharmacology*, vol. 2, pp. 57–66, 2013.

[36] J. H. Kang and D. S. Yim, "Effect of isoimperatorin on the proliferation of prostate cancer cell line DU145 cells," *Biomolecules & Therapeutics*, vol. 13, 189, no. 185, 2005.

[37] J. S. Lopez-Gonzalez, H. Prado-Garcia, D. Aguilar-Cazares, J. A. Molina-Guarneros, J. Morales-Fuentes, and J. J. Mandoki, "Apoptosis and cell cycle disturbances induced by coumarin and 7-hydroxycoumarin on human lung carcinoma cell lines," *Lung Cancer*, vol. 43, no. 3, pp. 275–283, 2004.

[38] M. E. Riveiro, R. Vazquez, A. Moglioni et al., "Biochemical mechanisms underlying the pro-apoptotic activity of 7,8-dihydroxy-4-methylcoumarin in human leukemic cells," *Biochemical Pharmacology*, vol. 75, no. 3, pp. 725–736, 2008.

[39] M. E. Riveiro, D. Maes, R. Vázquez et al., "Toward establishing structure-activity relationships for oxygenated coumarins as differentiation inducers of promonocytic leukemic cells," *Bioorganic and Medicinal Chemistry*, vol. 17, no. 18, pp. 6547–6559, 2009.

[40] R. Vázquez, M. E. Riveiro, M. Vermeulen et al., "Structure-anti-leukemic activity relationship study of ortho- dihydroxycoumarins in U-937 cells: Key role of the δ-lactone ring in determining differentiation-inducing potency and selective pro-apoptotic action," *Bioorganic and Medicinal Chemistry*, vol. 20, no. 18, pp. 5537–5549, 2012.

[41] R. Vázquez, M. E. Riveiro, M. Vermeulen et al., "Toddaculin, a natural coumarin from *Toddalia asiatica*, induces differentiation and apoptosis in U-937 leukemic cells," *Phytomedicine*, vol. 19, no. 8-9, pp. 737–746, 2012.

13

Simple and Robust Analysis of Cefuroxime in Human Plasma by LC-MS/MS: Application to a Bioequivalence Study

Xingjiang Hu, Mingzhu Huang, Jian Liu, Junchun Chen, and Jianzhong Shentu

Research Center for Clinical Pharmacy, State Key Laboratory for Diagnosis and Treatment of Infectious Diseases,
First Affiliated Hospital, Zhejiang University, Qingchun Road 79, Hangzhou 310003, China

Correspondence should be addressed to Jianzhong Shentu; hhfhxj@163.com

Academic Editor: Brian R. Overholser

A simple, robust LC-MS/MS assay for quantifying cefuroxime in human plasma was developed. Cefuroxime and tazobactam, as internal standard (IS), were extracted from human plasma by methanol to precipitate protein. Separation was achieved on a Zorbax SB-Aq (4.6 × 250 mm, 5 μm) column under isocratic conditions. The calibration curve was linear in the concentration range of 0.0525–21.0 μg/mL (r = 0.9998). The accuracy was higher than 90.92%, while the intra- and interday precision were less than 6.26%. The extraction procedure provides recovery ranged from 89.44% to 92.32%, for both analyte and IS. Finally, the method was successfully applied to a bioequivalence study of a single 500 mg dose of cefuroxime axetil in 22 healthy Chinese male subjects under fasting condition. Bioequivalence was determined by calculating 90% CIs for the ratios of C_{max}, AUC_{0-t}, and $AUC_{0-\infty}$ values for the test and reference products, using logarithmic transformed data. The 90% CIs for the ratios of C_{max} (91.4%~104.2%), AUC_{0-t} (97.4%~110.9%), and $AUC_{0-\infty}$ (97.6%~111.1%) values were within the predetermined range. It was concluded that the two formulations (test for capsule, reference for tablet) analyzed were bioequivalent in terms of rate and extent of absorption and the method met the principle of quick and easy clinical analysis.

1. Introduction

Cefuroxime is a second-generation cephalosporin used against a variety of infections. Due to its low oral bioavailability, cefuroxime is administered orally as a prodrug in the form of cefuroxime axetil [1]. Upon administration, the acid-stable lipophilic prodrug undergoes hydrolysis to yield cefuroxime [2]. However, the oral bioavailability of this ester prodrug would be changed violently for suffering from many factors, such as food [3]. To be able to optimize the dosing, it is necessary to characterize the pharmacokinetics of cefuroxime which requires a selective and sensitive analytical method for cefuroxime in plasma.

Several methods, including HPLC-DAD, LC-MS/MS, and UPLC-MS/MS, had been reported for the determination of cefuroxime in human plasma. However, they all need a complicated and expensive sample pretreatment method, or solid-phase extraction [4–6], or protein precipitation combined with back-extraction [7, 8], or protein precipitation followed by supernatant evaporated [9], for cleanup and enrichment of plasma samples, so as to get a lower limit of quantification. To the best of our knowledge, there was only one method with LLOQ of 25 ng/mL using simple protein precipitation extraction [10]. Generally speaking, using LC-MS technique for quantification in biofluids, IS should have similar physical, chemical, and chromatographic properties as the analyte (ideally eluted at similar retention time) [11]. Nevertheless, in this literature, the retention time of cefuroxime and IS was far apart, as 8 min and 4.4 min, respectively. Thus, it could not compensate for the sample losses that might occur during the sample preparation and chromatographic steps as well as for matrix effects under certain conditions.

In this study, we designed a sensitive and robust LC-MS/MS method following simple protein precipitation extraction with tazobactam as IS for determination of cefuroxime in human plasma. This method was accurate, sensitive, robust, and simple and was successfully applied to a bioequivalence study of a single 500 mg dose of cefuroxime axetil formulations (test and reference) in 22 healthy Chinese male subjects under fasting condition.

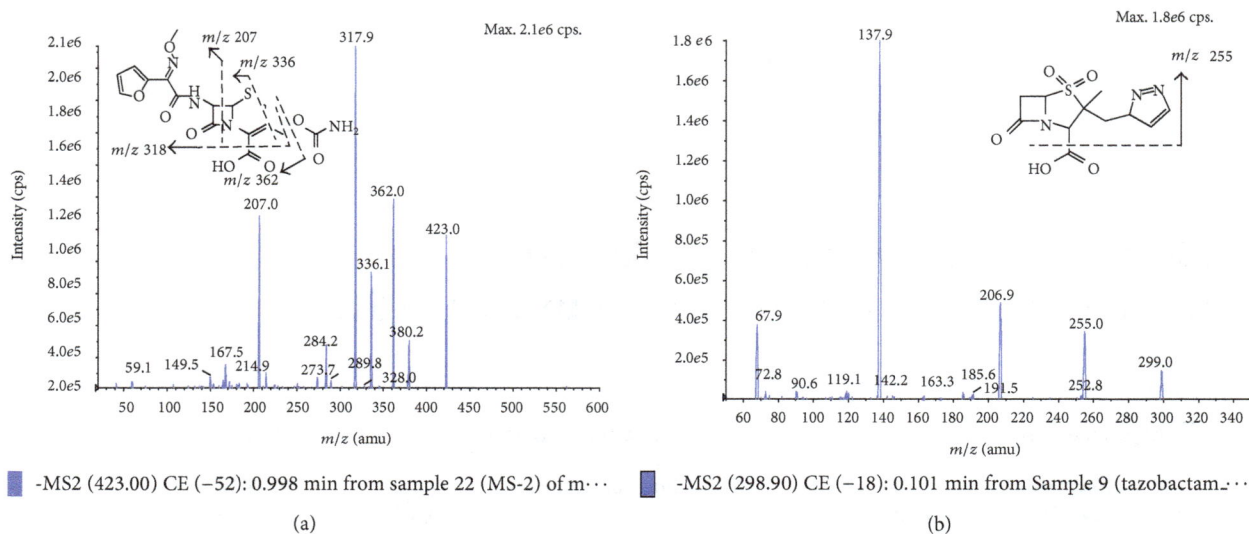

FIGURE 1: The structures and MS spectrums of cefuroxime (a) and IS (b).

2. Experimental

2.1. Chemicals and Reagents.
Cefuroxime (*Batch No. 130493-200704, purity 91.4%*) and tazobactam (IS) (*Batch No. 130511-200402, purity 99.1%*) were supplied by the National Pharmaceutical Institute of China. The chemical structures are shown in Figure 1. HPLC grade methanol, acetonitrile were purchased from Merck KGaA Company (Darmstadt, Germany). Water was purified using a Milli-Q system (Milford, MA, USA). HPLC grade ammonium formate and formic acid were purchased from Sigma (St. Louis, MO, USA). Human plasma was obtained from the Blood Center of Zhejiang Province (Hangzhou, China).

2.2. Instruments.
The HPLC was performed on an Agilent 1200 system equipped with a G1367C autosampler, a G1379B degasser, a G1316B thermostatted column, and a G1312B binary pump (Agilent, Waldbronn, Germany). The HPLC system was coupled with an API 4000 triple-quadrupole mass spectrometer (Applied Biosystems, Concord, ON, Canada) via electrospray ionization interface for mass analysis and detection. Data acquisition was performed with Analyst 1.4.2 software (Applied Biosystems).

2.3. LC-MS/MS Conditions.
Separation was performed on an Agilent Zorbax SB-Aq (4.6 × 250 mm, 5 μm) at a column temperature of 30°C. An isocratic mobile phase consisting of methanol/0.05% formic acid in water (42 : 58, v/v) was used at a flow rate of 1 mL/min, with the injection volume of 2 μL. The autosampler was set at 4°C. A primary flow rate of 1 mL/min was split to 500 μL/min using a T-piece. All measurements were carried out with mass spectrometer operated under the negative ESI mode. The multiple reaction monitoring transitions were m/z 423.0 → 317.9 for cefuroxime and m/z 298.9 → 138.0 for IS. Other parameters were as follows: collision gas, curtain gas, ion source gas 1 and ion source gas 2 (nitrogen) 6, 15, 55, and 50 psi, respectively; dwell time 200 ms; ion spray voltage −4500 V; ion source temperature 400°C; declustering potential (DP) −40 V for cefuroxime and −34 V for IS; collision energy −10 V for cefuroxime and −22 V for IS; collision exit potential (CXP) −10 V for cefuroxime and −9 V IS; and entrance potential (EP) −10 V for cefuroxime and IS. Unit resolution was used for both Q1 and Q3 mass detection.

2.4. Preparation of Standard Solution and Quality Control (QC) Samples.
Stock solution (1.05 mg/mL) of cefuroxime was prepared in 50% methanol and was further diluted with 50% methanol to achieve standard working solutions at concentrations of 210, 105, 52.5, 21.0, 10.5, 5.25, 2.10, 1.05, and 0.525 μg/mL. The QC stock solutions (low: 0.840 μg/mL, medium: 16.8 μg/mL, and high: 168 μg/mL) were also prepared in the same way. Tazobactam (IS), stock solution 1.86 mg/mL prepared in 50% methanol, was diluted with 50% methanol to give a final concentration of 18.6 μg/mL. Both of these stock solutions were stored at 4°C avoiding light for using.

The standard working solutions (20 μL) were used to spike blank plasma samples (200 μL). The final concentrations of cefuroxime standard calibration plasma samples were 21.0, 10.5, 5.25, 2.10, 1.05, 0.525, 0.210, 0.105, and 0.0525 μg/mL, respectively. The QC samples were also prepared in the same way by adding 20 μL diluted QC stock solutions to 200 μL blank human plasma. The final concentrations of cefuroxime in the low-, medium-, and high-QC plasma samples were 0.0842 μg/mL, 1.68 μg/mL, and 16.8 μg/mL, respectively.

2.5. Sample Extraction Procedures.
After frozen human plasma samples were thawed at ambient temperature and adequately vortexed, a total of 200 μL aliquot plasma sample was added with 20 μL of 50% methanol (supplementary volume) and 20 μL IS (18.6 μg/mL) solution. After a thorough

vortex mixing for 30 s, mixtures were precipitated with 600 μL methanol, vortex-mixed for 30 s, and centrifuged at 13000 rpm for 5 min. Finally, 2 μL of supernatant was injected into the LC-MS/MS system.

2.6. Method Validation.

The current method was validated prior to the analysis of human plasma samples according to the guidance of bioanalytical method validation [12]. The selectivity, linearity, precision, accuracy, sensitivity, recovery, matrix effect, and stability of cefuroxime in plasma sample were assessed and investigated.

To evaluate selectivity, drug-free plasma samples from 6 individuals were analyzed to check for the presence of any interfering peaks at the elution times of both cefuroxime and IS. The calibration curves were constructed using 9 standards ranging in concentration from 0.0525 to 21.0 μg/mL. The validity of the linear regression equation was indicated by the correlation coefficient (r).

The intraday and interday precision and accuracy were evaluated by assessing QC samples at the following concentrations ($n = 6$): LLOQ (0.0525 μg/mL), low (0.0842 μg/mL), medium (1.68 μg/mL), and high (16.8 μg/mL).

The extraction recovery and matrix effect of cefuroxime for three concentrations of QC samples was determined by comparing the response of analyte spiked plasma after extraction to that of analyte spiked into the solution extracted from blank plasma and the response of analyte spiked after extraction to that of analyte dissolved in mobile phase, respectively.

Stability experiments involved leaving the untreated plasma sample at ambient temperature for 6 h without light, placing the treated plasma sample in an autosampler for 20 h, three freeze-thaw cycles from −20°C to 25°C, and storing for 145 days at −20°C, using three aliquots of each QC sample at three different concentrations.

2.7. Application of the Assay.

The method described in this paper was applied to a bioequivalence study of two oral formulations of cefuroxime axetil (test formulation, a 250 mg cefuroxime axetil capsule from a Chinese company; reference formulation, a 250 mg cefuroxime axetil tablet produced by GlaxoSmithKline, UK). The study followed a single dose, two-way randomized crossover design with a 1-week washout period between doses. After an overnight fast of at least 10 h, subjects received a single oral 500 mg dose of either the test or reference formulation with 240 mL of water. During both treatment periods, heparinized blood samples were collected at the following times: before (0.0 h) and at 0.33, 0.67, 1.0, 1.5, 2.0, 2.5, 3.0, 4.0, 5.0, 6.0, 8.0, and 10.0 h after dosing. The blood samples were centrifuged at 4000 rpm for 10 min, and plasma samples were separated and stored at −20°C until analyzed.

In addition to C_{max} and T_{max} obtained directly from the measured data, other PK parameters (AUC_{0-t}, $AUC_{0-\infty}$, and $t_{1/2}$) were calculated by noncompartmental analysis using Drug Statistics (DAS) software 2.1.1 (University of Science and Technology, Hefei, China). The relative bioavailability ($F\%$) of the tested formulation was calculated as follows: $F\% = AUC_{0-t}(\text{test})/AUC_{0-t}(\text{reference}) \times 100\%$. Analysis of variance

(ANOVA) using DAS 2.1.1 was performed on C_{max}, AUC_{0-t}, and $AUC_{0-\infty}$ values evaluating treatment, period, sequence, and subject within sequence effects. Their ratios (test *versus* reference) of log-transformed data were analyzed for relative bioavailability. The 90% CIs served as interval estimates and were determined by two 1-sided t-tests. If the differences in PK parameters between the two formulations were not statistically significant ($P > 0.05$) and the 90% CIs for the ratios of C_{max}, AUC_{0-t}, and $AUC_{0-\infty}$ are located within the bioequivalence criteria range (80~125% for AUC and 70~143% for C_{max}), then the two formulations were considered to have met the regulatory requirement for bioequivalence.

3. Results and Discussion

3.1. Method Development.

To optimize chromatography, stationary phase, the composition of mobile phase, and column temperature were investigated in the LC domain, so as to achieve optimal peak shape and good separation from the void volume. Because of their amphotericity of chemical properties, various available columns of different lengths and bonded phases (Zorbax SB-C$_{18}$, Zorbax SB-Aq, Hypersil GOLD Aq, and Atlantis T3) were carefully evaluated. Finally, Agilent SB-Aq column was chosen in the present study for its high efficiency and peak symmetry. Different mobile phases (methanol-water and acetonitrile-water with different additives, such as formic acid and ammonium formate) were examined to obtain efficient chromatography and relatively short run time for cefuroxime and IS. It was found that the addition of formic acid could remarkably improve the peak symmetry and ionization of cefuroxime and IS. When methanol was used as the organic phase, the peak of cefuroxime was further improved. Therefore, the mobile phase was selected as methanol-mixture of 0.05% formic acid in water to achieve better separation and less interference from other components in the plasma. The retention time for cefuroxime and IS was 6.8 and 5.9 min, respectively. The total chromatographic run time was 8.0 min (Figure 2).

3.2. Selectivity.

The typical MRM chromatograms of mixed blank plasma from six drug-free individuals, a spiked plasma sample with cefuroxime at LLOQ and IS, and a plasma sample from a healthy volunteer 0.67 h after an oral administration were shown in Figure 2. The results indicated that there was no apparent endogenous interference for the determination of cefuroxime.

3.3. Linearity of Calibration Curves and LLOQ.

The standard calibration curve for spiked human plasma containing cefuroxime was linear over the range 0.0525–21.0 μg/mL. Good linearity was observed for the analyte using a weighted ($1/x$) least squares linear regression analysis with a coefficient of determination $r = 0.9998$. Typical equations for the calibration curve were as follows: $Y = (0.186 \pm 0.002)X + (0.00024 \pm 0.00049)$ ($n = 3$), where X represents the plasma concentration of cefuroxime (μg/mL) and Y represents the ratios of cefuroxime peak area to that of IS. LLOQ under the optimized conditions was 0.0525 μg/mL for cefuroxime,

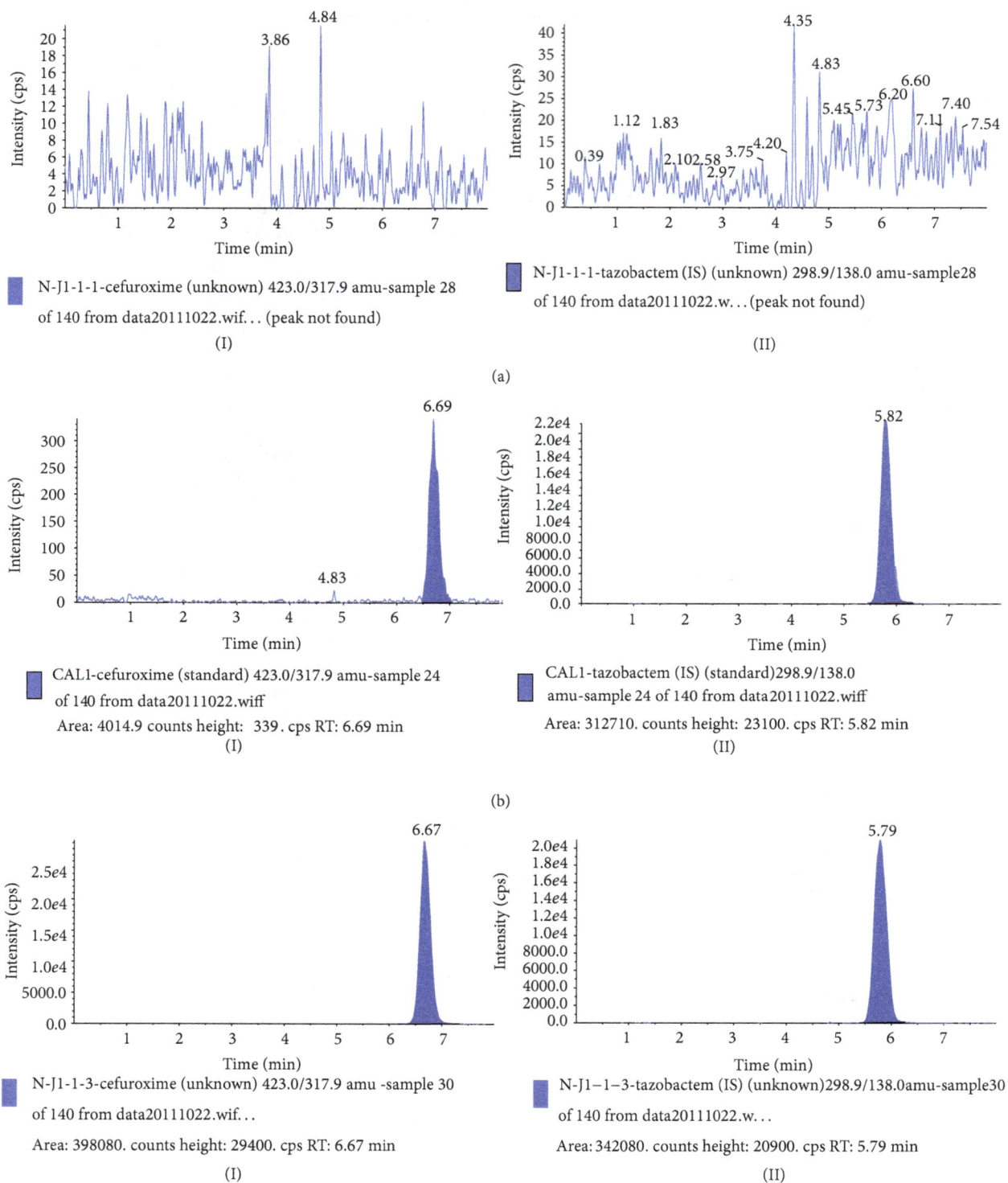

FIGURE 2: MRM chromatograms of cefuroxime (I) and IS (II) obtained from human plasma samples: (a) blank plasma, (b) blank plasma spiked with standard solution (LLOQ), and (c) plasma sample from a healthy subject 0.67 h after oral administration.

TABLE 1: Intraday and interday precision and accuracy of cefuroxime in human plasma.

	QC levels	Concentration (μg/mL)	Mean concentration found (μg/mL)	Precision (RSD%)	Accuracy (%)
Intraday (n = 6)	LLOQ	0.0525	0.0503	2.72	95.58
	L	0.0842	0.0766	2.84	90.92
	M	1.68	1.68	1.47	99.64
	H	16.8	16.7	1.40	99.43
Interday (3 days, n = 6)	L	0.0842	0.0851	6.26	101.1
	M	1.68	1.71	2.19	101.8
	H	16.8	16.8	2.09	100.1

which was judged from the fact that the precision and accuracy were less than 20% (Table 1) and the S/N ratios were much higher than 10. The LLOQ was sufficient for the bioequivalence study of cefuroxime following an oral administration.

3.4. Precision and Accuracy.

QC samples at three concentration levels were calculated over three validation runs (once a day). Six replicates of each QC level were determined in each run. Table 1 summarized the intraday and interday precision and accuracy for cefuroxime. In this assay, the intraday precision that was expressed by relative standard deviation (RSD) was no more than 2.84% for all tested concentrations (0.0842, 1.68, and 16.8 μg/mL), and the interday precision was less than 6.26%. The accuracy ranged from 90.92% to 101.8%. The above values were within the acceptable range, which demonstrated the good stability and repeatability of this described method.

3.5. Recovery and Matrix Effect.

The recoveries of the protein precipitation for cefuroxime were 89.44 ± 4.66%, 91.94 ± 0.94%, and 91.39 ± 1.67% at concentrations of 0.0842, 1.68, and 16.8 μg/mL, respectively. Mean recovery for the IS was 92.32 ± 0.90%. The RSDs for all recoveries were less than 5.21% throughout the entire concentration ranges, indicating assay consistency.

The matrix effect was evaluated to determine the influence of matrix components on analyte quantification. Average matrix effect values obtained were 110.6 ± 5.10%, 109.8 ± 1.58%, 111.4 ± 2.12%, and 108.8 ± 1.52% for QC samples at concentrations of 0.0842, 1.68, and 16.8 μg/mL, and IS. The results obtained were well within the acceptable limit [12] and indicated that the analysis of cefuroxime was not interfered with by endogenous substances in plasma.

3.6. Stability.

The stability experiment was performed by using QC samples at concentrations of 0.0842, 1.68 and 16.8 μg/mL, except for long-term stability for 0.105, 1.68 and 16.8 μg/mL. The results indicated that cefuroxime was stable in untreated plasma when placed in the short-term (6 h) at room temperature, repeated three freeze/thaw cycles and stored at −20°C for 145 days. In addition, it was found also stable in treated-plasma samples when placed in autosampler at 4°C for 20 h (Table 2).

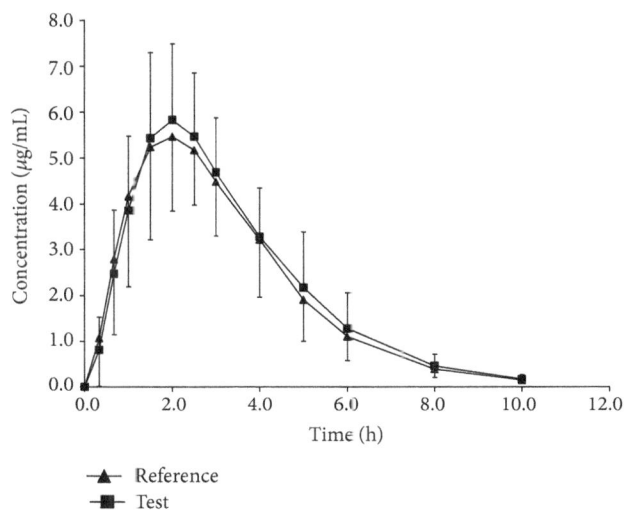

FIGURE 3: Mean plasma concentration-time profile of cefuroxime after oral administration of test and reference formulations to 22 healthy male subjects.

3.7. Bioequivalence Evaluation.

The mean plasma concentration-time curves of cefuroxime after oral administration of a single 500 mg dose of test and reference formulations in 22 healthy Chinese male volunteers were shown in Figure 3. The PK parameters of cefuroxime after oral administration of 500 mg test and reference formulations to 22 healthy volunteers were presented in Table 3. The results of the analysis of ANOVA for assessment of product, group, and period effects and 90% Cls for the ratio of C_{max}, AUC_{0-t}, and $AUC_{0-\infty}$ values of test and reference products, using logarithmic transformed data, were shown in Table 3. Power of statistical test was 97.6% for C_{max}, 103.9% for AUC_{0-t}, and 104.1% for $AUC_{0-\infty}$.

No significant differences in AUC_{0-t} or C_{max} were found between the test and reference formulations. The multivariate analysis accomplished through analysis of variance revealed the absence of period, group, and product effects for AUC_{0-t}, $AUC_{0-\infty}$, or C_{max}. The 90% Cls for the ratio of C_{max} (91.4%~104.2%), AUC_{0-t} (97.4%~110.9%), and $AUC_{0-\infty}$ (97.6%~111.1%) values for the test and reference products were all located within the bioequivalence criteria range (80~125% for AUC and 70~143% for C_{max}), proposed

TABLE 2: Summary of the stability of cefuroxime in human plasma on different conditions ($n = 3$).

Stability conditions	Concentration (μg/mL)	Calculated concentration		
		Mean ± SD (μg/mL)	Accuracy%	RSD%
Short-term (6 h, 25°C)	0.0842	0.0799 ± 0.0022	94.97	2.75
	1.68	1.70 ± 0.025	100.8	1.47
	16.8	16.4 ± 0.06	97.63	0.40
Long-term (145 days, −20°C)	0.105	0.103 ± 0.004	98.26	4.22
	1.68	1.73 ± 0.038	103.0	2.25
	16.8	16.77 ± 0.40	99.94	2.36
Autosampler (20 h, 4°C)	0.0842	0.0823 ± 0.0030	97.76	3.89
	1.68	1.71 ± 0.025	101.8	1.47
	16.8	16.6 ± 0.27	98.79	1.63
Three freeze-thaw cycles (from 25°C to −20°C)	0.0842	0.0837 ± 0.0048	99.46	5.76
	1.68	1.72 ± 0.032	102.1	1.84
	16.8	16.6 ± 0.36	98.65	2.15

TABLE 3: Mean pharmacokinetic parameters for cefuroxime after oral administration of 500 mg of test and reference formulations to healthy human volunteers under fasting condition ($n = 22$).

Parameters (units)	Reference formulation Mean ± SD	Test formulation Mean ± SD	Point estimate (90% Cls)
T_{max} (h)	2.14 ± 0.85	2.25 ± 0.95	—
C_{max} (μg/mL)	6.42 ± 1.19	6.31 ± 1.45	97.6 (91.42–104.2)
$T_{1/2}$ (h)	1.33 ± 0.10	1.38 ± 0.16	—
AUC_{0-t} (μg·h/mL)	22.01 ± 3.95	23.02 ± 4.78	103.9 (97.4–110.9)
$AUC_{0-\infty}$ (μg·h/mL)	22.30 ± 4.00	23.36 ± 4.87	104.1 (97.6–111.1)

by China Food and Drug Administration [13]. It was concluded that the two formulations analyzed were bioequivalent in terms of rate and extent of absorption and, thus, may be used interchangeably, with no effect on therapeutic effect.

4. Conclusion

A simple and sensitive LC-MS/MS method for the quantification of cefuroxime in human plasma was developed. Method validation has been demonstrated by a variety of tests for selectivity, linearity, sensitivity, precision, recovery, matrix effect, and stability. This method is attractive for the pharmacokinetic and bioequivalence analysis of cefuroxime, because of its high sensitivity and accuracy.

Conflict of Interests

The authors declare that there is no conflict of interests regarding the publication of this paper.

Acknowledgment

This research was funded by the Key Technologies R&D Program of 12th Five-Year Plan of China (no. 2011ZX09302-003-03).

References

[1] R. D. Foord, "Cefuroxime: human pharmacokinetics," *Antimicrobial Agents and Chemotherapy*, vol. 9, no. 5, pp. 741–747, 1976.

[2] S. M. Harding, P. E. O. Williams, and J. Ayrton, "Pharmacology of cefuroxime as the 1-acetoxyethyl ester in volunteers," *Antimicrobial Agents and Chemotherapy*, vol. 25, no. 1, pp. 78–82, 1984.

[3] A. Finn, A. Straughn, M. Meyer, and J. Chubb, "Effect of dose and food on the bioavailability of cefuroxime axetil," *Biopharmaceutics and Drug Disposition*, vol. 8, no. 6, pp. 519–526, 1987.

[4] R. Denooz and C. Charlier, "Simultaneous determination of five β-lactam antibiotics (cefepim, ceftazidim, cefuroxim, meropenem and piperacillin) in human plasma by high-performance liquid chromatography with ultraviolet detection," *Journal of Chromatography B: Analytical Technologies in the Biomedical and Life Sciences*, vol. 864, no. 1-2, pp. 161–167, 2008.

[5] P. Partani, S. Gurule, A. Khuroo, T. Monif, and S. Bhardwaj, "Liquid chromatography/electrospray tandem mass spectrometry method for the determination of cefuroxime in human plasma: Application to a pharmacokinetic study," *Journal of Chromatography B: Analytical Technologies in the Biomedical and Life Sciences*, vol. 878, no. 3-4, pp. 428–434, 2010.

[6] P. Colin, L. D. Bock, H. Tjollyn et al., "Development and validation of a fast and uniform approach to quantify beta-lactam antibiotics in human plasma by solid phase extraction-liquid chromatography-electrospray-tandem mass spectrometry," *Talanta*, vol. 103, pp. 285–293, 2013.

[7] J. B. Bulitta, C. B. Landersdorfer, M. Kinzig, U. Holzgrabe, and F. Sorgel, "New semiphysiological absorption model to assess the pharmacodynamic profile of cefuroxime axetil using nonparametric and parametric population pharmacokinetics," *Antimicrobial Agents and Chemotherapy*, vol. 53, no. 8, pp. 3462–3471, 2009.

[8] M. Carlier, V. Stove, J. A. Roberts et al., "Quantification of seven beta-lactam antibiotics and two beta-lactamase inhibitors in human plasma using a validated UPLC-MS/MS method," *International Journal of Antimicrobial Agents*, vol. 40, no. 5, pp. 416–422, 2012.

[9] F. Wolff, G. Deprez, L. Seyler et al., "Rapid quantification of six beta-lactams to optimize dosage regimens in severely septic patients," *Talanta*, vol. 103, pp. 153–160, 2013.

[10] A. Viberg, M. Sandström, and B. Jansson. "Determination of cefuroxime in human serum or plasma by liquid chromatography with electrospray tandem mass spectrometry," *Rapid Communications in Mass Spectrometry*, vol. 18, no. 6, pp. 707–710, 2004.

[11] L. Novakova, "Challenges in the development of bioanalytical liquid chromatography-mass spectrometry method with emphasis on fast analysis," *Journal of Chromatography A*, vol. 1292, pp. 25–37, 2013.

[12] FDA Guidance for Industry, Bioanalytical Method Validation, U.S. Department of Health and Human Services, Food and Drug Administration, Center for Drug Evaluation and Research (CDER), Center for Veterinary Medicine (CVM), 2001, http://www.fda.gov/downloads/drugs/guidancecomplianceregulatoryinformation/guidances/ucm070107.pdf.

[13] China Food and Drug Administration, Center for Drug Evaluation, "Guideline for bioavailability and bioequivalence studies of generic drug products," 2005 (Chinese), http://www.sfda.gov.cn/directory/web/WS01/images/u6Rp9KpzuWxrzByMvM5cn6zuA+9PDtsi6zcn6zu+1yNCr0NTR0L6vLzK9da4tbzUrdTyLnBkZg==.pdf.

14

Development of Mass Spectrometry Selected Reaction Monitoring Method for Quantitation and Pharmacokinetic Study of Stepharine in Rabbit Plasma

Arthur T. Kopylov,[1] Ksenia G. Kuznetsova,[1] Olga M. Mikhailova,[2] Andrey G. Moshkin,[2] Vladimir V. Turkin,[2] and Andrei A. Alimov[2]

[1] Institute of Biomedical Chemistry, 10 Pogodinskaya Street, Moscow 119121, Russia
[2] Institute of Applied Biochemistry JSC "Biochimmash," 4 Klara Tsetkin Street, Moscow 127299, Russia

Correspondence should be addressed to Arthur T. Kopylov; a.t.kopylov@gmail.com

Academic Editor: Robert Gogal

Highly sensitive liquid chromatography mass spectrometry method on triple quadrupole (QQQ) mass spectrometer was successfully applied for pharmacokinetic study of stepharine in rabbit plasma. Specific ion transitions of stepharine protonated precursor ion were selected and recorded in the certain retention time employing dynamic selected reaction monitoring mode. The developed method facilitated quantitative measurements of stepharine in plasma samples in linear range of five orders of magnitude with high accuracy and low standard deviation coefficient and pharmacokinetics parameters were calculated. The apparent volume of stepharine distribution (estimated as ratio of clearance to elimination rate constant, data not shown) allows us to assume that stepharine was extensively distributed throughout the body.

1. Introduction

Stephaglabrine sulfate is a sulfate of isoquinoline proaporphinealkaloid extracted from tuber roots of *Stephania glabra (Roxb.)* of the family Menispermaceae. Stephaglabrinesulfate has the chemical formula $(C_{18}H_{19}NO_3)_2 \cdot 1/2H_2SO_4$ (Figure 1) and is a white crystal powder with the melting point in the range of 243-244°C, with the subsequent decomposition, soluble in water and aqueous alcohol [1, 2]. Since stephaglabrine sulfate is the dimeric salt, it dissociates to stepharine base with molecular weight 297.1359, which is possible to detect as protonated ion [3].

It has been shown that intramuscular injection of stephaglabrine sulfate in dose of 0.1 mg/kg to rabbits significantly decreases intensity of trophic disturbances of denervated extremities at traumatic injuries of sciatic nerve. Stephaglabrine assists histological neogenesis and regeneration, electrophysiological and functional recovery of nerves after injury [4, 5]. However pharmacokinetic study of the stephaglabrine sulfate still remains poorly investigated.

The main aim of this study is to establish a valid method for detection of stepharine in rabbit plasma after intramuscular administration of the drug. For this purpose, quantitative assay of stepharine has been developed using selected reaction monitoring (SRM). The procedure consists of extraction of stepharine from rabbit plasma, detection by liquid chromatography/tandem mass spectrometry (LC-MS/MS), and measurements of the concentration of stepharine in plasma samples eliciting on the detection of characteristic fragment ions at certain retention time.

Based on the obtained data pharmacokinetic parameters of stepharine were calculated.

2. Material and Methods

2.1. Materials. Acetonitrile HPLC grade was purchased from Acros (USA), glacial acetic acid was purchased from Merck (Germany), ammonium formate chromatography grade was purchased from Fluka (Germany), ammonia hydroxide was

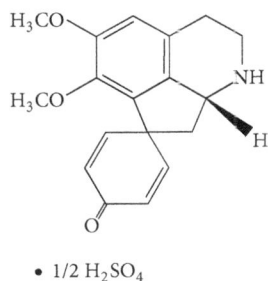

FIGURE 1: Structural chemical formula of stephaglabrine sulfate (image is adopted from PubChem Compound source).

purchased from Acros (USA), chloroform was purchased from Merck (Germany), and deionized water $18.2\,m\Omega*cm^2$ was obtained from MilliQ Elix 3 system.

For routine assay calibration, plasma pooled from three rabbits was used. The samples were aliquoted and stored at $-80°C$. For the matrix effect experiments, plasma pooled from five rabbits was obtained.

2.2. Compound. Stephaglabrine sulfate (powder) as analytical compound was obtained from "BioGene Technologies" (Russian Federation).

2.3. Animals and Administration of Stephaglabrine Sulfate. All experimental procedures with animals were carried out according the Animal Experimentation Ethics Committee and Veterinary Committee of the RSAU-MTAA (Russian State Agrarian University, Moscow, Russia) guidelines. The Approval Certificate verifying animal experimentation issued by the Animal Experimentation Ethics Committee is number E038-6.176RSAU, issued from November 29. 2012; the Veterinary certificate verifying animal keeping issued by Veterinary Committee is number V812-6.255RSAU, issued from November 26, 2012. The study was acquired on outbred, nonpregnant rabbits aged one year (weight range: 4-5 kg). All animals were kept in a standard animal holding room at Animal Center of RSAU-MTAA. Before the experimental procedure the selected animals were under veterinary supervision for seven days. All rabbits were kept at a standard animal holding room at a temperature of $20 \pm 2°C$, a relative humidity $65 \pm 10\%$, daylight duration 14-17 hours, and lighting 50–70 luxes. Water and food were *ad libitum*.

The selected rabbits were administrated intramuscular with stephaglabrine sulfate at doses 0.1 mg/kg as it was established before [4]. Each animal received a single dose.

2.4. Analytical Instruments and Conditions. Stephaglabrine is the dimeric salt; therefore detection of stepharine compound only (dissociated salt) with $m/z = 298.4$ is available LS-MS approach [3]. LC-MS and liquid chromatography with tandem mass spectrometry (LC-MS/MS) analysis were performed on Agilent 6520 Q-TOF mass spectrometer (Agilent, USA) equipped with 1200 HPLC system (Agilent Technologies) nanoflow liquid chromatography system and 6490 Triple Quad mass spectrometer interfaced with 1200 HPLC system microflow liquid chromatography. Evaluation of the

compound purity, identity, and full fragment ions spectra was performed on Q-TOF mass spectrometry coupled with chromatographic separation on Zorbax C-18 SB 80 column ($75\,\mu m \times 43$ mm, $5\,\mu m$ particle size, 80 A pore size). One μL of stephrine sulfate solution (0.1 $\mu g/mL$) loaded at flow rate of $2\,\mu L/min$ in the mobile phase A (12 mM ammonia formate with pH adjusted to 4.55 with glacial acetic acid) for 3.5 minutes. The elution of stepharine was carried out at flow rate of $0.3\,\mu L/min$ with the gradient of solvents A and B (acetonitrile) starting and maintained at 5% of mobile phase B for 2 minutes and increasing to 95% of solvent B at 20 minutes. Analytical column was washed with 100% of mobile phase B for 7 minutes followed by column equilibration at starting gradient conditions of solvent A-solvent B system (20 : 1, v/v) for 10 minutes. The 6520 Q-TOF mass spectrometer was operated in electrospray ionization at positive mode equipped with HPLC-Chip ion source interface at temperature 340°C. The drying gas (nitrogen) flow rate was 4 L/min, capillary voltage −1952 V, scan rate 3.225 scan/sec at 4 GHz mode, and scan range 100–700 m/z.

Quantitative analysis was acquired in SRM (selected reactions monitoring) mode on Agilent 6490 triple quadrupole mass spectrometer (Agilent, USA) operated in the positive mode and equipped with Jet Stream ESI ion source. Stepharine was detected in the scheduled selected reaction monitoring (SRM) with unit resolution at both first (Q1) and third (Q3) quadrupoles. The retention time point of stepharine was determined as 9.8 with isolation width of 1 minute for the scheduled SRM method application. The optimal conditions of the analysis were achieved as follows: capillary voltage was −4500 V, nozzle voltage was set at −1200 V, flow rate of drying gas (N_2) was 16 L/min, flow rate of sheath gas (N_2) was 8 L/min, temperature of drying gas was set at 340°C, temperature of sheath gas was set at 290°C, and nebulizer gas was operated at 20 psi. The transitions for protonated stepharine $[M+H]^+$ 298.4 → 161.2, 192.1, 238.2 were selected for SRM analysis. The isolation window for the fragment ions was set at 0.27 amu, the optimum fragmentor voltage was adjusted to 310 V and collision energy −19 eV. All the samples including calibration points were analyzed in three replications. 30 μL of the samples was injected and loaded on chromatographic column. Calibration was performed on standard samples solution prepared in 20% acetonitrile with concentration of stepharine from 10^{-4} $\mu g/mL$ to 100 $\mu g/mL$. Chromatographic separation was performed on Thermo Hypersil-Keystone ODS column (Thermo Scientific, USA) 100 × 2.1 mm, 5 μm particle size, at flow rate of 200 $\mu L/min$ and with the following elution conditions: loading onto the column at maintained 20% of mobile phase B for 3 minutes, increasing the gradient to 50% of B at 5 minutes following increasing the gradient to 100% of mobile phase B at 15 minutes. The column was washed and maintained at 100% mobile phase B from 15 to 22 minutes and the composition was decreased to 20% of solvent B at 23 minute. The column was reequilibrated at starting conditions of solvent A-solvent B system (5 : 1, v/v) for 10 minutes at flow 200 $\mu L/min$.

2.5. Preparation of the Standard Samples of the Stepharine and Determination of LOD and LOQ. The stock solution of stephaglabrine sulfate (1 mg/mL) was prepared by dissolving weighted reference compound in appropriate volume of water-acetonitrile 20% solution. Calibration standards in range of 100, 10, 1, 0.1, 0.01, 0.001, and 0.0001 μg/mL were prepared by dilution of the working solution (100 μg/mL) in of 20% acetonitrile to determine limit of detection (LOD), linearity, and limit of quantitation (LOQ). Each standard sample was analyzed in 10 replicates using developed scheduled SRM method. The fragment ion of stepharine with $m/z = 161.2$ was considered as ion quantifier, while fragment ions with $m/z = 192.1$ and $m/z = 238.2$ were considered as ion qualifiers. Calibration curve was plotted in linear regression fashion. Peaks with signal-to-noise ratio (SNR) more than 7.0 (calculated according to root-mean-square algorithm) and relative standard deviation (RSD) less than 15% were allowed to fit the calibration curve.

2.6. Extraction of Stepharine from Rabbit Plasma Samples.

0.5 mL of blood samples from each animal was collected from ear vein in the tubes with EDTA before administration and at 15, 30, 60, 90, 120, 180, 480, 720, and 1440 minutes after drug ingestion. Blood samples were immediately put on ice and centrifuged at 5000 g for 10 minutes at 4°C within one hour after blood collection. The obtained plasma was placed in sterile tube and kept at −20°C until analysis.

Plasma proteins were precipitated with acetonitrile. For this purpose, two volumes of acetonitrile were added to 100 μL of rabbit plasma into 1.5 mL plastic tube and 30% ammonia hydroxide was added to adjust the pH to 10. After vortex-mixing for 15 minutes at ambient temperature one volume of chloroform was added three times consequently for 2 hours and incubated at 30°C under regular stirring at 900 rpm at each occasion. The first fraction of upper organic layer was collected after 2 hours of incubation, the second and the third fractions of chloroform extract were collected after additional 30 and 60 minutes of incubation, respectively. The collected fractions were combined and transferred to a new tube and dried under vacuum at 30°C. The resulting pellet was resuspended in 100 μL of 20% water-acetonitrile solution and centrifuged at 14000 rpm for 15 minutes immediately before use. The obtained solution was used for LC-MS analysis.

2.7. Selectivity.

Selectivity was investigated on serum obtained from 5 different rabbits, which were not administrated with stephaglabrine sulfate (5 blank samples). Rabbit serum samples were treated as described for staphaglabrine sulfate extraction and analyzed in scheduled SRM mode in 10 replicates for possible interfering compounds. Selectivity was evaluated as confident if response level was less than 20% of summarized response of limit of detection and limit of quantitation.

2.8. Assessment of Matrix Effect and Extraction Efficiency.

Matrix effect was evaluated as ion suppression or ion enhancement. Matrix effect was investigated in plasma by measuring the peak intensities of stepharine in 5 different samples (100 μL) enriched with 0.03 μg/mL of stepharine by postextraction addition in five technical replicates. Samples

of rabbit plasma were treated as described for extraction procedure. The obtained organic solvent fractions were dried and resuspended in 100 μL of 20% acetonitrile-water solution. Stephaglabrine was spiked in matrix extracts to give final concentrations of 30 ng/mL and analyzed using scheduled SRM method. Matrtix effect of 15% was accepted. Peak areas of the compound of interest in matrixes with spiked stephaglabrine were compared with peak areas of stepharine of the same concentrations prepared in 20% acetonitrile. Matrix-influence factor f has been calculated as

$$f = \frac{A_{\text{add}} - A_{\text{end}}}{A_{\text{aq}}} \times 100, \tag{1}$$

where A_{add} is the peak area of the compound added in plasma, A_{end} the peak area of the endogenous compound, and A_{aq} the peak area of the standard compound in water-acetonitrile solution.

The recovery efficiency was evaluated in five different surrogate rabbit plasma samples. Each rabbit plasma was divided in three equal volumes of 100 μL. To one hundred μL of portion of rabbit plasma were added 3, 50, and 100 ng/mL of stepharine to final concentration. Plasma samples were treated with acetonitrile/chloroform solvent system for deproteinization. The resulting extract was dried and resuspended in 100 μL of 20% acetonitrile solution. The recovered amount of stepharine extracted from plasma was measured in 5 replicates. Recovery was estimated by comparison of peak areas of extracted stepharine and peak areas of stepharine measured in standard solutions with the same concentrations. The recovery was calculated according to the formula:

$$R\,(\%) = \frac{C_m}{C_a} \times 100, \tag{2}$$

where C_m is the measured concentration of stepharine after extraction; C_a is the known initial concentration of stephaglabrine added in rabbit plasma.

2.9. Sample Stability.

Freeze-thaw stability of stephaglabrine sulfate solution was evaluated because samples were stored at −20°C. The stability of stephaglabrine pool solutions (in water-acetonitrile 20%) at concentrations of 10 μg/mL, 50 μg/mL, and 100 μg/mL was evaluated after three cycles of overnight freezing following 3 hours of bench thaw at ambient temperature. The loss of stepharine was evaluated by comparison with freshly prepared standard solutions of the same concentrations. Loss of 10% and less was accepted.

2.10. Pharmacokinetics Model Design.

Calibration curve and pharmacokinetics parameters such as area under the plasma concentration-time curve (AUC) were estimated using trapeziodal method for the observed data and extrapolated to infinity from the last data point using the elimination constant (K_{el}); the values reported as the maximum plasma concentration (C_{max}) and the time corresponding to maximum plasma concentration (t_{max}) are the actual observed ones; the elimination constant (K_{el}) was calculated as the negative

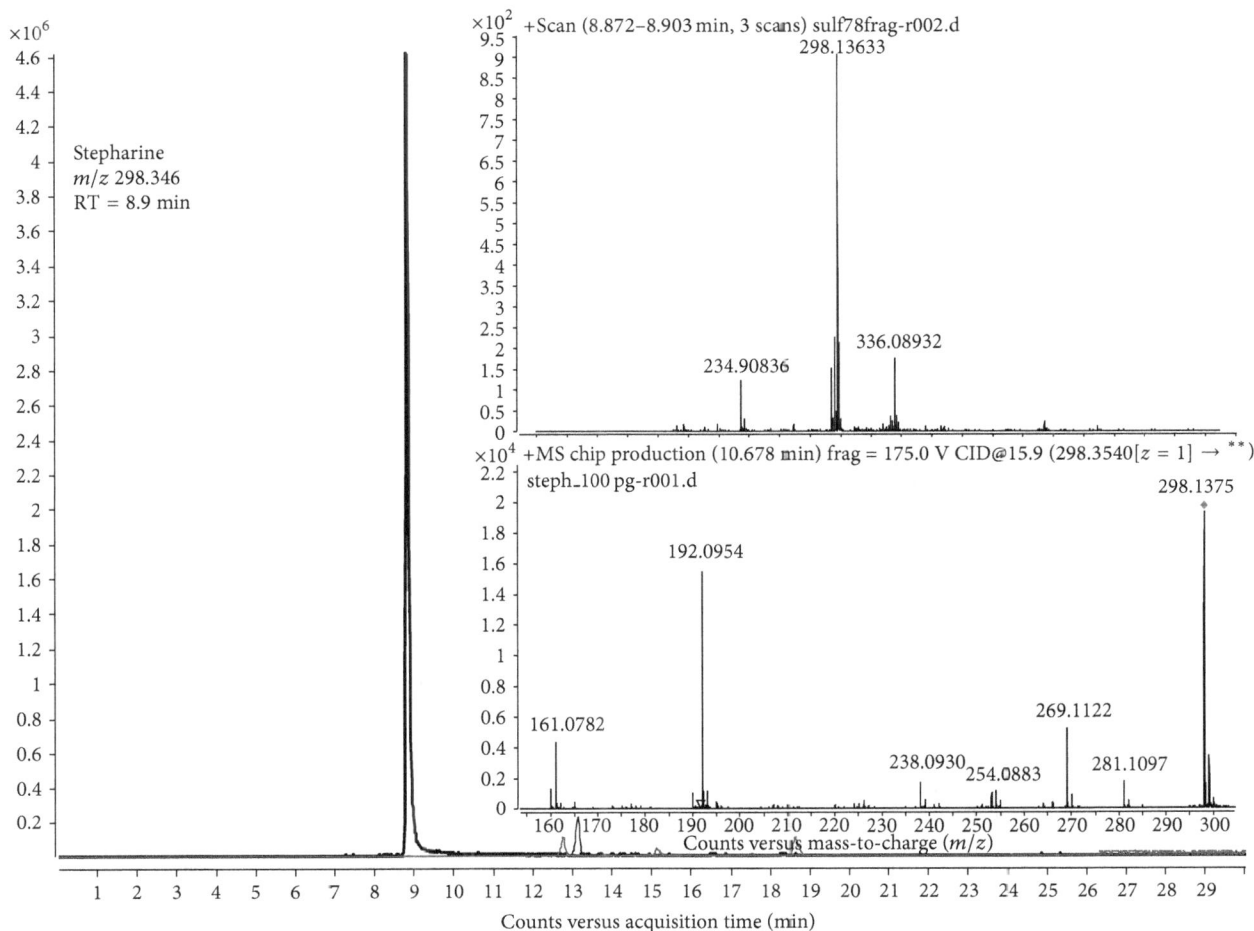

FIGURE 2: Extracted ion chromatography of stepharine ($m/z = 298.346$, retention time 8.9 minutes) precursor registered on high resolution Q-TOF mass spectrometer.

slope of the logarithmic-linear final portion of the plasma concentration-time curve by using linear regression. Half-time of absorption ($t_{1/2}$) was determined using elimination constant ($\ln(2)/K_{el}$). All the parameters were calculated in Mass Hunter Quantitative Analysis B03.02 (Agilent), Sigma Plot (version 9.0), and Microsoft Excel software

$$\int_{15}^{T_{max}} C_0 \left(1 - e^{-k_1 t}\right) dt + \int_{T_{max}}^{\infty} C_0 e^{-k_e t} dt$$

$$= C_0 \left[(T_{max} - 15) + \left(\frac{\left(e^{-k_1 T_{max}} - e^{-15 k_1}\right)}{k_1} \right) \right. \qquad (3)$$

$$\left. + \frac{e^{-k_{el} T_{max}}}{k_{el}} \right].$$

3. Results and Discussion

3.1. Method Development

3.1.1. Mass Spectrometry Determination of Stepharine. Stephaglabrine sulfate is well-known alkaloid compound

originated from plants substrates and represented as the dimeric salt of stepharine [3]. Chemical structure and properties of this molecule were mostly investigated by spectroscopy and spectrophotometry methods [2, 6]. Only a small portion of researches were accomplished using mass spectrometry analysis [7, 8] and no one reported considerate quantitative analysis of stepharine.

In this study the commercially available stephaglabrine sulfate was analyzed on a high resolution quadrupole time-of-flight mass spectrometer. The obtained data of 100 ng of the compound loaded onto the column demonstrates identification of protonated stepharine precursor ion [M+H]$^+$ with high accuracy mass measurements (error 2 ppm) and with $m/z = 298.346$ (Figure 2). The content of stepharine in sample makes a total of more than 97.5%, while the traced amount of 2.5% was assigned to auxiliary substances in the regions of 12.7, 15.2, and 18.7 minutes with $m/z = 234.909$, 284.183, and 279.153. At the certain chromatographic conditions the retention time point for stapharine was determined as 10.6 minutes.

Fragment ions spectra of stepharine were obtained for confident approval of the certain compound. Solvents adducts corresponding to [M+NH$_4$]$^+$ or [M+CH$_3$COO]$^+$

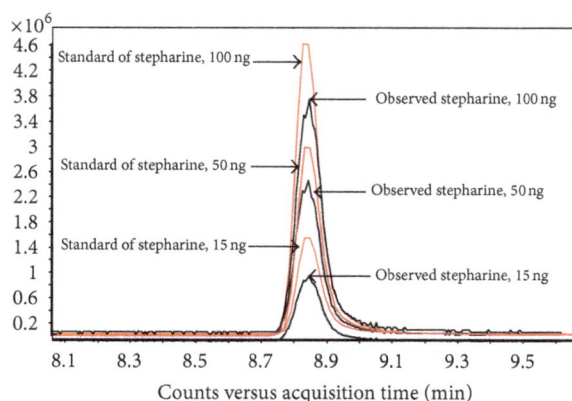

FIGURE 3: Comparison of peak areas of the spiked standard solutions of stepharine in amounts 15, 50, and 100 ng (solid lines) and observed amount of stepharine after extraction from rabbit plasma (dashed lines). The chromatograms demonstrate peaks of the most abundant fragment ion with $m/z = 161.2$.

TABLE 1: Stepharine extraction recovery from rabbit plasma using acetonitrile and methanol.

Extracting organic solvent	Concentration of stepharine in preextracted plasma, $\mu g/mL$	Postextraction recovery, % ± RSD
Acetonitrile	3	85.4 ± 5.2
	50	87.8 ± 3.3
	100	92.2 ± 3.7
Methanol	3	67.1 ± 4.7
	50	66.3 ± 6.1
	100	69.1 ± 4.9

*The results are averaged on five replicates ($n = 5$).

were not observed. Thus, as identity and purity of the obtained commercial compound were determined, we used it further to prepare standard calibration samples and injection form of stepharine for animals. Based on the obtained data of stepharine structure and its fragment ions behavior, the method of quantitative assay on triple quadrupole mass spectrometer was further developed.

3.1.2. Optimization and Validation of Stephaglabrine Extraction. Efficient extraction of stepharine from rabbit plasma needs to be applied for pharmacokinetic study. There is a little information related to isolation of stepharine from plant tissues and organs [3, 6, 9, 10]. Obviously, these protocols poorly fit the isolation procedure from animal tissues and liquids. In this research we have proposed deproteination of rabbit plasma using acetonitrile/chloroform solvents system highly alkalinized with ammonia hydroxide. To evaluate the recovery of stepharine after extraction, amount of stepharine was added to one hundred μL of rabbit plasma sample to give final concentrations of 3, 50, and 100 ng/mL. Prior assessment of the rabbit plasma was performed to find no interferences with the compound of interest. Stepharine was extracted and the recovery of the extract from rabbit plasma stepharine was evaluated on triple quadrupole mass spectrometer by comparison with peak area of spiked standard stepharine solutions (3, 50, and 100 ng/mL) (Figure 3).

Among several organic solvents which were tested (acetonitrile, methanol, hexane, and dichloromethane), acetonitrile has demonstrated the best recovery yielded at the level of 88.46 ± 4.07% in five replicates ($n = 5$) of each tested sample (Table 1).

As a result, the extracted compound was found as stepharine with $m/z = 298.34$ and charge state $z = 1+$. Efficiency of stepharine extraction in methanol solution with pH adjusted to 10 was appreciated at a close level of acetonitrile extraction and yielded 67.5 ± 5.23%. Treatment with dichloromethane and hexane as extracting solvents was depauperated and made mean recovery of 24.4 ± 6.3% (data not shown) which

is in consequence of low solubility of stepharine sulfate in highly nonpolar solvents. Thus, based on the successful yield we choose the alkalinized acetonitrile/chloroform solvents system for liquid extraction of stepharine from rabbit plasma. Matrix (rabbit plasma with spiked stepharine) was observed to have no significant ion suppressing effect and consisted of matrix-influence factor f in range from −0.07 to −0.09 with maximum RSD = 12.17% in three replicates among all matrix samples. Stability of stepharine demonstrates loss of less than 6% during over three freeze-thaw cycles and mean sample stability was estimated 94.6%.

3.1.3. Development of SRM for Stepharine Quantitative Analysis. Since the chromatographic conditions attributed to analysis on triple quadrupole LC-MS system have been changed as described in Section 2.4, the retention time of stepharine is also shifted and defined at 11.6 ± 0.3 minute. Combination of low pH maintained at 4.55 by addition of acetic acid in association with proton-capturing ammonium formate and rapid increasing the gradient to composition of water/acetonitrile with relatively strong hydrophobic properties caused best reproducibility, peak sharpness, and intensity of the stepharine chromatographic peak. Scheduled selected reactions monitoring (SRM) mode was used for stepharine detection on triple quadrupole which is allowed targeted scanning of stepharine compound. The precursor ion of stepharine compound with $m/z = 298.34$ and its fragment ions produced after collision-induced dissociation were monitored at the certain retention time (11.5 ± 1 minute) with narrow isolation width (±0.27 amu) in standard samples (solutions of stephaglabrine in acetonitrile) as well as after extraction from rabbit plasma. The collision energy at the level of −19 eV and fragmentor voltage at −310V were adjusted for the transitions ($298.34^{1+} \rightarrow 161.2^{1+}$, 192.1^{1+}, and 238.2^{1+}) to attain high sensitivity, reproducibility, and stability of the signal. Three fragment ions (161.2^{1+}, 192.1^{1+}, 238.2^{1+}) obtained from stepharine precursor ion with $m/z = 298.34^{1+}$ after collision-induced dissociation were recorded on triple quadrupole mass spectrometer for the quantitative analysis and pharmacokinetic characterization. Selection of the defined fragment ions was based on absence of solvent adducts, and SNR was exceeding 7.0 for all the fragment ions

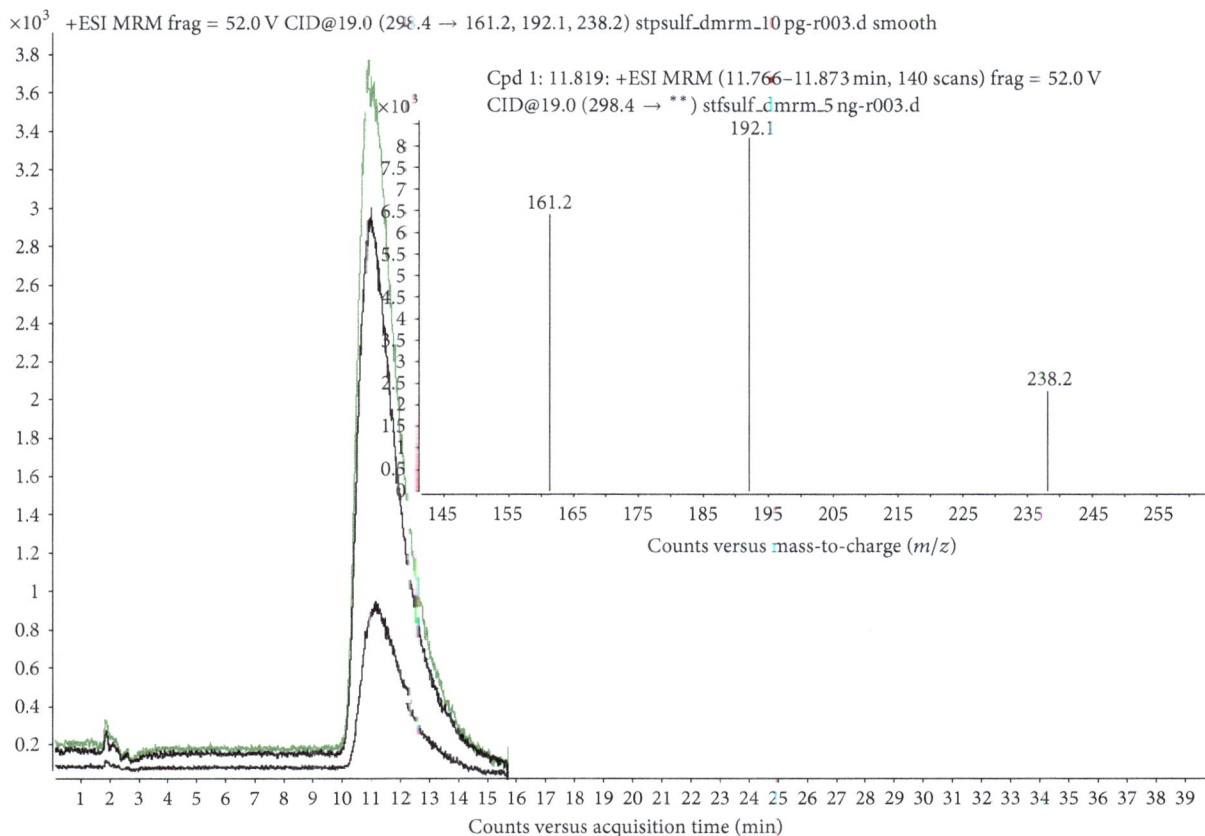

FIGURE 4: Extracted ion chromatogram (XIC) and SRM-spectrum of 10 pg of stepharine transitions $298.4^{1+} \rightarrow 161.2^{1+}, 192.1^{1+}, 238.2^{1+}$ registered in dynamic selected monitoring mode at the retention time 11.76 minutes.

and made 16.7, 12.1, and 13.3 for m/z 161.2, 192.1, and 238.2, respectively (Figure 4).

At the certain conditions, lowest limit of detection was obtained at the level of concentration 10^{-4} μg/mL. However, at the lowest limit of detection the RSD consisted of more than 27%: therefore we used concentration point of 0.001 μg/mL for quantitative analysis. Thus, a range of five orders of magnitude from 10^{-3} μg/mL to 100 μg/mL was considered for calibration curve plotting and the lowest limit of quantitation was attributed to 0.001 μg/mL with RSD of 2 39%.

Since no significant intercepts and curvatures were observed within the inspected concentration range, we applied linear model to fit the calibration curve. Heteroscedasticity was evaluated by comparison of covariance of the lowest (0.001 μg/mL) and the highest calibrators (100 μg/mL) and the best fit of linearity was achieved at weighting factor $1/x$. The achieved linearity of the dependence of peak area of stepharine on concentration in standard samples is demonstrated in Figure 5.

Each calibration point measurement was averaged on five replicates of each standard sample. The Pearson's correlation coefficient within this range was $r^2 = 0.99984$. Reproducibility of precursor peak area (RSD 9.3%, replicates $n = 5$, and concentration 0.001 μg/mL) was achieved while injecting stepharine onto the column equilibrated with 20% of mobile phase B (acetonitrile) and followed by a rapid increase of

acetonitrile to 50% which caused early elution of nonpolar compounds coextracting with stepharine from crude rabbit plasma extract. Quantitative assessment was accomplished with fragment ion $m/z = 161.2$, which was assigned as ion-quantifier.

The concentration of stepharine in rabbit plasma samples after intramuscular administration was determined using calibration curve plotted in linear regression fashion. Content of stepharine extracted from rabbit plasma was analyzed in five replicates of each sample before and after administration.

3.2. Pharmacokinetic Parameters of Stepharine Sulfate. Stephaglabrine sulfate affects the synaptic transmission and diminishes frequency of miniature endplate potential at low concentration [10]. It also inhibits cholinesterase and pseudocholinesterase in vitro [11] and possesses antihypertensive activity without side effects such as α- or β-adrenergic blockade, sedative or depressant effect. Pharmacokinetic parameters of stephaglabrine after intramuscular administration were determined. Animals were treated with stephaglabrine sulfate in dose of 0.1 mg/kg and 0.5 mL blood samples were collected subsequently before and after administration of drug as described in experimental section. Measurements of the stepharine in plasma were made immediately after extraction and utilized calibration curve extrapolated in the same testing day. The concentrations of stepharine measured

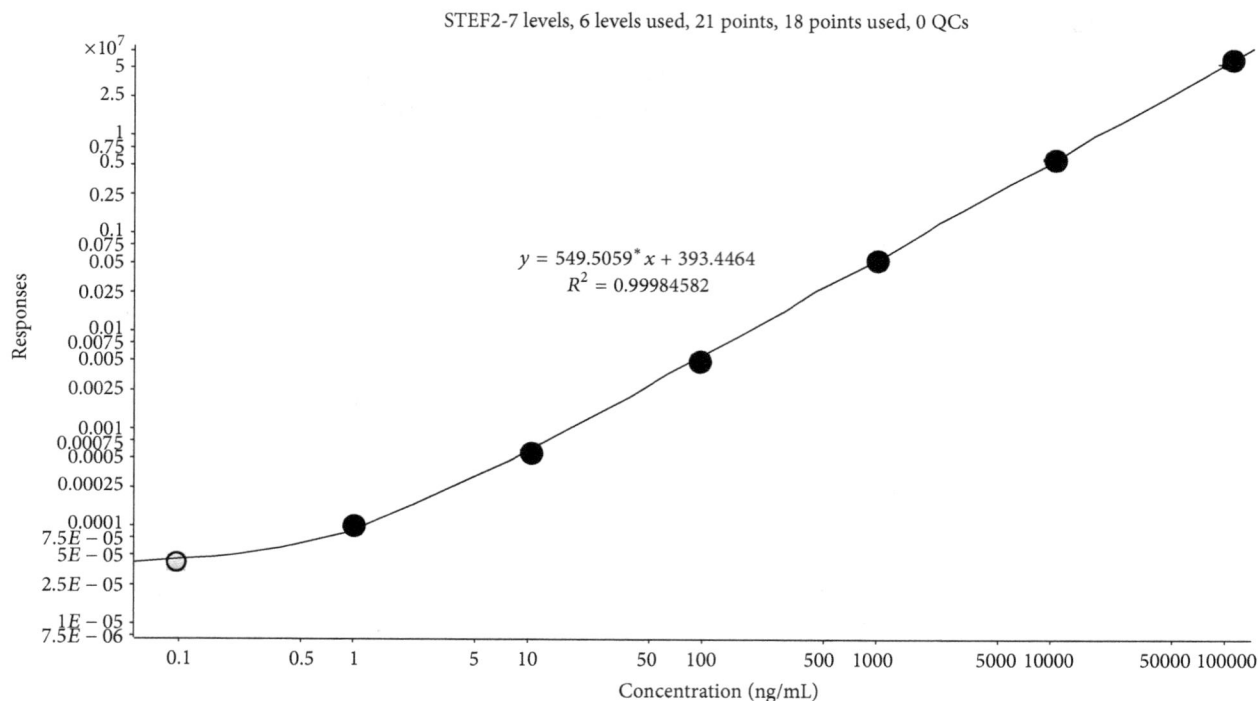

STEF2-7 levels, 6 levels used, 21 points, 18 points used, 0 QCs

$$y = 549.5059^* x + 393.4464$$
$$R^2 = 0.99984582$$

FIGURE 5: Calibration curve of stepharine plotted in the range of 100 pg/mL to 100 μg/mL. Calibration curve was weighted with $1/x$ factor and the correlation coefficient made $r^2 > 0.99$. Each data point averaged on three replicates.

TABLE 2: Concentration of stepharine in rabbit plasma after intramuscular administration*.

Time after administration, minutes	Animal internal ID					
	ST01	ST02	ST03	ST04	ST05	ST06
	Measured mean concentration of stephaglabrin in plasma, ng/mL					
0	0	0	0	0	0	0
15	8.1 ± 0.6	7.9 ± 0.2	6.8 ± 0.4	5.7 ± 0.2	6.3 ± 0.2	7.0 ± 0.3
30	9.4 ± 0.5	16.5 ± 0.8	14.8 ± 0.2	7.3 ± 0.3	12.7 ± 0.3	13.9 ± 0.2
60	10.0 ± 0.3	29.3 ± 2.2	19.5 ± 0.6	9.5 ± 0.5	18.5 ± 0.2	20.4 ± 0.2
90	13.9 ± 0.9	33.9 ± 2.8	20.4 ± 1.7	14.2 ± 0.2	21.2 ± 0.2	25.8 ± 0.1
120	5.8 ± 0.1	10.4 ± 0.5	6.5 ± 0.1	9.7 ± 0.2	5.1 ± 0.3	7.6 ± 0.09
180	3.8 ± 0.1	7.8 ± 0.3	n/a	2.8 ± 0.2	2.9 ± 0.07	3.3 ± 0.08
480	1.8 ± 0.02	1.2 ± 0.02	n/a	0.7 ± 0.01	1.4 ± 0.08	1.2 ± 0.08
720	1.5 ± 0.02	1.3 ± 0.01	n/a	0.6 ± 0.01	0.9 ± 0.04	0.7 ± 0.02
1440	0	0	n/a	0	0	0

*Measurements were made up by using calibration curve and averaged on five replicates.

in rabbit plasma at the defined time points are given in Table 2.

The effect of stephaglabrine injection on the rabbit plasma is demonstrated on the tracking time-concentration curves (Figure 6). The concentration-time curves show that plasma concentration of alkaloid varied more than 10-fold from the baseline. It should be noted that among all the studied animals stepharine varied in narrow concentration ranged from 5.7 to 8.1 ng/mL in first fifteen minutes after administration. The maximum concentration (C_{max}) of the drug was observed at 90 minutes in all cases. Registered

maximum concentration fluctuated in a few more wide limits: from 13.9 to 33.9 ng/mL that apparently related with the individual particularities of the animals. However, the minimum concentration of the substance was discovered through 12 hours in all analyzed cases.

The observed close values of elimination rate constants (K_{eq}) suggested the common mechanism of excretion. After 24 hours of intramuscular administration stepharine was not found in plasma samples. Thus, considering stated generality in maximum concentration reached and declination fashion one can assume that stepharine was rapidly cleared from

TABLE 3: Pharmacokinetic parameters of stephaglabrine in rabbit plasma samples after intramuscular injection.

Animal (ID)	Dosage, mg	C_{max}, ng/mL	T_{max}, min	K_1, min^{-1}	K_{el}, min^{-1}	$T_{1/2}$, min	C_0, ng/mL	AUC$_{15}$, ng*min/mL
ST01	0.50	13.9 ± 0.9	90	0.01	0.005	139	10.57	1661
ST02	0.50	33.9 ± 2.8	90	0.025	0.006	115	21.4	3187
ST03	0.45	20.4 ± 1.7	90	0.02	n/a	n/a	n/a	n/a
ST04	0.45	14.2 ± 0.2	90	0.013	0.007	99	22.5	2516
ST05	0.50	21.2 ± 0.2	90	0.02	0.006	118	15.3	2217
ST06	0.50	25.8 ± 0.1	90	0.023	0.007	121	17.1	2769

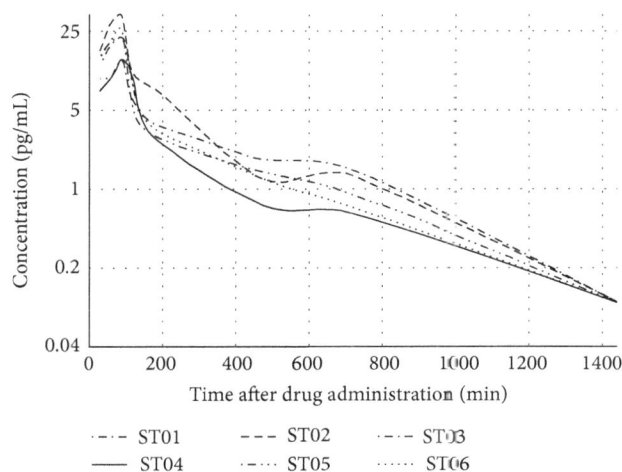

FIGURE 6: Concentration-time tracking curve of the observed in rabbit plasma stephaglabrine after intramuscular administration.

the body. The pharmacokinetic parameters of stephaglabrine sulfate are shown in Table 3.

Determination of the initial concentration (C_0) of stepharine in plasma showed that after intramuscular administration of stephaglabrine sulfate the absolute values may vary among the tested rabbits, which is probably caused by the individual particularities of the animals, in part, due to differences in absorption rate (K_1). The total body clearance (CL) was calculated as the ratio of injected dose to AUC$_{15 \to \infty}$ value and ranged from 118 to 226 mL/min in case complete stepharine absorption is assumed.

The estimated terminal phase half-life ($T_{1/2}$) ranged from 99 to 139 minutes. Half-life estimation is sensitive to the number of data points, as well as to the final point of time in the terminal stages. In part, half-life depends on the type of distribution throughout the body. Although, little is known about the metabolic pathways of stepharine, but an affinity of the drug to serum proteins can be assumed [12]. The apparent volume of stepharine distribution (estimated as ratio of clearance to elimination rate constant, data not shown) allows us to assume that stepharine was extensively distributed throughout the body.

4. Conclusion

In this research we have developed and validated highly sensitive liquid chromatography/tandem mass spectrometry

method for detection and quantization of stepharine in rabbit plasma after intramuscular administration and designed pharmacokinetic model. The extraction of stepharine from plasma samples was optimized and yielded more than 66% of stepharine. The identity of the parent drug extracted from plasma was confirmed by high resolution Q-TOF (quadrupole time-of-flight) and quantitative analysis was assessed by selected reactions monitoring on QQQ mass spectrometers by three characteristic transitions (298.4 → 161.2, 192.1, 238.2) of stepharine protonated precursor ion. Calibration curve of stepharine peak areas against its concentration was plotted in the range from 0.001 μg/mL to 100 μg/mL with standard deviation ±3%. The obtained pharmacokinetics data suggested that stepharine exhibits extensive distribution and rapidly cleared from the body.

Conflict of Interests

The authors declare that there is no conflict of interests regarding the publication of this paper.

References

[1] D. S. Bhakuni and S. Gupta, "The alkaloids of Stephania glabra," Journal of Natural Products, vol. 45, no. 4, pp. 407–411, 1982.

[2] M. Zhang, G. Liang, J. Yu, and W. Pan, "Aporphine alkaloids from the roots of Stephania viridiflavens," Natural Product Research, vol. 24, no. 13, pp. 1243–1247, 2010.

[3] W. Y. Huang, C. H. Su, and S. J. Sheu, "Separation and identification of the constituents in Fangchi Radix of different origins," Journal of Food and Drug Analysis, vol. 14, no. 4, pp. 357–367, 2006.

[4] J. Kuznecov, E. Arzamascev, and C. Malinovskaja, "Pharmacological properties and toxicologic characteristics of stefaglabrin sulphate," in Medicines Plant Origin in Modern Therapy, vol. 2, p. 71, 1989.

[5] I. I. Schelchkova, T. N. Il'inskaya, and A. D. Kuzovkov, "The alkaloids of Stephania glabra," Chemistry of Natural Compounds, vol. 1, no. 4, pp. 210–212, 1965.

[6] M. V. Titova, E. A. Berkovich, O. V. Reshetnyak, I. E. Kulichenko, A. V. Oreshnikov, and A. M. Nosov, "Respiration activity of suspension cell culture of Polyscias filicifolia bailey, Stephania glabra (Roxb.) miers, and Dioscorea deltoidea wall," Applied Biochemistry and Microbiology, vol. 47, no. 1, pp. 87–92, 2011.

[7] M. Tomita, A. Kato, T. Ibuka, H. Furukawa, and M. Kozuka, "Mass spectra of pronuciferine and stepharine," Tetrahedron Letters, vol. 6, no. 32, pp. 2825–2829, 1965.

[8] X. Dai, R. Hu, C. Sun, and Y. Pan, "Comprehensive separation and analysis of alkaloids from Stephania yunnanensis by counter-current chromatography coupled with liquid chromatography tandem mass spectrometry analysis," *Journal of Chromatography A*, vol. 1226, pp. 18–23, 2012.

[9] B. O. Sowemimo, J. L. Beal, R. W. Doskotch, and G. H. Svoboda, "The isolation of stepharine and coclaurine from Sarcopetalum harveyanum," *Lloydia*, vol. 35, no. 1, pp. 90–91, 1972.

[10] V. V. Bitkov, Z. M. Khashaev Kh., L. A. Pronevich, V. A. Nenashev, and S. G. Batrakov, "Effects of berberine, glaucine, stephaglabrine and sanguirythrine on the synaptic transmission," *Neirofiziologiya*, vol. 23, no. 2, pp. 131–135, 1991.

[11] V. V. Berezhinskaya, S. S. Nikittna, and E. A. Trutneva, "Medicinal plants pharmacology and chemotherapy," *Trudy Vsesoyuznogo Nauchno-Issledovatel'skogo Instituta Lekarstvenny Rastenii*, vol. 14, pp. 66–69, 1971.

[12] F. Q. Alali, X. X. Liu, and J. L. McLaughlin, "Annonaceous acetogenins: recent progress," *Journal of Natural Products*, vol. 62, no. 3, pp. 504–540, 1999.

15

Hemozoin Inhibition and Control of Clinical Malaria

Chibueze Peter Ihekwereme,[1] **Charles Okechukwu Esimone,**[2]
and Edward Chieke Nwanegbo[1]

[1] *Department of Pharmacology and Toxicology, Faculty of Pharmaceutical Sciences, Nnamdi Azikiwe University, Awka 420281, Nigeria*
[2] *Department of Pharmaceutical Microbiology and Biotechnology, Faculty of Pharmaceutical Sciences, Nnamdi Azikiwe University, Awka 420281, Nigeria*

Correspondence should be addressed to Chibueze Peter Ihekwereme; chibuezep@yahoo.com

Academic Editor: Steven Holladay

Malaria has a negative impact on health and social and economic life of residents of endemic countries. The ultimate goals of designing new treatment for malaria are to prevent clinical infection, reduce morbidity, and decrease mortality. There are great advances in the understanding of the parasite-host interaction through studies by various scientists. In some of these studies, attempts were made to evaluate the roles of malaria pigment or toxins in the pathogenesis of malaria. Hemozoin is a key metabolite associated with severe malaria anemia (SMA), immunosuppression, and cytokine dysfunction. Targeting of this pigment may be necessary in the design of new therapeutic products against malaria. In this review, the roles of hemozoin in the morbidity and mortality of malaria are highlighted as an essential target in the quest for effective control of clinical malaria.

1. Introduction

Malaria has plagued humankind since ancient times and is still a significant threat to half of the world's population [1]. Malaria is the fifth most common cause of death from infectious diseases worldwide (after respiratory infections, HIV/AIDS, diarrheal diseases, and tuberculosis) and the second in Africa, after HIV/AIDS [2]. Recent estimates show that as many as 3.3 billion people live in areas at risk of malaria in 109 countries or territories [3]. In addition to its health toll, malaria puts a heavy economic burden on endemic countries and contributes to the cycle of poverty people face in many countries. For example, it is estimated to have in Africa alone contemporaneous costs of at least US$12 billion per year in direct losses (e.g., illness, treatment, and premature death), but many times more than that in lost economic growth [4]. Malaria continues to be a major global health concern, with an estimated 243 million cases of malaria worldwide [5]. The vast majority of cases (85%) were in the African region, followed by Southeast Asia (10%) and Eastern Mediterranean regions (4%) [5]. Malaria accounted for an estimated 863 000 deaths in 2008 [5]. Malaria is a leading cause of child mortality in Africa, claiming a life nearly every 30 seconds [6]. Children are at highest risk for severe malarial illness and death during the first five years of life while their immune systems are developing [5]. Malaria causes anemia in pregnancy and is associated with a higher HIV-1 viral load in pregnant women [7, 8]. In Sub-Saharan Africa, *Plasmodium falciparum* is responsible for most cases of malaria.

The parasite's life cycle includes a cycle of asexual division in the human liver, another cycle of pigment-producing asexual division in red blood cells (RBCs), and a sporogenic development in the female anopheles mosquito. During the erythrocytic stage of development, the malaria parasite develops into a trophozoite form in a vacuole formed by the internal membrane of the host red cells. The trophozoite feeds on hemoglobin (Hb) by ingesting small amounts of red cell cytoplasm. The globin component is further digested into amino acids for the parasite's metabolic needs. However, heme is toxic to the parasite and is thus aggregated into the insoluble dark-brown crystal called hemozoin (Hz) which can accumulate in the parasitized red blood cell (pRBC). Both circulating and resident phagocytes acquire Hz through phagocytosis of pRBCs or free Hz crystals released after schizont rupture [9]. The presence of Hz disturbs normal cellular function and physiology of host whereas the parasite is less affected by it. The mechanism of inhibition of cellular function by Hz is thought to be the production of lipoperoxides from arachidonic acid [10, 11]. These compounds have been identified from Hz-fed macrophages and shown to inhibit macrophage function *in vitro* [12]. Furthermore, several studies have demonstrated that acquisition of malarial pigment by circulating monocytes and neutrophils is significantly associated with disease severity [13–16]. The Hz-monocyte complex has been associated with severe malaria anemia (SMA) [17], immunosuppression [9, 16], and cytokine dysregulation [18–20]. These findings demonstrate the pathological roles of Hz during malaria parasitaemia. However, recently researchers demonstrated that Hz may be an effective adjuvant for malaria vaccine [21–25]. This is because Hz was found to be a good ligand for Toll-like receptor 9 (TLR9) and induced both humoral and cellular immune responses in animals immunized with crude extract of Hz [21, 22].

Taken together, these findings suggest that Hz may be involved in both induction of immunity against malaria and the pathogenesis of the disease. In this brief review, we will evaluate reported roles of this pigment in the pathogenesis of malaria and provide the rationale for its targeting in antimalaria therapeutics development.

2. Hemozoin and Anemia

Structural abnormalities and extensive deposition of Hz were observed in the livers and bone marrows of children with SMA [26–28]. The abnormalities in these tissues indicate the pathological role of Hz in the development of SMA. Although there are many unexplained complex factors involved in the development of anemia during malaria infection, three mechanisms appear to be responsible for the problem, namely, direct destruction of infected red blood cells, increased destruction of unparasitized blood cells, and marrow suppression. Hz plays crucial roles in these three mechanisms.

2.1. Removal of Parasitized RBC. Anemia from *P. falciparum* malaria infection is usually responsible for severe morbidity and mortality in children and pregnant women in Sub-Saharan Africa. *P. falciparum* invades red cells of all ages [29] and digests Hb using parasite proteases [30] into small fragments consisting of about 20 different amino acids and free ferrous protoporphyrin IX, which is rapidly oxidized to heme [31]. Free toxic heme is rapidly oxidized to hematin and sequestered into inert, nontoxic crystalline Hz, which is present in the pRBC [32]. The presence of Hz in RBC results in appearance of antigenic molecules on membranes of these cells [33]. Recognition of Hz-containing RBC results in phagocytosis by circulating macrophages and removal from circulation. A study of the antigens exposed on the surface of pRBCs with different isolates of *P. falciparum* showed that the surface antigens could induce isolate-specific immunity [34]. Parasite-derived erythrocyte membrane protein

(PfEMP1) facilitates rosetting and mediates the binding of pRBC to endothelial cells [35]. In another study which described clinically relevant cytoadhesive phenotypes of *P. vivax* isolates, it was observed that the intensity of rosetting was higher among anaemic individuals compared to non-anaemic and decreased with increasing haematocrit and haemoglobin levels [36]. Consequently, the study concluded that rosetting may contribute to development of anaemia. Previous studies involving *P. falciparum* suggest that rosetting and cytoadhesion contribute to anaemia [37, 38]. In a study in Kenya, the presence of Hz-containing monocytes in children infected with *P. falciparum* was shown to be associated with SMA [17].

2.2. Hemolysis of Unparasitized RBC. Trophozoites in the RBC grow and develop into schizonts which rupture the cell releasing merozoites and free Hz into blood circulation [39]. Circulating free Hz released after rupture of the RBC may be deposited on unparasitized RBC and cause lipid peroxidation of RBC membranes resulting in loss of deformability of the cell [40–42]. This change in membrane predisposes unparasitized RBC to increased sequestration and lysis in the spleen and other reticuloendothelial organs. A study investigating the mechanisms behind the structural and functional effects of haem products on infected and uninfected red cells showed that hemolysis induced by haematin was dose and time dependent [41]. Since red cells preincubated with haematin were more sensitive to haemolysis induced by hypotonic shock, low pH, H_2O_2, or haematin itself, the study concludes that the destabilising effect of haem products (haematin and beta-haematin) on red cell membrane may not result from oxidative damage of membrane lipids but from direct binding or incorporation to membrane. Furthermore, direct binding or incorporation of haem products to npRBC membrane is expected to initiate immunological responses and phagocytosis of npRBC.

Another mechanism involves 4-hydroxynonenal (4-HNE). Rosetting is a specialized form of cytoadherence of late hemozoin-containing pRBCs to npRBCs [43]. The aldehyde 4-HNE is synthesized in the parasite when iron, present in Hz, peroxidizes polyunsaturated fatty acids [42]. Uyoga et al. (2012) having studied the role of transfer of 4-HNE from parasitized to nonparasitized erythrocytes in rosettes concluded that the transfer plays a role in the phagocytic removal of large numbers of npRBCs and may be key to the SMA found in malaria patients [43].

2.3. Marrow Suppression. Hz has also been associated with direct inhibition of reticulocyte formation [15, 44]. Previous autopsy investigation in children that died from severe malaria demonstrated large deposition of Hz in bone marrow suggesting direct inhibition of erythropoiesis [28]. In addition, dyserythropoietic changes, including multinuclear erythroblasts, karyorrhexis, incomplete and unequal amitotic nuclear divisions, and cytoplasmic bridging, were also noted by Abdalla and colleagues in children with SMA in 1980 [45]. Similarly, proinflammatory cytokines such as TNF-α have been shown to inhibit all stages of erythropoiesis [46, 47].

Hz increases the secretion of TNF-α in both human and animal malaria infection [48–50].

In all, Hz directly promotes SMA through enhancing increased hemolysis of RBC and inhibition of erythropoiesis. It also indirectly promotes SMA by triggering production of inflammatory cytokines such as TNF-α and nitric oxide (see below).

3. Hemozoin, Cytokine, and Chemokine Dysfunction

Previous investigations had shown that ingestion of Hz by monocytes may enhance malarial pathogenesis by causing dysregulation in the production of cytokines, chemokines, and effector molecules, including TNF-α, interleukin IL-12, IL-10, macrophage inflammatory protein (MIP)-1α, MIP-1β, nitric oxide (NO), and prostaglandin (PG)-E$_2$ [18–20, 33].

3.1. Tumor Necrosis Factor-Alpha. Systemic symptoms of malaria like fever occur after the rupture of malaria schizont [51, 52] and are caused by the release of proinflammatory cytokine TNF-α [35]. In both human and animal studies, Hz ingestion by mononuclear cells enhances production of TNF-α [48–50, 53] and nitric oxide [54, 55]. High systemic level of TNF-α is seen in acute *P. falciparum* malaria [56] and is believed to be protective by restricting parasitaemia [57]. However it also inhibits all stages of erythropoiesis and is associated with increased malaria pathogenesis [46, 58]. Similarly, inhibition of bone marrow and RBC destruction as a result of high TNF-α was reported in murine malaria [59, 60]. Higher TNF-α was also reported in fatal compared to nonfatal cerebral malaria in African children [61]. Similarly, higher TNF-α was seen in cerebral malaria compared to uncomplicated malaria [62]. In addition, elevated serum TNF-α level was associated with abortions [58, 63, 64]. Taken together, transient elevation of TNF may be beneficial since it enhances parasite clearance while sustained release of TNF in severe malaria is associated with increased malaria morbidity and perhaps mortality.

3.2. Nitric Oxide. Hz and pro-inflammatory cytokines including TNF-α increases the expression of nitric oxide synthase 2 (NOS$_2$) gene and generation of nitric oxide (NO). Initial high levels of NO appear to be protective against severe malaria [65, 66]. However sustained high levels are associated with *P. falciparum* malaria anemia in children [55] by inhibiting erythropoiesis [67, 68].

3.3. Prostaglandins. In children with acute malaria, plasma prostaglandin E$_2$ and COX-2 gene expression by PBMC are significantly reduced [69]. This is partly due to Hz ingested by PBMCs [70]. PGE$_2$ inhibits TNF-α [71] and appears to decrease malaria severity. It also enhances erythropoiesis by inducing burst forming unit erythroid formation [72]. Inhibitors of PGE$_2$ synthesis such as Hz, acetaminophen, and salicylates are associated with high levels of TNF-α and increased malaria severity and mortality [73–75]. In addition low circulating bicyclo-PG$_2$/TNF-α is associated

with decreased Hb concentration [55]. Hz has also been known to affect serum levels of IL-10 [33, 76] and IL-12 [77]. IL-10 may be increased in severe malaria while low IL-12 was also reported to be associated with increased malaria disease severity in children [13, 78].

In summary, Hz appears to trigger pathological levels of pro-inflammatory cytokines and chemokines like TNF-α, NO and at the same time reducing the level of more beneficial IL-12 and prostaglandin E$_2$. The role of anti-inflammatory cytokine IL-10 in malaria appears to enhance parasitemia since the Th1 immunological responses against the parasite are inhibited and IL-12 secretion is also suppressed by this cytokine. Taken together, Hz plays important role in deregulation of pro- and anti-inflammatory cytokines during malaria resulting in altered immunological responses to the disease, anemia, and host tissue damage.

4. Immunosuppression

Suppression of innate immune response during malaria infection has been reported in previous studies [9, 79]. One of the reported mechanisms is the suppression of dendritic cell (DC) function [33]. Dendritic cells play important roles in innate and adaptive immune responses. In contact with pathogen, these cells phagocytize the antigen, undergo a process of maturation, upregulate the requisite molecules and present to NK cells and naive and memory T and B lymphocytes. Ingestion of pRBC by DCs has been reported to impair the natural ability of DCs to stimulate both allogenic and antigen-specific T-cell immunity [80, 81]. This inhibition of DCs function is probably partially due to phagocytized Hz in pRBC. Moreover, Hz direct inhibition of DC maturation [33, 82] and suppression of general leucocytes proliferative responses [76] were also reported in previous studies. Similarly, ingestion of Hz by monocytes, macrophages, and neutrophils had been known to affect the functions of these cells resulting in defective phagocytosis and expression of MHC Class II, CD54, and CD11c [9, 79]. Specifically, decrease in IL-12 during malaria may be partly responsible for decreased immunity to the parasite. As mentioned above, low IL-12 has been associated with severe malaria infection in children [13, 78]. The derangement in the innate immune responses ultimately results in defective adaptive immune responses. As mentioned earlier, suppression of DC function is associated with failure of adequate priming and presentation of malaria antigens to CD4+ and CD8+ cells for appropriate Th1 and Th2 immune responses.

The suppression of immunity during malaria infection may be responsible for associated clinical problems. For instance, studies have demonstrated increased viral load in HIV patients [83] as a result of suppression of CD8+ function. Otieno et al. demonstrated increased SMA in HIV-1 positive infants and children in Kenya [84]. Also ineffective CD8+ function during malaria was linked to the association of Burkitt's lymphoma and endemic malaria [85, 86]. In addition, frequent association of bacteremia in children with clinical malaria was reported previously [87–89]. In all, presence of circulating malaria pigment in macrophages and neutrophils was associated with poor prognosis [90] or increased morbidity [91, 92].

On account of the global inhibition of innate and adaptive immune responses, Hz was described in previous studies as a potent immunosuppressant [93, 94]. However, these findings have been challenged by recent reports that demonstrated the potent immunogenicity of crude extract of Hz. These studies reported that Hz is an effective TLR9 ligand and can enhance immunity against malaria [50, 95].

5. Other Harmful Effects of Hemozoin

A number of harmful effects have been documented or associated with Hz. Hz compromises the functions of human monocytes, as previously noted, and this dysfunction has been related to its lipoperoxidation products, namely, 15-hydroxyeicosatetraenoic acid (15-HETE) and 4-HNE [96]. Hz has also been associated with malaria-associated acute respiratory distress syndrome (MA-ARDS). By quantifying Hz in the lungs and measuring the disease parameters of MA-ARDS, a highly significant correlation between pulmonary Hz concentrations, lung weights, and alveolar edema was demonstrated [97]. Another study has shown that Hz is implicated in cerebral malaria since it modulates matrix metalloproteinases and induces morphological changes in human microvascular endothelium [98]. Histological examination in the study revealed that human microvascular endothelial cell line (HMEC-1) treated with natural Hz appeared elongated instead of polygonal and formed microtubule-like vessels on synthetic basement membrane.

6. Summary

One of the factors responsible for malaria pathogenesis is the suppression of host immune responses. This suppression enhances parasitemia and diminishes the host immune response to malaria-expressed proteins and other pathogens. Hz plays both direct and indirect roles in orchestrating this immunosuppression which may be important for the survival of the parasite and completion of its life cycle in the human host [99]. Blocking of Hz formation will ultimately increase immune mediated parasite clearance and can prevent formation and transmission of the gametocytes. The host can also maintain immunological surveillance to other pathogens. Development of new chemotherapeutic agents that will prevent the formation of the pigment in pRBC may greatly reduce morbidity associated with malaria. Association of Hz and SMA has been demonstrated in several previous studies (see above).

Use of agents that will prevent formation of the pigment will prevent Hz-induced inhibition of erythroid precursors and also reduce the production of other mediators of SMA. Chloroquine, quinine, and artemisinin block the formation of Hz from heme [21, 22, 95]. Perhaps, reduction of morbidity and mortality with these drugs may be attributable to decreased circulating levels of Hz. In developing countries where malaria is endemic, effective targeting of Hz may greatly reduce high morbidity and mortality presently associated with the disease. In this regard, development of new therapeutics that will block formation of Hz by the parasite will be necessary. Modification of quinine, chloroquine, or artemether to overcome parasite resistance may also achieve the same goal. Furthermore, it may be important to investigate the prevalence of anti-Hz immunity in healthy, mild, and severe malaria in people living in malaria endemic regions. Similarly, evaluation of crude extract of Hz as an adjuvant for human application requires further studies. This may provide the rationale for the inclusion of Hz as a component of candidate malaria vaccines. The applications of these potential Hz targeting measures warrant further studies.

Conflict of Interests

The authors have neither financial issues nor conflict of interests to disclose.

References

[1] Roll Back Malaria, "Global malaria action plan," Roll Back Malaria, 2008, http://rbm.who.int/gmap/gmap.pdf.

[2] World Health Organisation, Global Burden of Disease Estimates, World Health Organisation, Geneva, Switzerland, 2002.

[3] World Health Organization, World Malaria Report, World Health Organization, Geneva, Switzerland, 2008.

[4] J. L. Gallup and J. D. Sachs, "The economic burden of malaria," American Journal of Tropical Medicine and Hygiene, vol. 64, no. 1-2, pp. 85–96, 2001.

[5] World Health Organization, World Malaria Report, World Health Organization, Geneva, Switzerland, 2009.

[6] R. W. Snow, M. Craig, U. Deichmann, and K. Marsh, "Estimating mortality, morbidity and disability due to malaria among Africa's non-pregnant population," Bulletin of the World Health Organization, vol. 77, no. 8, pp. 624–640, 1999.

[7] L. Molineaux, "Malaria and mortality: some epidemiological considerations," Annals of Tropical Medicine and Parasitology, vol. 91, no. 7, pp. 811–825, 1997.

[8] J. A. G. Whitworth and K. A. Hewitt, "Effect of malaria on HIV-1 progression and transmission," The Lancet, vol. 365, no. 9455, pp. 196–197, 2005.

[9] E. Schwarzer, F. Turrini, D. Ulliers, G. Giribaldi, H. Ginsburg, and P. Arese, "Impairment of macrophage functions after ingestion of Plasmodium falciparum-infected erythrocytes or isolated malarial pigment," The Journal of Experimental Medicine, vol. 176, no. 4, pp. 1033–1041, 1992.

[10] E. Schwarzer, P. Ludwig, E. Valente, and P. Arese, "15(S)-hydroxyeicosatetraenoic acid (15-HETE), a product of arachidonic acid peroxidation, is an active component of hemozoin toxicity to monocytes," Parassitologia, vol. 41, no. 1–3, pp. 199–202, 1999.

[11] E. Schwarzer, O. Müller, P. Arese, W. G. Siems, and T. Grune, "Increased levels of 4-hydroxynonenal in human monocytes fed with malarial pigment hemozoin. A possible clue for hemozoin toxicity," FEBS Letters, vol. 388, no. 2-3, pp. 119–122, 1996.

[12] B. C. Urban and D. J. Roberts, "Malaria, monocytes, macrophages and myeloid dendritic cells: sticking of infected erythrocytes switches off host cells," Current Opinion in Immunology, vol. 14, no. 4, pp. 458–465, 2002.

[13] A. J. F. Luty, D. J. Perkins, B. Lell et al., "Low interleukin-12 activity in severe *Plasmodium falciparum* malaria," *Infection and Immunity*, vol. 68, no. 7, pp. 3909–3915, 2000.

[14] K. E. Lyke, D. A. Diallo, A. Dicko et al., "Association of intraleukocytic *Plasmodium falciparum* malaria pigment with disease severity, clinical manifestations, and prognosis in severe malaria," *The American Journal of Tropical Medicine and Hygiene*, vol. 69, no. 3, pp. 253–259, 2003.

[15] C. Casals-Pascual, O. Kai, J. O. P. Cheung et al., "Suppression of erythropoiesis in malarial anemia is associated with hemozoin in vitro and in vivo," *Blood*, vol. 108, no. 8, pp. 2569–2577, 2006.

[16] P. Arese and E. Schwarzer, "Malarial pigment (haemozoin): a very active "inert" substance," *Annals of Tropical Medicine and Parasitology*, vol. 91, no. 5, pp. 501–516, 1997.

[17] E. M. Novelli, J. B. Hittner, G. C. Davenport et al., "Clinical predictors of severe malarial anaemia in a holoendemic *Plasmodium falciparum* transmission area: research paper," *British Journal of Haematology*, vol. 149, no. 5, pp. 711–721, 2010.

[18] D. O. Ochiel, G. A. Awandare, C. C. Keller et al., "Differential regulation of β-chemokines in children with *Plasmodium falciparum* malaria," *Infection and Immunity*, vol. 73, no. 7, pp. 4190–4197, 2005.

[19] C. C. Keller, G. C. Davenport, K. R. Dickman et al., "Suppression of prostaglandin E2 by malaria parasite products and antipyretics promotes overproduction of tumor necrosis factor-α: association with the pathogenesis of childhood malarial anemia," *Journal of Infectious Diseases*, vol. 193, no. 10, pp. 1384–1393, 2006.

[20] C. C. Keller, O. Yamo, C. Ouma et al., "Acquisition of hemozoin by monocytes down-regulates interleukin-12 p40 (IL-12p40) transcripts and circulating IL-12p70 through an IL-10-dependent mechanism: in vivo and in vitro findings in severe malarial anemia," *Infection and Immunity*, vol. 74, no. 9, pp. 5249–5260, 2006.

[21] C. Coban, M. Yagi, K. Ohata et al., "The malarial metabolite hemozoin and its potential use as a vaccine adjuvant," *Allergology International*, vol. 59, no. 2, pp. 115–124, 2010.

[22] H. Wagner, "Hemozoin: malaria's "built-In" adjuvant and TLR9 agonist," *Cell Host and Microbe*, vol. 7, no. 1, pp. 5–6, 2010.

[23] M. Jaramillo, M.-J. Bellemare, C. Martel et al., "Synthetic Plasmodium-like hemozoin activates the immune response: a morphology—function study," *PLoS ONE*, vol. 4, no. 9, Article ID e6957, 2009.

[24] C.-C. Hou, M. J. Day, T. J. Nuttall, and P. B. Hill, "Evaluation of IgG subclass responses against Dermatophagoides farinae allergens in healthy and atopic dogs," *Veterinary Dermatology*, vol. 17, no. 2, pp. 103–110, 2006.

[25] C. Coban, K. J. Ishii, D. J. Sullivan, and N. Kumar, "Purified malaria pigment (hemozoin) enhances dendritic cell maturation and modulates the isotype of antibodies induced by a DNA vaccine," *Infection and Immunity*, vol. 70, no. 7, pp. 3939–3943, 2002.

[26] S. H. Abdalla, "Hematopoiesis in human malaria," *Blood Cells*, vol. 16, no. 2-3, pp. 401–416, 1990.

[27] S. N. Wickramasinghe and S. H. Abdalla, "Blood and bone marrow changes in malaria," *Bailliere's Best Practice and Research in Clinical Haematology*, vol. 13, no. 2, pp. 277–299, 2000.

[28] G. Giribaldi, D. Ulliers, E. Schwarzer, I. Roberts, W. Piacibello, and P. Arese, "Hemozoin- and 4-hydroxynonenal-mediated inhibition of erythropoiesis. Possible role in malarial dyserythropoiesis and anemia," *Haematologica*, vol. 89, no. 4, pp. 492–493, 2004.

[29] P. A. Tamez, H. Liu, S. Fernandez-Pol, K. Haldar, and A. Wickrema, "Stage-specific susceptibility of human erythroblasts to Plasmodium falciparum malaria infection," *Blood*, vol. 114, no. 17, pp. 3652–3655, 2009.

[30] R. Banerjee, J. Liu, W. Beatty, L. Pelosof, M. Klemba, and D. E. Goldberg, "Four plasmepsins are active in the Plasmodium falciparum food vacuole, including a protease with an active-site histidine," *Proceedings of the National Academy of Sciences of the United States of America*, vol. 99, no. 2, pp. 990–995, 2002.

[31] N. T. Huy, Y. Shima, A. Maeda et al., "Phospholipid membrane-mediated hemozoin formation: the effects of physical properties and evidence of membrane surrounding hemozoin," *PLoS One*, vol. 8, no 7, 2013.

[32] A. K. Tripathi, S. K. Garg, and B. L. Tekwani, "A physiochemical mechanism of hemozoin (β-hematin) synthesis by malaria parasite," *Biochemical and Biophysical Research Communications*, vol. 290, no. 1, pp. 595–601, 2002.

[33] P. Giusti, B. C. Urban, G. Frascaroli et al., "Plasmodium falciparum-Infected erythrocytes and β-hematin induce partial maturation of human dendritic cells and increase their migratory ability in response to lymphoid chemokines," *Infection and Immunity*, vol. 79, no. 7, pp. 2727–2736, 2011.

[34] N. Kalantari and S. Ghaffari, "Identification and characterization of the antigens expressed on the surface of human erythrocytes infected with *Plasmodium falciparum*," *Iranian Journal of Parasitology*, vol. 8, no. 2, pp. 197–206, 2013.

[35] J. Alexandra Rowe, J. M. Moulds, C. I. Newbold, and L. H. Miller, "*P. falciparum* rosetting mediated by a parasite-variant erythrocyte membrane protein and complement-receptor 1," *Nature*, vol. 388, no. 6639, pp. 292–295, 1997.

[36] A. Marín-Menéndez, A. Bardají, F. E. Martínez-Espinosa et al., "Rosetting in *Plasmodium vivax*: a cytoadhesion phenotype associated with anaemia," *PLOS Neglected Tropical Diseases*, vol. 7, no. 4, 2013.

[37] A. Mayor, A. Hafiz, Q. Bassat et al., "Association of severe malaria outcomes with platelet-mediated clumping and adhesion to a novel host receptor," *PLoS ONE*, vol. 6, no. 4, Article ID e19422, 2011.

[38] J. A. Rowe, J. Shafi, O. K. Kai, K. Marsh, and A. Raza, "Non-immune IgM but not IgG binds to the surface of *Plasmodium falciparum*-infected erythrocytes and correlates with rosetting and severe malaria," *American Journal of Tropical Medicine and Hygiene*, vol. 66, no. 6, pp. 692–699, 2002.

[39] R. Stiebler, J. B. R. C. Soares, B. L. Timm et al., "On the mechanisms involved in biological heme crystallization," *Journal of Bioenergetics and Biomembranes*, vol. 43, no. 1, pp. 93–99, 2011.

[40] K. Mohan, M. L. Dubey, N. K. Ganguly, and R. C. Mahajan, "*Plasmodium falciparum*: role of activated blood monocytes in erythrocyte membrane damage and red cell loss during malaria," *Experimental Parasitology*, vol. 80, no. 1, pp. 54–63, 1995.

[41] F. Omodeo-Salè, A. Motti, A. Dondorp, N. J. White, and D. Taramelli, "Destabilisation and subsequent lysis of human erythrocytes induced by *Plasmodium falciparum* haem products," *European Journal of Haematology*, vol. 74, no. 4, pp. 324–332, 2005.

[42] O. A. Skorokhod, L. Caione, T. Marrocco et al., "Inhibition of erythropoiesis in malaria anemia: role of hemozoin and hemozoin-generated 4-hydroxynonenal," *Blood*, vol. 116, no. 20, pp. 4328–4337, 2010.

[43] S. Uyoga, O. A. Skorokhod, M. Opiyo et al., "Transfer of 4-hydroxynonenal from parasitized to non-parasitized erythrocytes in rosettes. Proposed role in severe malaria anemia," *British Journal of Haematology*, vol. 157, no. 1, pp. 116–124, 2012.

[44] A. A. Lamikanra, M. Theron, T. W. Kooij, and D. J. Roberts, "Hemozoin (malarial pigment) directly promotes apoptosis of erythroid precursors," *PLoS One*, vol. 4, no. 12, Article ID e8446, 2009.

[45] S. Abdalla, D. J. Weatherall, S. N. Wickramasinghe, and M. Hughes, "The anaemia of P. falciparum malaria," *British Journal of Haematology*, vol. 46, no. 2, pp. 171–183, 1980.

[46] C. Dufour, A. Corcione, J. Svahn et al., "TNF-alpha and IFN-gamma are overexpressed in the bone marrow of Fanconi anemia patients and TNF-alpha suppresses erythropoiesis in vitro," *Blood*, vol. 102, no. 6, pp. 2053–2059, 2003.

[47] C. Grigorakaki, F. Morceau, S. Chateauvieux, M. Dicato, and M. Diederich, "Tumor necrosis factor alpha-mediated inhibition of erythropoiesis involves GATA-1/GATA-2 balance impairment and PU. 1 over-expression," *Biochemical Pharmacology*, vol. 82, no. 2, pp. 156–166, 2011.

[48] B. Mordmüller, F. Turrini, H. Long, P. G. Kremsner, and P. Arese, "Neutrophils and monocytes from subjects with the Mediterranean G6PD variant: effect of Plasmodium falciparum hemozoin on G6PD activity, oxidative burst and cytokine production," *European Cytokine Network*, vol. 9, no. 3, pp. 239–245, 1998.

[49] S. Biswas, M. Karmarkar, and Y. Sharma, "Antibodies detected against Plasmodium falciparum haemozoin with inhibitory properties to cytokine production," *FEMS Microbiology Letters*, vol. 194, no. 2, pp. 175–179, 2001.

[50] C. Coban, K. Ishii, T. Kawai et al., "Toll-like receptor 9 mediates innate immune activation by the malaria pigment hemozoin," *The Journal of Experimental Medicine*, vol. 201, no. 1, pp. 19–25, 2005.

[51] D. Kwiatkowski, J. G. Cannon, K. R. Manogue, A. Cerami, C. A. Dinarello, and B. M. Greenwood, "Tumour necrosis factor production in Falciparum malaria and its association with schizont rupture," *Clinical and Experimental Immunology*, vol. 77, no. 3, pp. 361–366, 1989.

[52] D. Kwiatkowski and P. Perlman, *Inflammatory Processes in the Pathogenesis of Malaria*, Harwood Academic Publishers, 1999.

[53] B. A. Sherry, G. Alava, K. J. Tracey, J. Martiney, A. Cerami, and A. F. G. Slater, "Malaria-specific metabolite hemozoin mediates the release of several potent endogenous pyrogens (TNF, MIP-1α, and MIP-1β) in vitro, and altered thermoregulation in vivo," *Journal of Inflammation*, vol. 45, no. 2, pp. 85–96, 1995.

[54] M. Jaramillo, D. C. Gowda, D. Radzioch, and M. Olivier, "Hemozoin increases IFN-γ-inducible macrophage nitric oxide generation through extracellular signal-regulated kinase- and NF-κB-dependent pathways," *Journal of Immunology*, vol. 171, no. 8, pp. 4243–4253, 2003.

[55] C. C. Keller, P. G. Kremsner, J. B. Hittner, M. A. Misukonis, J. B. Weinberg, and D. J. Perkins, "Elevated nitric oxide production in children with malarial anemia: hemozoin-induced nitric oxide synthase type 2 transcripts and nitric oxide in blood mononuclear cells," *Infection and Immunity*, vol. 72, no. 8, pp. 4868–4873, 2004.

[56] M. Odeh, "The role of tumour necrosis factor-α in the pathogenesis of complicated Falciparum malaria," *Cytokine*, vol. 14, no. 1, pp. 11–18, 2001.

[57] P. G. Kremsner, S. Winkler, C. Brandts et al., "Prediction of accelerated cure in Plasmodium falciparum malaria by the elevated capacity of tumor necrosis factor production," *American Journal of Tropical Medicine and Hygiene*, vol. 53, no. 5, pp. 532–538, 1995.

[58] I. A. Clark and G. Chaudhri, "The balance of useful and harmful effects of TNF, with special reference to malaria," *Annales de l'Institut Pasteur. Immunologie*, vol. 139, no. 3, pp. 305–306, 1988.

[59] J. Taverne, N. Sheikh, J. B. de Souza, J. H. L. Playfair, L. Probert, and G. Kollias, "Anaemia and resistance to malaria in transgenic mice expressing human tumour necrosis factor," *Immunology*, vol. 82, no. 3, pp. 397–403, 1994.

[60] I. A. Clark and G. Chaudhri, "Tumour necrosis factor may contribute to the anaemia of malaria by causing dyserythropoiesis and erythrophagocytosis," *British Journal of Haematology*, vol. 70, no. 1, pp. 99–103, 1988.

[61] G. E. Grau, P.-F. Piquet, P. Vassalli, and P.-H. Lambert, "Tumor-necrosis factor and other cytokines in cerebral malaria: experimental and clinical data," *Immunological Reviews*, no. 112, pp. 49–70, 1989.

[62] D. Kwiatkowski, A. V. S. Hill, I. Sambou et al., "TNF concentration in fatal cerebral, non-fatal cerebral, and uncomplicated *Plasmodium falciparum* malaria," *The Lancet*, vol. 336, no. 8725, pp. 1201–1204, 1990.

[63] G. Entrican, "Immune regulation during pregnancy and host-pathogen interactions in infectious abortion," *Journal of Comparative Pathology*, vol. 126, no. 2-3, pp. 79–94, 2002.

[64] N. Y. Kim, H. J. Cho, H. Y. Kim et al., "Thyroid autoimmunity and its association with cellular and humoral immunity in women with reproductive failures," *American Journal of Reproductive Immunology*, vol. 65, no. 1, pp. 78–87, 2011.

[65] D. J. Perkins, P. G. Kremsner, D. Schmid, M. A. Misukonis, M. A. Kelly, and J. B. Weinberg, "Blood mononuclear cell nitric oxide production and plasma cytokine levels in healthy gabonese children with prior mild or severe malaria," *Infection and Immunity*, vol. 67, no. 9, pp. 4977–4981, 1999.

[66] J. F. Kun, B. Mordmüller, D. J. Perkins et al., "Nitric oxide synthase 2Lambaréné (G-954C), increased nitric oxide production, and protection against malaria," *Journal of Infectious Diseases*, vol. 184, no. 3, pp. 330–336, 2001.

[67] P. J. Shami and J. B. Weinberg, "Differential effects of nitric oxide on erythroid and myeloid colony growth from CD34+ human bone marrow cells," *Blood*, vol. 87, no. 3, pp. 977–982, 1996.

[68] S. Reykdal, C. Abboud, and J. Liesveld, "Effect of nitric oxide production and oxygen tension on progenitor preservation in ex vivo culture," *Experimental Hematology*, vol. 27, no. 3, pp. 441–450, 1999.

[69] D. J. Perkins, P. G. Kremsner, and J. Brice Weinberg, "Inverse relationship of plasma prostaglandin E2 and blood mononuclear cell cyclooxygenase-2 with disease severity in children with Plasmodium falciparum malaria," *Journal of Infectious Diseases*, vol. 183, no. 1, pp. 113–118, 2001.

[70] C. C. Keller, J. B. Hittner, B. K. Nti, J. B. Weinberg, P. G. Kremsner, and D. J. Perkins, "Reduced peripheral PGE2 biosynthesis in *Plasmodium falciparum malaria* occurs through hemozoin-induced suppression of blood mononuclear cell cyclooxygenase-2 gene expression via an interleukin-10-independent mechanism," *Molecular Medicine*, vol. 10, no. 1–6, pp. 45–54, 2004.

[71] S. L. Kunkel, M. Spengler, M. A. May, R. Spengler, J. Larrick, and D. Remick, "Prostaglandin E2 regulates macrophage-derived

tumor necrosis factor gene expression," *The Journal of Biological Chemistry*, vol. 263, no. 11, pp. 5380–5384, 1988.

[72] F. Dupuis, N. Gachard, A. Allegraud, C. Du ery, V. Praloran, and Y. Denizot, "Effect of platelet-activating factor on the growth of human erythroid and myeloid CD34+ progenitors," *Mediators of Inflammation*, vol. 7, no. 2, pp. 99–103, 1998.

[73] M. English, V. Marsh, E. Amukoye, B. Lowe, S. Murphy, and K. Marsh, "Chronic salicylate poisoning and severe malaria," *The Lancet*, vol. 347, no. 9017, pp. 1736–1737, 1996.

[74] H. J. Ball, H. G. MacDougall, I. S. McGregor, and N. H. Hunt, "Cyclooxygenase-2 in the pathogenesis of murine cerebral malaria," *Journal of Infectious Diseases*, vol. 189, no. 4, pp. 751–758, 2004.

[75] L. Xiao, P. S. Patterson, C. Yang, and A. A. Lal, "Role of eicosanoids in the pathogenesis of murine cerebral malaria," *American Journal of Tropical Medicine and Hygiene*, vol. 60, no. 4, pp. 668–673, 1999.

[76] P. Deshpande and P. Shastry, "Modulation of cytokine profiles by malaria pigment—Hemozoin: role of IL-10 in suppression of proliferative responses of mitogen stimulated human PBMC," *Cytokine*, vol. 28, no. 6, pp. 205–213, 2004.

[77] M. Cambos, S. Bazinet, E. Abed et al., "The IL-12p70/IL-10 interplay is differentially regulated by free heme and hemozoin in murine bone-marrow-derived macrophages," *International Journal for Parasitology*, vol. 40, no. 9, pp. 1003–1012, 2010.

[78] D. J. Perkins, J. B. Weinberg, and P. G. Kremsner, "Reduced interleukin-12 and transforming growth factor-β1 in severe childhood malaria: relationship of cytokine balance with disease severity," *Journal of Infectious Diseases*, vol. 182, no. 3, pp. 988–992, 2000.

[79] E. Schwarzer, H. Kühn, E. Valente, and P. Arese, "Malaria-parasitized erythrocytes and hemozoin nonenzymatically generate large amounts of hydroxy fatty acids that inhibit monocyte functions," *Blood*, vol. 101, no. 2, pp. 722–723, 2003.

[80] B. C. Urban, D. J. P. Ferguson, A. Pain et al., "Plasmodium falciparuminfected erythrocytes modulate the maturation of dendritic cells," *Nature*, vol. 400, no. 6739, pp. 73–77, 1999.

[81] M. F. Good and D. L. Doolan, "Immune effector mechanisms in malaria," *Current Opinion in Immunology*, vol. 11, no. 4, pp. 412–419, 1999.

[82] O. A. Skorokhod, M. Alessio, B. Mordmüller, P. Arese, and E. Schwarzer, "Hemozoin (malarial pigment) inhibits differentiation and maturation of human monocyte-derived dendritic cells: a peroxisome proliferator-activated receptor-γ-mediated effect," *Journal of Immunology*, vol. 173, no. 6, pp. 4066–4074, 2004.

[83] I. F. Hoffman, C. S. Jere, T. E. Taylor et al., "The effect of Plasmodium falciparum malaria on HIV-1 RNA blood plasma concentration," *AIDS*, vol. 13, no. 4, pp. 487–494, 1999.

[84] R. O. Otieno, C. Ouma, J. M. Ong'echa et al., "Increased severe anemia in HIV-1-exposed and HIV-1-positive infants and children during acute malaria," *AIDS*, vol. 20, no. 2, pp. 275–280, 2006.

[85] D. Burkitt, "A sarcoma of the jaw in African children," *British Journal of Surgery*, vol. 46, pp. 218–223, 1958.

[86] A. Chene, D. Donati, J. Orem et al., "Endemic Burkitt's lymphoma as a polymicrobial disease. New insights on the interaction between Plasmodium falciparum and Epstein-Barr virus," *Seminars in Cancer Biology*, vol. 19, no. 6, pp. 411–420, 2009.

[87] J. Berkley, S. Mwarumba, K. Bramham, B. Lowe, and K. Marsh, "Bacteraemia complicating severe malaria in children," *Transactions of the Royal Society of Tropical Medicine and Hygiene*, vol. 93, no. 3, pp. 283–286, 1999.

[88] Q. Bassat, C. Guinovart, B. Sigaúque et al., "Severe malaria and concomitant bacteraemia in children admitted to a rural Mozambican hospital," *Tropical Medicine and International Health*, vol. 14, no. 9, pp. 1011–1019, 2009.

[89] T. Were, G. C. Davenport, J. B. Hittner et al., "Bacteremia in Kenyan children presenting with malaria," *Journal of Clinical Microbiology*, vol. 49, no. 2, pp. 671–676, 2011.

[90] N. H. Phu, N. Day, P. T. Diep, D. J. P. Ferguson, and N. J. White, "Intraleucocytic malaria pigment and prognosis in severe malaria," *Transactions of the Royal Society of Tropical Medicine and Hygiene*, vol. 89, no. 2, pp. 200–204, 1995.

[91] W. G. Metzger, B. G. Mordmuller, and P. G. Kremsner, "Malaria pigment in leucocytes," *Transactions of the Royal Society of Tropical Medicine and Hygiene*, vol. 89, no. 6, pp. 637–638, 1995.

[92] O. K. Amodu, A. A. Adeyemo, F. E. Olumese, and R. A. Gbadegesin, "Intraleucocytic malaria pigment and clinical severity of malaria in children," *Transactions of the Royal Society of Tropical Medicine and Hygiene*, vol. 92, no. 1, pp. 54–56, 1998.

[93] N. Morakote and D. E. Justus, "Immunosuppression in malaria: effect of hemozoin produced by *Plasmodium berghei* and *Plasmodium falciparum*," *International Archives of Allergy and Applied Immunology*, vol. 86, no. 1, pp. 28–34, 1988.

[94] T. Scorza, S. Magez, L. Brys, and P. de Baetselier, "Hemozoin is a key factor in the induction of malaria-associated immunosuppression," *Parasite Immunology*, vol. 21, no. 11, pp. 545–554, 1999.

[95] C. Coban, Y. Igari, M. Yagi et al., "Immunogenicity of whole-parasite vaccines against *Plasmodium falciparum* involves Malarial Hemozoin and host TLR9," *Cell Host and Microbe*, vol. 7, no. 1, pp. 50–61, 2010.

[96] M. Polimeni, E. Valente, E. Aldieri, A. Khadjavi, G. Giribaldi, and M. Prato, "Role of 15-hydroxyeicosatetraenoic acid in hemozoin-induced lysozyme release from human adherent monocytes," *Biofactors*, vol. 39, no. 3, pp. 304–314, 2013.

[97] K. Deroost, A. Tyberghein, N. Lays et al., "Hemozoin induces lung inflammation and correlates with malaria-associated acute respiratory distress syndrome," *American Journal of Respiratory Cell and Molecular Biology*, vol. 48, no. 5, pp. 589–600, 2013.

[98] M. Prato, S. D'Alessandro, P. E. van den Steen et al., "Natural haemozoin modulates matrix metalloproteinases and induces morphological changes in human microvascular endothelium," *Cellular Microbiology*, vol. 13, no. 8, pp. 1275–1285, 2011.

[99] B. C. Urban and D. J. Roberts, "Inhibition of T cell function during malaria: implications for immunology and vaccinology," *The Journal of Experimental Medicine*, vol. 197, no. 2, pp. 137–141, 2003.

16

Teratogenic Effects of Coadministration of Fluoxetine and Olanzapine on Rat Fetuses

Azam Bakhtiarian,[1] **Nasrin Takzare,**[2] **Mehdi Sheykhi,**[3] **Narges Sistany,**[4] **Farahnaz Jazaeri,**[1] **Mario Giorgi,**[5] **and Vahid Nikoui**[1]

[1] *Department of Pharmacology, School of Medicine, Tehran University of Medical Sciences, Pour Sina Street, Qods Street, Keshavarz Boulevard, Tehran 1417613151, Iran*
[2] *Department of Anatomy, School of Medicine, Tehran University of Medical Sciences, Tehran 1417613146, Iran*
[3] *School of Medicine, Tehran University of Medical Sciences, Tehran 1417613110, Iran*
[4] *Department of Neurosurgery, Shariati Hospital, Tehran University of Medical Sciences, Tehran, Iran*
[5] *Department of Veterinary Sciences, University of Pisa, San Piero a Grado, Pisa 56122, Italy*

Correspondence should be addressed to Vahid Nikoui; nikoui@razi.tums.ac.ir

Academic Editor: Todd C. Skaar

Objective. Depression during pregnancy is a relatively common problem. Since little is known about the teratogenic effects of concomitant administration of fluoxetine and olanzapine during the organogenesis period, the aim of the present study was to evaluate the teratogenic effects of coadministration of fluoxetine and olanzapine on rat fetuses. *Method*. Forty-two pregnant rats were divided into seven groups, randomly. The first group received 0.5 mL of normal saline as the control. The second and third groups received fluoxetine at doses of 9 mg/kg and 18 mg/kg, respectively. Olanzapine was injected at 3 mg/kg and 6 mg/kg to the fourth and fifth groups, respectively. The sixth group received 9 mg/kg fluoxetine and 3 mg/kg olanzapine. Finally, the seventh group was administrated with fluoxetine and olanzapine at 18 mg/kg and 6 mg/kg, respectively. Drugs were injected intraperitoneally between day eight and day 15 of the pregnancy. On the 17th day of pregnancy, the fetuses were removed and micro-/macroscopically studied. *Results*. Fetuses of rats receiving high doses of these drugs showed a significant rate of cleft palate development, premature eyelid opening and torsion anomalies, compared to the control group ($P \leq 0.01$). It is concluded that these drugs can lead to teratogenicity, so their concomitant use during pregnancy should be avoided, or if necessary their doses must be decreased.

1. Introduction

One of the most used antidepressant drugs is fluoxetine. This active ingredient belongs to the SSRIs (selective serotonin reuptake inhibitors) class. It increases serotonin levels in synaptic clefts and is used for treatment of depression [1]. It is also used for obsessive-compulsive disorder (OCD), a prevalent disease of enhanced anxiety that has been diagnosed in around 2% of world population. Estrogen and progesterone imbalance and its influence on cerebrospinal fluid partly explain the incidence of psychological problems including OCD during pregnancy [2, 3]. Researchers have shown that OCD can be triggered during fertility periods like menstruation, pregnancy, or postparturition times. Its rate can be decreased by early diagnosis and appropriate treatment [4]. Maina and colleagues have demonstrated the precipitating effect that pregnancy and parturition can have for OCD which leads to postparturition problems for both mother and baby [5]. Leckman and colleagues found that oxytocin secretion during pregnancy increases intracerebral pressure (ICP) and can also lead to OCD [6].

Olanzapine is an atypical antipsychotic drug for treating schizophrenia and other manic syndromes. In 2013, Dubovsky reported that coadministration of fluoxetine and olanzapine has a potentiating impact on the treatment of depression due to their synergic effects [7]. The explanation for this phenomenon is that olanzapine stabilises serotonin levels already increased by fluoxetine treatment. Coadministration of olanzapine and fluoxetine shows synergistic effects on intracellular survival pathways that allow for persistence of the molecules [8]. Administration of prescription drugs during pregnancy should be avoided so as not to detrimentally effect fetal development; however sometimes this is not possible. Following the thalidomide disaster, there has been a significant increase in attention paid to teratogenic properties of drugs during pregnancy. Although drug prescription in pregnancy has decreased, some medications still may be used in pregnant women and could result in problems in development of the fetus [9, 10].

In some cases, pregnant mothers are not aware of their pregnancy in the early months, if they have been prescribed fluoxetine and olanzapine, they would be taking it, oblivious to the possible dangers. The aim of this study is to investigate the teratogenic effects of administration of either olanzapine or fluoxetine or their use in combination at different doses on fetal development in pregnant rats.

2. Materials and Methods

2.1. Animals. Healthy adult female and male NMRI (Naval Medical Research Institute) rats with an average age of approximately three months and weighing 250–300 grams were randomly selected. They were kept at a temperature of $22 \pm 2°C$ and humidity of 70% and exposed to 12 hours of daylight per day with *ad libitum* access to food and water. After mating and ensuring successful conception, forty-two pregnant rats were randomly divided into seven groups ($n = 6$). All experiments were conducted in Tehran University of Medical Sciences according to the recommendations of the Ethics Committee on Animal Experimentation of the Medical School.

2.2. Drugs. Drugs were purchased from Sigma-aldrich Company, USA. Predetermined doses of the drugs were injected intraperitoneally daily, between the eighth and fifteenth day of pregnancy. The first group received 0.5 mL of normal saline as the control. The second and third groups received fluoxetine at doses of 9 mg/kg and 18 mg/kg, respectively. Olanzapine was injected at 3 mg/kg and 6 mg/kg to the fourth and fifth groups, respectively. The sixth group received 9 mg/kg fluoxetine and 3 mg/kg olanzapine. Finally, the seventh group was administered with fluoxetine and olanzapine at 18 mg/kg and 6 mg/kg, respectively. On the 17th day of pregnancy, the animals were euthanized by inhalation of CO_2 and the fetuses were removed by caesarean section.

2.3. Macroscopic and Microscopic Studies. The fetuses were examined for macroscopic abnormalities. Histopathological slides from fetuses were also prepared. After hematoxylin and eosin staining, any microscopic changes in fetuses were noted using an optical microscope. Positional anomalies (abnormal body shape or non-C-shaped), limb abnormalities (bent limbs), and structural defects (unilateral or bilateral cleft palates and nonfused eyelids) were considered as abnormal fetuses [11].

2.4. Statistical Analysis. Data were analysed using statistical software GraphPad Prism version 5. Fisher's exact test was used to ascertain the significance of variations between the numbers of abnormal fetuses in different groups. Differences were considered significant at $P \leq 0.01$.

3. Results

No abnormal limbs were noted in the control group; however, in the other groups, multiple fetuses had obvious abnormalities of their limbs and body. Abnormalities in other tissues such as the ear, neck, and tail were not observed in the control, low dose (9 mg/kg) fluoxetine, and high dose (18 mg/kg) fluoxetine groups; however, in the groups treated with low dose (3 mg/kg) olanzapine, high dose (6 mg/kg) olanzapine, combination of fluoxetine and olanzapine in low doses, and combination of fluoxetine and olanzapine in high doses groups, several anomalies were seen. The number of total and abnormal fetuses and litters in different groups are shown in Table 1. Fisher's exact statistical analysis showed that the differences in the number of apparent anomalies between the control group and those that received low dose of olanzapine (3 mg/kg), high dose of olanzapine (6 mg/kg), and combination of fluoxetine and olanzapine in low and high doses are significant ($P \leq 0.01$). We also found a significant difference in the number of apparent anomalies between groups injected with low and high doses of olanzapine as compared to those treated with a combination of fluoxetine and olanzapine in low and high doses ($P \leq 0.01$). In the morphological exam, 17-day-old fetuses of the control group had formed their normal C-shaped body with normal extremities. (Figure 1(a)). In the group receiving the highest doses of fluoxetine and olanzapine, fetuses had an abnormal body shape and short limbs (Figure 1(b)). Histopathological slides from frontal sections of control group fetal heads showed that the wall of the nose (nasal septum) was located in the middle of the nasal cavity and was connected to the roof of the mouth. The oral cavity was completely isolated from the nasal cavity (Figure 2(a)). Eyelids were fused together and the cellular layers of eyeball were normal (Figure 3(a)). Microscopic slides of frontal skull sections in the groups receiving the high dose of fluoxetine and a combination of fluoxetine and olanzapine revealed unilateral cleft palates in some samples (Figure 2(b)). In addition, eyelids were not fused together in these groups (Figure 3(b)).

4. Discussion

After the thalidomide tragedy, scientists became aware of the importance of considering the teratogenic effects of drugs administered during pregnancy [10]. Drugs with low teratogenicity have no impact on most pregnant women but can be harmful in some cases. The rate of depression increases during pregnancy, and fluoxetine use may be considered.

In the present experiment, we used fluoxetine at doses of 9 mg/kg and 18 mg/kg and olanzapine at doses of 3 mg/kg and 6 mg/kg. Pohland et al. reported that fluoxetine at a dose of 12.5 mg/kg could pass through the placenta and distribute within the fetus during periods of organogenesis in rats [11]. Vorhees et al. have shown that administering fluoxetine at

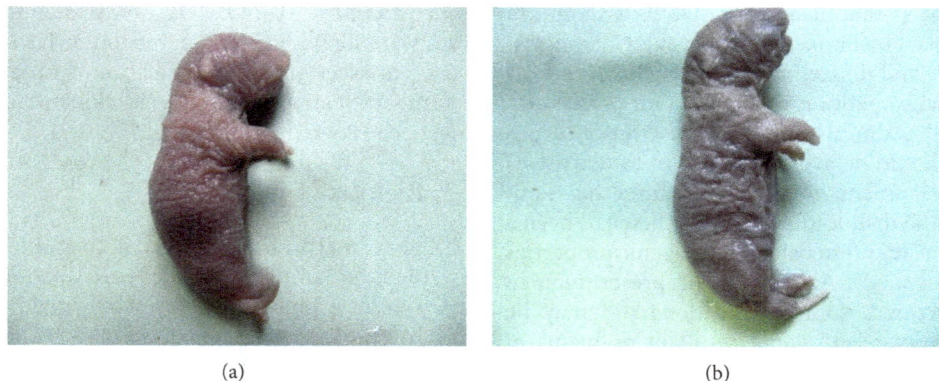

(a)   (b)

FIGURE 1: Macroscopic view of 17 days fetuses of control (a) and the group received high doses of fluoxetine and olanzapine (b). In the control group fetus, the body is C-shaped and upper and lower extremities are in their normal locations (a). In the fetus from the group that received high doses of fluoxetine and olanzapine, the body is not fully C-shaped and the forelimbs are not symmetrical (b).

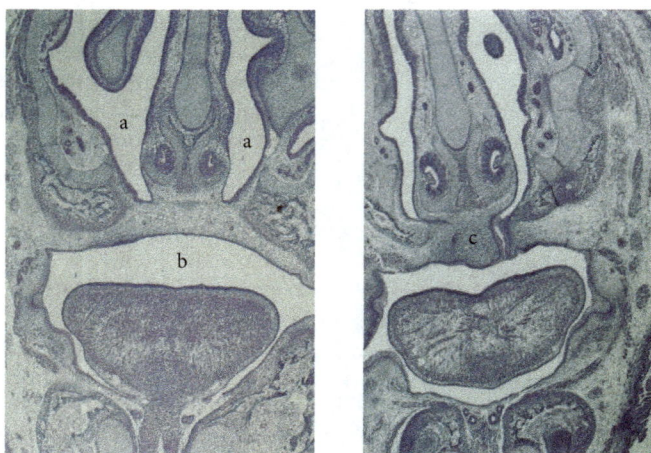

FIGURE 2: Histopathological slides of the frontal section of the head, 17-day fetuses in the control (left) and the group received high doses of fluoxetine and olanzapine (right) (H&E staining, 4x). In the control group (left), the nasal septum is attached to the roof of the mouth and nostrils (a) are completely separated from the oral cavity (b). In the fetus from the group that received high doses of fluoxetine and olanzapine (right), there is unilateral clefting of the palate (c).

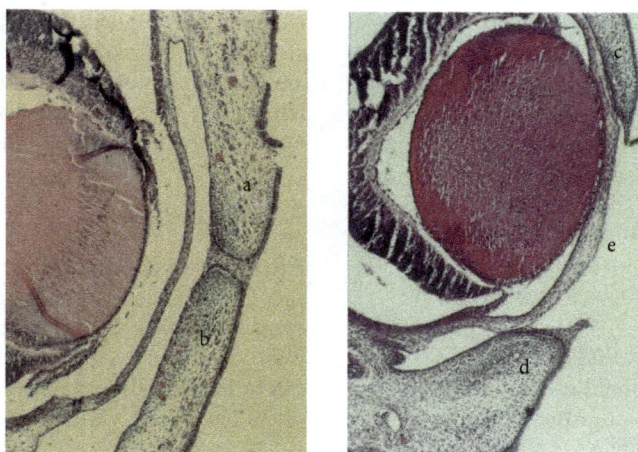

FIGURE 3: Histopathological slides of the eyes from 17 days fetuses in control (left) and the group received high doses of fluoxetine and olanzapine (right) (H&E staining, 10x). In control group fetus (left), the upper (a) and lower (b) eyelids are joined completely. In the fetus from the group that received high doses of fluoxetine and olanzapine (right), the upper (c) and lower (d) eyelids were separated completely and the cornea (e) is exposed.

TABLE 1: The number of total and abnormal fetuses and litters in the different groups (F: fluoxetine with doses of 9 and 18 mg/kg and O: olanzapine with doses of 3 and 6 mg/kg).

Groups			Anomalies				
	Total fetuses	Abnormal fetuses	Litters with at least one abnormal fetus	Bent limbs	Non-C-shaped body	Cleft palate	Nonfused eyelids
Control	58	1	1	0	1	0	0
F9	56	2	1	0	0	0	2
F18	59	4	3	4	0	1	4
O3	58	6*	2	3	1	0	2
O6	54	16*	6	7	4	0	7
F9 + O3	57	40*†	6	17	14	4	11
F18 + O6	60	48*†	6	15	17	9	20

Fisher's exact test. *Significant with abnormal fetuses of control group ($P \leq 0.01$). †Significant with abnormal fetuses of O3 and O6 groups ($P \leq 0.01$).

dose of 12 mg/kg caused maternal weight loss during pregnancy, reduced litter sizes at birth, and increased neonatal mortality [12]. Cabrera-Vera et al. showed that prenatal exposure to fluoxetine (10 mg/kg) could produce limited changes in brain serotoninergic neurons in rats [13]. Conversely, Byrd and Markham did not find any teratogenicity in fetuses of rats who had been given fluoxetine at doses of 12.5 mg/kg and lower [14]. In our experiment, we chose the doses of 9 and 18 mg/kg for fluoxetine, based on the above studies.

In 2002, Rosengarten and Quartermain administered olanzapine at a therapeutic dose of 2 mg/kg/day to pregnant rats [15]. In 1998, Li et al. demonstrated that olanzapine at doses of 0.5, 3, and 10 mg/kg administered subcutaneously exerted pharmacological effects through elevation of extracellular dopamine and norepinephrine levels in rat brains [16]. Aravagiri et al. in 1999 studied the pharmacokinetics and tissue distribution of olanzapine in rats. They performed their experiment with the standard doses of 0.25, 1, 3, and 6 mg/kg/day intraperitoneally [17]. The doses of 3 and 6 mg/kg of olanzapine in this study were chosen based on previous experiments, and these doses caused some anomalies in rat fetuses. Therapeutic doses of fluoxetine and olanzapine for human use are 0.25 to 1 mg/kg/day and 0.1 to 0.25 mg/kg/day, respectively. Since the metabolism of rats is much more efficient than that of humans, we used higher doses than would be used in humans.

Goldstein et al. in 1997 and Oberlander et al. in 2004 reported that most selective serotonin reuptake inhibitors, especially medical doses of fluoxetine, have no teratogenic effects [18, 19]. Many clinical assays have shown similar results [20, 21]. We also found no specific effect of fluoxetine in the present study.

Moses-Kolko et al. in 2005 published a literature review on the fetotoxic effects of some SSRIs [22]. Casper et al. in 2003, Cissoko and colleagues in 2005, and Gentile in 2005 have also mentioned these teratogenic effects [23–25]. Some assays reported that high doses of SSRIs like fluoxetine have potential harmful effects on fetus maturation, but they did not provide sufficient information about the onset and duration of these adverse effects [26–29]. Research has indicated

that coadministration of fluoxetine and olanzapine is useful for treating resistant depression [30]. The long half-life of fluoxetine and its active metabolite (dimethyl fluoxetine) increases the chance of drug interaction even after treatment is discontinued [31–33].

Metabolism of the drugs is catalysed by selective cytochrome P_{450} (CYP) isoenzymes. Fluoxetine and its metabolite norfluoxetine are potent inhibitors of the cytochrome CYP2D6 pathway [34], and olanzapine metabolism is dependent on this path [35], so it is possible that fluoxetine increases olanzapine persistence. Drug interactions, especially those involving metabolism, should be considered as an important matter. We have previously shown that coadministration of caffeine and clomipramine during pregnancy could potentiate the teratogenic effects of caffeine in rats [36]. This finding can be attributed to the inhibitory influence of clomipramine on caffeine metabolism via CYP1A2 [37]. It has been established that benzodiazepines, including alprazolam, also cause teratogenic effects, and drug interactions can be involved in this phenomenon too [38]. We observed that groups coadministered with fluoxetine and olanzapine showed more teratogenic features in comparison to groups were administered by fluoxetine alone, and abnormal limb rotations were much more frequent in these combined therapy groups (Table 1). Fluoxetine and olanzapine are categorised in group C of pregnancy medications [39, 40]. So maybe the benefits of using these drugs during pregnancy outweigh their possible risks. Anyway, cautions in their concomitant use during pregnancy should be considered.

5. Study Limitations

Since the individual pups are not independent, but belong to litters, the problem of dependence within litters can be considered as a limitation of the present study. Future studies with larger sample sizes using a hierarchic analysis of between-litter and within-litter variances could result in more reliable outcome. Metabolism differences between rats and humans and consequence dosage dissimilarities among these species are also a restriction of this experiment.

6. Conclusions

The present research has been carried out in rats, so caution should be used in extrapolating this data to human beings. With this caveat, it might be concluded that because of the potential teratogenic effects of fluoxetine and olanzapine and also the inhibitory effects of fluoxetine on metabolism and elimination of olanzapine, coadministration of these drugs during pregnancy should be avoided, or if necessary their doses must be decreased.

Conflict of Interests

None of the authors of this paper has a financial or personal relationship with other people or organizations that could inappropriately influence or bias the content of the paper.

Acknowledgments

This study has been founded and supported by Tehran University of Medical Sciences (TUMS), Grant no. 15614-61-04-90. Thanks are due to Dr. H. Owen (University of Queensland) for her invaluable editorial assistance.

References

[1] S. H. Preskorn, R. Ross, and C. Stanga, "Selective serotonin reuptake inhibitors," in *Antidepressants: Past, Present and Future*, vol. 157 of *Handbook of Experimental Pharmacology*, pp. 241–262, Springer, New York, NY, USA, 2004.

[2] L. M. Arnold, "A case series of women with postpartum-onset obsessive-compulsive disorder," *Primary Care Companion to the Journal of Clinical Psychiatry*, vol. 1, no. 4, pp. 103–108, 1999.

[3] K. L. Wisner, K. S. Peindl, T. Gigliotti, and B. H. Hanusa, "Obsessions and compulsions in women with postpartum depression," *Journal of Clinical Psychiatry*, vol. 60, no. 3, pp. 176–180, 1999.

[4] K. E. Williams and L. M. Koran, "Obsessive-compulsive disorder in pregnancy, the puerperium, and the premenstruum," *Journal of Clinical Psychiatry*, vol. 58, no. 7, pp. 330–334, 1997.

[5] G. Maina, U. Albert, F. Bogetto, P. Vaschetto, and L. Ravizza, "Recent life events and obsessive-compulsive disorder (OCD): the role of pregnancy/delivery," *Psychiatry Research*, vol. 89, no. 1, pp. 49–58, 1999.

[6] J. F. Leckman, W. K. Goodman, W. G. North et al., "Elevated cerebrospinal fluid levels of oxytocin in obsessive-compulsive disorder: comparison with Tourette's syndrome and healthy controls," *Archives of General Psychiatry*, vol. 51, no. 10, pp. 782–792, 1994.

[7] S. L. Dubovsky, "Pharmacokinetic evaluation of olanzapine + fluoxetine for the treatment of bipolar depression," *Expert Opinion on Drug Metabolism and Toxicology*, vol. 9, no. 2, pp. 207–214, 2013.

[8] G. Z. Reus, H. M. Abelaira, F. R. Agostinho et al., "The administration of olanzapine and fluoxetine has synergistic effects on intracellular survival pathways in the rat brain," *Journal of Psychiatric Research*, vol. 46, no. 8, pp. 1029–1035, 2012.

[9] P. R. McElhatton, "The effects of benzodiazepine use during pregnancy and lactation," *Reproductive Toxicology*, vol. 8, no. 6, pp. 461–475, 1994.

[10] P. F. Brain, J. S. Ajarem, and V. V. Petkov, "The application of ethopharmacological techniques to behavioural teratology: preliminary investigations," *Acta Physiologica et Pharmacologica Bulgarica*, vol. 12, no. 4, pp. 3–11, 1986.

[11] R. C. Pohland, T. K. Byrd, M. Hamilton, and J. R. Koons, "Placental transfer and fetal distribution of fluoxetine in the rat," *Toxicology and Applied Pharmacology*, vol. 98, no. 2, pp. 198–205, 1989.

[12] C. V. Vorhees, K. D. Acuff-Smith, M. A. Schilling, J. E. Fisher, M. S. Moran, and J. Buelke-Sam, "A developmental neurotoxicity evaluation of the effects of prenatal exposure to fluoxetine in rats," *Fundamental and Applied Toxicology*, vol. 23, no. 2, pp. 194–205, 1994.

[13] T. M. Cabrera-Vera, F. Garcia, W. Pinto, and G. Battaglia, "Effect of prenatal fluoxetine (prozac) exposure on brain serotonin neurons in prepubescent and adult male rat offspring," *Journal of Pharmacology and Experimental Therapeutics*, vol. 280, no. 1, pp. 138–145, 1997.

[14] R. A. Byrd and J. K. Markham, "Developmental toxicology studies of fluoxetine hydrochloride administered orally to rats and rabbits," *Fundamental and Applied Toxicology*, vol. 22, no. 4, pp. 511–518, 1994.

[15] H. Rosengarten and D. Quartermain, "Effect of prenatal administration of haloperidol, risperidone, quetiapine and olanzapine on spatial learning and retention in adult rats," *Pharmacology Biochemistry and Behavior*, vol. 72, no. 3, pp. 575–579, 2002.

[16] X. M. Li, K. W. Perry, D. T. Wong, and F. P. Bymaster, "Olanzapine increases in vivo dopamine and norepinephrine release in rat prefrontal cortex, nucleus accumbens and striatum," *Psychopharmacology*, vol. 136, no. 2, pp. 153–161, 1998.

[17] M. Aravagiri, Y. Teper, and S. R. Marder, "Pharmacokinetics and tissue distribution of olanzapine in rats," *Biopharmaceutics and Drug Disposition*, vol. 20, no. 8, pp. 369–377, 1999.

[18] D. J. Goldstein, K. L. Sundell, and L. A. Corbin, "Birth outcomes in pregnant women taking fluoxetine," *The New England Journal of Medicine*, vol. 336, no. 12, pp. 872–873, 1997.

[19] T. F. Oberlander, S. Misri, C. E. Fitzgerald, X. Kostaras, D. Rurak, and W. Riggs, "Pharmacologic factors associated with transient neonatal symptoms following prenatal psychotropic medication exposure," *Journal of Clinical Psychiatry*, vol. 65, no. 2, pp. 230–237, 2004.

[20] A. Einarson, B. Fatoye, M. Sarkar et al., "Pregnancy outcome following gestational exposure to venlafaxine: a multicenter prospective controlled study," *The American Journal of Psychiatry*, vol. 158, no. 10, pp. 1728–1730, 2001.

[21] A. Pastuszak, B. Schick-Boschetto, C. Zuber et al., "Pregnancy outcome following first-trimester exposure to fluoxetine (Prozac)," *The Journal of the American Medical Association*, vol. 269, no. 17, pp. 2246–2248, 1993.

[22] E. L. Moses-Kolko, D. Bogen, J. Perel et al., "Neonatal signs after late in utero exposure to serotonin reuptake inhibitors: literature review and implications for clinical applications," *The Journal of the American Medical Association*, vol. 293, no. 19, pp. 2372–2383, 2005.

[23] R. C. Casper, B. E. Fleisher, J. C. Lee-Ancajas et al., "Follow-up of children of depressed mothers exposed or not exposed to antidepressant drugs during pregnancy," *Journal of Pediatrics*, vol. 142, no. 4, pp. 402–408, 2003.

[24] H. Cissoko, D. Swortfiguer, B. Giraudeau, A. Jonville-Béra, and E. Autret-Leca, "Neonatal outcome after exposure to selective serotonin reuptake inhibitors late in pregnancy," *Archives de Pediatrie*, vol. 12, no. 7, pp. 1081–1084, 2005.

[25] S. Gentile, "The safety of newer antidepressants in pregnancy and breastfeeding," *Drug Safety*, vol. 28, no. 2, pp. 137–152, 2005.

[26] C. D. Chambers, K. A. Johnson, L. M. Dick, R. J. Felix, and K. L. Jones, "Birth outcomes in pregnant women taking fluoxetine," *The New England Journal of Medicine*, vol. 335, no. 14, pp. 1010–1015, 1996.

[27] L. S. Cohen, V. L. Heller, J. W. Bailey, L. Grush, J. S. Ablon, and S. M. Bouffard, "Birth outcomes following prenatal exposure to fluoxetine," *Biological Psychiatry*, vol. 48, no. 10, pp. 996–1000, 2000.

[28] A. M. Costei, E. Kozer, T. Ho, S. Ito, and G. Koren, "Perinatal outcome following third trimester exposure to paroxetine," *Archives of Pediatrics and Adolescent Medicine*, vol. 156, no. 11, pp. 1129–1132, 2002.

[29] D. J. Goldstein, "Effects of third trimester fluoxetine exposure on the newborn," *Journal of Clinical Psychopharmacology*, vol. 15, no. 6, pp. 417–420, 1995.

[30] S. Dodd and M. Berk, "Olanzapine/fluoxetine combination for treatment-resistant depression: efficacy and clinical utility," *Expert Review of Neurotherapeutics*, vol. 8, no. 9, pp. 1299–1306, 2008.

[31] W. J. Burke, S. E. Hendricks, D. McArthur-Miller et al., "Weekly dosing of fluoxetine for the continuation phase of treatment of major depression: results of a placebo-controlled, randomized clinical trial," *Journal of Clinical Psychopharmacology*, vol. 20, no. 4, pp. 423–427, 2000.

[32] V. Pérez, D. Puigdemont, I. Gilaberte, E. Alvarez, and F. Artigas, "Augmentation of fluoxetine's antidepressant action by pindolol: analysis of clinical, pharmacokinetic, and methodologic factors," *Journal of Clinical Psychopharmacology*, vol. 21, no. 1, pp. 36–45, 2001.

[33] D. J. Brunswick, J. D. Amsterdam, J. Fawcett et al., "Fluoxetine and norfluoxetine plasma concentrations during relapse-prevention treatment," *Journal of Affective Disorders*, vol. 68, no. 2-3, pp. 243–249, 2002.

[34] H. K. Crewe, M. S. Lennard, G. T. Tucker, F. R. Woods, and R. E. Haddock, "The effect of selective serotonin re-uptake inhibitors on cytochrome P4502D6 (CYP2D6) activity in human liver microsomes," *The British Journal of Clinical Pharmacology*, vol. 34, no. 3, pp. 262–265, 1992.

[35] J. A. Carrillo, A. G. Herráiz, S. I. Ramos, G. Gervasini, S. Vizcaíno, and J. Benítez, "Role of the smoking-induced cytochrome P450 (CYP)1A2 and polymorphic CYP2D6 in steady-state concentration of olanzapine," *Journal of Clinical Psychopharmacology*, vol. 23, no. 2, pp. 119–127, 2003.

[36] N. Takzare, V. Nikoui, S. Ostadhadi, S. M. A. Nabavi, and A. Bakhtiarian, "Teratogenic effects of caffeine and clomipramine on rat fetus," *Tehran University Medical Journal*, vol. 70, no. 6, pp. 335–339, 2012.

[37] J. A. Carrillo and J. Benitez, "Clinically significant pharmacokinetic interactions between dietary caffeine and medications," *Clinical Pharmacokinetics*, vol. 39, no. 2, pp. 127–153, 2000.

[38] N. Takzare, A. Bakhtiarian, E. Saeedi, and V. Nekoui, "The teratogenic effects of alprazolam intake on rat fetus," *Tehran University Medical Journal*, vol. 68, no. 10, pp. 578–582, 2011.

[39] S. W. Wen, Q. Yang, P. Garner et al., "Selective serotonin reuptake inhibitors and adverse pregnancy outcomes," *The American Journal of Obstetrics and Gynecology*, vol. 194, no. 4, pp. 961–966, 2006.

[40] P. Malek-Ahmadi, "Olanzapine in pregnancy," *Annals of Pharmacotherapy*, vol. 35, no. 10, pp. 1294–1295, 2001.

17

Antisecretory Action of the Extract of the Aerial Parts of *Eremomastax speciosa (Acanthaceae)* Occurs through Antihistaminic and Anticholinergic Pathways

Amang André Perfusion,[1,2] **Paul V. Tan,**[1] **Nkwengoua Ernestine,**[3] **and Nyasse Barthélemy**[3]

[1] *Department of Animal Biology & Physiology, Faculty of Science, P.O. Box 812, University of Yaoundé I, Yaoundé, Cameroon*
[2] *Department of Biological Sciences, Faculty of Science, P.O. Box 46, University of Maroua, Maroua, Cameroon*
[3] *Department of Organic Chemistry, Faculty of Science, P.O. Box 812, University of Yaoundé I, Yaoundé, Cameroon*

Correspondence should be addressed to Paul V. Tan; pvernyuy@yahoo.com

Academic Editor: Masahiro Oike

Objective. The objective of this study was to find out the possible antiulcer mechanism of action of *Eremomastax speciosa*. *Method.* Carbachol- and histamine-induced hypersecretion, associated with the pylorus ligation technique, were used in rats. Gastric mucosal ulceration, mucus production, pH, gastric volume, and acidity were measured. *Results.* Histamine and carbachol raised gastric acidity to 86.50 and 84.80 mEq/L, respectively, in the control rats, and the extracts (200 mg/kg) reduced gastric acidity to 34.60 and 39.00 mEq/L, respectively. Intraduodenal aqueous extract (400 mg/kg) in histamine- and carbachol-treated rats produced significant ($P < 0.001$) decreases in acid secretion to 28.50 and 28.80 mEq/L, respectively, and 100 percent inhibition of gastric ulceration. Augmented histamine-induced gastric acid secretion (90.20 mEq/L) was significantly reduced to 52.60 and 27.50 mEq/L by the 200 and 400 mg/kg doses of the aqueous extract, respectively. The extract significantly reduced ($P < 0.001$) the volume of gastric secretion and significantly increased mucus production. The ulcer inhibition potential of the extract significantly dropped to 25–44% (oral extract) and to 29–37% (duodenal extract) in carbachol/indomethacin-treated rats. *Conclusion.* The aqueous extract of *E. speciosa* has both cytoprotective and antisecretory effects. The antisecretory effect may involve a mechanism common to both cholinergic and histaminergic pathways.

1. Introduction

The central role of gastric acid hypersecretion in the etiology of gastroduodenal ulcers, gastrooesophageal reflux disease and gastric cancer is well known. Thus, while ulcers are almost always present in patients with Zollinger-Ellison syndrome, which is characterised by excessively high gastric acid secretion, they are absent in achlorhydric patients. The gastric acid hypersecretion can be of stress or genetic origin but can as well result from the interaction between a genetic component with environmental factors [1, 2]. Outstanding findings in the understanding of peptic ulcer etiology include the discovery histamine H_2-receptors, the H^+K^+-ATPase-driven parietal cell pump by the end of the 1970s, and the more recent discovery of the role of *Helicobacter pylori* in the development

of duodenal ulcer by [3]. Corresponding breakthroughs in the treatment of acid-peptic disorders include the discovery of the prototypical H_2 antagonist, cimetidine, developed by Smith, Kline; and French (now GlaxoSmithKline) in the mid-to-late 1960s [4], the development of proton pump inhibitors [5, 6], and the development of the *H. pylori* triple therapy eradication regimens [7, 8].

The FDA-approved triple therapy regimen includes a proton pump inhibitor (Omeprazole, Lansoprazole, or pantoprazole) + Clarithromycin and Metronidazole (or Amoxicillin) or a H_2-receptor antagonist (Cimetidine or Ranitidine) + Bismuth and antibiotics (Clarithromycin and Metronidazole (or Amoxicillin)) [9–11]. Unfortunately, *H. pylori* strains resistant to the commonly prescribed antibiotics have emerged. In addition, the high cost of the triple therapy regimen, especially for patients in poor countries, and the adverse effects associated with the antibiotics and antisecretory agents have been at the root of low patient compliance, treatment failures, and recurrence of treated ulcers [12–15]. For example, the reported adverse effects in patients taking Cimetidine involve various organ systems including the gastrointestinal system (diarrhea, constipation), central nervous system (psychosis, depression, and anxiety especially in the elderly), endocrine system (gynecomastia, reversible impotence), hepatobiliary system (dose-related increase in serum transaminases, occasional liver injury), renal system (dose-related increase in plasma creatinine) and cardiovascular system (rare cases of bradycardia and tachycardia). The three well-known disease interactions with Tagamet include liver disease, hemodialysis, and renal dysfunction, while drug interactions with Tagamet include 18 major, 336 moderate, and 317 minor ones. This litany of possible side effects associated with the most prescribed antisecretory agent underlines the current need to intensify the search for antisecretory materials from local medicinal plant sources. Other workers [16] have given a detailed description of the roles of extracellular calcium, histamine and H_2 receptors, and acetylcholine and muscarinic (M_3) receptors in the mechanism of gastric secretion, and our previous work [17] describes many medicinal plants with proven antisecretory activities. Some of the plants have provided active extracts, fractions, and compounds with anticholinergic or antihistaminic activity. Botanical compounds with antiulcer activity include flavonoids (i.e., quercetin, naringin, silymarin, anthocyanosides, and sophoradin derivatives), saponins (i.e., from *Panax japonicus* and *Kochia scoparia*), tannins (i.e., from *Linderae umbellatae*), gums, and mucilages (i.e., gum guar and myrrh). Among herbal drugs, liquorice, aloe gel, and capsicum (chilli) have been used extensively and their clinical efficacy documented. The cytoprotective, antioxidant, anti-inflammatory, and antiulcer activities of flavonoids, alkaloids, triterpenoids, and polyphenols have been demonstrated experimentally [17–20]. Comparative phytochemical screening of two species of *Eremomastax* revealed the presence of flavonoids, alkaloids, phenols, tannins, terpenes, and saponins [21]. A comprehensive review of drugs derived from botanical sources more commonly used or extensively studied in the world for peptic ulcer has been published [22].

Eremomastax speciosa (Hochst.) Cufod. (*Acanthaceae*) is widespread from West Africa through Central African Republic and N Congo-Kinshasa to S Sudan and SW Ethiopia, Madagascar. The plant is widely distributed in tropical Africa and is the only species of the genus *Eremomastax* (syn.: *Paulowilhelmia* (Lindau) and *Ruellia* (S. Moore)) [23]. It is a robust, polymorphous shrub that grows to 2 m high and has a characteristic quadrangular stem and violate underside of the leaves which has earned for it the local name *Pang nyemshe*, meaning "red on one side" in the Bamileke region of Cameroon.

The plant is commonly referred to in Cameroon as "blood plant" due to its reputed use in the treatment of cases of anemia. It is also used in Cameroonian ethnomedicine for the treatment of various stomach complaints and information from tradipractitioners suggested that it possesses antiulcer

effects. The antidiarrhoeal activity of *E. speciosa* leaf aqueous extract has been reported [24]. The leaf extract is used for the treatment of male infertility among the *Ifa Nkari* People of Akwa Ibom State, Nigeria (where it is known commonly as "golden seal;" "African blood tonic plant;" local name, *Edera Ididout, Ndana-edem*) [25]. Its widelyclaimed antianaemic activity has been experimentally demonstrated by workers [26] who also showed anti-microbial actions against pure clinical cultures of *Staphylococcus aureus*, *E. coli*, *Candida albicans*, and *Aspergillus niger*. The Douala people of Cameroon employ *E. speciosa* variously for malaria, kidney pain, scabies anaemia diabetes, and nerves pain [27]. *E. speciosa* has been cited for its local use in the treatment of female infertility in the west region of Cameroon [28], as well as for its use in the treatment of irregular menstruation by the Aguambu-Bamumbu people of the Lebialem highlands in the South West Region of Cameroon [29]. The plant has also been cited [30] for the treatment of menstrual pains, gonorrhea, appendicitis, and dry burns and as an antipoison, and to increase and purify blood in the mount Cameroon region.

In spite of the wide gastrointestinal ethnopharmacological potential of *E. speciosa*, the only literature report to date on its antiulcer activity is the preliminary study [31] which showed that the water extract significantly inhibited the formation of HCl/ethanol-inflicted gastric lesions in rats. Recently, we have demonstrated the activity of the methanol extract against various experimental ulcer models including HCl/ethanol, absolute ethanol, cold/restraint stress, and indomethacin [32]. In the present experiment we employed the pylorus ligated technique in a series of secretagogue-induced hypersecretion models in order to study the possible mechanism of action of *E. speciosa*.

2. Material and Methods

2.1. Material

2.1.1. Animals. Male albino Wistar rats (180–220 g) raised in the Animal house of the Animal Physiology laboratory, Faculty of Science, University of Yaounde I, were used. They were fed a standard laboratory diet (supplied by SPC Ltd., Bafoussam, Cameroon) and given tap water *ad libitum*. The animals were deprived of food prior to experimentation but access to water was maintained. Prior authorization for the use of laboratory animals in this study was obtained from the Cameroon National Ethics Committee (Reg. no. FWA-IRB00001954). The use, handling, and care of animals were done in adherence to the European Convention (Strasbourg, 18.III.1986) for the protection of vertebrate animals used for experimental and other purposes (ETS-123), with particular attention to Part III, articles 7, 8, and 9.

2.2. Methods

2.2.1. Preparation of the Plant Extracts and Fractions. The aerial parts of *E. speciosa* were collected in May/June 2012 in Yaounde (centre region) and identified botanically by Paul Mezili of the Cameroon National Herbarium (by comparison with existing voucher specimen N° HNC/136984). They were chopped, rapidly dried under room temperature (25°C) for one week, and transformed into powder. 3796 g of powder was macerated in 15 L of a 2 : 1 (v/v) mixture of methanol and methylene chloride, which was the highest yielding out of the five extraction solvents tested for 72 h at room temperature. After filtration through Wattman filter paper number 3 and sequential evaporation at 40°C and 65°C in a rotavapor to remove the methylene chloride and methanol, respectively, 318 g of crude extract was obtained (8.4% yield). 159 g of crude extract was fractionated with hexane (1 L), methylene chloride (0.5 L), ethyl acetate (0.25 L), and methanol (0.125 L), respectively, to obtain 39.3 g of hexane fraction (24.7% yield), 30.5 g of methylene chloride fraction (19.2% yield), 5.6 g of ethyl acetate fraction (3.52% yield), and 3.3 g of methanol fraction (2.1% yield).

Aqueous Extract. 500 g of ground powder was extracted by infusion in 4 litres of boiled water for 15 minutes. After filtration through Wattman filter paper number 3, the filtrate was evaporated using a *Raven* convection air oven (Jencons-PLS, UK). The brownish solid obtained (77.7 g (15.5% yield)) was stored at 4°C. The crude extracts and fractions dissolved readily in distilled water which was used as vehicle in the subsequent experiments.

2.2.2. Phytochemical Tests. Phytochemical tests for major secondary metabolites of the extracts and fractions were performed. They were screened for the presence of biologically active compounds such as alkaloids, anthocyanins, and cardiac glycosides [33]; phenols and flavonoids [34]; triterpenes and sterols [35]; saponins [36]; anthraquinones, hydrolysable, and condensed tannins [37]; and coumarins [38]. Based on the intensity of coloration or the precipitate formed during the test, secondary metabolites proportion was characterized as strongly present (+++), present (++), weakly present (+), and absent (−) when the test result was negative; it was characterized as strongly present (+++), present (++), weakly present (+) and absent (−) when the test result was negative.

2.2.3. Pylorus Ligated Gastric Secretion: Screening of Extracts and Fractions for Antisecretory Activity. Fifty male rats (5 per group) were used to screen the aqueous, methanol, and methanol/methylene chloride (Me-CH$_2$Cl$_2$) extracts and the methylene chloride (CH$_2$Cl$_2$), ethyl acetate, and hexane fractions for their antisecretory potential. Following a 48 h fast, the extracts, fractions, and vehicle were administered by oral route to the test and control rats, respectively, before the experiment. One hour later, laparotomy was performed under light ether anaesthesia and the pylorus of each rat was tied and the abdominal incisions were closed. The rats were sacrificed 6 h later and the gastric juice produced by each was collected, centrifuged, and the volume measured. The ulcers formed in the glandular region of the stomachs were scored as previously described [39].

2.2.4. Secretagogue-Induced Gastric Hypersecretion. Following the screening experiment, the aqueous extract, CH$_2$Cl$_2$

fraction, and MeOH-CH$_2$Cl$_2$ extract, which induced the highly significant reductions in gastric acidity, were retained for the next set of experiments. Thus, the two extracts and CH$_2$Cl$_2$ fraction (200 mg/kg) were administered by oral route and tested on gastric secretion induced in pylorus ligated rats by histamine (2.5 mg/kg, s.c.) or carbachol (1 mg/kg, s.c.) injected 1 h after pylorus ligature [39]. The animals were sacrificed 4 h after secretagogue administration and gastric juice was collected and ulcer indices measured. The hypersecretory effects of the secretagogues were also challenged by the aqueous extract alone (200–400 mg/kg) administered by intraduodenal route. After laparotomy and pylorus ligation, the extract was introduced into the duodenal lumen using a syringe. The stomach incisions were closed and histamine (2.5 mg/kg) or carbachol (1 mg/kg) were administered 1 h later by subcutaneous route [40]. The animals were sacrificed 4 h after secretagogue administration. Gastric juice was collected and mucus production and ulcer indices were measured.

2.2.5. Augmented Histamine-Induced Gastric Secretion. A modification of the classic augmented histamine test was used to study the effect of the aqueous extract of *E. speciosa* (200 and 400 mg/kg) in rats challenged with prolonged maximal circulating levels of histamine. The test and control rats were given the extract and vehicle, respectively, by oral route 30 minutes before pylorus ligation. The positive control rats received ranitidine (100 mg/kg). Histamine dihydrochloride (1 mg/kg, s.c) was administered 4 times at hourly intervals. The gastric juice was collected 1 h after the last histamine injection and prepared for gastric acid analysis.

2.2.6. Nonsteroidal Anti-Inflammatory Drug (NSAID)-Induced Gastric Ulcers in Carbachol-Treated Rats. A modification of the method of Rainsford [41] was used. Gastric ulcers were induced, following a 24 h fast, using indomethacin (30 mg/kg, s.c.) and carbachol (0.5 mg/kg, s.c.) in pylorus ligated rats. The aqueous extract of *E. speciosa* (200–400 mg/kg), ranitidine (100 mg/kg), and vehicle were administered orally 30 minutes before pylorus ligation. An hour after pylorus ligation, indomethacin (30 mg/kg, s.c.) and carbachol (0.5 mg/kg, s.c.) were administered. After 4 h the animals were sacrificed by deep ether anesthesia and the gastric secretion was collected and gastric ulceration and mucus production measured. In a second experiment, the effect of the extract administered by duodenal route was tested: immediately following pylorus ligation, the extract (200–400 mg/kg) was injected into the duodenal lumen, the abdomen stitched up, and indomethacin (30 mg/kg, s.c.) and carbachol (0.5 mg/kg, s.c.) were injected an hour later. Another 4 h later, the animals were sacrificed and the gastric secretion, gastric ulceration, and mucus production were measured.

2.2.7. Measurement of Gastric Acidity. Samples of centrifuged gastric juice (1 mL) were analysed for hydrogen ion concentration by pH-metric titration with 0.1 N NaOH solution

TABLE 1: Preliminary phytochemical analysis of the aqueous and MeOH/CH$_2$CL$_2$ extracts, hexane, methylene chloride, ethyl acetate, and methanol fractions of E. speciosa.

	Aqueous extract	MeOH/CH$_2$CL$_2$ extract	Hexane fraction	CH$_2$CL$_2$ fraction	Ethyl acetate fraction	MeOH fraction
Tannins	+	−	−	−	−	−
Alkaloids	+++	++	−	+	−	+
Resins	++	−	−	−	−	−
Saponins	−	−	−	−	−	−
Flavonoids	+++	+++	++	++	+	+
Anthocyanins	+++	−	−	−	−	−
Phenols	+	−	−	+	−	−
Quinones	+++	++	−	++	+	−
Acids	−	+	+	+	+	−
Sugars	−	−	−	−	−	−
Oils	+	+	−	−	++	+
Coumarins	−	+	−	−	−	+
Sterols	+	++	+	++	++	−
Triterpenoids	+	+++	+	++	++	−
Glycosides	+	++	++	++	+	−
Amino acids	+	+	−	+	+	−
Proteins	+++	−	−	++	++	−

Strongly present: +++; present: ++; weakly present: + absent: −.

using a digital pH meter. The acid content was expressed as mEq/L.

2.2.8. Mucus Production Assessment.
The mucus covering of each stomach was gently scraped using a glass slide and the mucus weighed carefully using a sensitive digital electronic balance. The same experimenter performed this exercise each time.

2.2.9. Statistical Analysis.
Results were analysed using the one-way ANOVA followed by the Student-Newman-Keuls posttest for comparison of treatment means. $P < 0.05$ was considered significant. Values in tables are given as arithmetic means ± standard error of the mean (S.E.M).

3. Results

Table 1 shows the phytochemical analysis of the aqueous and MeOH/CH$_2$CL$_2$ extracts, hexane, methylene chloride, ethyl acetate, and methanol fractions of E. speciosa. The major classes of compounds present included alkaloids, flavonoids, triterpenoids, glycosides, anthocyanins, quinones, and proteins which were distributed in the different extracts and fractions.

Table 2 shows the results obtained after screening the crude extracts and the various fractions for antisecretory and cytoprotective effects. At the dose of 100 mg/kg, only the crude MeOH-CH$_2$Cl$_2$ and the CH$_2$Cl$_2$ fractions significantly reduced gastric acidity. When tested at the higher dose of 200 mg/kg, they showed significant dose-dependent reductions in gastric acidity (51 and 45% reduction, resp.) compared with the aqueous extract (49% reduction) at the same dose. Cimetidine (50 mg/kg) reduced gastric acidity by

58 percent. The low acid concentrations were accompanied by highly significant reductions ($P < 0.001$) in the volumes of gastric secretions, and significant cytoprotection was evident from the highly significant increases in mucus production compared with the controls. The MeOH-CH$_2$Cl$_2$ extract, the CH$_2$Cl$_2$ fraction, and the aqueous extract were, thus, retained for the next set of experiments.

Tables 3 and 4 show the results obtained when, in addition to pylorus ligation, gastric hypersecretion was provoked by the administration of the secretagogues, histamine, and carbachol, respectively. Administration of histamine to the control animals raised gastric acidity to 86.50 ± 2.98 mEq/L (Table 3) while carbachol-induced secretion was 84.80 ± 3.57 mEq/L (Table 4). Treatment with the extracts (200 mg/kg) and cimetidine (100 mg/kg) resulted in highly significant reductions in gastric acidity ranging from 34.60 ± 3.33 to 59.00 ± 4.08 mEq/L in the histamine-treated rats (Table 3) and from 39.00 ± 5.34 to 59.80 ± 4.49 mEq/L in the carbachol-treated rats (Table 4). The extract-induced reductions in acid secretion were accompanied by highly significant reductions in volumes of gastric juice and ulcer indices and increases in mucus production both in the histamine- and carbachol-treated rats. Due to the similarity of the results between the extracts and the high presence of chlorophyll and the residual methanol in the MeOH-CH$_2$Cl$_2$ extract and CH$_2$Cl$_2$ fraction, the aqueous extract was retained for further experimentation.

Intraduodenal administration of E. speciosa aqueous extract (200 and 400 mg/kg) to pylorus ligated rats subjected to histamine-induced hypersecretion produced a highly significant ($P < 0.001$) dose-related decrease of acid secretion to 28.50 ± 1.30 mEq/L and volume of gastric juice to 2.54 ± 0.13 mL for the 400 mg/kg dose. pH values increased up to 4.83 ± 0.11 for the same dose. The high dose of aqueous extract

TABLE 2: Effects of *E. speciosa* extracts and fractions on gastric acid secretion and ulceration in pylorus ligated rats.

Treatment	Dose (mg/kg)	Ulcer index	% Inhibition	Gastric mucus (mg)	Gastric juice (mL)	Gastric pH	Gastric acidity (mE/L)
Control	—	3.88 ± 0.21	—	45.04 ± 5.09	5.07 ± 0.20	2.66 ± 0.15	79.40 ± 5.63
CH_3OH/CH_2CL_2	100	2.35 ± 0.05	39.43	$78.20 \pm 3.53^{***}$	$2.04 \pm 0.29^{**}$	$3.95 \pm 0.16^{***}$	$46.00 \pm 6.33^{**}$
CH_3OH/CH_2CL_2	200	$0.00 \pm 0.00^{***}$	100	$98.47 \pm 3.67^{***}$	$1.81 \pm 0.13^{***}$	$4.01 \pm 0.17^{***}$	$38.60 \pm 3.90^{***}$
CH_2CL_2 fraction	100	3.20 ± 0.17	17.53	51.13 ± 2.95	$2.14 \pm 0.32^{***}$	$3.54 \pm 0.19^{**}$	$55.60 \pm 6.57^{*}$
CH_2CL_2 fraction	200	$1.30 \pm 0.37^{***}$	66.49	$84.74 \pm 6.06^{***}$	$1.96 \pm 0.10^{***}$	$3.94 \pm 0.09^{***}$	$43.20 \pm 3.65^{***}$
Eth. Acet. fraction	100	3.40 ± 0.19	12.37	$60.70 \pm 2.83^{**}$	5.30 ± 0.26	2.94 ± 0.06	71.60 ± 4.06
Eth. Acet. fraction	200	$2.30 \pm 0.38^{*}$	40.72	$65.90 \pm 2.33^{**}$	4.93 ± 0.36	3.40 ± 0.09	59.70 ± 3.58
Hexane fraction	100	$2.77 \pm 0.16^{*}$	28.60	$70.72 \pm 2.73^{***}$	4.54 ± 0.21	$3.45 \pm 0.24^{**}$	64.20 ± 6.91
Hexane fraction	200	2.40 ± 0.20	38.14	$79.89 \pm 3.89^{***}$	4.01 ± 0.32	$3.52 \pm 0.39^{**}$	54.90 ± 5.92
CH_3OH fraction	100	3.43 ± 0.16	11.60	$65.87 \pm 2.70^{***}$	5.16 ± 0.21	3.06 ± 0.13	67.00 ± 6.12
CH_3OH fraction	200	2.90 ± 0.19	25.25	$67.33 \pm 2.00^{***}$	5.01 ± 0.19	$3.40 \pm 0.25^{**}$	$62.22 \pm 5.76^{*}$
Aqueous extract	100	$1.46 \pm 0.06^{***}$	62.37	$79.20 \pm 3.24^{***}$	4.70 ± 0.30	$3.01 \pm 0.15^{**}$	$63.40 \pm 4.10^{*}$
Aqueous extract	200	$1.00 \pm 0.27^{***}$	74.23	$92.19 \pm 3.05^{***}$	$2.10 \pm 0.17^{***}$	$3.97 \pm 0.13^{***}$	$40.02 \pm 2.56^{***}$
Cimetidine	50	$1.60 \pm 0.43^{***}$	58.76	$87.47 \pm 3.76^{***}$	$2.06 \pm 0.28^{***}$	$4.31 \pm 0.15^{***}$	$33.40 \pm 4.32^{***}$

$N = 5$ rats per treatment; $^{*}P < 0.05$, statistically significant relative to control; $^{**}P < 0.01$, statistically highly significant relative to control; $^{***}P < 0.001$, statistically very highly significant relative to control.

TABLE 3: Effects of orally administered *E. speciosa* on histamine-induced gastric ulcers and gastric secretion in rats.

Treatment	Dose (mg/kg)	Ulcer index (mean + SEM)	% Inhibition	Mucus production (mg) (mean + SEM)	Volume of gastric juice (mL) (mean + SEM)	Gastric pH (mean + SEM)	Gastric acidity (mEq/L) (mean + SEM)
Control	—	4.12 ± 0.16	—	52.83 ± 2.96	6.87 ± 0.31	2.37 ± 0.04	86.50 ± 2.98
CH_3OH/CH_2Cl_2	200	$0.00 \pm 0.00^{***}$	100.00	$92.13 \pm 2.89^{***}$	$3.07 \pm 0.18^{***}$	$4.74 \pm 0.34^{***}$	$39.50 \pm 3.19^{***}$
CH_2Cl_2 fraction	200	$1.57 \pm 0,65^{***}$	61.89	$87.32 \pm 6.91^{***}$	$3.32 \pm 0.38^{***}$	$4.47 \pm 0.27^{***}$	$49.80 \pm 4.14^{***}$
Aqueous extract	200	$1.90 \pm 0.29^{***}$	53.88	$85.05 \pm 4.21^{***}$	$3.50 \pm 0.45^{***}$	$4.33 \pm 0.23^{***}$	$59.00 \pm 4.08^{***}$
Cimetidine	100	$0.0 \pm 0.00^{***}$	100.00	$88.8 \pm 3.62^{***}$	$2.28 \pm 0.20^{***}$	$4.96 \pm 0.24^{***}$	$34.60 \pm 3.33^{***}$

$N = 5$ rats per treatment; $^{*}P < 0.05$, statistically significant relative to control; $^{**}P < 0.01$, statistically highly significant relative to control; $^{***}P < 0.001$, statistically very highly significant relative to control.

also produced 100 percent inhibition of gastric ulceration and increased mucus production to 101.69 ± 3.89 mg compared with 56.36 ± 3.35 mg for the controls (Table 5). When the aqueous extract (200 and 400 mg/kg) was administered intraduodenally to pylorus ligated rats treated with carbachol, similar dose-dependent reduction in gastric acid production to 28.80 ± 1.30 mEq/L was obtained for the 400 mg/kg dose. Gastric juice pH increased to 5.26 ± 0.12 and volume of gastric juice reduced to 2.37 ± 0.15 for the same dose. Ulcer formation was totally inhibited and gastric mucus production increased significantly for the dose of 400 mg/kg (Table 6).

Repeated histamine injection to the control rats (augmented histamine test) further raised the basal gastric acid levels to 90.20 ± 2.71 mEq/L. Pretreatment with a single oral dose of aqueous extract (200 and 400 mg/kg) prevented the histamine effect by reducing the acid secretion to values significantly below basal levels (52.60 ± 2.96 and 27.50 ± 1.29 mEq/L, resp.). pH and volume of gastric juice at the dose of 400 mg/kg were 5.02 ± 0.17 and $2.06 + 0.18$ mL compared to 2.29 ± 0.06 and 7.42 ± 0.26 mL, respectively, for the controls. There was complete inhibition of ulcer formation associated

with significant increase in mucus production for cimetidine (100 mg/kg) and extract (400 mg/kg) (Table 7).

The effects of the extract when administered to carbachol/indomethacin-treated rats are shown in Table 8. Coadministration of carbachol and indomethacin significantly reduced the ulcer inhibition capacity of the oral aqueous extract (200–400 mg/kg) to 25–44 % compared with 70–100 % inhibition (for carbachol alone, Table 4). This was accompanied by a drop in mucus production both for the controls and extract-treated rats. In addition, the volume of gastric juice (3.96–5.09 mL) and gastric acidity (59.5 ± 4.36–44.00 ± 4.08 mEq/L) remained high in response to the extract. When the extract was administered by duodenal route, the values of ulcer index, pH, and volumes of gastric juice remained largely unchanged, and gastric acidity reduced significantly only for the 400 mg/kg dose (Table 9).

4. Discussion

In a preliminary study [39] we found that the water extract of *E. speciosa* had possible cytoprotective and antisecretory

TABLE 4: Effects of orally administered *E. speciosa* on carbachol-induced gastric ulcers and gastric secretion in rats.

Treatment	Dose (mg/kg)	Ulcer index (mean + SEM)	% Inhibition	Mucus production (mg) (mean + SEM)	Volume of gastric juice (mL) (mean + SEM)	Gastric pH (mean + SEM)	Gastric acidity (mEq/L) (mean + SEM)
Control	—	4.03 ± 0.13	—	49.34 ± 3.20	6.89 ± 0.22	2.59 ± 0.04	84.80 ± 3.57
CH_3OH/CH_2Cl_2	200	$1.43 \pm 0.37^{***}$	64.52	$78.82 \pm 3.64^{**}$	$3.57 \pm 0.30^{***}$	$4.35 \pm 0.12^{***}$	$54.00 \pm 4.30^{**}$
CH_2Cl_2 fraction	200	$1.73 \pm 0.50^{***}$	57.07	$76.08 \pm 2.83^{**}$	$3.71 \pm 0.25^{***}$	$4.12 \pm 0.14^{***}$	$59.80 \pm 4.49^{**}$
Aqueous extract	200	$1.20 \pm 0.34^{***}$	70.22	$79.19 \pm 3.66^{**}$	$3.99 \pm 0.27^{***}$	$4.24 \pm 0.22^{***}$	$50.00 \pm 4.26^{***}$
Cimetidine	50	$1.10 \pm 0.46^{***}$	72.71	$69.42 \pm 3.42^{*}$	$2.76 \pm 0.37^{***}$	$5.48 \pm 0.17^{***}$	$39.00 \pm 5.34^{***}$

$N = 5$ rats per treatment; $^{*}P < 0.05$, statistically significant relative to control; $^{**}P < 0.01$, statistically highly significant relative to control; $^{***}P < 0.001$, statistically very highly significant relative to control.

TABLE 5: Effects of duodenally administered aqueous extract of *E. speciosa* on gastric ulceration and secretion induced by histamine in rats.

Treatment	Dose (mg/kg)	Ulcer index (mean + SEM)	% Inhibition	Mucus production (mg) (mean + SEM)	Volume of gastric juice (mL) (mean + SEM)	Gastric pH (mean + SEM)	Gastric acidity (mEq/L) (mean + SEM)
Control	—	4.07 ± 0.22	—	59.06 ± 2.30	6.54 ± 0.24	2.29 ± 0.06	88.30 ± 3.56
E. speciosa	200	$2.40 \pm 0.19^{***}$	41.03	$84.82 \pm 2.69^{***}$	$4.54 \pm 0.21^{***}$	$3.99 \pm 0.16^{***}$	$54.60 \pm 2.70^{***}$
E. speciosa	400	$0.00 \pm 0.00^{***}$	100.00	$101.69 \pm 3.89^{***}$	$2.54 \pm 0.13^{***}$	$4.65 \pm 0.10^{***}$	$28.50 \pm 1.30^{***}$
Ranitidine	100	$1.91 \pm 0.33^{***}$	53.00	$89.87 \pm 2.01^{***}$	$2.02 \pm 0.15^{***}$	$5.02 \pm 0.17^{***}$	$36.36 \pm 1.46^{***}$

$N = 5$ rats per treatment; $^{***}P < 0.001$; statistically very highly significant relative to control.

TABLE 6: Effects of duodenally administered aqueous extract of *E. speciosa* on gastric ulceration and secretion induced by carbachol in rats.

Treatment	Dose (mg/kg)	Ulcer index (mean + SEM)	% Inhibition	Mucus production (mg) (mean + SEM)	Volume of gastric juice (mL) (mean + SEM)	Gastric pH (mean + SEM)	Gastric acidity (mEq/L) (mean + SEM)
Control	—	3.90 ± 0.19	—	56.36 ± 3.35	6.71 ± 0.19	2.72 ± 0.07	85.50 ± 2.31
E. speciosa	200	$2.02 \pm 0.20^{***}$	48.21	$77.60 \pm 2.78^{***}$	$3.97 \pm 0.25^{***}$	$4.15 \pm 0.12^{***}$	$51.40 \pm 3.97^{***}$
E. speciosa	400	$0.00 \pm 0.00^{***}$	100.00	$103.20 \pm 3.19^{***}$	$2.37 \pm 0.15^{***}$	$5.26 \pm 0.12^{***}$	$28.80 \pm 1.38^{***}$
Ranitidine	100	$1.76 \pm 0.23^{***}$	55.00	$82.34 \pm 3.48^{***}$	$2.48 \pm 0.19^{***}$	$4.96 \pm 0.28^{***}$	$34.20 \pm 1.42^{***}$

$N = 5$ rats per treatment; $^{***}P < 0.001$; statistically very highly significant relative to control.

TABLE 7: Effects of orally administered aqueous extract of *E. speciosa* on gastric ulceration and secretion in rats submitted to the augmented histamine test.

Treatment	Dose (mg/kg)	Ulcer index (mean + SEM)	% Inhibition	Mucus production (mg) (mean + SEM)	Volume of gastric juice (mL) (mean + SEM)	Gastric pH (mean + SEM)	Gastric acidity (mEq/L) (mean + SEM)
Control	—	4.33 ± 0.17	—	52.84 ± 2.42	7.42 ± 0.26	2.29 ± 0.06	90.20 ± 2.71
E. speciosa	200	$2.27 \pm 0.19^{***}$	47.58	$82.20 \pm 2.82^{***}$	$3.76 \pm 0.26^{***}$	$3.99 = 0.16^{***}$	$52.60 \pm 2.96^{***}$
E. speciosa	400	$0.00 \pm 0.0^{***}$	100.00	$96.51 \pm 3.12^{***}$	$2.20 \pm 0.27^{***}$	$4.65 = 0.10^{***}$	$27.50 \pm 1.29^{***}$
Ranitidine	100	$0.00 \pm 0.00^{***}$	100.00	$73.21 \pm 2.43^{***}$	$2.06 \pm 0.18^{***}$	$5.02 = 0.17^{***}$	$19.20 \pm 1.68^{***}$

$N = 5$ rats per treatment; $^{***}P < 0.001$; statistically very highly significant relative to control.

TABLE 8: Effects of orally administered aqueous extract of *E. speciosa* on gastric ulceration and secretion in pylorus-ligated rats treated with indomethacin/carbachol.

Treatment	Dose (mg/kg)	Ulcer index (mean + SEM)	% Inhibition	Mucus production (mg) (mean + SEM)	Volume of gastric juice (mL) (mean + SEM)	Gastric pH (mean + SEM)	Gastric acidity (mEq/L) (mean + SEM)
Control	—	4.13 ± 0.21	—	38.87 ± 4.59	7.32 ± 0.26	2.64 ± 0.15	92.10 ± 4.39
E. speciosa	200	$3.10 \pm 0.25^{**}$	24.94	$60.63 \pm 5.67^{*}$	$5.14 \pm 0.29^{***}$	$3.96 \pm 0.08^{***}$	$59.50 \pm 4.36^{***}$
E. speciosa	400	$2.31 \pm 0.13^{***}$	44.07	$74.01 \pm 6.90^{**}$	$4.16 \pm 0.31^{***}$	$4.77 \pm 0.07^{***}$	$44.00 \pm 4.08^{***}$
Ranitidine	100	$2.03 \pm 0.20^{***}$	50.85	49.02 ± 5.31	$3.64 \pm 0.30^{***}$	$5.09 \pm 0.25^{***}$	$35.05 \pm 3.03^{***}$

$N = 5$ rats per treatment; $^{*}P < 0.05$, statistically significant relative to control; $^{**}P < 0.01$, statistically highly significant relative to control; $^{***}P < 0.001$, statistically very highly significant relative to control.

TABLE 9: Effects of duodenally administered aqueous extract of *E. speciosa* on gastric ulceration and secretion in pylorus-ligated rats treated with indomethacin/carbachol.

Treatment	Dose (mg/kg)	Ulcer index (mean + SEM)	% Inhibition	Mucus production (mg) (mean + SEM)	Volume of gastric juice (mL) (mean + SEM)	Gastric pH (mean + SEM)	Gastric acidity (mEq/L) (mean + SEM)
Control	—	3.80 ± 0.13	—	44.39 ± 4.82	6.91 ± 0.15	2.72 ± 0.11	88.50 ± 5.10
E. speciosa	200	$2.68 \pm 0.23^{***}$	29.47	59.43 ± 4.45	$5.02 \pm 0.42^{***}$	$4.02 \pm 0.12^{***}$	$60.50 \pm 4.36^{***}$
E. speciosa	400	$2.40 \pm 0.10^{***}$	36.84	$66.73 \pm 5.44^{*}$	$4.48 \pm 0.25^{***}$	$4.60 \pm 0.15^{***}$	$34.50 \pm 3.57^{***}$
Ranitidine	100	$2.03 \pm 0.20^{***}$	50.85	49.02 ± 5.31	$3.64 \pm 0.30^{***}$	$5.09 \pm 0.25^{***}$	$35.05 \pm 3.03^{***}$

$N = 5$ rats per treatment; $^{*}P < 0.05$, statistically significant relative to control; $^{***}P < 0.001$, statistically very highly significant relative to control.

effects but no study has been carried out to explore the possible mechanism of action. In the present study, several extracts and unpurified fractions were screened for comparative antisecretory effects. The MeOH-CH$_2$Cl$_2$ and aqueous extracts and the CH$_2$Cl$_2$ fraction showed significant antisecretory activity at the lower dose of 100 mg/kg and significant dose-dependent activity at 200 mg/kg and were further screened for their response to secretagogue-induced gastric acid secretion. The three products (200 mg/kg) showed highly significant reductions in acid secretion induced by histamine (31–54%) and carbachol (29–41%). However, the MeOH-CH$_2$Cl$_2$ extract had higher antisecretory activity against histamine-induced secretion, while the aqueous extract showed higher antisecretory effects against carbachol-induced gastric acid secretion.

The pylorus ligation technique usually causes accumulation of gastric acid in the stomach and agents that reduce acid secretion and/or increase mucus secretion are effective in inhibiting ulcer formation by this method. The accumulated acid, in addition to its corrosive action on gastric glandular epithelium, provides the optimum pH (1.6–3.2) for the conversion of pepsinogen to pepsin. Both HCl and pepsin are important ingredients for the formation of pylorus ligated ulcers [42]. The MeOH-CH$_2$Cl$_2$ and aqueous extracts and the CH$_2$Cl$_2$ fraction significantly reduced the volume and acidity of gastric secretions and increased pH of gastric juice compared with the controls. This, in addition to the significant increases in gastric mucus production, contributed to the significant inhibition of gastric ulceration (Table 2). In Shay ligated rats, gastric acid levels of 40 mEq/L and above have been associated with severe ulceration of the rat gastric mucosa [39, 43, 44]. In the present study, the extracts reduced gastric acidity from 79.4 mEq/L in the controls down to between 38.6 and 40.2 mEq/L, while inhibition of ulcer formation ranged between 74 and 100%. These results underline the protective role of the increased gastric mucus secretion in extract-treated rats (92.19–98.47 g) compared with the controls (45.04 g) (Table 1). Pepsin inactivation occurs at about pH 6. Between pH 4 and 6, pepsin is still stable but inactive [45]. Gastric pH values obtained in all the experiments in response to extract administration ranged between 3.97 and 5.26, suggesting that the extract may deactivate gastric pepsin and interfere with protein digestion.

Neural, endocrine, and paracrine systems are responsible for the physiological control of gastric secretion. Acetylcholine and histamine directly activate acid secretion but by different pathways. While acetylcholine binds to M$_3$-muscarinic receptors causing an increase in parietal cell intracellular calcium, histamine binds to H$_2$-receptors and provokes an elevation of both intracellular calcium and of cyclic AMP. Cimetidine, which is a well-known H$_2$-receptor antagonist, inhibits the activation of adenyl cyclase, thus, blocking the formation of cyclic AMP that is necessary for HCl production. Carbachol is a cholinomimetic drug which, like acetylcholine, increases free intracellular calcium. The resulting activation of protein kinase by phosphorylation leads to increased HCl production. Degranulation of peritoneal mast cells to release histamine is critically dependent on extracellular calcium concentration. Agents like verapamil and ranitidine, that block T-type low voltage-sensitive calcium channel opening and calcium influx through interference with H$^+$K$^+$ ATPase from the luminal side of the stomach, reduce both the volume and acidity of gastric secretions [46–50]. Calcium channel blockers exert their inhibitory effects on histamine, gastrin, carbachol, and cyclic AMP-induced stimulation of gastric acid secretion [51].

In our study, the CH$_2$Cl$_2$ fraction, the MeOH-CH$_2$Cl$_2$ and aqueous extracts (200 mg/kg), and cimetidine significantly raised gastric pH and reduced the volume and secretion of gastric acid in both histamine- and carbachol-treated rats. Further experimentation with the aqueous extract (200–400 mg/kg) yielded highly significant dose-dependent reduction of volume and acidity of gastric secretion when the extract was administered by intraduodenal route. These results suggest that the observed reductions in gastric acidity could be due to an H$_2$-receptor blocking mechanism similar to cimetidine as well as M-3 muscarinic receptor blocking activity similar to verapamil. Since carbachol- and histamine-activated acid secretions occur by separate mechanisms, the extract of *E. speciosa* may contain two or more antisecretory ingredients acting separately and synergistically. This may, therefore, explain the highly significant acid reduction observed in the secretagogue-treated rats. It is worth noting that even in histamine-treated rats, the laparotomy- and pylorus ligation-induced pain constitutes a source of stress which contributes to acid secretion through the cholinergic pathway. When histaminergic and cholinergic stimulations of gastric acid secretion were similarly reduced by the aqueous extract of *Stachytarpheta cayennensis*, it was suggested [40] that the extract could be acting through the inhibition of common steps in both pathways, possibly at the level of histamine release/H$_2$-receptor interaction or at the proton pump. In addition, the effects of *E. speciosa* aqueous extract may not be attributed to a gastric luminal topical activity alone since the extract was also active when administered by intraduodenal route. The striking similarity in acid reduction capacity when the aqueous extract (200 mg/kg) was administered by oral and duodenal route both for histamine- (59.00 ± 4.08 and 54.62 ± 2.70 mEq/L, resp.) and carbachol- (50.00 ± 4.26 and 51.40 ± 3.97 mEq/L, resp.) induced secretion is suggestive of the involvement of an active secondary metabolite.

The antiulcerogenic and antisecretory effects of *E. speciosa* aqueous extract dropped when carbachol was coadministered with indomethacin. Indomethacin, an NSAID, is well-known for its ability to suppress prostaglandin synthesis, bicarbonate secretion, and gastric mucosal blood flow in animals [52–54]. These effects increase gastric mucosal susceptibility to injury and exacerbate, in synergy with carbachol, the ulcerogenic effects of increased acid, and pepsin secretion in the stomach [41, 55]. The vital role that prostaglandins play in gastric mucosal protection is well-known. When the cytoprotective effect of an antiulcer agent is significantly reduced by pretreatment with indomethacin, it is usually interpreted that the cytoprotection is mediated by endogenous prostaglandins.

In the present study, histamine-induced basal acid secretion was higher (86.5–88.3 mEq/L) compared to carbachol-induced basal secretions (84.5–85.2 mEq/L), and histamine-induced basal secretion rose to 90.2 mEq/L in the augmented histamine test. These results are in agreement with previous findings [55] which showed that carbachol-induced secretion by parietal cells is fast, small, and transient, whereas histamine-provoked secretion is slow, large, and sustained. The large sustained secretion induced by the augmented histamine test (90.20 ± 2.71 mEq/L) was reduced to very low levels by 400 mg/kg of *E. speciosa* aqueous extract (27.50 ± 1.29 mEq/L) and by 100 mg/kg of cimetidine (19.2 ± 1.68 mEq/L). Similar levels of gastric acidity (25 mEq/L) have previously been observed [39] not to cause gastric mucosal ulceration in pylorus ligated rats. Our results are similar to findings that cimetidine significantly reduces both the volume and acidity of gastric secretions. They also demonstrate the strong antisecretory and antiulcer actions of *E. speciosa* aqueous extract at 400 mg/kg similar to *Myristica fragrans* [56] and *Hibiscus rosasinensis* [7] aqueous extracts (500 mg/kg) against secretagogue-induced hyperacidity. Phytochemical screening of the extracts and fractions (Table 1) showed the predominant presence of alkaloids, triterpenes, flavonoids, and phenols which are well-known for their gastric antisecretory and cytoprotective activities [17–20].

5. Conclusion

In conclusion, the water and MeOH-CH$_2$Cl$_2$ extracts and the CH$_2$Cl$_2$ fraction of *E. speciosa* protected the rat gastric mucosa and inhibited gastric acid secretion. In addition to increased mucus production, the aqueous extract offers cytoprotection through a mechanism that involves the physicochemical reenforcement of the gastric mucous layer or by

effects similar to endogenous prostaglandins. The antisecretory effect of the aqueous extract may involve a mechanism common to both cholinergic and histaminergic pathways. This may be attributed to the various bioactive compounds present in the extract. The results lend credence to the wide traditional use of *E. speciosa* in the management of complaints symptomatic of peptic ulcer disease.

Conflict of Interests

The authors declare that there is no conflict of interests regarding the publication of this paper.

References

[1] M. I. Grossman, Ed., *Peptic Ulcer: A Guide for the Practicing Physician*, Year book Medical, Chicago, Ill, USA, 1981.

[2] C. R. W. Edward, I. A. D. Bouchier, and C. Haslett, "Diseases of the stomach," in *Davison's Principles and Practice of Medicine*, pp. 425–434, Churchill Livingstone, London, UK, 1995.

[3] B. J. Marshall and J. R. Warren, "Unidentified curved bacilli in the stomach of patients with gastritis and peptic ulceration," *The Lancet*, vol. 1, no. 8390, pp. 1311–1314, 1984.

[4] J. W. Black, W. A. M. Duncan, C. J. Durant, C. R. Ganellin, and E. M. Parsons, "Definition and antagonism of histamine H2-receptors," *Nature*, vol. 236, no. 5347, pp. 385–390, 1972.

[5] E. Fellenius, T. Berglindh, and G. Sachs, "Substituted benzimidazoles inhibit gastric acid secretion by blocking (H+ + K+)ATPase," *Nature*, vol. 290, no. 5802, pp. 159–161, 1981.

[6] J. M. Wolosin and J. G. Forte, "Stimulation of oxyntic cell triggers K+ and Cl− conductances in apical H+−K+−ATPase membrane," *American Journal of Physiology*, vol. 15, no. 3, pp. C537–C545, 1984.

[7] M. F. Dixon, R. M. Genta, J. H. Yardley et al., "Classification and grading of Gastritis: the updated Sydney system," *American Journal of Surgical Pathology*, vol. 20, no. 10, pp. 1161–1181, 1996.

[8] K. E. L. McColl, E. El-Omar, and D. Gillen, "Interactions between *Helicobacter pylori* infection, gastric acid secretion and anti-secretory therapy," *British Medical Bulletin*, vol. 54, no. 1, pp. 121–138, 1998.

[9] K. A. Ryan, L.-J. Van Doorn, A. P. Moran, M. Glennon, T. Smith, and M. Maher, "Evaluation of clarithromycin resistance and cagA and vacA genotyping of *Helicobacter pylori* strains from the west of Ireland using line probe assays," *Journal of Clinical Microbiology*, vol. 39, no. 5, pp. 1978–1980, 2001.

[10] I. L. P. Beales, "Efficacy of *Helicobacter pylori* eradication therapies: a single centre observational study," *BMC Gastroenterology*, vol. 1, article 7, 2001.

[11] S. Suerbaum and P. Michetti, "Helicobacter pylori infection," *The New England Journal of Medicine*, vol. 347, no. 15, pp. 1175–1186, 2002.

[12] M. B. Skirrow, "Campylobacter and helicobacter; enteritis; gastritis," in *Medical Microbiology*, D. Greenwood et al., Ed., pp. 353–361, Churchill Livingstone, 14th edition, 1992.

[13] J. L. Fauchere, "Bacteriological characteristics and diagnosis of *Helicobacter pylori*," *Laborama*, vol. 6, pp. 10–14, 1999.

[14] M. Kato, Y. Yamaoka, J. J. Kim et al., "Regional differences in metronidazole resistance and increasing clarithromycin resistance among *Helicobacter pylori*, isolates from Japan," *Antimicrobial Agents and Chemotherapy*, vol. 44, no. 8, pp. 2214–2216, 2000.

[15] T. Okamoto, H. Yoshiyama, T. Nakazawa et al., "A change in PBP1 is involved in amoxicillin resistance of clinical isolates of *Helicobacter pylori*," *Journal of Antimicrobial Chemotherapy*, vol. 50, no. 6, pp. 849–856, 2002.

[16] M. L. Schubert and D. A. Peura, "Control of gastric acid secretion in health and disease," *Gastroenterology*, vol. 134, no. 7, pp. 1842–1860, 2008.

[17] A. Favier, "Le stress oxydant: intérêt conceptuel et expérimental dans la compréhension des mécanismes des maladies et potentiel thérapeutique. Dans: Mécanismes Biochimiques," *L'Actualité Chimique*, pp. 108–115, 2003.

[18] M. B. Gupta, R. Nath, G. P. Gupta, and K. P. Bhargava, "Antiulcer activity of some plant triterpenoids," *Indian Journal of Medical Research*, vol. 73, no. 4, pp. 649–652, 1981.

[19] P. V. Tan and B. Nyasse, "Anti-ulcer compound from *Voacanga africana* with possible histamine H_2 receptor blocking activity," *Phytomedicine*, vol. 7, no. 6, pp. 509–515, 2000.

[20] P. V. Tan, B. Nyasse, G. E. Enow-Orock, P. Wafo, and E. A. Forcha, "Prophylactic and healing properties of a new anti-ulcer compound from *Enantia chlorantha* in rats," *Phytomedicine*, vol. 7, no. 4, pp. 291–296, 2000.

[21] O. E. Mboso, E. U. Eyong, M. O. Odey, and E. Osakwe, "Comparative phytochemical screening of *Ereromastax speciosa* and *Ereromastax polysperma*," *Journal of Natural Product and Plant Resources*, no. 2, pp. 37–41, 2013.

[22] F. Borrelli and A. A. Izzo, "The plant kingdom as a source of anti-ulcer remedies," *Phytotherapy Research*, vol. 14, pp. 581–591, 2000.

[23] H. Heine, "Acanthacees," in *Flore Du Gabon*, vol. 3, pp. 29–32, Museum Nationale d'Histoire Naturelle, Paris, France, 1966.

[24] J. E. Oben, S. E. Assi, G. A. Agbor, and D. F. Musoro, "Effect of Eremomastax speciosa on experimental diarrhoea," *African Journal of Traditional, Complementary and Alternative Medicines*, vol. 3, no. 1, pp. 95–100, 2006.

[25] J. O. Erhabor, M. Idu, and F. O. Udo, "Ethnomedicinal survey of medicinal plants used in the treatment of male infertilty among the IFA Nkari People of Ini Local Government area of Akwa Ibom State, Nigeria," *Research Journal of Recent Sciences*, vol. 2, pp. 5–11, 2013.

[26] J. E. Okokon, B. S. Antia, A. E. Udoh, and M. M. Akpan, "Antianaemic and antimicrobial activity of *Eremomastax speciosa*," *Journal of Pharmacology and Toxicology*, vol. 2, pp. 196–199, 2007.

[27] S. D. Dibong, M. E. Mpondo, A. Ngoye, and R. J. Priso, "Modalities of exploitation of medicinal plants in Douala's region," *American Journal of Food and Nutrition*, vol. 1, no. 2, pp. 67–73, 2011.

[28] P. B. Telefo, M. C. Lemfack, B. Bayala et al., "Ethnopharmacological survey of medicinal plants used in women infertility treatment in Fossong-Wentcheng and Foto villages, Western Region of Cameroon," *Phytotherapie*, vol. 10, no. 1, pp. 25–34, 2012.

[29] D. A. Focho, W. T. Ndam, and B. A. Fonge, "Medicinal plants of Aguambu—Bamumbu in the Lebialem highlands, southwest province of Cameroon," *African Journal of Pharmacy and Pharmacology*, vol. 3, no. 1, pp. 001–013, 2009.

[30] E. N. Ndenecho, "Herbalism and resources for the development of ethnopharmacology in Mount Cameroon region," *African Journal of Pharmacy and Pharmacology*, vol. 3, no. 3, pp. 078–086, 2009.

[31] P. V. Tan, N. G. Nditafon, M. P. Yewah, T. Dimo, and F. J. Ayafor, "Eremomastax speciosa: effects of leaf aqueous extract on ulcer formation and gastric secretion in rats," *Journal of Ethnopharmacology*, vol. 54, no. 2-3, pp. 139–142, 1996.

[32] P. A. Amang, P. V. Tan, S. A. Patamaken, and M. N. Mefe, "Cytoprotective and antioxidant effects of the methanol extract of *Eremomastax speciosa* in rats," *African Journal of Traditional, Complementary and Alternative Medicines*, vol. 11, no. 1, pp. 165–171, 2014.

[33] O. O. Odebiyi and E. A. Sofowora, "Phytochemical screening of Nigerian medicinal plants II," *Lloydia*, vol. 41, no. 3, pp. 234–246, 1978.

[34] J. B. Harbone, *Phytochemical Methods. A Guide to Modern Techniques of Plant Analysis*, Chapman and Hall, London, UK, 1976.

[35] C. V. Schoppe, *Chemistry of the Steroids*, Butterworth, London, UK, 2nd edition, 1964.

[36] M. E. Wall, C. R. Eddy, M. L. McClennan, and M. E. Klumpp, "Detection and estimation of steroidal sapogenins in plant tissue," *Analytical Chemistry*, vol. 24, no. 8, pp. 1337–1341, 1952.

[37] G. E. Trease and W. C. Evans, *A Textbook of Pharmacognosy*, Bailliere Tindall, London, UK, 13th edition, 1989.

[38] E. E. Kovac-Besovi and K. Duri, "Thin layer Chromatography-application in qualitative analysis on presence of coumarins and flavonoids in plant material," *Bosnian Journal of Basic Medical Sciences*, vol. 3, no. 3, pp. 19–26, 2003.

[39] S. M. Vela, C. Souccar, M. T. R. Lima-Landman, and A. J. Lapa, "Inhibition of gastric acid secretion by the aqueous extract and purified extracts of *Stachytarpheta cayennensis*," *Planta Medica*, vol. 63, no. 1, pp. 36–39, 1997.

[40] K. D. Rainsford, "Gastric ulcerogenicity of non-steroidal anti-inflamatory drugs in mice with mucosa sensitized by choli-nomimetic treatment," *Biochemical Pharmacology*, vol. 27, pp. 1281–1289, 1978.

[41] J. P. Shay, S. A. Komarov, S. S. Fels, D. Meranze, M. Grunstein, and H. Simpler, "A simple method for the uniform production of gastric ulceration in the rat," *Gastroenterology*, vol. 5, pp. 43–61, 1945.

[42] M. J. Martin, E. Marhuenda, C. Perez-Guerrero, and J. M. Franco, "Antiulcer effect of naringin on gastric lesions induced by ethanol in rats," *Pharmacology*, vol. 49, no. 3, pp. 144–150, 1994.

[43] E. Marhuenda, M. J. Martin, and C. Alarcon De La Lastra, "Antiulcerogenic activity of aescine in different experimental models," *Phytotherapy Research*, vol. 7, no. 1, pp. 13–16, 1993.

[44] J. Vatier and T. Vallot, "Antacides," in *Pharmacologie. Des Concceptes Fondamentaux Aux Applications Therapeutiques*, pp. 555–565, Frison-Roche, Paris, France, 1998.

[45] J. F. Perez-Zoghbi, A. Mayora, M. C. Ruiz, and F. Michelangeli, "Heterogeneity of acid secretion induced by carbachol and histamine along the gastric gland axis and its relationship to $[Ca^{2+}]_i$," *American Journal of Physiology*, vol. 295, no. 4, pp. G671–G681, 2008.

[46] R. J. Mandade, S. A. Sreenivas, D. M. Sakarkar, and A. Choudhury, "Pharmacological effects of aqueous-ethanolic extract of Hibiscus rosasinensis on volume and acidity of stimulated gastric secretion," *Asian Pacific Journal of Tropical Medicine*, vol. 4, no. 11, pp. 883–888, 2011.

[47] P. A. Negulescu and T. E. Matchen, "Intracelluar calcium regulation during secretagogue stimulation of the parietal cells," *American Journal of Physiology*, vol. 254, pp. 130–138, 1998.

[48] R. Brage, J. Cortjio, and J. Esplugues, "Effects of calcium channel blockers on gastric emptying and acid secretion of the rat in vivo," *British Journal of Pharmacology*, vol. 89, no. 4, pp. 627–633, 1986.

[49] B. Kadalmani, M. Saravana Kumar, P. Revathi, and K. Prakash Shyam, "Gastric ulcer protective property of calcium channel Blockers in male albino rats," *International Journal of Pharma and Bio Sciences*, vol. 2, no. 1, pp. 629–636, 2011.

[50] K. F. Sewing and H. Hannemann, "Calcium channel antagonists verapamil and gallopamil are powerful inhibitors of acid secretion in isolated and enriched guinea pig parietal cells," *Pharmacology*, vol. 27, no. 1, pp. 9–14, 1983.

[51] G. Flemstrom, A. Garner, and O. Nylander, "Surface epithelial HCO_3 transport by mammalian duodenum in vivo," *American Journal of Physiology*, vol. 6, no. 5, pp. G343–G358, 1982.

[52] B. J. R. Whittle, "Mechanisms underlying gastric mucosal damage induced by indomethacin and bile salts, and the actions of prostaglandins," *British Journal of Pharmacology*, vol. 60, no. 3, pp. 455–460, 1977.

[53] J. A. Selling, D. L. Hogan, and A. Aly, "Indomethacin inhibits duodenal mucosal bicarbonate secretion and endogenous prostaglandin E2 output in human subjects," *Annals of Internal Medicine*, vol. 106, no. 3, pp. 368–371, 1987.

[54] W. Toma, J. D. S. Gracioso, F. D. P. De Andrade, C. A. Hiruma-Lima, W. Vilegas, and A. R. M. Souza Brito, "Antiulcerogenic activity of four extracts obtained from the bark wood of *Quassia amara* L. (Simaroubaceae)," *Biological and Pharmaceutical Bulletin*, vol. 25, no. 9, pp. 1151–1155, 2002.

[55] J. F. Pérez, M. C. Ruiz, and F. Michelangeli, "Simultaneous measurement and imaging of intracellular Ca^{2+} and H^+ transport in isolated rabbit gastric glands," *Journal of Physiology*, vol. 537, no. 3, pp. 735–745, 2001.

[56] M. Jan, A. Hussain, S. M. Naeem, S. A. Malik, R. Masood ur, and M. Hassan, "Comparison between the effects of of the extract of *Myristica fragrans* and cimetidine on the volume and acidity of carbachol-induced gastric secretion in fasting rabbits," *Pakistan Journal of Medical Sciences*, vol. 43, no. 4, pp. 191–194, 2004.

18

Liver Fibrosis and Protection Mechanisms Action of Medicinal Plants Targeting Apoptosis of Hepatocytes and Hepatic Stellate Cells

Florent Duval,[1] **Jorge E. Moreno-Cuevas,**[1] **Maria Teresa González-Garza,**[1] **Carlos Rodríguez-Montalvo,**[2] **and Delia Elva Cruz-Vega**[1]

[1] *Catedra de Terapia Celular, Escuela de Medicina, Tecnológico de Monterrey, Avenida Morones Prieto 3000 Pte., 64710 Monterrey, NL, Mexico*
[2] *Centro de Enfermedades Hepáticas-Digestivas y Nutrición, Hospital San José, Avenida Morones Prieto 3000, 64710 Monterrey, NL, Mexico*

Correspondence should be addressed to Delia Elva Cruz-Vega; cruzvegade@gmail.com

Academic Editor: Eduardo Munoz

Following chronic liver injury, hepatocytes undergo apoptosis leading to activation of hepatic stellate cells (HSC). Consequently, activated HSC proliferate and produce excessive extracellular matrix, responsible for the scar formation. The pandemic trend of obesity, combined with the high incidence of alcohol intake and viral hepatitis infections, highlights the urgent need to find accessible antifibrotic therapies. Treatment strategies should take into account the versatility of its pathogenesis and act on all the cell lines involved to reduce liver fibrosis. Medicinal plants are achieving popularity as antifibrotic agents, supported by their safety, cost-effectiveness, and versatility. This review will describe the role of hepatocytes and HSC in the pathogenesis of liver fibrosis and detail the mechanisms of modulation of apoptosis of both cell lines by twelve known hepatoprotective plants in order to reduce liver fibrosis.

1. Introduction

Fibrosis is an inappropriate tissue repair of the liver resulting from almost all of the chronic liver injuries including alcohol induced damage, chronic viral hepatitis, autoimmune, parasitic, and metabolic diseases and less frequent, toxic, or drugs exposure [1]. When fibrosis is not controlled, it can further progress into cirrhosis. In contrast with the traditional idea that cirrhosis is an irreversible state, there is solid evidence indicating that fibrosis even cirrhosis could be reversible [2].

Liver fibrosis is an important public health concern with significant morbidity and mortality [3]. Hundreds of millions of people worldwide suffer from cirrhosis [4]. Chronic viral hepatitis B and C, alcoholic liver diseases, and nonalcoholic fatty liver diseases are the three most common causes [5]. Prevalence of chronic liver diseases, hence hepatic fibrosis-cirrhosis, is predicted to increase, due in part to the rising prevalence of obesity and metabolic syndrome, especially in developed countries [6].

Pathogenesis of liver fibrosis is complex and varies between the different kinds of hepatic injuries. Usually after an acute liver damage, parenchymal cells regenerate and replace the necrotic and apoptotic cells; this process is associated with an inflammatory response and a limited deposition of extracellular matrix (ECM). When the injury persists, eventually the regenerative response fails and the hepatocytes are substituted by abundant ECM mainly composed by collagen type I-III-IV, fibronectin, elastin, laminin, and proteoglycans. Hepatic stellate cells (HSC) are the main sources of ECM [7].

There is no standard treatment for liver fibrosis, although it is known that reducing liver injury events, such as interruption of alcohol intake or successful treatment of viral hepatitis, contributes to the control of the process. Nevertheless,

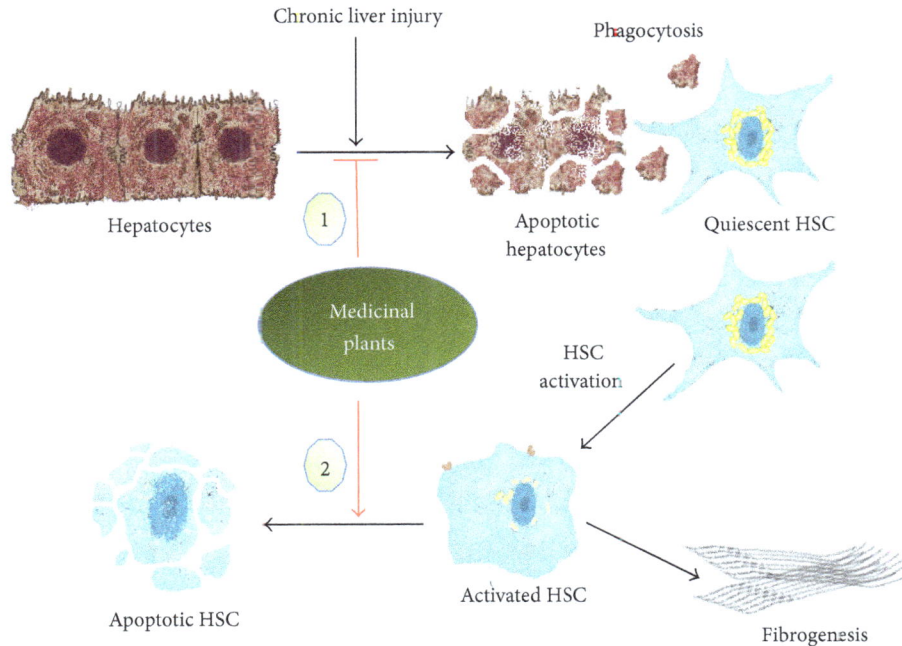

FIGURE 1: Anti-liver fibrosis of medicinal plants targeting apoptosis of hepatocytes and hepatic stellate cells. (1) *C. longa, S. marianum, G. biloba, S. miltiorrhiza, G. glabra, S. baicalensis, Phyllanthus* species, *B. aristata, P. kurroa, Ginseng* species, *A. paniculata*. (2) *C. longa, G. biloba, S. miltiorrhiza, G. glabra, S. baicalensis, E. falcatum,* and *Ginseng* species.

these actions do not seem to be sufficient, in the vast majority of patients, to avoid progression to cirrhosis [8]. Even though important advances have been made in the knowledge of the pathogenesis of hepatic fibrosis for the past 20 years, there are still important gaps to translate this basic information into efficient antifibrotic drugs. Treatment strategies for liver fibrosis should take into account the versatility of its pathogenesis and acting on all the cell lines involved starting with HSC and hepatocytes.

Supported by their safety, cost-effectiveness, and versatility, medicinal plants enjoy a growing popularity as antifibrotic agents. We already reviewed how medicinal plants reduce liver fibrosis by inhibiting HSC activation and reducing ECM deposition [9]. However, other antifibrotic mechanisms could explain this activity such as modulation of apoptosis of different cell lines. This review focuses on two more ways by which the bioactive compounds from twelve known hepatoprotective plants, including *Curcuma longa, Silybum marianum, Ginkgo biloba, Salvia miltiorrhiza, Glycyrrhiza glabra, Scutellaria baicalensis, Bupleurum falcatum, Phyllanthus* species, *Berberis aristata, Picrorhiza kurroa, Ginseng* species, and *Andrographis paniculata*, reduce liver fibrosis by targeting apoptosis: the induction of HSC apoptosis and the protection of hepatocytes from apoptosis (Figure 1).

2. Induction of HSC Apoptosis

2.1. Role of HSC in the Pathogenesis of Liver Fibrosis. Quiescent HSC act as the major vitamin A-storing cells located in the perisinusoidal space of Disse between the basolateral

surface of hepatocytes and the antiluminal side of sinusoidal endothelial cells [10]. HSC are the key effectors in the development of liver fibrosis.

The process of liver fibrosis initiates with HSC activation; this is mainly due to several mediators' effects, like reactive oxygen species (ROS), lipid peroxidation (LPO) products, and fibrogenic cytokines such as transforming growth factor beta (TGF-β1) and platelet derived growth factor (PDGF). These substances come from damaged hepatocytes, as we detailed below, and/or activated Kupffer cells, macrophages, and platelets following hepatic injury [11, 12]. Activated HSC acquire different phenotypes such as enhanced production of ECM, expression of contractile smooth muscle α-actin (α-SMA), enhanced proliferation, secretion of pro-inflammatory cytokines, and release of matrix-degrading enzymes and their inhibitors [13]. Activated HSC remain the main contributors of major and minor matrix proteins of the fibrotic liver including types I, III, and IV collagens, fibronectin, laminin, and proteoglycans [11, 14] even though many other cells, including portal fibroblasts, circulating cells from the bone marrow, hepatocytes, and biliary epithelial cells that undergo an epithelial to mesenchymal transition, also produce ECM [15].

Activated HSC are also characterized by an enhanced survival. Hepatic macrophages promote the survival of activated HSC in a nuclear factor-kappaB- (NF-κB-) dependent manner and thereby promote liver fibrosis [16]. However, inhibition of NF-κB pathway reverses hepatic fibrosis by stimulating HSC apoptosis [17], thereby highlighting selective induction of HSC apoptosis as a promising strategy to treat liver fibrosis [4, 18–21].

TABLE 1: Mechanisms of induction of hepatic stellate cells apoptosis by medicinal plants.

Plants	Bioactive compounds and/or extracts	Types of study	Cell lines/animals used (fibrogenic inducers)	Mechanisms of induction of HSC apoptosis
C. longa	Curcumin	I [25]	PCR-HSC	↑caspase-3, ↓Bcl-2, ↑PPAR-γ and ↓NF-κB
		I [26]	PCR-HSC	↑PPAR-γ, ↑Bax, ↓Bcl-2 and ↑caspase-3
		I [27]	PCR-HSC	↑PPAR-γ
		I [28]	PCR-HSC	↑Bax, ↓Bcl-2, ↑PPAR-γ, ↓ERK, ↓JNK and ↓PI-3K/AKT
		I [29]	PCR-HSC	↑PPAR-γ, ↑Bax, ↓Bcl-2 and ↓NF-κB p65
		I, II [30]	PCR-HSC and SD rats (CCl₄)	↑caspase-3
		I [31]	HSC-T6 (TGF-β1)	↑cytochrome *c* release
		I [32]	Human telomerase reverse transcriptase HSC	Modulate BAX and FLIP and ↓Wnt signaling pathway components AXIN2 and FRA1
S. miltiorrhiza	IH764-3	I [33]	CFSC	↑caspase-3
		I [34]	HSC (H₂O₂)	↓ERK
		II [35]	SD rats (BDL)	↓FAK, ↓p-FAK, ↓ERK and ↓p-ERK
	Tanshinone I	I [36]	T-HSC/Cl-6	↑caspase-3, ↑PARP, ↑cytochrome *c* release and ↓MMP
	Tanshinone IIA	I [37]	T-HSC/Cl-6	↑caspase-3, ↑PARP, ↑cytochrome *c* release, ↑Bax, ↓Bcl-2 and ↓MMP
		I, II [38]	HSC-T6 and Wistar rats (DMN)	↑prohibitin, ↑C-Raf membrane tanslocation, ↑pERK, ↓AKT phosphorylation, ↑Bax, ↓Bcl-2, ↑cytochrome *c* release, ↑caspase-3, ↑caspase-9 and ↑PARP cleavage.
	Salvianolic acid A	I [39]	HSC-T6 (PDGF-BB)	↓AKT phosphorylation, ↑caspase-3 and ↓Bcl-2
	PF2401-SF	I, II [40]	T-HSC/Cl-6 and SD rats (CCl₄)	↑caspase-3, ↑caspase-8, ↑caspase-9, ↑PARP cleavage, ↑Bax and ↓Bcl-2
	Root of *S. miltiorrhiza*	I [41]	HSC-T6	↑Bax, ↑Fas and ↓Bcl-XL
G. glabra	18α-glycyrrhizin	I, II [23]	CFSC and SD rats (CCl₄)	↓NF-κB
B. falcatum	Saikosaponin A and D	I [42]	HSC-T6	↓ERK
P. notoginseng	20-O-beta-D-glucopyranosyl-20(S)-protopanaxadiol	I [43]	T-HSC/Cl-6	↓MMP, ↑caspase-3 and ↑PARP cleavage
	25-OCH₃-PPD	I [44]	T-HSC/Cl-6 (TNF-α)	↑caspase-3, ↓survivin, ↓Bcl-2, ↑c-FLIP_L, ↓c-FLIP_S, ↓XIAP, ↑NF-κB p65 nuclear translocation and ↓IκB-α

Abbreviations: ↑: inductor effect; ↓: inhibitor effect; I: *in vitro*; II: *in vivo*; AKT: protein kinase B; Bax: Bcl-2-associated X protein; Bcl-2: B-cell lymphoma 2; Bcl-XL: B-cell lymphoma-extralarge; BDL: bile duct ligation; c-FLIP_L: cellular FLICE (FADD-like IL-1β-converting enzyme)-inhibitory protein (isoform L); c-FLIP_S: cellular FLICE- (FADD-like IL-1β-converting enzyme-) inhibitory protein (isoform S); CCl₄: carbon tetrachloride; CFSC: hepatic stellate cell line; DMN: dimethylnitrosamine; ERK: extracellular signal-regulated kinases; FAK: focal adhesion kinase; H₂O₂: hydrogen peroxide; HSC: hepatic stellate cells; HSC-T6: immortalized rat liver stellate cell line; IκB-α: inhibitor of nuclear factor kappa B alpha; JNK: c-Jun N-terminal kinases; MMP: mitochondrial membrane potential; NF-κB: nuclear factor kappaB; NF-κB p65: p65 subunit of nuclear factor kappaB; p-ERK: phosphorylated extracellular signal-regulated kinases; p-FAK: phosphorylated focal adhesion kinase; PARP: poly ADP ribose polymerase; PCR-HSC: primary cultured rat hepatic stellate cells; PDGF-BB: platelet derived growth factor-BB; PI-3K/AKT: phosphatidylinositide 3-kinases/protein kinase B; PPAR-γ: peroxisome proliferator-activated receptor gamma; SD: Sprague-Dawley; TGF-β1: transforming growth factor beta 1; T-HSC/Cl-6: rat hepatic stellate cells transformed by simian virus 40; TNF-α: tumor necrosis factor alpha; XIAP: X-linked inhibitor of apoptosis protein.

2.2. Hepatic Stellate Cells as Targets of Antifibrotic Medicinal Plants. Twenty-three articles were chosen (Table 1). Curcumin from *C. longa* and bioactive compounds from *S. miltiorrhiza*, including IH764-3, tanshinones I and IIA, and salvianolic acid A, are by far the most investigated, followed by compounds extracted from *Ginseng* species. Consequently, their mechanisms of induction of HSC apoptosis have been well characterized. On the opposite, apoptosis induction by *G. biloba* extract [22], 18α-glycyrrhizin from *G. glabra* [23], baicalin from *S. baicalensis*, and saponins from *B. falcatum* [24] have only been observed; thus, their mechanisms need to be clarified. No proof that *S. marianum*, *Phyllanthus* species, *B. aristata*, *P. kurroa*, and *A. paniculata* produce compounds that induce HSC apoptosis exists. The apoptotic events induced by medicinal plants present similarities since they all act by modulating mitochondrial caspases cascade. However, different targets have been identified upstream to the apoptotic cascade.

Curcumin increases and decreases Bcl-2-associated X protein (Bax) and B-cell lymphoma 2 (Bcl-2) expressions, respectively [25, 26, 28, 29], promotes cytochrome c release from mitochondria into cytoplasm [31], and increases caspase-3 activity [25, 26, 30] in primary cultured rat HSC. Induction of apoptosis by curcumin correlates with its inhibitory effect on NF-κB [29], which involves the stimulation of gene expression of peroxisome proliferator-activated receptor gamma (PPARγ) [25–29] by blocking TGF-β, PDGF, and epidermal growth factor (EGF) signaling pathways through interruption of extracellular signal-regulated kinases (ERK), c-Jun N-terminal kinases (JNK), and phosphatidylinositide 3-kinases/protein kinase B (PI-3K/AKT) pathways [28]. Additionally, modulation of BAX and cellular FADD-like IL-1β-converting enzyme- (FLICE-) like inhibitory protein (c-FLIP) (CASP8 and FADD-like apoptosis regulator) expressions and reduction of the expression of Wnt signaling pathway components, axis inhibition protein 2 (AXIN2), and FOS-like antigen 1 (FRA1) mediate induction of HSC apoptosis by curcumin in human telomerase reverse transcriptase HSC [32].

Root of *S. miltiorrhiza* promotes HSC apoptosis by increasing Bax and Fas expressions and decreasing B-cell lymphoma-extralarge (Bcl-XL) expression *in vitro* in HSC-T6 cells [41]. Monomer IH764-3, tanshinone I, tanshinone IIA, salvianolic acid A, and fraction PF2401-SF (tanshinone I, tanshinone IIA, and cryptotanshinone) mediate proapoptotic effects of *S. miltiorrhiza* root. Like curcumin, they act via increasing Bax/Bcl-2 ratio [37–40], decreasing mitochondrial membrane potential (MMP) [36, 37], inducing cytochrome c release [36–38], stimulating poly ADP ribose polymerase (PARP) cleavage [36–38, 40], and enhancing caspase-3 and 9 activities [33, 36–40]. IH764-3 downregulates the expression of focal adhesion kinase (FAK) and phosphorylated FAK, ERK, and phosphorylated ERK to promote HSC apoptosis [34, 35]. Tanshinone IIA acts by enhancing prohibitin expression, inducing intracellular translocation of the cytosolic C-Raf protein to the membrane, increasing p-ERK, and suppressing AKT phosphorylation, thereby indicating that tanshinone IIA induces apoptotic cell by promoting binding between prohibitin and C-Raf which in turn activates mitogen activated protein kinases (MAPK) pathway and consequently Bax/caspase cascade [38]. Interestingly, salvianolic acid A also reduces AKT phosphorylation [39].

Saponins from *P. notoginseng* induce HSC of apoptosis *in vitro* but their mechanisms have not been investigated [24]. 20-O-Beta-D-glucopyranosyl-20(S)-protopanaxadiol, a ginsenoside metabolite, triggers apoptosis in activated HSC by reducing MMP and increasing caspase-3 activity and PARP cleavage [43]. Moreover, 25-OCH3-PPD, a dammarane-type triterpene isolated from *P. notoginseng*, induces the apoptosis of HSC activated by tumor necrosis factor alpha (TNF-α). 25-OCH3-PPD increases the level of cleaved caspase-3, downregulates the ratio of Bcl-2/Bax, and the expression of caspase-3 inhibitor survivin. This effect takes place through

increasing the expression of c-FLIPL and decreasing c-FLIPs and X-linked inhibitor of apoptosis protein (XIAP) expressions, which lead to NF-κB activation via degradation and phosphorylation of inhibitor of NF-κB alpha (IκBα) and translocation of p65 subunit into the nucleus [44].

3. Protection of Hepatocytes from Apoptosis

3.1. Role of Hepatocytes in the Pathogenesis of Liver Fibrosis. Hepatocytes account for about 80% of the liver. Under chronic liver injury, hepatocytes undergo apoptosis liberating hepatocyte-derived apoptotic bodies [45]. This initial event is no longer viewed as a silent consequence of liver injury but rather as a potent inductor of liver fibrosis [46]. Profibrogenic response following hepatocytes apoptosis is enabled by the capacity of HSC to perform phagocytic function [46, 47]. Phagocytosis of the hepatocyte-derived apoptotic bodies directly induces HSC activation and matrix deposition as it up-regulates TGF-β1 and induces collagen α1(I) through PI-3K and p38MAPK pathways [46, 48, 49]. This profibrogenic event requires nicotinamide adenine dinucleotide phosphate reduced (NADPH) oxidase activation [46, 50]. Concurrently, an indirect signal mediated by the generation of damage-associated molecular patterns (DAMPs) results in HSC activation [49]. DNA from apoptotic hepatocytes induces HSC differentiation by upregulating TGF-β1 and collagen expression and inhibiting chemotaxis of HSC, so mobile HSC stop when they reach an area of apoptosing hepatocytes, via toll-like receptor 9 (TLR9) [51]. Adenosine, another product of apoptosing hepatocytes, has been identified also as a mediator of fibrogenic cascade [52]. In addition, phagocytosis of apoptotic bodies promotes HSC survival through Janus kinase/signal transducer and activator of transcription (JAK/STAT) and AKT/NF-κB-dependent pathways, contributing to progression of liver fibrosis [53]. Thus therapeutic strategies, which aim to protect hepatocytes from apoptosis, could be useful to reverse liver fibrosis [54].

3.2. Hepatocytes as Targets of Antifibrotic Medicinal Plants. Thirty-two articles were selected (Table 2). It has been demonstrated that all the reviewed plants, except *B. falcatum*, produce compounds that inhibit apoptosis of hepatocytes induced by a wide range of agents, including ethanol, iron, carbon tetrachloride (CCl₄), tert-butylhydroperoxide (t-BHP), toxic bile salts (glycochenodeoxycholic acid [GCDC]), thioacetamide (TAA), lipopolysaccharide (LPS) with D-galactosamine (D-GalN), concanavalin A (Con A), high free fatty acids (HFFAs), and so forth. Most investigated compounds are those of *C. longa*, *G. biloba*, *S. miltiorrhiza*, and *G. glabra*. Almost all the bioactive components from reviewed plants act similarly by inhibiting mitochondrial pathway of apoptosis and reducing oxidative stress.

Curcumin inhibits ethanol-, iron-, and HFFAs-induced apoptosis in primary cultured rat hepatocytes [55–57]. Curcumin regulates mitochondrial biogenesis [57], inhibits LPO [55] and RCS synthesis [56, 57], downregulates Bcl-2 and Bcl-XL expressions [56], inhibits cytochrome c release [55], restores MMP [57], and suppresses caspase-3 activity [56].

TABLE 2: Mechanisms of protection of hepatocytes from apoptosis by medicinal plants.

Plants	Bioactive compounds and/or extracts	Types of study	Cell lines/animals used	Apoptosis inducers	Mechanisms of protection of hepatocytes from apoptosis
C. longa	Curcumin	I [55]	PCRH	Ethanol	↓LPO, ↓cytochrome c release
		I [56]	PCRH	FeNTA	↓Bcl-2, ↓Bcl-XL, ↓ROS, ↓caspase-3 and ↓NF-κB
		I [57]	PCRH	HFFAs	↓ROS, ↑ATP, ↓PEPCK, ↓G6Pase, ↑mtDNA copy number, ↑PGCIα, ↑NRF1, ↑Tfam, ↑MMP and ↓NF-κB p65
S. marianum	Silymarin	I [58]	PCRH	t-BHP	↑NOS-2 and ↓HO-1
G. biloba	G. biloba extract	II [59]	Rats	CCl4	↓LPO
	G. biloba extract	II [60]	SD rats	Ethanol	↑GSH, ↓LPO, ↑SOD, ↑GPx, ↑CAT and ↑HO-1
	G. biloba	II [61]	Wistar rats	99mTc	↑P53/Bcl-2 ratio and ↓LPO
S. miltiorrhiza	Tanshinone IIA	I [62]	PCRH	LPS and ethanol	↓ROS, ↓RNS, ↓fatty acid synthesis, ↑fatty acid oxidation, ↓SCD1 and ↑RXR-α
		II [63]	Kunming mice	TAA	↓IGFBP7
	Danshen	I [64]	PCRH	CCl4	↑MMP
		II [65]	Kunming mice	Iron dextran	↓LPO, ↑GPx and ↑SOD
	PF2401-SF, tanshinone IIA, cryptotanshinone	I [66]	PCRH	GDCD	↓ROS, ↓JNK phosphorylation and ↓p38 phosphorylation
	PF2401-SF and cryptotanshinone	I [67]	PCRH	LPS and ethanol	↓lipid accumulation and activation, ↓SREBP1 nuclear translocation
	Extract of S. miltiorrhiza	I [68]	SD rats	BDL	↑p53 cytoplasmic sequestration, ↓Bax and ↑Bcl-2
	salvianolic acid B	I, II [69]	Mice and HL-7702	Death receptor (I) and LPS + D-GalN (II)	↓TNFRI, ↑Bcl-2, ↓cytochrome c release and ↓caspase-3
G. glabra	Glycyrrhizin	I [70]	PCRH	t-BHP	↑GSH, ↓ROS, ↑SOD, ↓LPO, ↑MMP, ↓cytochrome c release, ↓caspase-3 and ↓caspase-9
		II [71]	SD rats	CCl4	↓caspase-3, ↓p53, ↓Bax/Bcl-2 ratio, ↓caspase-9, ↓Smac, ↓cytochrome c release and ↓Smac release
		I [72]	PCRH	BCG vaccine + LPS	↓NO and ↓ICAM-1
		II [73]	Wistar rats	LPS	↓caspase-3 and ↓cytochrome c release
		II [74]	Balb/c mice	LPS + D-GalN	↓IL-18
	18β-glycyrrhetinic acid	I [75]	Huh-BAT	HMGB1	↓cytochrome c release and ↓p38 activation
		I [76]	PCRH	GDCD	↓ROS, ↓caspase-3, ↓caspase-9, ↓caspase-10, ↓PARP cleavage, ↓JNK, ↑MMP and ↓cytochrome c release
		I, II [77]	HepG2 and SD rats	HFFAs (I) and HFD (II)	Stabilize lysosomal membrane, ↓cathepsin B, ↓cytochrome c release and ↓oxidative stress
S. baicalensis	Baicalin	I, II [78]	PCRH and Balb/c mice	TNF-α + (Act D) (I) and Con A (II)	↓TNF-α, ↓IFN-γ, ↓IL-6, ↓MPO, ↓LPO and ↓SOD
	35kD P. niruri protein	I [79]	PCMH	FeSO4	↑GSH, ↓GSSG, ↓SOD, ↓CAT, ↓GST, ↓GR, ↓GPx, ↓protein carbonylation, ↓LPO, ↑MMP, ↓cytochrome c release, ↓caspase, ↓PARP cleavage, ↑PI3k/Akt, ↓NF-κB phosphorylation, ↓MAPK and ↓ERK
Phyllanthus species	Geraniin and amariin from P. amarus	II [80]	Cultured liver slices of mice	Ethanol	↓LPO, ↓protein carbonylation, ↓CAT, ↓SOD, ↑GPx, ↑GR, ↓PARP cleavage, ↓Bax and ↑Bcl-2
	Protein from P. niruri	I [81]	PCMH	t-BHP	↑SOD ↑GSH/GSSG ratio, ↑MMP, ↓Bax, ↑Bcl-2, ↓caspase-3, ↓caspase-9 and ↓cytochrome c release

TABLE 2: Continued.

Plants	Bioactive compounds and/or extracts	Types of study	Cell lines/animals used	Apoptosis inducers	Mechanisms of protection of hepatocytes from apoptosis
B. aristata	Berberine	I [82]	L02	H_2O_2	↓caspase-3, ↓PARP, ↑FasL, ↓Bim and ↑SIRT1
P. kurroa	Picroside II	II [83]	Kunming mice	CCl_4, D-GalN and AP	↓LPO, ↑SOD, ↑GPx, ↑ATPase, ↓swelling extent of mitochondria
		I, II [84]	PCRH and Kunming mice	TNF-α + Act D (I) and LPS + D-GalN	↓LPO, ↑SOD, ↑Bcl-2 and ↓Bax
Ginseng species	Ginseng extract from P. ginseng Meyer	II [85]	SD rats	AFB_1	↑SOD, ↑CAT, ↑GPx and ↓LPO
A. paniculata	Andrographolide	II [86]	C57BL/6 mice	Con A	↓LDH, ↓MPO, ↓COX2, ↓Glut1, ↓HIF-1α, ↓HO-1, ↑SOD1, ↓iNOS and ↓TNF-α

Abbreviations: ↑: inductor effect; ↓: inhibitor effect; I: *in vitro*; II: *in vivo*; ^{99m}Tc: technetium ^{99m}Tc; Act D: actinone D; AFB_1: aflatoxin B_1; AP: acetaminophen; ATP: adenosine triphosphate; ATPase: adenosinetriphosphatase; BDL: bile duct ligation; Bim: Bcl-2-interacting mediator; CAT: catalase; CCl_4: carbon tetrachloride; Con A: concanavalin A; COX2: cyclooxygenase 2; D-GalN: D-galactosamine; FasL: Fas ligand; FeNTA: ferric nitrilotriacetate; $FeSO_4$: iron (II) sulfate; G6Pase: glucose-6-phosphatase; GDCD: glycochenodeoxycholic acid; Glut1: glucose transporter 1; GPx: gluthatione peroxidase; GR: glutathione reductase; GSH: glutathione; GSSG: glutathione disulfide; GST: glutathione S-transferase; H_2O_2: hydrogen peroxide; HFD: high fat diet; HFFAs: high free fatty acids; HIF-1α: hypoxia-inducible factor 1-alpha; HMGR: high-mobility group box 1; HO-1: heme oxygenase 1; ICAM-1: intercelular adhesion molecule 1; IFN-γ: interferon-gamma; IGFBP7: insulin-like growth factor binding protein 7; IL-6: interleukine-6; IL-18: interleukine-18; iNOS: inducible nitric oxide synthase; JNK: c-Jun-NH2-terminal kinase; LDH: lactate dehydrogenase; LPO: lipid peroxidation; LPS: lipopolysaccharide; MAPK: mitogen activated protein kinases; MMP: mitochondrial membrane potential; MPO: myeloperoxidase; mtDNA: mitochondrial DNA; NF-κB: nuclear factor kappaB; NO: nitric oxide; NOS-2: nitric oxide synthase 2; NRF1: nuclear respiratory factor 1; PARP: poly ADP ribose polymerase; PCMH: primary cultured mouse hepatocytes; PCRH: primary cultured rat hepatocytes; PEPCK: phosphoenol pyruvate carboxykinase; PGC1α: peroxisome proliferator-activated receptor gamma coactivator 1 alpha; PI3k/Akt: phosphatidylinositide 3-kinases/protein kinase B; RNS: reactive nitrosative species; ROS: reactive oxygen species; RXR-α: retinoid-X receptor-alpha; SCD1: stearoyl-CoA desaturase-1; SD: Sprague-Dawley; SIRT1: sirtuin 1; Smac: second mitochondria derived activator of caspases; SOD: superoxide dismutase; SREBP1: sterol regulatory element binding protein-1; t-BHP: tert-butylhydroperoxide; TAA: thioacetamide; Tfam: mitocondrial transcription factor A; TNF-α: tumor necrosis factor alpha; TNFRI: tumor necrosis factor alpha receptor type 1.

Cytoprotective effects of curcumin are mediated by downregulation of NF-κB activity [56], especially p65 subunit [57].

Glycyrrhizin, also known as glycyrrhizin acid, is the main bioactive component from *G. glabra*. Glycyrrhizin protects hepatocytes from apoptosis *in vitro* and *in vivo*. *In vitro*, it prevents glutathione depletion, decreases ROS generation and LPO, and increases superoxide dismutase (SOD) activity, highlighting the importance of its antioxidant properties to inhibit hepatocytes apoptosis [70]. It also inhibits MMP, cytochrome c release, p38 activation, and caspases-3 and -9 activities [70, 75]. Additionally, it decreases nitric oxide (NO) and intercellular adhesion molecule 1 (ICAM-1) expression [72]. Involvement of caspases pathway inhibition has also been observed *in vivo* [71, 73]. Nevertheless, protection of hepatocytes could also occur through caspases-independent pathway related to the inhibition of the release of interleukin-18 [74].

S. miltiorrhiza bioactive components include tanshinones and salvianolic acids. PF2401, a standardized fraction of root of *S. miltiorrhiza*, and its components tanshinone I, tanshinone IIA, and cryptotanshinone, protect primary cultured rat hepatocytes from GCDC-, LPS-, and ethanol-induced apoptosis by inhibiting MAPK pathway via blockage of JNK and p38 phosphorylations [66], lipid accumulation, and activation and transactivation of genes involved in fatty acid biosynthesis through suppression of the nuclear translocation of sterol regulatory element binding protein-1 (SREBP-1) [67]. Besides, tanshinone IIA inhibits synthesis of ROS and reactive nitrogen species, fatty acid synthesis, and the opening of mitochondrial permeability transition and stimulates fatty acid oxidation by decreasing and increasing stearoyl-CoA desaturase-1 (SCD1) and retinoid-X receptor-alpha (RXR-α), respectively, in LPS-, ethanol-, and CCl4-treated primary cultured rat hepatocytes [62, 64]. *In vivo*, its antiapoptotic properties have been related to the downregulation of insulin-like growth factor-binding protein 7 (IGFBP7) [63]. Finally, protection of hepatocytes from apoptosis by salvianolic acid B is associated with its ability to reduce the expression of tumor necrosis factor alpha receptor type 1 (TNFR1), balance the expression of Bcl-2 family members, decrease release of cytochrome c, and inhibit caspase-3 *in vitro* and *in vivo* [69].

Bioactive extract of *G. biloba* (EGB) is composed of 6% of terpenes and 24% of flavonols heterosides. EGB inhibits technetium 99mTc-, ethanol-, and CCl$_4$-induced apoptosis in rats principally by reducing oxidative stress via inhibiting LPO [59–61], glutathione depletion, promoting SOD, glutathione peroxidase (GPx), and catalase (CAT) activities and upregulating heme oxygenase-1 (HO-1) expression and activity [60]. It also reduces p53/Bcl-2 ratio [61].

4. Highlights

In this review, we highlighted the polyvalence of *C. longa*, *S. marianum*, *G. biloba*, *S. miltiorrhiza*, *G. glabra*, *S. baicalensis*, *B. falcatum*, *Phyllanthus* species, *B. aristata*, *P. kurroa*, *Ginseng* species, and *A. paniculata* and respective bioactive compounds and extracts to reduce liver fibrosis targeting apoptosis of hepatocytes and activated HSC. By protecting hepatocytes from apoptosis, medicinal plants are able to inhibit

the liberation of hepatocyte-derived apoptotic bodies and DAMPs, some of the initial profibrogenic stimuli that converge to activation and survival of HSC, while inducing apoptosis of activated HSC; they eliminate the main source of ECM. Regulation of mitochondrial pathways of apoptosis by vegetal compounds mainly explains the induction and protection of apoptosis *in vitro* and *in vivo*.

To induce apoptosis of activated HSC, medicinal plants increase proapoptotic proteins, such as Bax and Fas, and decrease antiapoptotic proteins, like Bcl-2 and Bcl-xl. The increase in Bax/Bcl-2 ratio stimulates the release of cytochrome c from mitochondria into cytosol through MMP. The release activates initiator caspases (caspases-8 and -9) which leads to activation of executioner caspases such as caspase-3, responsible for the apoptotic process eventually through cleavage of PARP, a protein involved in repairing DNA damage. Opposite effects mediate the antiapoptotic properties of medicinal plants to protect hepatocytes.

NF-κB, a transcription factor involved in inflammatory and apoptotic response, seems to play an intermediary role in the modulation of apoptosis of activated HSC and hepatocytes. Interestingly, inhibition of NF-κB activity results in opposite effects in activated HSC and hepatocytes. Medicinal plants downregulate NF-κB activity in activated HSC leading to inhibition of survival and promotion of apoptosis. On the contrary, inhibition of NF-κB activity results in the protection from cell death in hepatocytes. Involvement of NF-κB in both antifibrotic activities suggests a common stimulus of activation of this transcriptional factor between medicinal plants. Antioxidant properties of bioactive compounds from reviewed plants could explain such a similarity. Indeed, NF-κB is regulated by the intracellular redox state thereby implying that antioxidant compounds of reviewed medicinal plants reduce chronic liver injury-induced oxidative stress which is sensed by NF-κB resulting in modulation of apoptosis in hepatocytes and HSC [87].

Antiliver fibrosis mechanisms of medicinal plants have been mostly studied in liver fibrosis models *in vitro* and *in vivo*. Clinical studies are sparse and mainly use chronic hepatitis B and C patients to assess the hepatoprotective effects of medicinal plants. Consequently, more clinical investigations on fibrosis induced by other agents than HBV and HCV are urgently needed. Silymarin, glycyrrhizin, and *Salvia miltiorrhiza* have been more or less successfully tested. Glycyrrhizin could benefit patients with chronic hepatitis C nonresponders or unlikely respond to interferon therapy by decreasing alanine transaminase and improving necroinflammation [88–91]. Silymarin has also been tested in patients infected with HCV. However, contradictory results, as well as its low bioavailability, have not been able to conclude about its clinical efficacy [92–95]. Finally, *Salvia miltiorrhiza* injection and one of his bioactive compounds, salvianolic acid B, could be relevant in the treatment of hepatitis B [96–99].

Besides HSC and hepatocytes, inflammatory and immune cells take part actively in the fibrogenic response. In addition, important events, including HSC activation, ECM deposition, inflammation, and oxidative stress, are involved in the pathogenesis of liver fibrosis. Such targets could be relevant to reducing hepatic fibrosis. The extensive literature search made as part of this review evidenced other mechanisms besides the ones described here, by which medicinal plants reduce liver fibrosis, including previously reviewed inhibition of HSC activation and reduction of ECM deposition [9], as well as lowering of oxidative stress and suppression of inflammation and immune response.

5. Conclusion

Medicinal plants could be a source of polyvalent antiliver fibrosis compounds targeting apoptosis of hepatocytes and activated HSC. The importance of knowing the main mechanisms, by which medicinal plants act as antifibrotic agents, provides options for the development of pharmaceutical compounds and their subsequent use in medical practices.

Conflict of Interests

The authors declare that there is no conflict of interests regarding the publication of this paper.

Acknowledgments

This paper is supported by CONACYT for the Ph.D. student grant. This work was partially funded by endowments from the Tecnológico de Monterrey (cat-134) and the Zambrano-Hellion Foundation.

References

[1] E. Mormone, J. George, and N. Nieto, "Molecular pathogenesis of hepatic fibrosis and current therapeutic approaches," *Chemico-Biological Interactions*, vol. 193, no. 3, pp. 225–231, 2011.

[2] E. L. Ellis and D. A. Mann, "Clinical evidence for the regression of liver fibrosis," *Journal of Hepatology*, vol. 56, no. 5, pp. 1171–1180, 2012.

[3] V. Sánchez-Valle, N. C. Chávez-Tapia, M. Uribe, and N. Méndez-Sánchez, "Role of oxidative stress and molecular changes in liver fibrosis: a review," *Current Medicinal Chemistry*, vol. 19, no. 28, pp. 4850–4860, 2012.

[4] S. L. Friedman, "Liver fibrosis—from bench to bedside," *Journal of Hepatology*, vol. 38, supplement 1, pp. S38–S53, 2003.

[5] T. Poynard, P. Mathurin, C.-L. Lai et al., "A comparison of fibrosis progression in chronic liver diseases," *Journal of Hepatology*, vol. 38, no. 3, pp. 257–265, 2003.

[6] Y.-S. Lim and W. R. Kim, "The global impact of hepatic fibrosis and end-stage liver disease," *Clinics in Liver Disease*, vol. 12, no. 4, pp. 733–746, 2008.

[7] H. L. Reeves and S. L. Friedman, "Activation of hepatic stellate cells—a key issue in liver fibrosis," *Frontiers in Bioscience*, vol. 7, pp. d808–d826, 2002.

[8] N. C. Henderson and J. P. Iredale, "Liver fibrosis: cellular mechanisms of progression and resolution," *Clinical Science*, vol. 112, no. 5-6, pp. 265–280, 2007.

[9] F. Duval, J. E. Moreno-Cuevas, M. T. González-Garza, C. Rodríguez-Montalvo, and D. E. Cruz-Vega, "Liver fibrosis and mechanisms of the protective action of medicinal plants—targeting hepatic stellate cell activation and extracellular matrix deposition," *Chinese Medicine*. In press.

[10] S. L. Friedman, "Hepatic stellate cells: protean, multifunctional, and enigmatic cells of the liver," *Physiological Reviews*, vol. 88, no. 1, pp. 125–172, 2008.

[11] S. L. Friedman, "Mechanisms of hepatic fibrogenesis," *Gastroenterology*, vol. 134, no. 6, pp. 1655–1669, 2008.

[12] D. A. Mann and F. Marra, "Fibrogenic signalling in hepatic stellate cells," *Journal of Hepatology*, vol. 52, no. 6, pp. 949–950, 2010.

[13] D. C. Rockey, "Translating an understanding of the pathogenesis of hepatic fibrosis to novel therapies," *Clinical Gastroenterology and Hepatology*, vol. 11, no. 3, pp. 224.e5–231.e5, 2013.

[14] D. C. Rockey, "Current and future anti-fibrotic therapies for chronic liver disease," *Clinics in Liver Disease*, vol. 12, no. 4, pp. 939–962, 2008.

[15] R. G. Wells, "Cellular sources of extracellular matrix in hepatic fibrosis," *Clinics in Liver Disease*, vol. 12, no. 4, pp. 759–768, 2008.

[16] J.-P. Pradere, J. Kluwe, S. de Minicis et al., "Hepatic macrophages but not dendritic cells contribute to liver fibrosis by promoting the survival of activated hepatic stellate cells in mice," *Hepatology*, vol. 58, no. 4, pp. 1461–1473, 2013.

[17] F. Oakley, M. Meso, J. P. Iredale et al., "Inhibition of inhibitor of κb kinases stimulates hepatic stellate cell apoptosis and accelerated recovery from rat liver fibrosis," *Gastroenterology*, vol. 128, no. 1, pp. 108–120, 2005.

[18] A. M. Elsharkawy, F. Oakley, and D. A. Mann, "The role and regulation of hepatic stellate cell apoptosis in reversal of liver fibrosis," *Apoptosis*, vol. 10, no. 5, pp. 927–939, 2005.

[19] J. P. Iredale, R. C. Benyon, J. Pickering et al., "Mechanisms of spontaneous resolution of rat liver fibrosis: hepatic stellate cell apoptosis and reduced hepatic expression of metalloproteinase inhibitors," *The Journal of Clinical Investigation*, vol. 102, no. 3, pp. 538–549, 1998.

[20] F. R. Murphy, R. Issa, X. Zhou et al., "Inhibition of apoptosis of activated hepatic stellate cells by tissue inhibitor of metalloproteinase-1 is mediated via effects on matrix metalloproteinase inhibition. Implications for reversibility of liver fibrosis," *The Journal of Biological Chemistry*, vol. 277, no. 13, pp. 11069–11076, 2002.

[21] J. A. Fallowfield, "Therapeutic targets in liver fibrosis," *The American Journal of Physiology- Gastrointestinal and Liver Physiology*, vol. 300, no. 5, pp. G709–G715, 2011.

[22] Y.-J. Luo, J.-P. Yu, Z.-H. Shi, and L. Wang, "Ginkgo biloba extract reverses CCl4-induced liver fibrosis in rats," *World Journal of Gastroenterology*, vol. 10, no. 7, pp. 1037–1042, 2004.

[23] Y. Qu, W.-H. Chen, L. Zong, M.-Y. Xu, and L.-G. Lu, "18α-Glycyrrhizin induces apoptosis and suppresses activation of rat hepatic stellate cells," *Medical Science Monitor*, vol. 18, no. 1, pp. BR24–BR32, 2012.

[24] X. Li, X.-D. Peng, W.-L. Zhang, and L.-L. Dai, "Inhibiting effects of danshensu, baicalin, astragalus and Panax notoginseng saponins on hepatic fibrosis and their possible mechanisms," *Zhonghua Gan Zang Bing Za Zhi*, vol. 16, no. 3, pp. 193–197, 2008.

[25] J. Xu, Y. Fu, and A. Chen, "Activation of peroxisome proliferator-activated receptor-γ contributes to the inhibitory effects of curcumin on rat hepatic stellate cell growth," *The American Journal of Physiology—Gastrointestinal and Liver Physiology*, vol. 285, no. 1, pp. G20–G30, 2003.

[26] S. Zheng and A. Chen, "Activation of PPARγ is required for curcumin to induce apoptosis and to inhibit the expression of extracellular matrix genes in hepatic stellate cells in vitro," *Biochemical Journal*, vol. 384, no. 1, pp. 149–157, 2004.

[27] S. Zheng and A. Chen, "Disruption of transforming growth factor-β signaling by curcumin induces gene expression of peroxisome proliferator-activated receptor-γ in rat hepatic stellate cells," *The American Journal of Physiology: Gastrointestinal and Liver Physiology*, vol. 292, no. 1, pp. G113–G123, 2007.

[28] Y. Zhou, S. Zheng, J. Lin, Q.-J. Zhang, and A. Chen, "The interruption of the PDGF and EGF signaling pathways by curcumin stimulates gene expression of PPARγ in rat activated hepatic stellate cell in vitro," *Laboratory Investigation*, vol. 87, no. 5, pp. 488–498, 2007.

[29] Y. Cheng, J. Ping, and L.-M. Xu, "Effects of curcumin on peroxisome proliferator-activated receptor γ expression and nuclear translocation/redistribution in culture-activated rat hepatic stellate cells," *Chinese Medical Journal*, vol. 120, no. 9, pp. 794–801, 2007.

[30] S. Priya and P. R. Sudhakaran, "Curcumin-induced recovery from hepatic injury involves induction of apoptosis of activated hepatic stellate cells," *Indian Journal of Biochemistry and Biophysics*, vol. 45, no. 5, pp. 317–325, 2008.

[31] Y.-L. Lin, C.-Y. Lin, N.-W. Chi, and Y.-T. Huang, "Study on antifibrotic effects of curcumin in rat hepatic stellate cells," *Phytotherapy Research*, vol. 23, no. 7, pp. 927–932, 2009.

[32] H. W. Shin, S. Y. Park, K. B. Lee, and J.-J. Jang, "Down-regulation of Wnt signaling during apoptosis of human hepatic stellate cells," *Hepato-Gastroenterology*, vol. 56, no. 89, pp. 208–212, 2009.

[33] X.-L. Zhang, L. Liu, and H.-Q. Jiang, "Salvia miltiorrhiza monomer IH764-3 induces hepatic stellate cell apoptosis via caspase-3 activation," *World Journal of Gastroenterology*, vol. 8, no. 3, pp. 515–519, 2002.

[34] S.-M. Fang, C.-S. Li, J.-Y. An et al., "The role of extracellular signal-regulated kinase in induction of apoptosis with salvia miltiorrhiza monomer IH764-3 in hepatic stellate cells," *Zhongguo Ying Yong Sheng Li Xue Za Zhi*, vol. 27, no. 4, pp. 402–406, 2011.

[35] L. Liu, J. Wei, X. Huo et al., "The Salvia miltiorrhiza monomer IH764-3 induces apoptosis of hepatic stellate cells in vivo in a bile duct ligation-induced model of liver fibrosis," *Molecular Medicine Reports*, vol. 6, no. 6, pp. 1231–1238, 2012.

[36] J. Y. Kim, K. M. Kim, J.-X. Nan et al., "Induction of apoptosis by tanshinone I via cytochrome c release in activated hepatic stellate cells," *Pharmacology and Toxicology*, vol. 92, no. 4, pp. 195–200, 2003.

[37] X.-H. Che, E.-J. Park, Y.-Z. Zhao, W.-H. Kim, and D. H. Sohn, "Tanshinone II A induces apoptosis and s phase cell cycle arrest in activated rat hepatic stellate cells," *Basic and Clinical Pharmacology and Toxicology*, vol. 106, no. 1, pp. 30–37, 2010.

[38] T.-L. Pan and P.-W. Wang, "Explore the molecular mechanism of apoptosis induced by tanshinone IIA on activated rat hepatic stellate cells," *Evidence-Based Complementary and Alternative Medicine*, vol. 2012, Article ID 734987, 15 pages, 2012.

[39] Y.-L. Lin, T.-F. Lee, Y.-J. Huang, and Y.-T. Huang, "Antiproliferative effect of salvianolic acid A on rat hepatic stellate cells," *Journal of Pharmacy and Pharmacology*, vol. 58, no. 7, pp. 933–939, 2006.

[40] D. R. Parajuli, E.-J. Park, X.-H. Che et al., "PF2401-SF, standardized fraction of *Salvia miltiorrhiza*, induces apoptosis of activated hepatic stellate cells in vitro and in vivo," *Molecules*, vol. 18, no. 2, pp. 2122–2134, 2013.

[41] S. Y. Chor, A. Y. Hui, K. F. To et al., "Anti-proliferative and pro-apoptotic effects of herbal medicine on hepatic stellate cell,"

[42] M. F. Chen, C. C. Huang, P. S. Liu, C. H. Chen, and L. Y. Shiu, "Saikosaponin a and saikosaponin d inhibit proliferation and migratory activity of rat HSC-T6 cells," *Journal of Medicinal Food*, vol. 16, no. 9, pp. 793–800, 2013.

[43] E.-J. Park, Y.-Z. Zhao, J. Kim, and D. H. Sohn, "A ginsenoside metabolite, 20-O-β-D-glucopyranosyl-20(S)- protopanaxadiol, triggers apoptosis in activated rat hepatic stellate cells via caspase-3 activation," *Planta Medica*, vol. 72, no. 13, pp. 1250–1253, 2006.

[44] Y. L. Wu, Y. Wan, X. J. Jin et al., "25-OCH3-PPD induces the apoptosis of activated t-HSC/Cl-6 cells via c-FLIP-mediated NF-κB activation," *Chemico-Biological Interactions*, vol. 194, no. 2-3, pp. 106–112, 2011.

[45] H. Malhi and G. J. Gores, "Cellular and molecular mechanisms of liver injury," *Gastroenterology*, vol. 134, no. 6, pp. 1641–1654, 2008.

[46] S.-S. Zhan, J. X. Jiang, J. Wu et al., "Phagocytosis of apoptotic bodies by hepatic stellate cells induces NADPH oxidase and is associated with liver fibrosis in vivo," *Hepatology*, vol. 43, no. 3, pp. 435–443, 2006.

[47] A. Canbay, S. Friedman, and G. J. Gores, "Apoptosis: the nexus of liver injury and fibrosis," *Hepatology*, vol. 39, no. 2, pp. 273–278, 2004.

[48] A. Canbay, P. Taimr, N. Torok, H. Higuchi, S. Friedman, and G. J. Gores, "Apoptotic body engulfment by a human stellate cell line is profibrogenic," *Laboratory Investigation*, vol. 83, no. 5, pp. 655–663, 2003.

[49] W. Mehal and A. Imaeda, "Cell death and fibrogenesis," *Seminars in Liver Disease*, vol. 30, no. 3, pp. 226–231, 2010.

[50] J. X. Jiang, S. Venugopal, N. Serizawa et al., "Reduced nicotinamide adenine dinucleotide phosphate oxidase 2 plays a key role in stellate cell activation and liver fibrogenesis in vivo," *Gastroenterology*, vol. 139, no. 4, pp. 1375–1384, 2010.

[51] A. Watanabe, A. Hashmi, D. A. Gomes et al., "Apoptotic hepatocyte DNA inhibits hepatic stellate cell chemotaxis via toll-like receptor 9," *Hepatology*, vol. 46, no. 5, pp. 1509–1518, 2007.

[52] M. A. Sohail, A. Z. Hashmi, W. Hakim et al., "Adenosine induces loss of actin stress fibers and inhibits contraction in hepatic stellate cells via Rho inhibition," *Hepatology*, vol. 49, no. 1, pp. 185–194, 2009.

[53] J. X. Jiang, K. Mikami, S. Venugopal, Y. Li, and N. J. Török, "Apoptotic body engulfment by hepatic stellate cells promotes their survival by the JAK/STAT and Akt/NF-κB-dependent pathways," *Journal of Hepatology*, vol. 51, no. 1, pp. 139–148, 2009.

[54] J. X. Jiang, X. Chen, N. Serizawa et al., "Liver fibrosis and hepatocyte apoptosis are attenuated by GKT137831, a novel NOX4/NOX1 inhibitor in vivo," *Free Radical Biology & Medicine*, vol. 53, no. 2, pp. 289–296, 2012.

[55] A. I. Ghoneim, "Effects of curcumin on ethanol-induced hepatocyte necrosis and apoptosis: implication of lipid peroxidation and cytochrome c," *Naunyn-Schmiedeberg's Archives of Pharmacology*, vol. 379, no. 1, pp. 47–60, 2009.

[56] J.-J. Qian, X.-G. Zhai, M.-H. Niu, Q. Zhou, and Y.-J. Zhou, "Curcumin inhibits iron overload-induced hepatocytic apoptosis and nuclear factor-κB activity," *National Medical Journal of China*, vol. 92, no. 28, pp. 1997–2001, 2012.

[57] J. J. Kuo, H. H. Chang, T. H. Tsai, and T. Y. Lee, "Curcumin ameliorates mitochondrial dysfunction associated with inhibition of gluconeogenesis in free fatty acid-mediated hepatic

Journal of Ethnopharmacology, vol. 100, no. 1-2, pp. 180–186, 2005.

lipoapoptosis," *International Journal of Molecular Medicine*, vol. 30, no. 3, pp. 643–649, 2012.

[58] D. Černý, N. K. Canová, J. Martínek et al., "Effects of resveratrol pretreatment on tert-butylhydroperoxide induced hepatocyte toxicity in immobilized perifused hepatocytes: involvement of inducible nitric oxide synthase and hemoxygenase-1," *Nitric Oxide—Biology and Chemistry*, vol. 20, no. 1, pp. 1–8, 2009.

[59] S. Ozenirler, S. Dincer, G. Akyol, C. Ozogul, and E. Oz, "The protective effect of Ginkgo biloba extract on CCI4-induced hepatic damage," *Acta Physiologica Hungarica*, vol. 85, no. 3, pp. 277–285, 1997.

[60] P. Yao, K. Li, F. Song et al., "Heme oxygenase-1 upregulated by Ginkgo biloba extract: potential protection against ethanol-induced oxidative liver damage," *Food and Chemical Toxicology*, vol. 45, no. 8, pp. 1333–1342, 2007.

[61] B. M. Raafat, A. Saleh, M. W. Shafaa, M. Khedr, and A. A. Ghafaar, "Ginkgo biloba and *Angelica archangelica* bring back an impartial hepatic apoptotic to anti-apoptotic protein ratio after exposure to technetium ^{99m}Tc," *Toxicology and Industrial Health*, vol. 29, no. 1, pp. 14–22, 2013.

[62] H.-Q. Yin, Y.-S. Kim, Y.-J. Choi et al., "Effects of tanshinone IIA on the hepatotoxicity and gene expression involved in alcoholic liver disease," *Archives of Pharmacal Research*, vol. 31, no. 5, pp. 659–665, 2008.

[63] R.-F. Sun, L.-X. Liu, and H.-Y. Zhang, "Effect of tanshinone II on hepatic fibrosis in mice," *Zhongguo Zhong Xi Yi Jie He Za Zhi*, vol. 29, no. 11, pp. 1012–1017, 2009.

[64] B. Zhu, Q. Zhai, and B. Yu, "Tanshinone IIA protects rat primary hepatocytes against carbon tetrachloride toxicity via inhibiting mitochondria permeability transition," *Pharmaceutical Biology*, vol. 48, no. 5, pp. 484–487, 2010.

[65] Y. Gao, N. Wang, Y. Zhang et al., "Mechanism of protective effects of Danshen against iron overload-induced injury in mice," *Journal of Ethnopharmacology*, vol. 145, no. 1, pp. 254–260, 2013.

[66] E. J. Park, Y. Z. Zhao, Y. C. Kim, and D. H. Sohn, "PF2401-SF, standardized fraction of *Salvia miltiorrhiza* and its constituents, tanshinone I, tanshinone IIA, and cryptotanshinone, protect primary cultured rat hepatocytes from bile acid-induced apoptosis by inhibiting JNK phosphorylation," *Food and Chemical Toxicology*, vol. 45, no. 10, pp. 1891–1898, 2007.

[67] H.-Q. Yin, Y.-J. Choi, Y.-C. Kim, D.-H. Sohn, S.-Y. Ryu, and B.-H. Lee, "Salvia miltiorrhiza Bunge and its active component cryptotanshinone protects primary cultured rat hepatocytes from acute ethanol-induced cytotoxicity and fatty infiltration," *Food and Chemical Toxicology*, vol. 47, no. 1, pp. 98–103, 2009.

[68] S.-H. Oh, J.-X. Nan, D.-H. Sohn, Y.-C. Kim, and B.-H. Lee, "Salvia miltiorrhiza inhibits biliary obstruction-induced hepatocyte apoptosis by cytoplasmic sequestration of p53," *Toxicology and Applied Pharmacology*, vol. 182, no. 1, pp. 27–33, 2002.

[69] X. Yan, T. Zhou, Y. Tao, Q. Wang, P. Liu, and C. Liu, "Salvianolic acid B attenuates hepatocyte apoptosis by regulating mediators in death receptor and mitochondrial pathways," *Experimental Biology and Medicine*, vol. 235, no. 5, pp. 623–632, 2010.

[70] M. Tripathi, B. K. Singh, and P. Kakkar, "Glycyrrhizic acid modulates t-BHP induced apoptosis in primary rat hepatocytes," *Food and Chemical Toxicology*, vol. 47, no. 2, pp. 339–347, 2009.

[71] X.-L. Guo, B. Liang, X.-W. Wang et al., "Glycyrrhizic acid attenuates CCl4-induced hepatocyte apoptosis in rats via a p53-mediated pathway," *World Journal of Gastroenterology*, vol. 19, no. 24, pp. 3781–3791, 2013.

[72] Q.-Z. Zheng and Y.-J. Lou, "Pathologic characteristics of immunologic injury in primary cultured rat hepatocytes and protective effect of glycyrrhizin in vitro," *Acta Pharmacologica Sinica*, vol. 24, no. 8, pp. 771–777, 2003.

[73] B. Tang, H. Qiao, F. Meng, and X. Sun, "Glycyrrhizin attenuates endotoxin-induced acute liver injury after partial hepatectomy in rats," *Brazilian Journal of Medical and Biological Research*, vol. 40, no. 12, pp. 1637–1646, 2007.

[74] T. Ikeda, K. Abe, N. Kuroda et al., "The inhibition of apoptosis by glycyrrhizin in hepatic injury induced by injection of lipopolysaccharide/D-galactosamine in mice," *Archives of Histology and Cytology*, vol. 71, no. 3, pp. 163–178, 2008.

[75] G.-Y. Gwak, T. G. Moon, D. H. Lee, and B. C. Yoo, "Glycyrrhizin attenuates HMGB1-induced hepatocyte apoptosis by inhibiting the p38-dependent mitochondrial pathway," *World Journal of Gastroenterology*, vol. 18, no. 7, pp. 679–684, 2012.

[76] E. Gumpricht, R. Dahl, M. W. Devereaux, and R. J. Sokol, "Licorice compounds glycyrrhizin and 18β-glycyrrhetinic acid are potent modulators of bile acid-induced cytotoxicity in rat hepatocytes," *Journal of Biological Chemistry*, vol. 280, no. 11, pp. 10556–10563, 2005.

[77] X. Wu, L. Zhang, E. Gurley et al., "Prevention of free fatty acid-induced hepatic lipotoxicity by 18beta-glycyrrhetinic acid through lysosomal and mitochondrial pathways," *Hepatology*, vol. 47, no. 6, pp. 1905–1915, 2008.

[78] L.-L. Liu, L.-K. Gong, H. Wang et al., "Baicalin protects mouse from Concanavalin A-induced liver injury through inhibition of cytokine production and hepatocyte apoptosis," *Liver International*, vol. 27, no. 4, pp. 582–591, 2007.

[79] S. Bhattacharyya, P. B. Pal, and P. C. Sil, "A 35kD Phyllanthus niruri protein modulates iron mediated oxidative impairment to hepatocytes via the inhibition of ERKs, p38 MAPKs and activation of PI3k/Akt pathway," *Food and Chemical Toxicology*, vol. 56, pp. 119–130, 2013.

[80] J. S. Londhe, T. P. A. Devasagayam, L. Y. Foo, P. Shastry, and S. S. Ghaskadbi, "Geraniin and amariin, ellagitannins from *Phyllanthus amarus*, protect liver cells against ethanol induced cytotoxicity," *Fitoterapia*, vol. 83, no. 8, pp. 1562–1568, 2012.

[81] M. K. Sarkar and P. C. Sil, "Prevention of tertiary butyl hydroperoxide induced oxidative impairment and cell death by a novel antioxidant protein molecule isolated from the herb, Phyllanthus niruri," *Toxicology in Vitro*, vol. 24, no. 6, pp. 1711–1719, 2010.

[82] X. Zhu, X. Guo, G. Mao et al., "Hepatoprotection of berberine against hydrogen peroxide-induced apoptosis by upregulation of sirtuin 1," *Phytotherapy Research*, vol. 27, no. 3, pp. 417–421, 2013.

[83] H. Gao and Y.-W. Zhou, "Anti-lipid peroxidation and protection of liver mitochondria against injuries by picroside II," *World Journal of Gastroenterology*, vol. 11, no. 24, pp. 3671–3674, 2005.

[84] H. Gao and Y.-W. Zhou, "Inhibitory effect of picroside II on hepatocyte apoptosis," *Acta Pharmacologica Sinica*, vol. 26, no. 6, pp. 729–736, 2005.

[85] Y.-S. Kim, Y.-H. Kim, J.-R. Noh, E.-S. Cho, J.-H. Park, and H.-Y. Son, "Protective effect of korean red ginseng against aflatoxin B1-induced hepatotoxicity in rat," *Journal of Ginseng Research*, vol. 35, no. 2, pp. 243–249, 2011.

[86] G. Shi, Z. Zhang, R. Zhang et al., "Protective effect of andrographolide against concanavalin A-induced liver injury," *Naunyn-Schmiedeberg's Archives of Pharmacology*, vol. 385, no. 1, pp. 69–79, 2012.

[87] R. van den Berg, G. R. M. M. Haenen, H. van den Berg, and A. Bast, "Transcription factor NF-κB as a potential biomarker for oxidative stress," *British Journal of Nutrition*, vol. 86, no. 1, pp. S121–S127, 2001.

[88] T. G. J. van Rossum, A. G. Vulto, W. C. J. Hop, J. T. Brouwer, H. G. M. Niesters, and S. W. Schalm, "Intravenous glycyrrhizin for the treatment of chronic hepatitis C: a double-blind, randomized, placebo-controlled phase I/II trial," *Journal of Gastroenterology and Hepatology (Australia)*, vol. 14, no. 11, pp. 1093–1099, 1999.

[89] T. G. J. van Rossum, A. G. Vulto, W. C. J. Hop, and S. W. Schalm, "Glycyrrhizin-induced reduction of ALT in European patients with chronic hepatitis C," *The American Journal of Gastroenterology*, vol. 96, no. 8, pp. 2432–2437, 2001.

[90] H. Orlent, B. E. Hansen, M. Willems et al., "Biochemical and histological effects of 26 weeks of glycyrrhizin treatment in chronic hepatitis C: a randomized phase II trial," *Journal of Hepatology*, vol. 45, no. 4, pp. 539–546, 2006.

[91] M. P. Manns, H. Wedemeyer, A. Singer et al., "Glycyrrhizin in patients who failed previous interferon alpha-based therapies: biochemical and histological effects after 52 weeks," *Journal of Viral Hepatitis*, vol. 19, no. 8, pp. 537–546, 2012.

[92] N. D. Freedman, T. M. Curto, C. Morishima et al., "Silymarin use and liver disease progression in the Hepatitis C Antiviral Long-Term Treatment against Cirrhosis trial," *Alimentary Pharmacology and Therapeutics*, vol. 33, no. 1, pp. 127–137, 2011.

[93] R. L. Hawke, S. J. Schrieber, T. A. Soule et al., "Silymarin ascending multiple oral dosing phase I study in noncirrhotic patients with chronic hepatitis C," *Journal of Clinical Pharmacology*, vol. 50, no. 4, pp. 434–449, 2010.

[94] S. J. Schrieber, R. L. Hawke, Z. Wen et al., "Differences in the disposition of silymarin between patients with nonalcoholic fatty liver disease and chronic hepatitis C," *Drug Metabolism and Disposition*, vol. 39, no. 12, pp. 2182–2190, 2011.

[95] M. W. Fried, V. J. Navarro, N. Afdhal et al., "Effect of silymarin (milk thistle) on liver disease in patients with chronic hepatitis C unsuccessfully treated with interferon therapy: a randomized controlled trial," *Journal of the American Medical Association*, vol. 308, no. 3, pp. 274–282, 2012.

[96] P. Liu, Y.-Y. Hu, C. Liu et al., "Clinical observation of salvianolic acid B in treatment of liver fibrosis in chronic hepatitis B," *World Journal of Gastroenterology*, vol. 8, no. 4, pp. 679–685, 2002.

[97] S.-F. She, X.-Z. Huang, and G.-D. Tong, "Clinical study on treatment of liver fibrosis by different dosages of Salvia injection," *Zhongguo Zhong Jie He Za Zhi*, vol. 24, no. 1, pp. 17–20, 2004.

[98] F. Ye, Y. Liu, G. Qiu, Y. Zhao, and M. Liu, "Clinical study on treatment of cirrhosis by different dosages of salvia injection," *Zhong Yao Cai*, vol. 28, no. 9, pp. 850–854, 2005.

[99] C.-X. Jin, J. Yang, and H.-F. Sun, "Comparative study of the clinical effects of salvia miltiorrhiza injection and shengmai injection on chronic hepatitis B," *Zhongguo Zhong Xi Yi Jie He Za Zhi*, vol. 26, no. 10, pp. 936–938, 2006.

19

Effects of Melatonin and Epiphyseal Proteins on Fluoride-Induced Adverse Changes in Antioxidant Status of Heart, Liver, and Kidney of Rats

Vijay K. Bharti,[1,2] R. S. Srivastava,[1] H. Kumar,[3] S. Bag,[1] A. C. Majumdar,[1] G. Singh,[1] S. R. Pandi-Perumal,[4] and Gregory M. Brown[5]

[1] Division of Physiology and Climatology, Indian Veterinary Research Institute (IVRI), Izatnagar, Uttar Pradesh 243122, India
[2] Nutrition and Toxicology Laboratory, Defence Institute of High Altitude Research (DIHAR),
  Defence Research and Development Organization (DRDO), Ministry of Defence, C/o- 56 APO, Leh 194101, India
[3] Division of Animal Reproduction, Indian Veterinary Research Institute (IVRI), Izatnagar, Uttar Pradesh 243122, India
[4] Somnogen Inc., College Street, Toronto, ON, Canada M6H 1C5
[5] Department of Psychiatry, Faculty of Medicine, University of Toronto and Centre for Addiction and Mental Health,
  250 College Street, Toronto, ON, Canada M5T 1R8

Correspondence should be addressed to Vijay K. Bharti; vijaykbharti@rediffmail.com

Academic Editor: Mustafa F. Lokhandwala

Several experimental and clinical reports indicated the oxidative stress-mediated adverse changes in vital organs of human and animal in fluoride (F) toxicity. Therefore, the present study was undertaken to evaluate the therapeutic effect of buffalo *(Bubalus bubalis)* epiphyseal (pineal) proteins (BEP) and melatonin (MEL) against F-induced oxidative stress in heart, liver, and kidney of experimental adult female rats. To accomplish this experimental objective, twenty-four adult female Wistar rats (123–143 g body weights) were divided into four groups, namely, control, F, F + BEP, and F + MEL and were administered sodium fluoride (NaF, 150 ppm elemental F in drinking water), MEL (10 mg/kg BW, i.p.), and BEP (100 μg/kg BW, i.p.) for 28 days. There were significantly ($P < 0.05$) high levels of lipid peroxidation and catalase and low levels of reduced glutathione, superoxide dismutase, glutathione reductase, and glutathione peroxidase in cardiac, hepatic, and renal tissues of F-treated rats. Administration of BEP and MEL in F-treated rats, however, significantly ($P < 0.05$) attenuated these adverse changes in all the target components of antioxidant defense system of cardiac, hepatic, and renal tissues. The present data suggest that F can induce oxidative stress in liver, heart, and kidney of female rats which may be a mechanism in F toxicity and these adverse effects can be ameliorated by buffalo *(Bubalus bubalis)* epiphyseal proteins and melatonin by upregulation of antioxidant defense system of heart, liver, and kidney of rats.

1. Introduction

Various animal diseases and toxicity are often associated with oxidative stress in vital organs, including the kidney, heart, and liver. This pathophysiological stress has multiple effects but is especially characterized by reductions in enzymatic activity, including that of catalase (CAT), superoxide dismutase (SOD), glutathione peroxidase (GPx), and glutathione reductase (GR) [1]. Every trace element is potentially toxic when the rate of exposure is excessive. Increased generation of reactive oxygen species (ROS) is implicated in the pathogenesis of many diseases and in the toxicity of a wide range of compounds, including fluoride (F) [2–4]. Fluoride was found to exert diverse effects on a number of cellular functions and physiological systems, including inhibition of a variety of enzymes [2]. Generation of free radicals, lipid peroxidation, and altered antioxidant defense systems are considered to play an important role in the toxic effects of fluoride [3, 5–7]. Free radicals participate in several reactions, which in turn can produce chain reaction byproducts that also act to damage cells. Oxidative stress results when free radical formation is unbalanced in proportion to the protective antioxidants [8]. Thus, excess free radical formations are associated with many disease states. With increased understanding both of the mechanisms of oxidative stress and the role of antioxidants, it has become apparent that antioxidant defense systems have a balanced coexistence with endogenous reactive oxygen species. Disruption of this balance, such as that which occurs in F toxicity, appears to be one of the major factors producing the oxidative stress associated with diseases involving degeneration of the kidney, heart, and liver [8, 9]. Although evidence regarding the therapeutic value of administering antioxidants in F toxicity is still inconclusive, some studies have nevertheless reported beneficial effects following this strategy [10, 11]. Therefore, evaluation of antioxidant enzymes activities and markers of free radical damage in the heart, liver, and kidney tissue are important for assessing F toxicity. Melatonin is known to have the ability to protect cells from free radical damage [12–14]. Previous studies have shown that melatonin [12, 15] and buffalo epiphyseal proteins (BEP) have various physiological functions that might protect against fluoride and as-induced oxidative stress [16–21]. In view of the cumulative evidence suggesting that antioxidant proteins in the epiphysis could possibly have therapeutic potential, we sought specifically to determine if BEP could protect the kidney, heart, and liver against the F-induced oxidative stress in rats. These findings may have significant implications in elucidating the therapeutic use of buffalo pineal proteins and melatonin as antioxidant drugs in the management of oxidative stress.

2. Materials and Methods

The present study was conducted at an altitude of 172 meters above the mean sea level at latitude of 28.20° north and longitude of 79.24° east. All the procedures, conducted on the experimental animals, were duly approved by the Institutional Animal Ethics Committee (IAEC) for the purpose of control and supervision of experiments on animals.

2.1. Chemicals. All chemicals used in the study were of analytical grade from HiMedia, Loba Chemie (Mumbai, India); SRL Chemicals, India. Melatonin was procured from Sigma Chemical Co., St. Louis, USA. Buffalo (*Bubalus bubalis*) epiphyseal proteins were supplied by the Neurophysiology Laboratory, Division of Physiology and Climatology, IVRI, Izatnagar.

2.2. Experimental Animals. The present study was carried out in adult female Wistar rats of 123–143 g body weights. On arrival at the laboratory all rats were examined for any abnormality or overt signs of ill health. The rats were housed in polypropylene cages and rice husk was used as the nesting material. After a 1-week-long acclimatization period, they were weighed and randomly assigned to four groups so as to give approximately equal initial group mean body weights. Animal room temperature and relative humidity were set at $21 \pm 2°C$ and $50 \pm 10\%$, respectively, and lighting was controlled to give 12 h light and 12 h darkness. All the animals had free access to standard laboratory animal diet and clean water. The animals were checked daily for the health and husbandry conditions.

2.3. Experimental Design, Doses, and Mode of Administration of Test Molecules. The experimental design for present study, including group assignment, doses, and route of exposure, is presented in Table 1. BEP and MEL were selected as treatment agents for comparative purposes since we have previously carried out and reported studies which have used these reagents. Appropriate dosages of BEP and MEL were optimized from experience in our previous work and thereafter were dissolved in a suitable vehicle (normal saline-based diluents, pH 7.4) before administration (intraperitoneal route) at exactly 16.00 hrs [18, 20–23]. Melatonin was dissolved in ethanol and further diluted with normal saline. The final concentrations of ethanol in solution were <1%. The F level in drinking water was calculated and thereafter the required concentration of F was made by addition of sodium fluoride daily to drinking water for 28 days [18, 20, 21]. Solutions for administration in experimental animals were prepared daily to minimize possible instability of the chemicals in the mixture. Food intake and water consumption were recorded daily.

2.4. Sample Collection. Daily observations were taken for the behavioral changes and mortality, if any, throughout the experimental period. The animals were euthanized, using ether, at the end of the experiment and kidney, heart, and liver were collected immediately. Thereafter, organs were cleaned, rinsed in chilled saline, blotted, and weighed. Then 200 mg of each tissue sample was weighed and placed in 2 mL of ice-cold saline. Another 200 mg of the sample was weighed separately and placed in 2 mL of 0.02 M EDTA for reduced glutathione estimation. Organ homogenates were prepared using an IKA homogenizer (Germany) under ice-cold conditions. Homogenates were collected and centrifuged for 10 min at 3000 rpm. Thereafter, cell free supernatant was collected and transferred to precooled microfuge tubes in duplicate and stored below −20°C. These supernatants were used for estimation of various biochemical parameters to assess body antioxidant defense systems.

2.5. Analytical Procedures. Cell free supernatants of tissue homogenates were taken for the analysis of total proteins (organs), lipid peroxidation (LPO), and different parameters of body antioxidant defense systems, in particular, catalase (CAT), superoxide dismutase (SOD), glutathione peroxidase (GPx), and glutathione reductase (GR) activity, as well as nonenzymatic reduced glutathione (GSH) concentration. Lipid peroxidation and GSH in renal, cardiac, and hepatic tissues were measured on the day of tissue collection. Absorbance of all the tissue biochemical estimations was read using Double Beam UV-VIS Spectrophotometer (UV 5704 SS, ECIL, India).

2.5.1. Lipid Peroxidation (LPO). Lipid peroxidation in tissues sample was determined in terms of malondialdehyde (MDA) production by the method of Rehman [24].

2.5.2. Reduced Glutathione (GSH). The concentration of GSH in the kidney, heart, and liver was estimated by evaluating

TABLE 1: Distribution of experimental rats to different treatments.

Group	Treatment	Dose	Mode of administration
Control	Normal saline		Intraperitoneal
F	Sodium fluoride + normal saline	150 ppm	Drinking water, intraperitoneal
F + BEP	Sodium fluoride + buffalo epiphyseal proteins (BEP)	150 ppm + 100 μg/kg BW	Drinking water, intraperitoneal
F + MEL	Sodium fluoride + melatonin (MEL)	150 ppm + 10 mg/kg BW	Drinking water, intraperitoneal

TABLE 2: Changes in lipid peroxidation (LPO), catalase (CAT), superoxide dismutase (SOD), glutathione reductase (GR), reduced glutathione (GSH), and glutathione peroxidase (GPx) in heart of female rats ($n = 6$; means ± S.E.).

Group	Parameter					
	LPO (nM MDA/mL)	CAT (nM/min/mg protein)	SOD (U)*	GR (nM/min/mg protein)	GPx (nM/min/mg protein)	GSH (μM/g tissue)
Control	$4.63^a \pm 0.09$	$141.19^a \pm 6.05$	$2.78^b \pm 0.15$	$28.33^{bc} \pm 1.66$	$46.40^b \pm 2.79$	$6.58^b \pm 0.20$
F	$16.24^c \pm 0.13$	$201.19^b \pm 10.52$	$1.26^a \pm 0.08$	$16.92^a \pm 1.31$	$30.06^a \pm 2.21$	$5.48^a \pm 0.25$
F + BEP	$5.66^b \pm 0.20$	$152.04^a \pm 8.81$	$2.72^b \pm 0.14$	$29.96^c \pm 1.64$	$54.47^b \pm 2.76$	$7.21^c \pm 0.19$
F + MEL	$5.03^a \pm 0.08$	$151.53^a \pm 2.27$	$2.61^b \pm 0.11$	$25.98^b \pm 1.28$	$50.56^b \pm 1.53$	$5.81^a \pm 0.21$

Comparisons are between the rows. Values in the same column bearing no common superscripts (a, b, and c) differ significantly ($P < 0.05$).
*The activity was expressed as U/g of protein [one unit of SOD is the amount (Δg) of protein required to inhibit the MTT reduction by 50%].

free-SH groups and using the DTNB method described by Sedlak and Lindsay [25].

2.5.3. Catalase (CAT). Activities of catalase enzymes were estimated by spectrophotometry as described by Bergmayer [26].

2.5.4. Superoxide Dismutase (SOD). Superoxide dismutase activities in liver, heart, and kidney were estimated as per the method described by Madesh and Balasubramanian [27].

2.5.5. Glutathione Peroxidase (GPx). Glutathione peroxidase activities were determined by the method of Paglia and Valentine [28].

2.5.6. Glutathione Reductase (GR). This enzyme activity was assayed by the method of Goldberg and Spooner [29].

2.5.7. Protein Assay. Protein contents in liver, heart, and kidney homogenates were determined and calculated by the method of Lowry et al. [30].

2.5.8. Statistical Analysis. Differences between groups were statistically analyzed by a one-way ANOVA, and the differences between the means of groups were separated by the least significant difference (LSD) test. All data were presented as mean ± standard error. Values of $P < 0.05$ were regarded as significant. A computer program (SPSS 10.01, SPSS Inc., Chicago, IL, USA) was used for statistical analysis.

3. Results

Cardiac, hepatic, and renal tissues oxidative stress in relation to fluoride treatment and antioxidant properties of melatonin (MEL) and buffalo epiphyseal proteins (BEP) were monitored

by the study of products of free radicals such as malondialdehyde (MDA) as well as the activity of enzymes including CAT, GPx, GR, SOD, and GSH levels. Cardiac, hepatic, and renal tissue LPO levels CAT activities were significantly ($P > 0.05$) increased on fluoride administration when compared with the control (Tables 2, 3, and 4). Fluoride treatment resulted in a significant ($P < 0.05$) diminution in the GSH level and activities of cardiac, hepatic, and renal SOD, GR, and GPx (Tables 2, 3, and 4). These data indicate F-induced augmentation of oxidative stress in cardiac, hepatic, and renal tissues.

In F + MEL- and F + BEP-treated animals, MDA (LPO) levels in cardiac, hepatic, and renal tissues were found to be reduced whereas CAT, SOD, GPx, and GR activities and GSH concentration were increased significantly ($P < 0.05$) (Tables 2, 3, and 4). Interestingly, cardiac GR and GSH were higher in F + BEP-treated animals as compared with F + MEL-administered animals (Table 2), whereas higher hepatic SOD activity was observed in F + MEL-administered animals as compared to F + BEP-administered animals (Table 3).

4. Discussion

Although some data on F-induced oxidative stress provide supportive evidence for the view that free radicals and oxidative stress are root causes of degenerative disease, there is only a limited amount of animal model data on this point. The present study provides evidence that our in vivo rat model of F-induced oxidative stress is a useful system for studying this pathological condition and in particular for evaluating potential antioxidant therapies such as melatonin and epiphyseal proteins.

Several enzymes are important in antioxidative defense and are basic for their actions in metabolizing either free radicals or reactive oxygen intermediates to no-radical products [31, 32]. Our results suggested that the F treatment

TABLE 3: Effect of different treatments on lipid peroxidation (LPO), catalase (CAT), superoxide dismutase (SOD), glutathione peroxidase (GPx), glutathione reductase (GR), and reduced glutathione (GSH) in liver of female rats ($n = 6$; means ± S.E.).

Group	Parameter					
	LPO (nM MDA/mL)	CAT (nM/min/mg protein)	SOD (U)*	GR (nM/min/mg protein)	GPx (nM/min/mg protein)	GSH (μM/g tissue)
Control	$4.61^a \pm 0.11$	$291.03^a \pm 14.93$	$6.15^b \pm 0.37$	$145.85^c \pm 7.33$	$25.67^b \pm 1.87$	$3.30^b \pm 0.06$
F	$12.21^c \pm 0.77$	$385.63^b \pm 13.50$	$2.58^a \pm 0.16$	$83.92^a \pm 10.10$	$14.87^a \pm 0.91$	$2.53^a \pm 0.14$
F + BEP	$6.33^b \pm 0.11$	$276.36^a \pm 12.12$	$5.53^b \pm 0.21$	$119.33^b \pm 7.69$	$25.88^b \pm 1.28$	$3.29^b \pm 0.06$
F + MEL	$6.28^b \pm 0.11$	$269.54^a \pm 14.38$	$7.81^c \pm 0.18$	$109.73^b \pm 7.82$	$27.14^b \pm 0.90$	$3.15^b \pm 0.10$

Comparisons are between the rows. Values in the same column bearing no common superscripts (a, b, and c) differ significantly ($P < 0.05$).
*The activity was expressed as U/g of protein [one unit of SOD is the amount (Δg) of protein required to inhibit the MTT reduction by 50%.].

TABLE 4: Effect of different treatments on lipid peroxidation (LPO), catalase (CAT), superoxide dismutase (SOD), glutathione peroxidase (GPx), glutathione reductase (GR), and reduced glutathione (GSH) in kidney of female rats ($n = 6$; means ± S.E.).

Group	Parameter					
	LPO (nM MDA/mL)	CAT (nM/min/mg protein)	SOD (U)*	GR (nM/min/mg protein)	GPx (nM/min/mg protein)	GSH (μM/g tissue)
Control	$4.99^a \pm 0.130$	$251.70^a \pm 4.58$	$5.98^b \pm 0.17$	$126.64^c \pm 8.47$	$20.13^b \pm 1.11$	$3.50^b \pm 0.06$
F	$16.62^c \pm 0.360$	$382.46^c \pm 14.89$	$2.56^a \pm 0.12$	$41.11^a \pm 5.40$	$14.38^a \pm 0.49$	$2.68^a \pm 0.09$
F + BEP	$6.90^b \pm 0.140$	$295.11^b \pm 4.22$	$5.64^b \pm 0.37$	$85.85^b \pm 3.97$	$20.18^b \pm 2.59$	$3.76^b \pm 0.08$
F + MEL	$6.88^b \pm 0.089$	$307.06^b \pm 5.24$	$5.96^b \pm 0.28$	$93.01^b \pm 7.78$	$18.43^b \pm 0.83$	$3.25^b \pm 0.10$

Comparisons are between the rows. Values in the same column bearing no common superscripts (a, b, and c) differ significantly ($P < 0.05$).
*The activity was expressed as U/g of protein [one unit of SOD is the amount (Δg) of protein required to inhibit the MTT reduction by 50%.].

depleted antioxidant enzymes and concomitantly increased levels of LPO differentially in rats' liver, heart, and kidney. The findings reported here are consistent with those of others in showing that, in F-treated rats, the combined effect of reductions in antioxidant enzyme activity plus high levels of LPO is associated with deleterious oxidative changes due to the accumulation of toxic products [3, 33, 34]. CAT was the only antioxidant enzyme whose activity was increased. Although GPx and CAT share the substrate H_2O_2, the glutathione redox cycle is a major protective mechanism against low levels of oxidant stress, whereas CAT becomes more important in protecting against severe oxidant stress [35]. Guo et al. [2] also reported that antioxidant enzymatic activity as well as overall amounts of antioxidants was reduced in the livers of animals treated with F, conditions which can promote the heavy accumulation of free radicals.

The decrease in the levels of GSH in heart, liver, and kidney observed in our study may have been due to the increased utilization of GSH by GPx in detoxification of H_2O_2 generated by F-induced oxidative stress. GSH serves as a reservoir for cysteines which in turn participate in detoxification reactions for xenobiotics and metabolism of numerous cellular compounds [36, 37]. The liver and kidney are the main target organs for attacks by excessive amount of F [38, 39]. Inasmuch as the liver is an important source of GSH, metabolism of xenobiotics in the liver, which can drastically deplete liver GSH, may also result in GSH depletion in other tissues [40]. He et al. [39] also reported that high-fluoride intake enhances oxidative stress in blood and liver, disturbing the antioxidant defense of rats. These events may

be implicated in the impaired organ function and poor health of both animals and humans under F-induced oxidative stress.

MEL functions as a free radical scavenger and antioxidant. Its wide range of actions is due in part to its amphiphilicity (it is neutral in cell membranes, i.e., it is neither hydrophobic nor hydrophilic) and thus it easily enters cells and subcellular compartments as well as important morphological barriers such as the blood-brain barrier [41]. In the present study, BEP and MEL reversed the adverse effect of oxidative stress by increasing antioxidant enzyme activity and reducing LPO in cardiac, hepatic, and renal tissues. These findings therefore support the hypothesis that BEP may have antioxidant properties and are also consistent with our earlier findings [18–21]. Additionally, the study demonstrated that the antioxidant activities of BEP were equal in potency and in some cases were superior to those of MEL, which is also produced by the pineal gland. Recently, pineal proteins have been shown to have a role in the stimulation of MEL production [16]. The occasionally superior effects of BEP on MEL may have been due in part to the fact that pineal proteins not only have direct antioxidant effects but also are able to stimulate MEL synthesis, expression of SOD, ceruloplasmin, and other antioxidant enzymes [42–44]. This might have been the reason for the selectively greater antioxidative effect on certain enzymes as compared to MEL action alone. Finally, the findings prove that BEP are effective antioxidants and may play a protective role against cardiac, renal, and hepatic damage induced by oxidative stress following F treatment.

5. Conclusions

These findings clearly demonstrate the importance of the pineal gland's neuroendocrine activity and, in particular, of its role as a promoter of antioxidant activity. The study has also elucidated the ameliorative effects of buffalo epiphyseal proteins and melatonin against fluoride-induced oxidative stress. Further, this study findings reveal that exogenous administration of melatonin and buffalo epiphyseal proteins may have therapeutic potential for reducing the fluoride-induced oxidative stress mediated pathogenesis and damage in cardiac, hepatic, and renal damage. However, further study is required to test these molecules in different animals and to know details of these proteins (structure of the individual proteins) with respect to their pharmacological role.

Conflict of Interests

The authors declare that there is no conflict of interests regarding the publication of this paper.

Acknowledgments

Research grant in the shape of Institute Senior Research Fellowship (Vijay K. Bharti) and facilities provided by Indian Veterinary Research Institute for conducting this study is duly acknowledged. The authors also acknowledge the tireless efforts of their lab and animal shed assistants.

References

[1] R. Rzeuski, D. Chlubek, and Z. Machoy, "Interactions between fluoride and biological free radical reactions," *Fluoride*, vol. 31, no. 1, pp. 43–45, 1998.

[2] X. Y. Guo, G. F. Sun, and Y. C. Sun, "Oxidative stress from fluoride-induced hepatotoxicity in rats," *Fluoride*, vol. 36, no. 1, pp. 25–29, 2003.

[3] D. Shanthakumari, S. Srinivasalu, and S. Subramanian, "Effect of fluoride intoxication on lipidperoxidation and antioxidant status in experimental rats," *Toxicology*, vol. 204, no. 2-3, pp. 219–228, 2004.

[4] X. Zhao, J. Wang, F. Wu et al. "Removal of fluoride from aqueous media by Fe3O4@Al(OH)3 magnetic nanoparticles," *Journal of Hazardous Materials*, vol. 173, no. 1–3, pp. 102–109, 2010.

[5] J. Gutiérrez-Salinas, J. A. Morales-González, E. Madrigal-Santillán et al., "Exposure to sodium fluoride produces signs of apoptosis in rat leukocytes," *International Journal of Molecular Sciences*, vol. 11, no. 9, pp. 3610–3622, 2010.

[6] J. A. Morales-González, J. Gutiérrez-Salinas, L. García-Ortiz et al., "Effect of sodium fluoride ingestion on malondialdehyde concentration and the activity of antioxidant enzymes in rat erythrocytes," *International Journal of Molecular Sciences*, vol. 11, no. 6, pp. 2443–2452, 2010.

[7] Y. M. Shivarajashankara, A. R. Shivashankara, P. Gopalakrishna Bhat, and S. Hanumanth Rao, "Effect of fluoride intoxication on lipid peroxidation and antioxidant systems in rats," *Fluoride*, vol. 34, no. 2, pp. 108–113, 2001.

[8] B. Halliwell, J. M. C. Gutteridge, and C. E. Cross, "Free radicals, antioxidants, and human disease: where are we now?" *Journal of Laboratory and Clinical Medicine*, vol. 119, no. 6, pp. 598–620, 1992.

[9] C. D. Filippo, S. Cuzzocrea, F. Rossi, R. Marfella, and M. D'Amico, "Oxidative stress as the leading cause of acute myocardial infarction in diabetics," *Cardiovascular Drug Reviews*, vol. 24, no. 2, pp. 77–87, 2006.

[10] N. J. Chinoy and M. R. Memon, "Beneficial effects of some vitamins and calcium on fluoride and aluminium toxicity on gastrocnemius muscle and liver of male mice," *Fluoride*, vol. 34, no. 1, pp. 21–33, 2001.

[11] A. K. Susheela, "Fluorosis management programme in India," *Current Science*, vol. 77, no. 10, pp. 1250–1256, 1999.

[12] V. Simonneaux and C. Ribelayga, "Generation of the melatonin endocrine message in mammals: a review of the complex regulation of melatonin synthesis by norepinephrine, peptides, and other pineal transmitters," *Pharmacological Reviews*, vol. 55, no. 2, pp. 325–395, 2003.

[13] S. Zhang, W. Li, Q. Gao, and T. Wei, "Effect of melatonin on the generation of nitric oxide in murine macrophages," *European Journal of Pharmacology*, vol. 501, no. 1–3, pp. 25–30, 2004.

[14] R. Huculeci, D. Dinu, A. C. Staicu, M. C. Munteanu, M. Costache, and A. Dinischiotu, "Malathion-induced alteration of the antioxidant defence system in kidney, gill, and intestine of Carassius auratus gibelio," *Environmental Toxicology*, vol. 24, no. 6, pp. 523–530, 2009.

[15] S. L. Chawla, R. Yadav, D. Shah, and M. V. Rao, "Protective action of melatonin against fluoride-induced hepatotoxicity in adult female mice," *Fluoride*, vol. 41, no. 1, pp. 44–51, 2008.

[16] V. Sejian, *Studies on pineal-adrenal relationship in goats (Capra hircus) under thermal stress [Ph.D. thesis]*, Indian Veterinary Research Institute, Izatnagar, India, 2006.

[17] M. Tandon, R. S. Srivastava, S. K. Meur, and M. Saini, "Proteins and peptides present in pineal gland and other brain structures of buffaloes," *Indian Journal of Animal Sciences*, vol. 76, no. 5, pp. 383–384, 2006.

[18] V. K. Bharti and R. S. Srivastava, "Fluoride-induced oxidative stress in rat's brain and its amelioration by buffalo (*Bubalus bubalis*) pineal proteins and melatonin," *Biological Trace Element Research*, vol. 130, no. 2, pp. 131–140, 2009.

[19] V. K. Bharti and R. S. Srivastava, "Protective role of buffalo pineal proteins on arsenic-induced oxidative stress in blood and kidney of rats," *Health*, vol. 1, no. 3, pp. 167–172, 2009.

[20] V. K. Bharti and R. S. Srivastava, "Effects of epiphyseal proteins and melatonin on blood biochemical parameters of fluoride-intoxicated rats," *Neurophysiology*, vol. 42, no. 4, pp. 258–264, 2011.

[21] V. K. Bharti and R. S. Srivastava, "Effect of pineal proteins at different dose level on fluoride-induced changes in plasma biochemicals and blood antioxidants enzymes in rats," *Biological Trace Element Research*, vol. 141, no. 1–3, pp. 275–282, 2011.

[22] V. K. Bharti, R. S. Srivastava, J. K. Malik, D. W. Spence, S. R. Pandi-Perumal, and G. M. Brown, "Evaluation of blood antioxidant defense and apoptosis in peripheral lymphocytes on exogenous administration of pineal proteins and melatonin in rats," *Journal of Physiology and Biochemistry*, vol. 68, no. 2, pp. 237–245, 2012.

[23] V. K. Bharti, R. S. Srivastava, B. Sharma, and J. K. Malik, "Buffalo (*Bubalus bubalis*) epiphyseal proteins counteract arsenic-induced oxidative stress in brain, heart, and liver of female rats," *Biological Trace Element Research*, vol. 146, no. 2, pp. 224–229, 2012.

[24] S.-U. Rehman, "Lead-induced regional lipid peroxidation in brain," *Toxicology Letters*, vol. 21, no. 3, pp. 333–337, 1984.

[25] J. Sedlak and R. H. Lindsay, "Estimation of total, protein-bound, and nonprotein sulfhydryl groups in tissue with Ellman's reagent," *Analytical Biochemistry C*, vol. 25, pp. 192–205, 1968.

[26] H. U. Bergmayer, "UV method of catalase assay," in *Methods of Enzymatic Analysis*, vol. 3rd, p. 273, Chemie, Weinheim, Germany, 1983.

[27] M. Madesh and K. A. Balasubramanian, "Microtiter plate assay for superoxide dismutase using MTT reduction by superoxide," *Indian Journal of Biochemistry and Biophysics*, vol. 35, no. 3, pp. 184–188, 1998.

[28] D. E. Paglia and W. N. Valentine, "Studies on the quantitative and qualitative characterization of erythrocyte glutathione peroxidase," *The Journal of Laboratory and Clinical Medicine*, vol. 70, no. 1, pp. 158–169, 1967.

[29] D. M. Goldberg and R. J. Spooner, "Glutathione reductase," in *Methods in Enzymatic Analysis*, J. Bergmeyer and M. Grassi, Eds., pp. 258–265, VCH, Weinheim, Germany, 1983.

[30] O. H. Lowry, N. J. Rosebrough, A. I. Farr, and R. J. Randall, "Protein measurement with the Folin phenol reagent," *The Journal of Biological Chemistry*, vol. 193, no. 1, pp. 265–275, 1951.

[31] N. J. Chinoy and T. N. Patel, "The influence of fluoride and/or aluminium on free radical toxicity in the brain of female mice and beneficial effects of some antidotes," *Fluoride*, vol. 33, p. 8, 2000.

[32] D. X. Tan, L. C. Manchester, M. P. Terron, L. J. Flores, and R. J. Reiter, "One molecule, many derivatives: a never-ending interaction of melatonin with reactive oxygen and nitrogen species?" *Journal of Pineal Research*, vol. 42, no. 1, pp. 28–42, 2007.

[33] Y. M. Shivarajashankara, A. R. Shivashankara, P. Gopalakrishna Bhat, and S. Hanumanth Rao, "Lipid peroxidation and antioxidant systems in the blood of young rats subjected to chronic fluoride toxicity," *Indian Journal of Experimental Biology*, vol. 41, no. 8, pp. 857–860, 2003.

[34] L. R. Chioca, I. M. Raupp, C. Da Cunha, E. M. Losso, and R. Andreatini, "Subchronic fluoride intake induces impairment in habituation and active avoidance tasks in rats," *European Journal of Pharmacology*, vol. 579, no. 1–3, pp. 196–201, 2008.

[35] H. Yan and J. J. Harding, "Glycation-induced inactivation and loss of antigenicity of catalase and superoxide dismutase," *Biochemical Journal*, vol. 328, no. 2, pp. 599–605, 1997.

[36] R. F. Burk, "Glutathione-dependent protection by rat liver microsomal protein against lipid peroxidation," *Biochimica et Biophysica Acta-General Subjects*, vol. 757, no. 1, pp. 21–28, 1983.

[37] D. A. Yahia, S. Madani, E. Prost, J. Prost, M. Bouchenak, and J. Belleville, "Tissue antioxidant status differs in spontaneously hypertensive rats fed fish protein or casein," *Journal of Nutrition*, vol. 133, no. 2, pp. 479–482, 2003.

[38] Y. N. Wang, K. Q. Xiao, J. L. Liu, G. Dallner, and Z. Z. Guan, "Effect of long term fluoride exposure on lipid composition in rat liver," *Toxicology*, vol. 146, no. 2-3, pp. 161–169, 2000.

[39] X. He, M. G. Chen, G. X. Lin, and Q. Ma, "Arsenic induces NAD(P)H-quinone oxidoreductase I by disrupting the Nrf2·Keap1·Cul3 complex and recruiting Nrf2·Maf to the antioxidant response element enhancer," *Journal of Biological Chemistry*, vol. 281, no. 33, pp. 23620–23631, 2006.

[40] S. M. Deneke, D. F. Baxter, D. T. Phelps, and B. L. Fanburg, "Increase in endothelial cell glutathione and precursor amino acid uptake by diethyl maleate and hyperoxia," *American Journal of Physiology-Lung Cellular and Molecular Physiology*, vol. 257, no. 3, pp. 265–271, 1989.

[41] R. J. Reiter, D. Melchiorri, E. Sewerynek, and B. Poeggler, "A review of the evidence supporting melatonin's role as an antioxidant," *Journal of Pineal Research*, vol. 18, no. 1, pp. 1–11, 1995.

[42] L. S. Kozina, A. V. Arutjunyan, S. L. Stvolinskii, M. S. Stepanova, M. G. Makletsova, and V. K. Khavinson, "Regulatory peptides protect brain neurons from hypoxia in vivo," *Doklady Biological Sciences*, vol. 418, no. 1, pp. 7–10, 2008.

[43] M. V. Rao and R. N. Bhatt, "Protective effect of melatonin on fluoride-induced oxidative stress and testicular dysfunction in rats," *Fluoride*, vol. 45, no. 2, pp. 116–124, 2012.

[44] M. V. Rao and S. B. Thakur, "Effects of melatonin and amla on F-induced genotoxicity in human peripheral blood lymphocytes," *Fluoride*, vol. 46, pp. 128–134, 2013.

20

The Therapeutic Potential of Medicinal Foods

Nelvana Ramalingum and M. Fawzi Mahomoodally

Department of Health Sciences, Faculty of Science, University of Mauritius, 230 Réduit, Mauritius

Correspondence should be addressed to M. Fawzi Mahomoodally; f.mahomoodally@uom.ac.mu

Academic Editor: Neal Davies

Pharmaceutical and nutritional sciences have recently witnessed a bloom in the scientific literature geared towards the use of food plants for their diversified health benefits and potential clinical applications. Health professionals now recognize that a synergism of drug therapy and nutrition might confer optimum outcomes in the fight against diseases. The prophylactic benefits of food plants are being investigated for potential use as novel medicinal remedies due to the presence of pharmacologically active compounds. Although the availability of scientific data is rapidly growing, there is still a paucity of updated compilation of data and concerns about the rationale of these health-foods still persist in the literature. This paper attempts to congregate the nutritional value, phytochemical composition, traditional uses, *in vitro* and *in vivo* studies of 10 common medicinal food plants used against chronic noncommunicable and infectious diseases. Food plants included were based on the criteria that they are consumed as a common food in a typical diet as either fruit or vegetable for their nutritive value but have also other parts which are in common use in folk medicine. The potential challenges of incorporating these medicinal foods in the diet which offers prospective opportunities for future drug development are also discussed.

1. Introduction

With the epidemic of chronic diseases and associated pathological complications, health has become the forefront of scientific research for finding novel foods and strategies to tackle such public health burden. The past years have witnessed significant challenges in the traditional concepts of nutrition and pharmaceuticals. Indeed, the classical notion of "adequate nutrition," that is, a diet that provides nutrients in sufficient quantities to satisfy particular organic needs, is being gradually replaced by the concept of "optimal nutrition." This concept portrays food components as having the potential to promote health, improve general well-being, and reduce the risk of developing certain illnesses [1]. Hence, while attempting to unravel the various mechanisms by which food provide protection to the body, health experts have identified the presence of a plethora of bioactive compounds which are referred to as phytochemicals. This was the thrust that drove the conception of the term "functional food," also expressed in a variety of terms like "pharmafoods," "medifoods," "vitafoods," or "medicinal foods" [2]. Medicinal food plants may be defined as those food plants whose

consumed parts receive recognition as therapeutic either in traditional medicine, ethnomedicine, or biomedicine [3].

A holistic approach of the concept of medicinal foods was drawn from the study that foods are not intended to satisfy hunger and only provide essential macro- and micronutrients to the body but also to supply it with bioactive ingredients that aid to decrease nutrition-related diseases and ensure physical and mental well-being [4]. In contrast, nutraceutical has been defined as "food or part of food that provide medical or health benefits, including the prevention and treatment of disease" [5]. The main difference is that nutraceuticals can be consumed in a nonfood matrix form as pills, capsules, or tablets, whereas functional or medicinal foods are taken as part of a normal food pattern [6]. The amount of intake and form of the medicinal food should be as it is normally expected for dietary purposes. Functional foods were first launched in Japan in the early 1980s as a food category called Foods for Specific Health Use (FOSHU) [4]. To date, there is no real unanimous definition for functional food. However, the EU project, Functional Food Science in Europe (FUFOSE), has come forward with the following statement: "A food can be

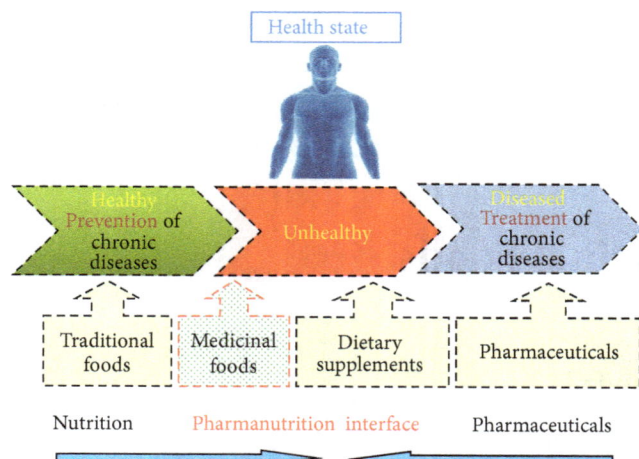

FIGURE 1: Pharmanutrition interface.

regarded as functional if it is satisfactorily demonstrated to affect beneficially one or more target functions in the body, beyond adequate nutritional effects, thus either improving the general physical conditions or/and decreasing the risk of the generation of diseases" [4]. In contrast, pharmaceuticals or drugs are especially formulated and developed to treat, cure, or prevent disease, which under normal conditions do not form part of our physiology [7]. Also, the pharmaceuticals have higher potency or biological activity compared to the phytochemicals which are normally ingested in insignificant amounts in diet and exert physiological effects only after long term use [6]. Therefore, a medicinal food can be considered to position itself between traditional foods and pharmaceuticals, termed as the "Pharmanutrition interface" (Figure 1) [8].

2. The Renaissance of Food Plants as Therapeutic Agents

Records of the use of plants for their therapeutic activities existed as early as from the Middle Paleolithic age [9]. From that point onwards, the value of this therapeutic approach has long been supported by traditional medicinal systems like Ayurveda, Unani, and Traditional Chinese Medicine. As defined by the World Health Organization (WHO), "traditional medicine is the sum total of knowledge, skills and practices based on the theories, beliefs and experiences indigenous to different cultures that are used to maintain health, as well as to prevent, diagnose, improve or treat physical and mental illnesses" [10]. Through generations, knowledge about botanicals and the savoir faire of preparing remedies have allowed humans to recognise the prophylactic benefits of certain plants and rely on their traditional *materia medica* for their healthcare needs [11]. Plants were administered mostly in their crude forms as infusions (herbal teas), tinctures (alcoholic extracts), decoctions (boiled extracts), and syrups (extracts of herbs made with syrup or honey) or applied externally as poultices, balms, and essential oils [11].

Among the earliest complete records which highlighted the use of over seven hundred herbs or plants as supplements were the Egyptian hieroglyphics. The Papyrus Ebers noted some of the herbs which are still in use today among which is *Aloe vera* L. [12]. A strong connection existed between food and pharmacology for maintaining health and treating various ailments. Indeed, Hippocrates, 500 BC stated the following: "Let food be your medicine and medicine be your food." For example, spices which normally are used as flavour or taste enhancers in food were described as "influencers of body metabolism" [13]. Traditionally used in Indian cooking, turmeric (*Curcuma longa*) contains the active ingredient curcumin which is considered to have antioxidant, anti-inflammatory, and anticarcinogenic properties [14]. This is thought to be mediated through inhibition of several cell-signalling pathways, inhibition of enzymes such as cyclooxygenases and glutathione S-transferases, immunomodulation, and effects on angiogenesis and cell-cell adhesion [15]. Garlic (*Allium sativum*), which can be eaten raw or cooked, contains allicin. It has been documented to have LDL cholesterol lowering effects while increasing HDL levels, antihypertensive effects, and caused improved circulation [16]. Peppermint (*Mentha piperita*) has long been used to treat digestive problems like bloating, abdominal distension, and difficulty in evacuation due to its smooth muscle relaxant effect [17], while thyme (*Thymus vulgaris*) and sage (*Salvia officinalis*) of the Lamiaceae family were used to cure spasmodic gastric-intestinal complaints, cough, bronchitis, laryngitis, and tonsillitis and used as a vermifuge in ancient Egypt [18].

With rapid advances in pharmacological research, active ingredients from plants served as prototype molecules for possible development of novel drugs, with aspirin being first produced in 1897, derived from salicylic acid [19]. Consequently, this discovery ushered in an epoch of pharmaceutical development, where most ailments were treated with synthetic drugs. Until recently, the pharmaceutical industry has been faced with a "research drought" [20]. The unprecedented challenges are due to factors like the rising costs of research and development (R&D) in drug discovery and development, concerns about the integrity and transparency of the industry, and the strict regulations exerted by the Food and Drug Administration (FDA) in drug approval [21]. Coupled with this, there has been the swelling of the devastating scourge of chronic diseases worldwide, accounting for 80% of deaths among low and middle income countries [22] as well as a rampant spread of drug resistant pathogens causing infectious diseases. For example, diabetes mellitus and its pathological complications are costly to manage both for affected individuals and healthcare systems around the world. Much resource has been invested in the screening of antidiabetic agents in the past decades. As the knowledge of heterogeneity of these diseases increases, many people are shifting back to natural products. Natural products have served as a major source of drugs such that they contribute to about half of the armamentarium of pharmaceuticals in use today. On the other hand, more people are aiming towards the concept of self-care and believe that natural foods are associated with fewer side effects and consequently safer for use [23]. Their uses for health management has stood the test of time and are often considered relatively cheaper compared to synthetic drugs [24].

The past decade has witnessed an explosion of clinical research to show specifically what health benefits individual foods can offer, identifying the various nutrients and phytochemicals associated with these benefits and how they can be incorporated in the diet. One of the major issues of the WHO was to deepen investigation of plants as a promising source of therapies for human disease management [25]. Rationally designed polyherbal preparations are progressively being developed as alternative for multitarget therapeutic and prophylactic usage. This has resulted in growing lines of evidence to show that old molecules are finding new applications through a better understanding of traditional knowledge and clinical observations [26]. Till date, a miscellany of phytochemicals has been identified in medicinal plants to have versatile profile of effectiveness [24]. One sole plant may, for example, contain bitter substances that stimulate digestion, anti-inflammatory compounds, polyphenols that can act as an antioxidant, and venotonics, antibacterial, and antifungal tannins that perform as natural antibiotics [26]. In certain cases, when a combination of medicinal foods or extracts is consumed at the same time or mixed in appropriate formulation, the therapeutic effects could be a result of total sum of different classes of compounds present within the foods [27]. Indeed, there have been reports highlighting that intake of whole medicinal food which have resulted in significantly better outcomes compared when an equivalent dose of single isolated active ingredient was given. Thus, it can be argued that synergism can occur when two or more compounds interact in ways that mutually enhance, amplify, or potentiate each other's effect [28].

The present paper reviews common medicinal food plants which appeared in the literature with potential for the management of chronic diseases like diabetes mellitus, hyperlipidemia, or cancer and infectious illnesses. An attempt has also been made to congregate the nutritional value, phytochemical composition, traditional uses, and *in vitro* and *in vivo* studies from various common medicinal food plants (edible and nonedible parts) used among various populations worldwide for the management of both chronic noncommunicable and infectious diseases. The different plants included were based on the criteria that they are consumed as a common food in a typical diet as either fruit or vegetable for their nutritive value but have also other parts which are in common use in folk medicine. Another inclusion criterion was those food plants that came from different families which have previously gained scientific momentum and demonstrated to have medicinal virtues against panoply of ailments. Thus, focus was laid on Annonaceae, Moraceae, Myrtaceae, Cucurbitaceae, Moringaceae, Solanaceae, and Punicaceae families from which important phytochemicals have been isolated and offer prospective opportunities for future drug development.

2.1. Annona squamosa Linn. (Annonaceae): Sugar Apple or Custard Apple.

Annona squamosa, also known as sugar apple or custard apple, is a small tropical tree which is native to South America and distributed throughout India and other tropical countries. The ripe fruit pulp contains around 88.9–95.7 g calories where the sugar content is 14.58%, amino acid lysine (54–69 mg), carotene (5–7 IU), and ascorbic acid (34.7–42.2 mg) [29]. The various chemical constituents isolated from leaves, stems, and roots of the plant include anonaine, aporphine, coryeline, isocorydine, norcorydine, and glaucine [30]. Folkloric record reports its use as an insecticidal and antitumor agent [31], antidiabetic [32], antioxidant, antilipidemic [33], and anti-inflammatory agent [34] which may be characterized due to the presence of the cyclic peptides [35]. An infusion with 2 handfuls of fresh leaves in 1 L of water is prepared to fight against heart failure and palpitations (1 cup after meal). This infusion is also effective for proper digestion and has antispasmodic activities [36]. The seeds are reported to have antiparasitic activities (against lice). A cream consisting of 3 cl bee wax, 12 cl almond oil, 3 cl coconut oil, 6 cl of water, 6 cl glycerin, and 1 handful of crushed *A. squamosa* seeds is prepared and heated over a water bath for 3 hours before applying to the hair [36]. In India the crushed leaves are applied on ulcers and wounds and a leaf decoction is taken in cases of dysentery [35]. In Aligarh district of Northern India, villagers used to consume a mixture of 4-5 newly grown young leaves of *A. squamosa* along with black pepper (*Piper nigrum*) for management of diabetes. It is documented that this may ensure up to 80% of the positive results with continued therapy [35]. The bark decoction is given as a tonic and to halt diarrhea. Throughout tropical America, a decoction of the leaves is imbibed either as an emmenagogue, febrifuge, tonic, cold remedy, digestive, or to clarify urine. The leaf decoction is also employed in baths to alleviate rheumatic pain [29].

The effect of aqueous and organic extracts from defatted seeds of *A. squamosa* was studied on a rat histolytic tumour cell line, AK-5. Both organic and aqueous extracts caused significant apoptotic tumour cell death with enhanced caspase-3 activity and downregulation of antiapoptotic genes Bcl-2 and Bcl-xl [37].

Chen et al. [38] have recently identified and quantified two main compounds, namely, annonaceous acetogenins from the ethanol extract of *A. squamosa* seeds. The extract was reported to exhibit an antitumor effect against H_{22} tumor cells line. Bullatacin, a bistetrahydrofuran annonaceous acetogenin is recognized as the most potent inhibitor of the mitochondrial respiratory chain complex I and was observed to be 300 times more active than taxol *in vivo* [39]. Water extracts of *A. squamosa* leaves also possess antioxidant activity as shown by increased activities of scavenging enzymes such as catalase, superoxide dismutase, reduced glutathione, and malondialdehyde levels present in various tissues [37]. Administration of the hot-water extract of leaves of *A. squamosa* at a dose 300 mg/kg body weight for 12 weeks to nephrectomized rats resulted in a significant decrease in the plasma urea and creatinine values with even partial restoration to normal values along with a significant rise in the activity of superoxide dismutase. Thus, custard apple shows potential for amelioration of renal failure [40]. Administration of the aqueous extract of the leaves also improved the activities of plasma insulin and lipid profile and reduced the levels of blood glucose and lipid peroxidation, indicating that the high levels of triglyceride and total cholesterol associated with diabetes can also be significantly managed with the extract [41, 42]. When petroleum ether, ethyl acetate and alcoholic extracts of *A. squamosa* fruit peel were administered orally (250 mg/kg body weight) for 21 days; the extracts showed a significant decrease of blood glucose level and lipid profile on streptozotocin (STZ) induced diabetic rats when compared to untreated diabetic control group [43]. *A. squamosa* were also found to promote increased enzymatic (catalase, superoxide dismutase, glutathione peroxidase, and glutathione S-transferase) and nonenzymatic (vitamin E and ascorbic acid) antioxidants levels and nitric oxide levels in wound tissues for better wound repair mechanism in normal and diabetic rats [44].

The chloroform, petroleum ether, and ethanol extracts of custard apple also demonstrated important antimicrobial properties against the gram positive microorganisms such as *Bacillus subtilis*, *Bacillus cereus*, *Bacillus megaterium*, *Staphylococcus aureus*, and *Sarcina lutea* and the gram negative bacteria such as *Escherichia coli*, *Shigella dysenteriae*, *Shigella shiga*, *Shigella flexneri*, *Shigella sonnei*, *Salmonella typhi*, *Pseudomonas aeruginosa*, and *Klebsiella* spp. [35]. Similar results were also reported from the methanolic extracts of custard apple [45].

2.2. Artocarpus altilis Parkinson Fosberg (Moraceae): Breadfruit. *Artocarpus altilis*, also known as breadfruit is a pantropical tree widely distributed throughout Southeast Asia and most Pacific Ocean islands. It is a staple crop and a primary component of traditional agroforestry systems in Oceania [46]. The nutritional composition of breadfruit varies among cultivars. The fresh fruit contains around 22.8–77.3 g of carbohydrates (among which 68% is starch) calcium (15.2–31.1 mg), potassium (352 mg), phosphorus (34.4–79 mg), and niacin (0.81–1.96 mg). It is estimated that 2 cups (500 g) of boiled breadfruit at lunch and dinner provide around 25 g of fibre, but a similar serving of white rice provides only 6.8 g. A wide range of provitamin A carotenoid levels were found in breadfruit cultivars; some containing very high levels of 295–868 mg/100 g in breadfruit edible portion [47]. The essential amino acids that were found in the greatest amounts were leucine (605 mg) and lysine (799 mg) during the ripe developmental stage. The essential fatty acids detected at the highest concentration in ripe fruits were linoleic acid (0.15 mg) and linolenic acid (2.13 mg) [48]. Breadfruit can be consumed ripe, boiled fried, or grilled and is now commonly used to replace starchy vegetables, pasta, or rice. In the Indian culture, it is usually cooked with a blend of spices [47].

Breadfruit is a rich source of prenylated phenolic compounds such as geranylated flavones. For instance, artocarpin, isolated from an extract of heartwood of *A. altilis*, possesses potent α-reductase inhibitory effect and superoxide anion-scavenging activity [49]. Cataplasm of the fruits is effective against rheumatic and muscular pain, while decoction of the leaves has been documented to be a good antidote against ingestion of toxic fish [36]. The native people of

Indonesia and Pacific islands use the fruit pulp as liver tonic, against liver cirrhosis and hypertension [50]. Most chitin-binding lectins have shown antifungal activity against phytopathogenic species, since chitin is the key component of the cell wall of these microorganisms. They have shown to affect fungal growth and development, disturbing the synthesis and/or deposition of chitin in the cell wall [51, 52]. The isolated chitin-binding lectins from the seeds of *A. altilis*, frutackin, promoted hemagglutination and growth inhibition against fungi *Fusarium moniliforme* and *Saccharomyces cerevisiae in vitro* [53].

Ethyl acetate and methanolic extracts of *A. altilis* have also demonstrated potential for significant antibacterial activities against various pathogenic organisms like *Staphylococcus aureus*, *Pseudomonas aeruginosa*, *Streptococcus mutans*, and *Enterococcus faecalis* [54]. Flavonoids present, inhibited 5-lipoxygenase of cultured mastocytoma cells *in vitro* [47] and prenylflavonoids showed antinephritis activity *in vivo* [55]. Aqueous extract of the leaves of *A. altilis* was found to exhibit negative chronotropic and hypotensive effects through α-adrenoceptor and Ca^{2+} channel antagonism and cause moderate inhibition of cytochrome P450s (CYP3A4 and CYP 2D6) [56]. A body of evidence suggests that advanced glycation endproducts (AGEs) play critical roles as pathogenic mediators of almost all diabetes complications, typically clustered as micro- or macrovascular lesions [57]. Diabetic inflammation is triggered by the engagement of the receptor for advanced glycation end products (RAGE) by AGEs on the surface of monocytes which subsequently induce the production of cytosolic reactive oxygen species and NF-κB activation to promote the release of proinflammatory cytokines and facilitates the transformation of monocytes into macrophage. Recently, Lin et al. [58] have evaluated the effects of the geranyl flavonoid derivatives isolated from the fruit on the human THP-1 monocyte (THP-1) activation stimulated by S100B, a ligand of RAGE. It was found that addition of the geranyl flavonoid derivatives of breadfruit inhibited the S100B-induced THP-1 morphological characteristics of inflammation. The geranyl flavonoid derivatives inhibited S100B-induced reactive oxygen species generation, mRNA expression of inflammatory mediators (COX-2, TNF-α, and IL-6) [58].

2.3. Artocarpus heterophyllus Lam. (Moraceae): Jackfruit. *Artocarpus heterophyllus* is a tropical tree native to Western Ghats of India, Malaysia, and also found in Central and Eastern Africa, South-eastern Asia, the Caribbean, and many Pacific Islands [59]. Depending on the variety of the jackfruit, the proximate nutritional composition per 100 g of ripe fruit has been shown to vary. The ripe fruit has a proximate energy value of 88–410 KJ and principally contains 1.2–1.9 g of protein, 0.1–0.4 g of fat, 16–25.4 g of carbohydrates, 175–540 IU of vitamin A, 7–10 mg of vitamin C, 20–37 mg of calcium, 38–41 mg of phosphorus, and 191–407 mg of potassium [60]. Reports suggest that almost all parts of the jackfruit tree are of use in the preparations of various Ayurvedic and Unani medicines [61, 62] and ripe fruits are consumed to prevent excessive formation of bile, to develop flesh, phlegm, to strength the body, and increases virility [60]. Aqueous extracts of mature leaves of A. heterophyllus are used by traditional medical practitioners in Sri Lanka and India for the treatment of diabetes [63]. Roots useful in treating various skin diseases, asthma, and diarrhea. An ash produced by burning bark is supposed to heal abscesses and ear problems [61]. The infusion of mature leaves and bark is supposed to be effective in the treatment of diabetes, gall stones, and to relieve asthma. In the Chinese system of medicine, jackfruit is found to be of use in overcoming the influence of alcohol [60]. Depending on the variety, jackfruit was shown to be rich in compounds like carotenoids, volatile acids sterols, tannins, and important compounds like morin, dihydromorin, cynomacurin, artocarpin, isoartocarpin, cyloartocarpin, artocarpesin, oxydihydroartocarpesin, artocarpetin, norartocarpetin, cycloartinone, and artocarpanone [60].

Recently, two new chalcones, artocarpusins A and B; one new flavone, artocarpusin C; one new 2-arylbenzofuran derivative, artocarstilene A, were isolated from the twigs of the plant [64]. Artocarpesin has been found to reduce obesity associated inflammation by suppressing production of nitric oxide and prostaglandin E2 in macrophage cells [65]. Artocarpin has the ability to reduce cell viability in dose-dependent manner, causes alteration in cell morphology, and induces apoptosis of T47D breast cancer cells [55]. Gemichalcones A and artocarpin were presented to have moderate inhibitory activity on the proliferation of the PC-3 and H460 cell line [64]. Methanol extract of A. heterophyllus has likewise been showed to be nontoxic to normal cells (HEK293) but toxic to tA549 cell line as determined by MTT and SRB cytotoxic assays [66]. Jacalin, from the seeds, was similarly reported for its anticarcinogenic effect [50]. Jacalin was found to be strongly mitogenic for human CD4+ T-lymphocytes. It is considered as an important constituent to be studied for the evaluation of the immune status of patients infected with human immunodeficiency virus HIV-1 [65].

A. heterophyllus was also found to inhibit α-amylase activity in vitro and in rat plasma [67]. In STZ-induced diabetic rats, chronic administration of the ethylacetate fraction of A. heterophyllus leaves daily (20 mg/kg) for 5 weeks resulted in a significant lowering of serum glucose (39%), cholesterol (23%) and triglyceride levels (<0%) compared to control group. Such results mediated by the extract were comparable with those produced by glibenclamide (0.6 mg/kg) [63]. Pressurized hot water extract of A. heterophyllus seeds was observed to possess a significant antiglycation activity [68]. Furthermore, similar investigation into the leaves of A. heterophyllus has indicated its efficiency in the attenuation of glycosylation of hemoglobin, enhancement in the transport of glucose across cells, stimulation of insulin release, and inhibition of cholesterol biosynthetic enzymes [63–69]. With regard to the antimicrobial activity, the butanol extracts of the root bark and fruits were found to be active against Bacillus cereus, Bacillus coagulans, Bacillus megaterium, Bacillus subtilis, Lactobacillus casei, Micrococcus luteus, Micrococcus roseus, Staphylococcus albus, Staphylococcus aureus, Staphylococcus epidermidis, Streptococcus faecalis, Streptococcus pneumoniae, Agrobacterium tumefaciens, Citrobacter freundii, Enterobacter aerogenes, Escherichia coli, Klebsiella

pneumonia, Neisseria gonorrhoeae, Proteus mirabilis, Proteus vulgaris, Pseudomonas aeruginosa, Salmonella typhi, Salmonella typhimurium, and Serratia marcescens as evaluated by the disc diffusion method [70].

2.4. Eugenia jambolana Lam. (Myrtaceae): Jambolan. Eugenia jambolana, commonly known as jambolan, black plum, or jamun, is a tropical plant native to India and produces oblong or ellipsoid fruits (berries) annually [71]. The ripe fruit contains around 60 Kcal of energy, water (83.13 g), vitamin A (3 IU), pantothenic acid (0.16 mg), vitamin C (14.3 mg), calcium (19 mg), phosphorus (17 mg), magnesium (15 mg), potassium (79 mg), sodium (14 mg), and iron (16.2 mg) [72]. A glycoside in the seed, jamboline, is considered to have antidiabetic properties. It a is also reported to be a rich source of ellagitannins, including corilagin, 3,6-hexa hydroxyl diphenoyl glucose and its isomer 4,6-hexahydroxy diphenoyl glucose, 1-galloyl glucose, 3-galloyl glucose, gallic acid, and ellagic acid [72]. Decoction of 5 g of grounded seeds in 15 cl of water is prepared against diabetes and taken 3 times daily. Infusion of the bark along with the bark of guava (Psidium guajava) can be taken against dysentery and diarrhoea in folk medicines [36]. According to the Unani system of medicine, the fruits are used as liver tonic, to enrich blood and strengthen teeth and gums [71]. In India, juice extracted from the leaves is mixed with cow's milk and taken orally twice a day after taking food for 3 months for control of diabetes. Fresh fruits are taken to get relief from stomach ache, colic, and other digestive complaints [73]. The juice from the stem bark is mixed with butter milk and taken orally every day before going to bed to treat constipation. The same recipe, when taken early in the morning on empty stomach, is claimed to stop blood discharge in faeces [74]. Juice from the bark is also given to women with a history of repeated abortions [75].

The antibacterial potential of the leaf essential oil, petroleum ether, chloroform, ethyl acetate, and methanol extracts of the leaves were studied against human pathogenic bacteria, namely, Bacillus cereus, Enterobacter faecalis, Salmonella paratyphi, Staphylococcus aureus, Escherichia coli, Proteus vulgaris, Klebsiella pneumoniae, Pseudomonas aeruginosa, and Serratia marcescens and were found to have activity quite comparable with the standard antibiotics [76]. Additionally, aqueous extract of leaf of jambolan was shown to be effective against clinical isolates of Citrobacter spp., Salmonella typhi, Salmonella typhimurium, Shigella boydii, Shigella sonnei, and Streptococcus faecalis [77]. Aqueous, methanolic, and hydromethanolic extracts of the leaf are also effective against cariogenic bacteria such as Streptococcus mutans, and to suppress plaque formation in vitro [71], whereas aqueous extract of the seed was also found to produce significant and dose dependent antidiarrhoeal, antimotility, and antisecretory effects [78].

The ethanolic extracts of the fruit pulp, kernel, and seed coat were evaluated with gallic acid, quercetin, and trolox as reference molecules. The kernel extract was observed to be better than the seed coat and pulp extracts in 2,2-diphenyl-1-picrylhydrazyl (DPPH), superoxide radical scavenging, and hydroxyl radical scavenging assays [79]. The anthocyanin rich pulp extract was shown to inhibit the iron-induced lipid peroxidation in the rat brain, liver mitochondria, testes, and human erythrocyte cells *in vitro* [80]. Many clinical and experimental studies suggest that different parts of the jambolan especially fruits and seeds possess promising activity against diabetes mellitus [81]. A recent review by Ayyanar et al. [81] has elaborated on the antidiabetic action of various parts of jambolan. Though the exact mechanisms of action in animals are not fully understood, it is suggested that jambolan exerts an action by mimicking sulphonylurea and biguanides. It is postulated that it exerts about its hypoglycaemic action by stimulating of surviving β cells of islets of Langerhans to release more insulin. Moreover, it has also been reported to modulate glucose-6-phosphatase content in liver which caused an overall increase in glucose influx. Incubation of the *E. jambolana* aqueous seed extract with rat everted gut sacs resulted in the inhibition of the transport of glucose across the membrane, showing hypoglycemic activities [82]. Jambolan fruit is associated with decreased risk of secondary complications of diabetes. It is reported that oral feeding of fruit extract might help in the prevention of cataract development and decrease the risk of diabetic patients developing atherosclerosis as it contains oleanolic acid. This natural triterpenoid is known for its antioxidant properties by hampering the chemical reactions that generate toxic free radicals and reduces the action of free radicals in atherosclerosis by 60–90% [81].

2.5. Eugenia uniflora Linn. (Myrtaceae): Pitanga Fruit or Cayenne Cherry.

Eugenia uniflora, a tropical fruit-bearing shrub, is native to Surinam and widely distributed throughout Brazil. The ripe fruit contains around calcium (9 mg), phosphorus (11 mg), carotene (1200–2000 IU), and ascorbic acid (20–30 mg) but is low in iron (0.2 mg) [83]. The phytochemical screening showed the presence of phenolics eugeniflorin D1 and eugeniflorin D2, tannins, triterpenes, heterosides, anthraquinones, flavonoids, and saponins [66]. The leaves yield essential oil containing citronellal, geranyl acetate, geraniol, cineole, terpinene, sesquiterpenes, and polyterpenes [84]. The Pitanga fruit contains 26 mg/100 g of total anthocyanins and the identification of anthocyanins revealed the presence of cyanidin-3-glucoside and delphinidin-3-glucoside [85]. Infusion of young leaves or young shoots together with leaves of lemongrass (*Cymbopogon citratus*) is prepared to fight against flu and soothe headache. The infusion is also effective against diarrhea [36] and against gingival bleedings [86]. In Nigeria, a decoction of the leaves, mixed with guava (*Psidium guajava*) and neem (*Azadirachta indica*), is taken against fever and gastrointestinal disturbances in infants [87]. Throughout Brazil the ripe fruit is used in popular medicine as a diuretic, antirheumatic, febrifuge, and anti-inflammatory agent and as a therapeutic agent for stomach diseases [88]. In Paraguay, water decoctions are used to lower cholesterol and blood pressure [89]. The essential oil showed antimicrobial activity against two important pathogenic bacteria, *Staphylococcus aureus* and *Listeria monocytogenes*, and against two fungi; *Candida lipolytica*

and *Candida Guilliermondii*. It was found to reduce lipid peroxidation in the kidney [88]. Acute oral administration of the essential oil did not cause lethality or toxicological effects in mice. Santos et al. [90] also described that *E. uniflora* presents anti-*Trypanosoma* activity, which might help to combat infectious diseases such as Chagas disease caused by the parasite *Trypanosoma cruzi*. Tannins present were shown to have an inhibitory effect on Epstein Barr Virus DNA polymerase. Epstein Barr Virus is a human B lymphotropic herpes virus which is known to be closely associated with nasopharyngeal carcinoma [55]. Ethanol extract of *E. uniflora* also showed hypoglycemic activity by inhibiting maltase and sucrase activities as well as help decrease plasma triglyceride levels by inhibiting lipase activity [91]. Besides, the essential oil of *E. uniflora* leaves was demonstrated to reduce acetaminophen induced lipid peroxidation and restored all of the biochemical parameters modified by the injury like nonprotein thiol content, δ-aminolevulinate dehydratase, and glutathione-S-transferase activities and plasma activities of aspartate aminotransferase and alanine aminotransferase [92].

2.6. Lagenaria siceraria (Molina) Standley (Cucurbitaceae): Bottle Gourd.

Lagenaria siceraria has a wide occurrence in India where both its bottle or bell-shaped fruits and aerial parts are consumed as a vegetable [93]. The gourd has low energy value (14 Kcal) and low fat content (0.02 g) [94] but is moderate in vitamin C (10 mg) and water (96%) [95]. The iron content of bottle gourd taken with the peel on is 11.87 mg. It is also a rich source of phosphorus (240 mg), potassium (3320 mg), and magnesium (162 mg) [95]. *L. siceraria* is rich in cardiac glycosides, alkaloids, saponins, tannins, and flavonoids [96]. The fruit contains good choline level-a lipotropic factor, known to be important in the treatment of mental disorders. It is also reported to contain triterpenoid cucurbitacins B, D, G, H, and 22-deoxycucurbitacin, the bitter principle of Cucurbitaceae [97]. A decoction of young tender fruits or infusion of young shoots is prepared to fight against diabetes and hypertension (2-3 cups per day), whilst decoction of the seeds is effective for cleaning the digestive system and against constipation [36]. A decoction of the peels is also consumed at a frequency of 1 cup for 3 days for the treatment of diabetes [98]. The pulp of the fruit is considered to have cooling effects, diuretic, and antibilious properties and is effective against cough, fever, asthma, and other bronchial disorders. Decoction of leaves of *L. siceraria* is taken against jaundice, while decoction of skin of young fruits is documented to be taken against uremia, albuminuria, inflammation, and diabetes [36]. A novel protein, langenin, was isolated from seeds and reported to have antitumor, antiviral, antiproliferative, and anti-HIV activities [99]. Langenin has been documented to be a ribosome-inactivating protein (RIP). RIPs catalytically cleave N-glycosidic bonds of adenine in a specific RNA sequence, resulting in inhibition of protein synthesis. The potential applications of RIPs include conjugation with antibodies to form immunotoxins for cancer therapy [100]. Hydroalcoholic extract of *L. siceraria* indeed showed strong and dose-dependent inhibition of cancer cell line of the lung (A549) [101].

Juice extract of the fresh fruits of *L siceraria* on rats caused significant decrease in the levels of serum cholesterol and triglyceride levels by inhibition of lipoprotein lipase and lecithin-cholesterol acyl-transferase activity making triglycerides available for uptake and metabolism by tissues. Serum biochemistry changes suggested that the juice extract has a tonic effect on the kidneys and the liver and these organs play a central role in drug metabolism [96]. The juice extract also shows potential diuretic activity comparable to that of furosemide (20 mg/kg) and might be important in management of hypertension [98]. *L. siceraria* fruit powder also shows cardioprotective effects on isoprenaline-induced toxicity [99]. Deshpande et al. [102] studied antihyperglycemic activity of *L. siceraria* fruit in rats with induced hyperglycemia by alloxan monohydrate. It was found that the extract effectively prevented biochemical changes of induced hyperglycemia. Similar results were also obtained in a more recent study [93], where methanol extracts of aerial parts of *L. siceraria* reduced significantly fasting blood glucose levels and improved the antioxidant and histologic observations of the pancreas, kidney, and liver in STZ-induced diabetic rats. Katare et al. [103] have studied the administration of freshly prepared bottle gourd juice (200 mL) to human participants on empty stomach for 90 consecutive days. A notable reduction in blood glucose levels along with a significant reduction in total cholesterol (17.8%), serum triglycerides (16–22%), and LDL-c (22.2%) and a considerable decrease in VLDL-c was observed in diabetic subjects on juice therapy. Juice administration also contributed to significant elevations in superoxide dismutase and catalase activities in both diabetic (40.5%) and normal healthy subjects. Additionally, *L. siceraria* fruit extract was shown to ameliorate fat amassment and serum TNF- in high-fat diet-induced obese rats [104].

2.7. Momordica charantia Linn. (Cucurbitaceae): Bitter Melon.
Momordica charantia or bitter melon, also known as balsam pear or karela, is a valuable vegetable worldwide and has been extensively used in folk medicine as a remedy against diabetes. Bitter melon is grown in tropical areas of Asia, the Amazon, East Africa, the Caribbean, and throughout South America [105]. The nutrient profile of *M. charantia* has been listed by Jeyadevi et al. [106] and Yuwai et al. [107]. The fruit (per 100 g) has an energy value of 60 Kcal and contains approximately 23 mg calcium, 171 mg potassium, 2.4 mg sodium, 119.92 mg magnesium, 5.97 mg iron, 38 mg phosphorus, 96 mg vitamin C, and 126 mg β-carotene. Depending on the varieties ranging from the wild type to the hybrid green or hybrid white, bitter gourd is documented to have negligible level of reducing sugar and a total amount of protein ranging from 1.17 to 2.4% [108].

Examination of the phytochemicals of this plant indicates the presence of various active components like momorcharins, momordenol, momordicilin, momordicins, momordicinin, momordin, momordolol, charantin, charine, cryptoxanthin, cucurbitins, cucurbitacins, cucurbitanes, cycloartenols, diosgenin, elaeostearic acids, erythrodiol, galacturonic acids, gentisic acid, goyaglycosides, goyasaponins, and multiflorenol [109]. In India it is used for abortions, birth control, constipation, diabetes, eczema, fat loss, food, fever, gout, hemorrhoids, hydrophobia, hyperglycemia, increasing milk flow, intestinal parasites, jaundice, kidney stones, leprosy, liver, menstrual disorders, pneumonia, psoriasis, rheumatism, snakebite, and vaginal discharge [110]. A decoction is prepared by adding bitter melon leaves to 2 glasses of water. Diabetic people traditionally consumed 1/3 cup of the decoction thrice a day for effective control of blood sugar level [110]. Indeed, various scientific studies validated that fresh juice of bitter melon can lower blood sugar values and keep insulin level under check. Hypoglycemic activity has been documented to be due to the mixture of phytoconstituents isolated and the charantins which are insulin-like peptides [111]. Polypeptide-p is one of the few active compounds in bitter melon which has been extensively studied [112]. Several possible modes of the hypoglycemic actions of *M. charantia* have been proposed. These include stimulation of peripheral and skeletal muscle glucose utilization, inhibition of intestinal glucose uptake, inhibition of adipocyte differentiation, suppression of key gluconeogenic enzymes, stimulation of key enzyme of hexose monophosphate pathway, enhancement of insulin secretion by the Islets of Langerhans, and regeneration and preservation of islet β cells and their functions [113]. Supplementation of STZ-induced diabetic rats with *M. charantia* extract indeed showed improved activity level of enzymes hepatic glucokinase, hexokinase, glucose-6-phosphatase, and glycogen synthase [114]. Acute intravenous administrations of whole-plant of *M. charantia* extract produced dose-dependent, significant reductions in systemic arterial blood pressure, and heart rates of both normal and hypertensive Dahl salt-sensitive rats [115]. A more recent study stated that *M. charantia* can also inhibit the proliferation of preadipocytes in a dose dependent manner [116]. Furthermore, the clinical potential of bitter melon has been examined in several human cell line experiments. Momordin increases the expression of peroxisome proliferator-activated receptor (PPAR) δ mRNA in hepatoblastoma cells (HepG2), which is important in the regulation of glucose metabolism and fatty acid storage. Bitter melon juice also has been reported to significantly reduce sterol regulatory element-binding protein 1c (SREBP-1c) when applied to primary preadipocytes, further highlighting the prospective benefit of this compound in glycemic control [112]. Moreover, owing to its free radical scavenging abilities, it showed hepatoprotective effects against xenobiotics [117] like cyclophosphamide, a chemotherapy drug [118]. Though the exact mechanisms need to be elucidated, *M. charantia* has also been shown to decrease serum/tissue lipid parameters in hyperammonemic rats [119]. High levels of ammonia are considered toxic, affecting the central nervous system by causing functional disturbances that could even lead to coma and death [119]. It was found that the levels of serum and tissue cholesterol, triglycerides, free fatty acids, and phospholipids were significantly increased in ammonium chloride-induced hyperammonemic rats. However, upon administration of ethanolic extract of *M. charantia* fruit all these changes were significantly restored to almost normal levels. Several phytochemicals isolated from *M. charantia* like alpha- and beta-momorcharin, lectin, and *Momordica* anti-HIV protein (MAP30) have been documented to have *in vitro* antiviral activity against Epstein-Barr, herpes, HIV, coxsackie virus B3, and polio viruses [120]. MAP30 is reported to be a ribosomal inactivating protein that inhibits the HIV-1 reverse transcription, integration, and syncytium formation between the infected and the new white blood cells. MAP30 also inhibits the viral core protein synthesis [120]. Hexane, ethyl acetate, and ethanol seed extracts also exhibited broad spectrum antimicrobial activity against *Escherichia coli*, *Candida albicans*, *Staphylococcus aureus*, *Staphylococcus epidermidis*, and *Klebsiella pneumonia* [121].

2.8. Moringa oleifera Lam. (Moringaceae): Drumstick Tree. *Moringa oleifera*, also known as drumstick tree or horseradish tree, is a pan-tropical species that is native to the sub-Himalayan tracts of India, Pakistan, Bangladesh, and Afghanistan. It has long been used in Ayurvedic and Unani systems of medicines [122]. Many parts of this plant including the leaves, pods, and flowers are edible and are used as a highly nutritive vegetable and have even been used to combat malnutrition [123]. Moringa has even been advocated as "natural nutrition for the tropics" [124]. In folk medicine, leaves are used as purgative, applied as poultice to sores, rubbed on the temples for headaches, against fevers, sore throat, bronchitis, eye, and ear infection. Leaf juice is reported to control glucose levels and is applied topically to reduce glandular swelling. In contrast, the juice from the root bark is put into ears to relieve ear aches [125]. In the Philippines, it is known as "mother's best friend" for its virtue of increasing breast milk production and is often recommended for anemia [126]. Moringa leaves have been reported "ounce for ounce" to contain more β-carotene than carrots, more calcium than milk, more iron than spinach, and more potassium than bananas, high quality proteins, and even more vitamin C than oranges [124]. Melo et al. [127] reported that *M. oleifera* leaves contained good level of protein (22.75 g), fiber (7.92 g), and soluble carbohydrates (51.66 g) per 100 g dry weight. Equally, a previous study [128] showed that the dried leaves had crude protein levels of 30.3% and 19 amino acids. Different mineral contents were also identified like calcium (3.65%), phosphorus (0.3%), magnesium (0.5%), potassium (1.5%), sodium (0.164%), sulphur (0.63%), zinc (13.03 mg/kg), copper (8.25%), manganese (86.8 mg/kg), iron (490 mg/kg), and selenium (363 mg/kg). Additionally, 17 fatty acids were found among which α-linolenic acid made up 44.57%.

Regarding the medicinal value of leaves of *M. oleifera*, it was described to have antihypertensive, anti-inflammatory, and antimicrobial effects due to the presence of specific components like 4-(4′-O-acetyl-α-L-rhamnopyranosyloxy)benzyl isothiocy-anate, 4-(α-L-rhamnopyranosyloxy) benzyl isothiocy-anate, niazimicin, pterygospermin, benzyl isothiocyanate, and 4-(α-L-rhamnopyranosyloxy) benzyl glucosinolate [129]. Isolated compounds, like niazinin and niazimicin, showed blood pressure lowering effect in rats,

possibly through calcium antagonist effect. Niazimicin has been as well stated to be chemoprotective in nature [125]. The alkaloid, morigine, isolated from seed extract has the ability to relax bronchioles which is beneficial in respiratory disorders [129].

Drumstick leaves also showed decrease in blood glucose level in STZ-mild induced diabetic rats in a dose-response relationship [130]. Similarly, treatment of methanol extracts of *M. oleifera* pods in STZ-induced diabetic albino rats resulted in significant reduction in the advancement of diabetes. There was a significant reduction in serum glucose and nitric oxide as well as parallel increases in serum insulin, protein levels, and a reduction in the degenerative changes in the β cells [131]. *M. oleifera* has also been described as a promising food plant in protecting the liver against acetaminophen-induced liver injury via restoration and elevation of glutathione level in the liver [132]. Hannan et al. [133] demonstrated that ethanol extract of *M. oleifera* leaf promoted neurite outgrowth in a concentration-dependent manner and significantly promoted the earlier stages of neuronal differentiation. Therefore, this subsequently increased the number and length of dendrites, the length of axon, and the number and length of both dendrite and axonal branches and facilitated synaptogenesis. Thus, this extract shows potential application in neuronal survival. Findings from another study [134] tend to suggest that the ethanol extract of *M. oleifera* leaves possesses CNS depressant and anticonvulsant activities. This might possibly be mediated through the enhancement of central inhibitory mechanism involving release γ-amino butyric acid (GABA) and thus supports its traditional use against epilepsy. Hydroalcoholic extract of *M. oleifera* leaves also displayed the potential to improve or prevent vascular intimal damage and atherogenesis and thus help in limiting cardiovascular complications [135]. For instance, oral administration of the extract (100 and 200 mg/kg/body weight) showed significant reduction in elevated levels of body weight, total cholesterol, triglycerides, low density lipoprotein, very low density lipoprotein, and parallel significant increase in high density lipoprotein level. Intravenous administration of the hydroalcoholic extract delayed the plasma recalcification time in rabbits and also inhibited ADP induced platelet aggregation *in vitro*, which was comparable to commercial heparin. Pertaining to antimicrobial activity, the aqueous and ethanolic extracts of the leaves showed high activity against *Candida albicans* and Gram positive bacteria such *Staphylococcus aureus* and *Enterococcus faecalis* but weak activity for Gram-negative bacteria such as *Escherichia coli*, *Salmonella typhimurium*, *Klebsiella pneumoniae*, and *Pseudomonas aeruginosa* [136]. Almost similar results were obtained from another study which tested the acetone extract of *M. oleifera* [137].

2.9. Punica granatum Linn. (Punicaceae): Pomegranate. *Punica granatum*, commonly known as pomegranate, granada (Spanish), and grenade (French), is native from Iran to and Northern India. It was cultivated and naturalized over the whole Mediterranean region since ancient times [138] and has been used in several systems of medicine for a variety of ailments. In the Ayurveda system of medicine, almost all parts (fruits, flowers, seeds, leaves, and bark) have been used for remedial purposes. For instance, it has been used as an antiparasitic agent and a blood tonic, against aphthae, diarrhea, and ulcers. In addition in the Unani system, it is used for the management of diabetes. It is also reported that decoction prepared with the bark and water in a ratio of 1:5 is recommended against intestinal worms. A decoction of the bark, cinnamon (*Cinnamomum verum*), and cloves (*Syzygium aromaticum*) is taken against diarrhea [36]. *Punica granatum* was referred to as "a pharmacy unto itself" [139]. The proximate nutritional value of raw pomegranate fruit per 100 g is as follows: water (77.93 g), protein (1.67 g), carbohydrate (18.70 g), total lipid (1.17 g), fibre (4 g), calcium (10 mg), iron (0.3 mg), magnesium (12 mg), and phosphorus (36 mg) [140]. Pomegranate aril juice provides about 16% of an adult's daily vitamin C requirement per 100 mL serving and is a good source of vitamin B5 (pantothenic acid) and potassium [139].

Phytochemical isolation and characterization revealed different functional components in various parts of the plant [141]. The pomegranate leaf extract was found to contain tannins like punicalin, pedunculagin, gallagic acid, and ellagic acid. The flowers are composed of ursolic acids, triterpenoids like oleanolic acid, maslinic acid, and asiatic acid. The pomegranate seeds are a rich source of conjugated fatty acids such as linoleic acid and linolenic acid and other lipids such as punicic acid, stearic acid, palmitic acid, and phytosterols. The juice is known to be a rich source of antioxidants from the polyphenols, tannins, anthocyanins, coenzyme Q10, and lipoic acid [141]. Studies have also looked at the beneficial effects of pomegranates antioxidant activity *in vivo* and *in vitro*. Bekir et al. [142] indeed confirmed the high level of total phenolics, flavonoids, and anthocyanins in the methanol extract of *P. granatum* leaves and also demonstrated good DPPH and ABTS radical scavenging potential and strong lipoxygenase inhibition activities. It was reported that pomegranate juice and seed extracts have 2-3 times the antioxidant capacity of either red wine or green tea [143]. Aviram et al. [144] analyzed *in vivo* and *in vitro* antiatherogenic properties of pomegranate fruit parts, that is, the peel, arils, seeds, and flower. All extracts were shown to possess antioxidative properties *in vitro*. After consumption of pomegranate juice, peels, arils, and flowers by e-deficient mice, the atherosclerotic lesion area was significantly decreased, as compared to placebotreated group. The pomegranate fruit extract consumption resulted in lower serum lipids and glucose levels by 18% to 25%. The uptake rates of oxidized-LDL by e-deficient-peritoneal macrophages were significantly reduced by approximately 15%. Pomegranate juice consumption causes a decrease in procarcinogen activation through CYP activity/expression (CYP1A2 and CYP3A) [145] and protects rat gastric mucosa from ethanol or aspirin toxicity [146]. Pomegranate fruit extract was shown to inhibit cell growth through modulations in the cyclin kinase inhibitor-cyclin-dependent kinase system, followed by apoptosis of highly aggressive human-prostate carcinoma PC3 cells. These events were associated with alterations in the levels of Bax and Bcl-2 shifting the Bax: Bcl-2 ratio in favour of apoptosis [147].

Pomegranate rind extract has also been shown to have topical anti-inflammatory and analgesic properties since it dose-dependently attenuated the inflammatory responses in acute and chronic models of inflammation [148]. The anti-inflammatory and analgesic effects were achieved through inhibiting the leukocyte in filtration and modulating the proinflammatory cytokines IL-β and TNF-α [148]. The anti-inflammatory and antimicrobial properties of pomegranate were furthermore assessed through a randomized controlled clinical trial which evaluated the effectiveness of mouth rinse with pomegranate and chamomile plant extracts, against chlorhexidine 0.12% in the gingiva bleeding condition [149]. It was found that the gingival bleeding index in the groups of patients with gingivitis and chronic periodontitis, who used pomegranate extract mouthwash, was as statistically significant as those observed in groups of chamomile and chlorhexidine 0.12%. The antimicrobial activity was confirmed by the study of Abdollahzadeh et al. [150]. The latter demonstrated that methanol extract of *P. granatum* peel could inhibit growth of certain pathogens involved in oral infections like *Streptococcus mutans, Staphylococcus aureus, Streptococcus salivarius, Streptococcus sanguinis, Staphylococcus epidermidis, Actinomyces viscosus, Lactobacillus acidophilus,* and *Candida albicans*.

2.10. Solanum nigrum Linn. (Solanaceae): Black Nightshade. *Solanum nigrum* usually grows as a weed in moist land and is semicultivated in a few countries in Africa and Indonesia. It is mainly utilized as a vegetable. The leaves have an energy value of 38 Kcal, calcium (99–442 mg), phosphorus (75 mg), iron (1–4.2 mg), and ascorbic acid (20 mg) but is also high in oxalate (around 58–90 mg) [151]. It has been found that *S. nigrum* contains glycoalkaloids such as solamargine, solasonine and solanidine, saponins, and glycoprotein, exhibiting antitumor activity [152]. In South India, fresh leaves cooked with onion bulbs and cumin seeds are taken against stomach ache. Cooked leaves are also recommended in cases of hypotension, anaemia, and to improve vision. Juice of fresh leaves, mixed with honey, is applied on painful lesions which appear on the buccal mucosa [153]. The juice may also be applied on burns. One handful of the leaves is boiled in 1L of water and used to reduce fever [36]. The leaves are used as poultice for rheumatic and gouty joints. Leaves are also used in dropsy, nausea, and nervous disorders [151]. Decoction of the plant depresses the CNS and reflexes of the spinal cord. The whole plant is used as anti-inflammatory, expectorant, cardiotonic, digestive, diuretic, and laxative, for swelling cough, and asthma. The plant is also effective against, haemorrhoids, nephropathy, ophthalmopathy, and general weakness [154]. Leaf decoction is given to drink once a day on an empty stomach for 7 days to manage stomach ulcers [155]. The water extract of *S. nigrum* shows protective effects against carbon tetrachloride induced chronic liver damage in rats and this hepatoprotective effect might be contributed to its modulation on detoxification enzymes and its antioxidant and free radical scavenger effects [156].

Aqueous plant extracts possess antiproliferative activity as demonstrated by growth inhibition of cervical carcinoma. The antiproliferative activity of solanine on transformed cell lines *in vitro* is mainly due to its ability to facilitate induction of apoptosis by inhibiting Bcl-2, an antiapoptotic protein [157]. *S. nigrum* also exhibits antiulcer activity through acid and peptic suppression in aspirin induced ulcerogenesis in rats [151].

Other compounds like solasonine, β1-solasonine, solamargine, and solanigroside P were also proved to have cytotoxicity to MGC-803 cells. It was established that compounds with three sugar units and α-L-rhamnopyranose at C-2 or a hydroxyl group on the steroidal backbone may be potential candidates for the treatment of gastric cancer. The mechanism of action may be related to the decrease of mutation p53, the increase of the ratio of Bax to Bcl-2, and the activation of caspase-3 to induce apoptosis. More specifically, solamargine induced an accumulation of cells in S phase with an increasing apoptotic rate, which indicated that solamargine induced apoptosis perhaps through S phase arrest [158]. However, another study revealed that solamargine could inhibit the growth of human hepatoma SMMC-7721 and HepG2 cells by inducing cell cycle arrest at the G2/M phase [159]. The petroleum extract of *S. nigrum* berries was tested for its therapeutic potential against asthma. The extract demonstrated ability to inhibit clonidine-induced catalepsy and increased leukocyte and eosinophilic count due to milk allergen significantly. It also showed maximum protection against mast cell degranulation caused by clonidine and demonstrate presence of antiasthmatic compound, β-sitosterol [160]. Results from the study of Sohrabipour et al. [161] showed that administration of 1 g/l of *S. nigrum* fruit extract to drinking water of diabetic animals for 8 weeks can decrease blood glucose levels. However the exact mechanism whereby this is accomplished is not well understood. Intraperitoneal glucose tolerance test revealed that *S. nigrum* extract leads to improvement in glucose intolerance in condition of chronic diabetes. The outcomes tend to suggest that *S. nigrum* may repair pancreas β cells and enhance insulin secretion or increase Glu4 translocation in the cell membrane, which then decreases blood glucose levels. *S. nigrum* also decreased calcium/magnesium ratio which might indicate a reduced atherogenic risk since Ca/Mg ratio is a marker of vascular tone, in which an increase represents increased vascular reactivity [161].

3. Discussion

Medicinal foods are the oldest form of therapies known to mankind and the traditional pharmacopeia of various populations has documented such practice [9, 162]. Various countries possess rich endemic flora and a rich milieu of biodiversity that still remain an untapped reservoir for prototype molecules or pharmacophores for the pharmaceutical industry. For instance, according to Gurib-Fakim [162], about 25% of the global biodiversity in plants are found in Indian Ocean Islands and Sub-Saharan Africa and represent key constituents in the traditional medicinal systems in this region, especially in rural areas. The common use of medicinal food plants to treat and/or manage diverse health problems, ranging from acute cold and flu, stress, and pain to more severe chronic illnesses has led to the term "phytotherapy" to describe such practices. The medicinal foods are often perceived by the patient community as being safe since they have been used by communities in various countries for generations and some are still being commonly consumed today [163]. With such notion there has been a steady growth of the world market for the functional foods and phytopharmaceuticals—the pharmaceuticals designed using traditional compounds derived from botanicals instead of chemicals [164]. Indeed, the emergence of this new market segment called "Health and Wellness" has provided potential benefits to consumers' diet and new business opportunities for producers [165] such that it is now known as the fastest growing food sector with a compound annual growth rate of 8.6% in the last 10 years to 2012 and a global value of US$ 625 billion in 2012 [166]. Even though such success of the functional food market and trade has been attributed to various factors like research-oriented collaborative networks or the onset of "industrial marriage," which is the joint efforts in sharing of resources and skills for functional food product development by pharmaceutical and food manufacturers, consumer acceptance remained the decisive factor in positive market response [166]. The challenge brought forward is that consumers want to eat healthily, with low calories and nutritionally added value but without missing the enjoyment and pleasure of eating from any modified food texture and quality [167]. Consequently, it seems clear that a collaborative work between food researchers, food technologists, nutritionists, and food designers might be crucial in the design of the functional food product especially in maintaining the bioavailability and functionality of added active ingredients. Currently, efforts are still being made in understanding the physiological or behavioural interactions between medicinal foods and pharmaceuticals, their pharmacokinetics, and pharmacodynamics. This still offers a challenge to the scientific community due to the complexity of plant matrix and bioactive molecules. Little is known about the processes through which the metabolites are absorbed into the body, reach their biological target, and are eliminated [168]. The risks for food-drug or nutrient drug interactions also exist. An interaction is considered significant from a clinical perspective if it alters the therapeutic response. Food-drug interactions can result in 2 main clinical effects: the decreased bioavailability of a drug, which predisposes to treatment failure, or an increased bioavailability, which increases the risk of adverse events and may even precipitate toxicities [168].

Many of the food plants presented here show very promising medicinal properties, but attention should be drawn on other issues such as possible food-drug interactions. For instance, studies highlighted the possible interaction between pomegranate juice and warfarin [169, 170]. Pomegranate juice was shown to inhibit cytochrome P450 enzymes involved in warfarin metabolism. Concomitant use of *M. charantia* with oral hypoglycaemic medication was also analysed. *M. charantia* was demonstrated to augment the hypoglycaemic effect of rosiglitazone, a PPAR-gamma agonist in STZ induced diabetic rats [171]. The enhanced hypoglycemic effect was also observed with combination of metformin and *M. charantia* juice compared when the drug alone was administered [172]. Thus, it can be suggested that *M. charantia* might produce synergistic effect when used along with hypoglycaemic drugs which may be either beneficial or harmful to patients and should be used under careful supervision.

The possibility of biotransformation which occurs in gastrointestinal tract or through hepatic metabolism in the patient should not be ruled out or ignored. This point is critically important in assessing the therapeutic benefits of purified compounds. This is because the active ingredient may not be present in the initial medicinal food but is only produced after absorption and metabolic transformation [163]. In this framework, current developments in the area of functional food design and technology have already been made to demonstrate that the bioavailability of the bioactive components can be improved by the proper selection and development a delivery and protection system such as use of microparticles. Microencapsulation is a process by which the functional ingredient (core) is packaged within a secondary material (encapsulant) to form a microcapsule (2 to 2000 μm) [173]. The encapsulant in the form of matrix or shell forms a protective coating around the core, isolating it from its surrounding environment (pH, water activity, time, pressure, physical force, or enzymatic action) until its release is triggered by changes in its environment [173]. This avoids undesirable interactions of the bioactive with other food components or chemical reactions that can lead to degradation of the bioactive, with the possible undesirable consequences on taste and odour as well as negative health effects [174]. Çam et al. [175] have reported the effects of microencapsulation conditions on product quality of pomegranate peel phenolics and found that addition of microencapsulated pomegranate peel phenolics showed significant improvement of the antioxidant and α-glucosidase inhibitory activities of the enriched ice creams compared with control sample. Besides, more than 75% of panelists involved in the study positively rated the phenolic enriched ice creams in sensory evaluation, which lends supports to such products for commercial introduction to the general public with the potential as functional food. This technology can be a decisive step forward towards solving problems regarding the targeting of active functional ingredients to its target site and controlling its delivery rate to a specific organ or tissue [175]. However, a more recent technological extension of microencapsulation involves the formation of active loaded particles with diameters ranging from 1 to 1000 nm, a process known as nanoencapsulation. Indeed, currently the second largest area of nanotechnology application is in the food sector [176]. For instance, application of nanoencapsulation has been studied for various functional food ingredients. Despite curcumin's multiple medicinal benefits, low bioavailability of curcumin continues to be highlighted as a major challenge in developing formulations for clinical efficacy [176]. This is because it has been found that low serum and tissue levels of curcumin are observed irrespective of the route of administration due to extensive intestinal and hepatic metabolism and rapid elimination thus restraining curcumin's bioavailability [177].

Moreover, curcumin is insoluble in water and degrades at neutral to basic pH conditions and found to be photosensitive and requires careful handling. In this view, nanoparticles have been developed where unlike free curcumin was shown to readily disperse in aqueous media and demonstrated comparable *in vitro* therapeutic efficacy to free curcumin against a panel of human pancreatic cancer cell lines [176]. Nevertheless, the toxicological aspect and risk assessment for such technologies are still unclear and should not be overlooked [177]. It is possible that such nanomaterial upon degradation of the structure to release the active ingredient will form compounds with other food material, interact with one another, solubilize on reaction with acid or digestive enzyme, or remain in a free state, while in the alimentary canal and how this will affect absorption of other nutrients is unknown [177].

Likewise, despite that plant bioactive constituents have proved to offer various health benefits, their potential risks should also be considered. Typically, ethnopharmacological surveys are used to describe uses, dosages, sources, and methods of preparation of traditional medicines of food plants. Nevertheless, their application in examining the adverse effects, authenticity, quality, contraindications, and other safety aspects of these preparations remains limited and should not be overlooked. Cravotto et al. [178] reported that about 12% of the plants currently on the Western market have no substantial published scientific studies on their properties, while about 1 in 200 were toxic or allergenic, such that their use ought to be discouraged or forbidden. The quality of medicinal foods can be affected by several factors both intrinsic and extrinsic. Species differences and seasonal variations are examples of intrinsic factors that can affect the qualitative and quantitative accumulation of the biologically active chemical constituents produced and accumulated in the plant [179]. Extrinsic factors include environmental conditions, agricultural practices, postharvest handling, storage, manufacturing, inadvertent contamination, substitution, and intentional adulteration [179]. Hence, continued use of medicinal foods for disease management presents risks of potential adverse effects, especially when being used in combination with synthetic drugs. Few plants have been subjected to randomized clinical trials under the International Conference on Harmonization (ICH) Good Clinical Practice Guidelines to determine their efficacy and safety [180].

Another challenge is legislation governing the trade and marketing of the medicinal or functional foods [181]. Individual countries have their own legislation on functional foods. While in USA, functional foods are regulated by the FDA and also encompass dietary supplements; in the E.U, there is no legislation operating on functional foods and there is no legal authority for its definition [181]. In order to protect public health, it was deemed essential to guarantee that such novel foods or functional food ingredients are subjected to a safety assessment through a community procedure before they are placed on the market along with a regulation on nutrition and health claims [181]. Health-related claims should be scientifically substantiated, valid for the food as it is consumed or in its future anticipated use to reach the minimal effective dose and communicated clearly, understandably, and truthfully to the consumer [181]. It is the European Food Safety Authority (EFSA) that has the objective of providing scientific opinion on the safety of food plants and its bioactive constituents. EFSA even requires RCT (Randomized Controlled Trial) giving proof of beneficial physiological effects of a compound on a healthy population. However, one problem which arises is that RCT might be of help only when purified compounds are analyzed but subsequently become practically impossible using whole food plants, where a plethora of bioactive compounds exist, which have different physiological targets. Also, phytochemical compositions vary greatly in hydrophilic and lipophilic nature and in different plant parts. Thus, traditional knowledge still remains an important aspect that should not be neglected at the expense of emerging science and technologies. It still remains crucial for safety assessment of functional foods in the E.U. countries where there are no proper legislations because it indicates us which parts of the plants were traditionally used, how the preparation is made (infusion, decoction or alcoholic extracts), and what are the specific conditions of use [181].

4. Conclusion

Medicinal foods have long been integrated in the cultural and habitual dietary pattern of various populations. Research has demonstrated that nutrition plays a crucial role in the prevention of chronic disease and now with the recognition that typical foods may provide prophylactic benefits, efforts are being directed towards promoting the "functional diet." The new concept of functional foods has been identified as a promising field to boost nutritional sciences to the forefront of preventive medicines for both existing and emerging diseases of man. However, the exact mechanisms of actions of isolated compounds of various traditionally used plant extracts still remain to be elucidated in many cases. The use of medicinal food plants as dietary adjuncts among patients on conventional pharmacological therapy should be carefully assessed due to possibility of food-drug interactions or herb-herb interactions. Hence, combined approaches of parallel preclinical studies involving *in vitro*, *in vivo* and *in silico* models and well-designed clinical studies are crucial to provide basic toxicological data to assess its suitability in this regard. The present review also draws attention on some active metabolites of the plants with the potential for new drugs development or improved plant medicines. The elucidation of the mechanisms of action of biologically active extracts and phytocompounds should be strengthened and given priority in future clinical investigations. In this view use of medicinal foods could provide phytotherapy a new dimension and enable their use to treat and/or manage diseases which have hitherto been treated using synthetic drugs alone with limited therapeutic window.

Conflict of Interests

The authors declare that there is no conflict of interests.

References

[1] M. F. Ramadan and A. Al-Ghamdi, "Bioactive compounds and health-promoting properties of royal jelly: a review," *Journal of Functional Foods*, vol. 4, no. 1, pp. 39–52, 2012.

[2] U. Krupa, "Main nutritional and anti-nutritional compounds of bean seeds—a review," *Polish Journal of Food and Nutrition Sciences*, vol. 58, no. 2, pp. 149–155, 2008.

[3] D. Rivera, C. Obon, C. Inocencio et al., "The ethnobotanical study of local mediterranean food plants as medicinal resources in southern Spain," *Journal of Physiology and Pharmacology*, vol. 56, no. 1, pp. 97–114, 2005.

[4] L. Siró, E. Kápolna, B. Kápolna, and A. Lugasi, "Functional food. Product development, marketing and consumer acceptance—a review," *Appetite*, vol. 51, pp. 456–476, 2008.

[5] V. Prakash and M. A. J. S. Van Boekel, "Nutraceuticals: possible future ingredients and food safety aspects," in *Ensuring Global Food Safety*, Chapter 19, pp. 333–338, Elsevier, 2010.

[6] J. Bernal, J. A. Mendiola, E. Ibáñez, and A. Cifuentes, "Advanced analysis of nutraceuticals," *Journal of Pharmaceutical and Biomedical Analysis*, vol. 55, no. 4, pp. 758–774, 2011.

[7] N. A. Georgiou, J. Garssen, and R. F. Witkamp, "Pharma-nutrition interface: the gap is narrowing," *European Journal of Pharmacology*, vol. 651, no. 1–3, pp. 1–8, 2011.

[8] S. R. B. M. Eussen, H. Verhagen, O. H. Klungel et al., "Functional foods and dietary supplements: products at the interface between pharma and nutrition," *European Journal of Pharmacology*, vol. 668, no. 1, pp. S2–S9, 2011.

[9] D. S. Fabricant and N. R. Farnsworth, "The value of plants used in traditional medicine for drug discovery," *Environmental Health Perspectives*, vol. 109, no. 1, pp. 69–75, 2001.

[10] World Health Organisation (WHO), "General guidelines for methodologies on research and evaluation of traditional medicine," EDM/TRM/1, 2000.

[11] A. Gurib-Fakim, "Medicinal plants: traditions of yesterday and drugs of tomorrow," *Molecular Aspects of Medicine*, vol. 27, no. 1, pp. 1–93, 2006.

[12] A. M. Abdel-Salam, "Functional foods: hopefulness to good health," *American Journal of Food Technology*, vol. 5, no. 2, pp. 86–99, 2010.

[13] K. Srinivasan, "Spices as influencers of body metabolism: an overview of three decades of research," *Food Research International*, vol. 38, no. 1, pp. 77–86, 2005.

[14] F. R. Saunders and H. M. Wallace, "On the natural chemoprevention of cancer," *Plant Physiology and Biochemistry*, vol. 48, no. 7, pp. 621–626, 2010.

[15] N. E. Thomas-Eapen, "Turmeric: the intriguing yellow spice with medicinal properties," *Explore*, vol. 5, no. 2, pp. 114–115, 2009.

[16] G. Dinelli, I. Marotti, S. Bosi, D. Di Gioia, B. Biavati, and P. Catizone, "Physiologically bioactive compounds of functional foods, herbs, and dietary supplements," in *Advances in Food Biochemistry*, pp. 239–289, CRC Press, 2009.

[17] S. M. Brierley and O. Kelber, "Use of natural products in gastrointestinal therapies," *Current Opinion in Pharmacology*, vol. 11, no. 6, pp. 604–611, 2011.

[18] M. H. H. Roby, M. A. Sarhan, K. A. Selim, and K. I. Khalel, "Evaluation of antioxidant activity, total phenols and phenolic compounds in thyme (*Thymus vulgaris* L.), sage (*Salvia officinalis* L.), and marjoram (*Origanum majorana* L.) extracts," *Industrial Crops and Products*, vol. 43, pp. 827–831, 2013.

[19] B. Schmidt, D. M. Ribnicky, A. Poulev, S. Logendra, W. T. Cefalu, and I. Raskin, "A natural history of botanical therapeutics," *Metabolism: Clinical and Experimental*, vol. 57, no. 1, pp. S3–S9, 2008.

[20] I. M. Cockburn, "Is the pharmaceutical industry in a productivity crisis?" in *Innovation Policy and the Economy, National Bureau of Economic Research*, J. Lerner and S. Stern, Eds., pp. 1–32, MIT Press, 2007.

[21] S. M. Paul, D. S. Mytelka, C. T. Dunwiddie et al., "How to improve RD productivity: the pharmaceutical industry's grand challenge," *Nature Reviews Drug Discovery*, vol. 9, no. 3, pp. 203–214, 2010.

[22] World Health Organisation (WHO), "Noncommunicable disease-media centre," WT/500, 2013.

[23] B. K. Tiwari, H. Tynsong, and S. Rani, "Medicinal plants and human health," in *Medicinal, Food and Aromatic Plants: Ethnobotany and Conservation Status*, pp 515–523, Elsevier, 2004.

[24] K. Konaté, A. Hilou, J. F. Mavoungou et al., "Antimicrobial activity of polyphenol-rich fractions from *Sidaalba* L. (Malvaceae) against cotrimoxazol-resistant bacteria strains," *Annals of Clinical Microbiology and Antimicrobials*, vol. 11, no. 5, pp. 1–6, 2012.

[25] E. J. T. Mbosso, S. Ngouela, J. C. A. Nguedia, V. P. Beng, M. Rohmer, and E. Tsamo, "In vitro antimicrobial activity of extracts and compounds of some selected medicinal plants from Cameroon," *Journal of Ethnopharmacology*, vol. 128, no. 2, pp. 476–481, 2010.

[26] A. Gurib-Fakim, "Traditional roles and future prospects for medicinal plants in health care," *Asian Biotechnology and Development Review*, vol. 13, no. 3, pp. 77–83, 2011.

[27] B. Ncube, J. F. Finnie, and J. Van Staden, "In vitro antimicrobial synergism within plant extract combinations from three South African medicinal bulbs," *Journal of Ethnopharmacology*, vol. 139, no. 1, pp. 81–89, 2012.

[28] E. M. Williamson, "Synergy and other interactions in phytomedicines," *Phytomedicine*, vol. 8, no. 5, pp. 401–409, 2001.

[29] J. Morton, "Sugar apple," in *Fruits of Warm Climates*, Miami, Fla, USA, 1987.

[30] N. Pandey and D. Barve, "Phytochemical and pharmacological review on *Annona squamosa* Linn," *International Journal of Research in Pharmaceutical and Biomedical Sciences*, vol. 2, no. 4, pp. 1404–1412, 2011.

[31] P. S. Cheema, R. S. Dixit, T. Koshi, and S. L. Perti, "Insecticidal properties of the seed oil of *Annona squamosa* L," *Journal of Scientific and Industrial Research*, vol. 17, pp. 132–136, 1985.

[32] A. Shirwaikar, K. Rajendran, and C. D. Kumar, "In vitro antioxidant studies of *Annona squamosa* Linn. Leaves," *Indian Journal of Experimental Biology*, vol. 42, no. 8, pp. 803–807, 2004.

[33] R. K. Gupta, A. N. Kesari, S. Diwakar et al., "In vivo evaluation of anti-oxidant and anti-lipidimic potential of *Annona squamosa* aqueous extract in Type 2 diabetic models," *Journal of Ethnopharmacology*, vol. 118, no. 1, pp. 21–25, 2008.

[34] Y.-L. Yang, K.-F. Hua, P.-H. Chuang et al., "New cyclic peptides from the seeds of *Annona squamosa* L. and their anti-inflammatory activities," *Journal of Agricultural and Food Chemistry*, vol. 56, no. 2, pp. 386–392, 2008.

[35] S. Gajalakshmi, R. Divya, V. Divya Deepika, S. Mythili, and A. Sathiavelu, "Pharmacological activities of *Annona squamosa*: a review," *International Journal of Pharmaceutical Sciences Review and Research*, vol. 10, no. 2, pp. 24–29, 2011.

[36] A. Gurib-Fakim, *Toutes les plantes qui soignent, plantes d'hier, médicaments d'ujourdhui*, Michel Lafon, Neuilly-sur-Seine, Hautes-de-Seine, France, 2008.

[37] B. V. V. Pardhasaradhi, M. Reddy, A. M. Ali, A. L. Kumari, and A. Khar, "Antitumour activity of *Annona squamosa* seed extracts is through the generation of free radicals and induction of apoptosis," *Indian Journal of Biochemistry and Biophysics*, vol. 41, no. 4, pp. 167–172, 2004.

[38] Y. Chen, S. Xu, J. Chen et al., "Anti-tumor activity of *Annona squamosa* seeds extract containing annonaceous acetogenin compounds," *Journal of Ethnopharmacology*, vol. 142, pp. 462–466, 2012.

[39] C.-C. Liaw, T.-Y. Wu, F.-R. Chang, and Y.-C. Wu, "Historic perspectives on Annonaceous acetogenins from the chemical bench to preclinical trials," *Planta Medica*, vol. 76, no. 13, pp. 1390–1404, 2010.

[40] A. B. Deshmukh and J. K. Patel, "Aqueous extract of *Annona squamosa* (L.) ameliorates renal failure induced by 5/6 nephrectomy in rat," *Indian Journal of Pharmacology*, vol. 43, no. 6, pp. 718–721, 2011.

[41] R. K. Gupta, A. N. Kesari, S. Diwakar et al., "In vivo evaluation of anti-oxidant and anti-lipidimic potential of *Annona squamosa* aqueous extract in Type 2 diabetic models," *Journal of Ethnopharmacology*, vol. 118, no. 1, pp. 21–25, 2008.

[42] M. Kaleem, M. Asif, Q. U. Ahmed, and B. Bano, "Antidiabetic and antioxidant activity of *Annona squamosa* extract in streptozotocin-induced diabetic rats," *Singapore Medical Journal*, vol. 47, no. 8, pp. 670–675, 2006.

[43] A. Sharma, T. Chand, M. Khardiya, K. Chand Yadav, R. Mangal, and A. K. Sharma, "Antidiabetic and antihyperlipidemic activity of *Annona squamosa* fruit peel in streptozotocin induced diabetic rats," *International Journal of Toxicological and Pharmacological Research*, vol. 5, no. 1, pp. 15–21, 2013.

[44] T. Ponrasu, M. K. Subamekala, M. Ganeshkumar, and L. Suguna, "Role of *Annona squamosal* on antioxidants during wound healing in streptozotocin nicotinamide induced diabetic rats," *Journal of Pharmacology and Phytochemistry*, vol. 2, no. 4, pp. 77–84, 2013.

[45] J. Aamir, A. Kumari, M. N. Khan, and S. K. Medam, "Evaluation of the combinational antimicrobial effect of *Annona Squamosa* and *Phoerix Dactylifera* seeds methanolic extract on standard microbial strains," *International Research Journal of Biological Sciences*, vol. 2, no. 5, pp. 68–73, 2013.

[46] D. Ragone, *Artocarpus Atilis-Species Profiles for Pacific Island Agroforestry*, 2006.

[47] N. Badrie and J. Broomes, "Beneficial uses of breadfruit (*Artocarpusaltilis*): nutritional, medicinal and other uses," in *c. actions of individual fruits in disease and cancer prevention and treatment-Bioactive Foods in Promoting Health: Fruits and Vegetables*, Elsevier, 2010.

[48] K. D. Golden and O. J. Williams, "The amino acid, fatty acid and carbohydrate content of *Artocarpus altilis* (breadfruit); the white heart cultivar from the west indies," *Acta Horticulturae*, vol. 757, pp. 201–208, 2007.

[49] W. C. Lan, C. W. Tzeng, C. C Lin, F. L. Yen, and H. H. Ko, "Prenylated flavonoids from *Artocarpus altilis*: antioxidant activities and inhibitory effects on melanin production," *Phytochemistry*, vol. 89, pp. 78–88, 2013.

[50] U. B. Jagtap and V. A. Bapat, "Artocarpus: a review of its traditional uses, phytochemistry and pharmacology," *Journal of Ethnopharmacology*, vol. 129, no. 2, pp. 142–166, 2010.

[51] C. P. Selitrennikoff, "Antifungal proteins," *Applied and Environmental Microbiology*, vol. 67, no. 7, pp. 2883–2894, 2001.

[52] T. B. Ng, "Antifungal proteins and peptides of leguminous and non-leguminous origins," *Peptides*, vol. 25, no. 7, pp. 1215–1222, 2004.

[53] M. B. Trindade, J. L. S. Lopes, A. Soares-Costa et al., "Structural characterization of novel chitin-binding lectins from the genus Artocarpus and their antifungal activity," *Biochimica et Biophysica Acta*, vol. 1764, no. 1, pp. 146–152, 2006.

[54] C. Pradhan, M. Mohanty, A. Rout, A. B. Das, K. B. Satyapathy, and H. K. Patra, "Phytoconstituent screening and comparative assessment of antimicrobial potentiality of *Artocarpus altilis* fruit extract," *International Journal of Pharmacy and Pharmaceutical Sciences*, vol. 5, no. 3, 2013.

[55] T. K. Lim, *Edible Medicinal and Non Medicinal Plants*, vol. 3 of *Fruits*, Springer, London, UK, 2012.

[56] C. R. Nwokocha, D. U. Owu, M. McLaren et al., "Possible mechanisms of action of the aqueous extract of *Artocarpus altilis* (breadfruit) leaves in producing hypotension in normotensive Sprague-Dawley rats," *Pharmaceutical Biology*, vol. 50, no. 9, pp. 1096–1102, 2012.

[57] A. Elosta, T. Ghous, and N. Ahmed, "Natural products as Antiglycation agents: possible therapeutic potential for diabetic complications," *Current Diabetes Reviews*, vol. 8, no. 2, pp. 92–108, 2012.

[58] J.-A. Lin, C.-H. Wu, S.-C. Fang, and G.-C. Yen, "Combining the observation of cell morphology with the evaluation of key inflammatory mediators to assess the anti-inflammatory effects of geranyl flavonoid derivatives in breadfruit," *Food Chemistry*, vol. 132, no. 4, pp. 2118–2125, 2012.

[59] M. Azizur Rahman, N. Nahar, A. Jabbar Mian, and M. Mosihuzzaman, "Variation of carbohydrate composition of two forms of fruit from jack tree (*Artocarpus heterophyllus* L.) with maturity and climatic conditions," *Food Chemistry*, vol. 65, no. 1, pp. 91–97, 1999.

[60] M. S. Baliga, A. R. Shivashankara, R. Haniadka, J. Dsouza, and H. P. Bhat, "Phytochemistry, nutritional and pharmacological properties of *Artocarpus heterophyllus* Lam (jackfruit): a review," *Food Research International*, vol. 44, pp. 1800–1811, 2011.

[61] K. Gupta and N. Tandon, *Review on Indian Medicinal Plants*, Indian Council of Medical Research, New Delhi, India, 1996.

[62] A. Saxena, A. S. Bawa, and P. S. Raju, "Phytochemical changes in fresh-cut jackfruit (*Artocarpus heterophyllus* L.) bulbs during modified atmosphere storage," *Food Chemistry*, vol. 115, no. 4, pp. 1443–1449, 2009.

[63] S. Chackrewarthy, M. Thabrew, M. K. B. Weerasuriya, and S. Jayasekera, "Evaluation of the hypoglycemic and hypolipidemic effects of an ethylacetate fraction of *Artocarpus heterophyllus* (jak) leaves in streptozotocin-induced diabetic rats," *Pharmacognosy Magazine*, vol. 6, no. 23, pp. 186–190, 2010.

[64] X. Di, S. Wang, B. Wang et al., "New phenolic compounds from the twigs of *Artocarpus heterophyllus*," *Drug Discoveries and Therapeutics*, vol. 7, no. 1, pp. 24–28, 2013.

[65] G. Pereira-Da-Silva, A. N. Moreno, F. Marques et al., "Neutrophil activation induced by the lectin KM+ involves binding to CXCR2," *Biochimica et Biophysica Acta*, vol. 1760, no. 1, pp. 86–94, 2006.

[66] R. M. Patel and S. K. Patel, "Cytotoxic activity of methanolic extract of *Artocarpus heterophyllus* against A549, Hela and MCF-7 cell lines," *Journal of Applied Pharmaceutical Science*, vol. 1, no. 7, pp. 167–171, 2011.

[67] M. I. Kotowaroo, M. F. Mahomoodally, A. Gurib-Fakim, and A. H. Subratty, "Screening of traditional antidiabetic medicinal plants of Mauritius for possible α-amylase inhibitory effects *in vitro*," *Phytotherapy Research*, vol. 20, no. 3, pp. 228–231, 2006.

[68] A. S. Deve, T. S. Kumar, K. Kumaresan, and V. S. Rapheal, "Extraction process optimization of polyphenols from Indian *Citrus sinensis* -as novel antiglycative agents in the management of diabetes mellitus," *Journal of Diabetes and Metabolic Disorders*, vol. 13, no. 11, pp. 2–10, 2014.

[69] S. S. Nair, V. Kavrekar, and A. Mishra, "*In vitro* studies on alpha amylase and alpha glucosidase inhibitory activities of selected plant extracts," *European Journal of Experimental Biology*, vol. 3, no. 1, pp. 128–131, 2013.

[70] M. R. Khan, A. D. Omoloso, and M. Kihara, "Antibacterial activity of *Artocarpus heterophyllus*," *Fitoterapia*, vol. 74, no. 5, pp. 501–505, 2003.

[71] M. S. Baliga, H. P. Bhat, B. R. V. Baliga, R. Wilson, and P. L. Palatty, "Phytochemistry, traditional uses and pharmacology of *Eugenia jambolana* Lam. (black plum): a review," *Food Research International*, vol. 44, no. 7, pp. 1776–1789, 2011.

[72] B. S. Shrikant, S. J. T. Nayan, M. P. Meghatai, and M. H. Parag, "Jamun (*Syzygium cumini* L.): a review of its food and medicinal uses," *Food and Nutrition Sciences*, vol. 3, pp. 1100–1117, 2012.

[73] M. Ayyanar, *Ethnobotanical wealth of Kani tribe in Tirunelveli hills [Ph.D. thesis]*, University of Madras, Chennai, India, 2008.

[74] M. J. Bhandary, K. R. Chandrashekar, and K. M. Kaveriappa, "Medical ethnobotany of the Siddis of Uttara Kannada district, Karnataka, India," *Journal of Ethnopharmacology*, vol. 47, no. 3, pp. 149–158, 1995.

[75] H. K. Sharma, L. Chhangte, and A. K. Dolui, "Traditional medicinal plants in Mizoram, India," *Fitoterapia*, vol. 72, no. 2, pp. 146–161, 2001.

[76] L. J. Reddy and B. Jose, "Evaluation of antibacterial and DPPH radical scavenging activities of the leaf extracts and leaf essential oil of *Syzygium cumini* Linn. from South India," *International Journal of Pharmacy and Pharmaceutical Sciences*, vol. 5, no. 3, pp. 1–5, 2013.

[77] S. Satish, M. P. Raghavendra, and K. A. Raveesha, "Evaluation of the antibacterial potential of some plants against human pathogenic bacteria," *Advances in Biological Research*, vol. 2, pp. 44–48, 2008.

[78] P. B. Shamkumar, D. P. Pawar, and S. S. Chauhan, "Antidiarrhoeal activity of seeds of *Syzygium cumini* L.," *Journal of Pharmacy Research*, vol. 5, no. 12, pp. 5537–5539, 2012.

[79] P. S. Benherlal and C. Arumughan, "Chemical composition and in vitro antioxidant studies on *Syzygium cumini* fruit," *Journal of the Science of Food and Agriculture*, vol. 87, no. 14, pp. 2560–2569, 2007.

[80] J. M. Veigas, M. S. Narayan, P. M. Laxman, and B. Neelwarne, "Chemical nature, stability and bioefficacies of anthocyanins from fruit peel of *Syzygium cumini* Skeels," *Food Chemistry*, vol. 105, no. 2, pp. 619–627, 2007.

[81] M. Ayyanar, P. Subash-Babu, and S. Ignacimuthu, "*Syzygium cumini* (L.) skeels., a novel therapeutic agent for diabetes: folk medicinal and pharmacological evidences," *Complementary Therapies in Medicine*, vol. 21, pp. 232–243, 2013.

[82] E. David, S. V. Therasa, J. Hemachandran, E. K. Elumalai, and T. Thirumalai, "*Eugenia jambolana* seed extract inhibit uptake of glucose across rat everted gut sacs *in vitro*," *International Journal of Pharmaceutical and Research Development*, vol. 2, no. 9, pp. 107–112, 2010.

[83] T. S. Fiúza, S. M. T. Sabóia-Morais, J. R. De Paula, L. M. F. Tresvenzol, and F. C. Pimenta, "Evaluation of antimicrobial activity of the crude ethanol extract of Eugenia uniflora L. leaves," Revista de Ciencias Farmaceuticas Basica e Aplicada, vol. 29, no. 3, pp. 245–250, 2008.

[84] J. Morton, "Surinam Cherry," in Fruits of Warm Climates, Miami, Fla, USA, 1987.

[85] A. G. V. Costa, D. F. Garçia-Diaz, P. Jimenez, and P. I. Silva, "Bioactive compounds and health benefits of exotic tropical red-black berries," Journal of Functional Foods, vol. 5, pp. 539–549, 2013.

[86] S. G. D. Oliveira, F. R. R. De Moura, F. F. Demarco, P. D. S. Nascente, F. A. B. D. Pino, and R. G. Lund, "An ethnomedicinal survey on phytotherapy with professionals and patients from Basic Care Units in the Brazilian Unified Health System," Journal of Ethnopharmacology, vol. 140, no. 2, pp. 428–437, 2012.

[87] M. O. Fadeyi and U. E. Akpan, "Antibacterial activities of the leaf extracts of Eugenia uniflora Linn. (Synonym stenocalyx michelli Linn.) Myrtaceae," Phytotherapy Research, vol. 3, no. 4, pp. 154–155, 1989.

[88] N. F. Victoria, J. E. Lenardão, L. Savegnago et al., "Essential oil of the leaves of Eugenia uniflora L.: antioxidant and antimicrobial properties," Food and Chemical Toxicology, vol. 50, pp. 2668–2674, 2012.

[89] E. Ferro, A. Schinini, M. Maldonado, J. Rosner, and G. S. Hirschmann, "Eugenia uniflora leaf extract and lipid metabolism in Cebus apella monkeys," Journal of Ethnopharmacology, vol. 24, no. 2-3, pp. 321–325, 1988.

[90] K. K. A. Santos, E. F. F. Matias, S. R. Tintino et al., "Anti-Trypanosoma cruzi and cytotoxic activities of Eugenia uniflora L.," Experimental Parasitology, vol. 131, no. 1, pp. 130–132, 2012.

[91] I. Arai, S. Amagaya, Y. Komatsu et al., "Improving effects of the extracts from Eugenia uniflora on hyperglycemia and hypertriglyceridemia in mice," Journal of Ethnopharmacology, vol. 68, no. 1-3, pp. 307–314, 1999.

[92] F. N. Victoria, R. G. Anversa, L. Savegnago, and E. J. Lenardaõ, "Essential oils of E. uniflora leaves protective rinjury induced by acetaminophen," Food Bioscience, vol. 4, pp. 50–57, 2013.

[93] P. Saha, U. K. Mazumder, P. K. Haldar, S. K. Sen, and S. Naskar, "Antihyperglycemic activity of Lagenaria siceraria aerial parts on streptozotocin induced diabetes in rats," Diabetologia Croatica, vol. 40, no. 2, pp. 49–60, 2011.

[94] Agricultural Research Service, USDA Nutrient Database For Standard Reference, Release 14. Nutrient Data Laboratory Home, 2009.

[95] M. Modgil, R. Modgil, and R. Kumar, "Carbohydrate and mineral content of chyote (Sechiumedule) and bottle gourd (Lagenaria siceraria)," Journal of Human Ecology, vol. 15, pp. 157–159, 2004.

[96] P. Nainwal, K. Dhamija, and S. Tripathi, "Study of antihyperlipidemic effect on the juice of the fresh fruits of Lagenaria siceraria," International Journal of Pharmacy and Pharmaceutical Sciences, vol. 3, no. 1, pp. 88–90, 2011.

[97] B. N. Shah, A. K. Seth, and R. V. Desai, "Phytophannacological profile of Ligenaria sicararia: a review," Asian Journal of Plant Sciences, vol. 9, no. 3, pp. 152–157, 2010.

[98] A. Mootoosamy and M. F. Mahomoodally, "Ethnomedicinal application of native remedies used against diabetes and related complications in Mauritius," Journal of Ethnopharmacology, vol. 10, pp. 413–444, 2014.

[99] B. V. Ghule, M. H. Ghante, A. N. Saoji, and P. G. Yeole, "Antihyperlipidemic effect of the methanolic extract from Lagenaria siceraria Stand. fruit in hyperlipidemic rats," Journal of Ethnopharmacology, vol. 124, no. 2, pp. 333–337, 2009.

[100] I. Ahmad, M. Irshad, and M. M. A. Rizvi, "Nutritional and medicinal potential of Lagenaria siceraria," International Journal of Vegetable Science, vol. 17, no. 2, pp. 157–170, 2011.

[101] M. Shokrzadeh, A. Parvaresh, S. Shahani, E. Habibi, and Z. Zalzar, "Cytotoxic effects of Lagenaria siceraria standl. extract on cancer cell line," Mazadaran University of Medical Sciences, vol. 23, no. 97, pp. 225–230, 2013.

[102] J. R. Deshpande, A. A. Choudhari, M. R. Mishra, V. S. Meghre, S. G. Wadodkar, and A. K. Dorle, "Beneficial effects of Lagenaria siceraria (Mol.) Standley fruit epicarp in animal models," Indian Journal of Experimental Biology, vol. 46, no. 4, pp. 234–242, 2008.

[103] C. Katare, S. Saxena, S. Agrawal, and G. B. K. S. Prasad, "Alleviation of diabetes induced dyslipidemia by Lagenaria siceraria fruit extract in human type 2 diabetes," Journal of Herbal Medicine, vol. 3, pp. 1–8, 2013.

[104] S. Nadeem, P. Dhore, M. Quazi, S. Pawar, and N. Raj, "Lagenaria siceraria fruit extract ameliorate fat amassment and serum TNF-in high-fat diet-induced obese rats," Asian Pacific Journal of Tropical Medicine, vol. 5, no. 9, pp. 698–702, 2012.

[105] A. H. Subratty, A. Gurib-Fakim, and F. Mahomoodally, "Bitter melon: an exotic vegetable with medicinal values," Nutrition and Food Science, vol. 35, no. 3, pp. 143–147, 2005.

[106] R. Jeyadevi, A. T. Sivasudha, A. Rameshkumar, B. Sangeetha, D. A. Ananth, and G. S. B. Aseervatham, "Nutritional constituents and medicinal values of Momordica cymbalaria (Athalakkai)—a review," Asian Pacific Journal of Tropical Biomedicine, pp. S456–S461, 2012.

[107] K. E. Yuwai, K. S. Rao, C. Kaluwin, G. P. Jones, and D. E. Rivett, "Chemical composition of Mcmordiea charantia L. Fruits," Journal of Agricultural and Food Chemistry, vol. 39, no. 10, pp. 1762–1763, 1991.

[108] M. Ullah, F. K. Chy, S. K. Sarkar, M. K. Islam, and N. Absar, "Nutrient and phytochemical analysis of four varieties of bitter gourd (Momordica charantia) grown in chittagong hill tracts, Bangladesh," Asian Journal of Agricultural Research, vol. 5, no. 3, pp. 186–193, 2011.

[109] A. J. Thenmozhi and P. Subramanian, "Antioxidant potential of Momordica charantia in ammonium chloride-induced hyperammonemic rats," Evidence-Based Complementary and Alternative Medicine, vol. 2011, Article ID 612023, 7 pages, 2011.

[110] K. P. S. Kumar and D. Bhowmik, "Traditional medicinal uses and therapeutic benefits of Momordica charantia Linn," International Journal of Pharmaceutical Sciences Review and Research, vol. 4, no. 3, pp. 23–28, 2010.

[111] J. K. Grover and S. P. Yadav, "Pharmacological actions and potential uses of Momordica charantia: a review," Journal of Ethnopharmacology, vol. 93, no. 1, pp. 123–132, 2004.

[112] J. T. Efird, Y. M. Choi, S. W. Davies, S. Mehra, E. J. Anderson, and L. A. Katunga, "Potential for improved glycemic control with dietary Momordica charantia in patients with insulin resistance and pre-diabetes," International Journal of Environmental Research and Public Health, vol. 11, pp. 2328–2345, 2014.

[113] B. Joseph and D. Jini, "Antidiabetic effects of Momordica charantia (bitter melon) and its medicinal potency," Asian Pacific Journal of Tropical Disease, vol. 3, no. 2, pp. 93–102, 2013.

[114] E. A. Lucas, G. G. Dumancas, B. J. Smith, S. L. Clarke, and B. H. Arjmandi, "Health benefits of bitter melon (Momordica

charantia)," in *Bioactive Foods in Promoting Health: Fruits and Vegetables*, Elsevier, 2010.

[115] J. A. O. Ojewole, S. O. Adewole, and G. Olayiwola, "Hypoglycaemic and hypotensive effects of *Momordica charantia* Linn (Cucurbitaceae) whole-plant aqueous extract in rats," *Cardiovascular Journal of South Africa*, vol. 17, no. 5, pp. 227–232, 2006.

[116] N. G. Sahib, A. A. Hamid, D. Kitts, M. Purnama, N. Saari, and F. Abas, "The effects of *Morinda citrifolia, Momordica charantia* and *Centella asiatica* extracts on lipoprotein lipase and 3T3-L1 preadipocytes," *Journal of Food Biochemistry*, vol. 35, no. 4, pp. 1186–1205, 2011.

[117] R. C. Agrawal and T. Beohar, "Chemopreventive and anticarcinogenic effects of *Momordica charantia* extract," *Asian Pacific Journal of Cancer Prevention*, vol. 11, no. 2, pp. 371–375, 2010.

[118] N. Nithya, K. Chandrakumar, V. Ganesan, and S. Senthilkumar, "Efficacy of *Momordica charantia* in attenuating hepatic abnormalities in cyclophosphamide intoxicated rats," *Journal of Pharmacology and Toxicology*, vol. 7, no. 1, pp. 38–45, 2012.

[119] A. J. Thenmozhi and P. Subramanian, "*Momordica charantia* (bitter melon)decreases serum/tissue lipid parameters in hyperammonemic rats," *International Journal of Nutrition, Pharmacology, Neurological Diseases*, vol. 3, no. 3, pp. 249–253, 2013.

[120] S. Palamthodi and S. S. Lele, "Nutraceutical applications of gourd family vegetables: *Benincasa hispida, Lagenaria siceraria* and *Momordica charantia*," *Biomedicine and Preventive Nutrition*, vol. 4, pp. 15–21, 2014.

[121] L. N. Oragwa, O. O. Efiom, and S. K. Okwute, "Phytochemicals, anti-microbial and free radical scavenging activities of *Momordica charantia* Linn (Palisota Reichb) seeds," *African Journal of Pure and Applied Chemistry*, vol. 7, no. 12, pp. 405–409, 2013.

[122] S. M. Divi, R. Bellamkonda, and S. K. Dasireddy, "Evaluation of antidiabetic and antihyperlipedemic potential of aqueous extract of *Moringa oleifera* in fructose fed insulin resistant and STZ induced diabetic wistar rats: a comparative study," *Asian Journal of Pharmaceutical and Clinical Research*, vol. 5, no. 1, pp. 67–72, 2012.

[123] F. Anwar and M. I. Bhanger, "Analytical characterization of *Moringa oleifera* seed oils grown in temperate regions of Pakistan," *Journal of Agricultural and Food Chemistry*, vol. 51, no. 22, pp. 6558–6563, 2003.

[124] J. W. Fahey, "*Moringa oleifera*: a review of the medical evidence for its nutritional," *Therapeutic, and Prophylactic Properties. Part 1, Trees For Life Journal*, vol. 1, no. 5, pp. 1–15, 2005.

[125] F. Anwar, S. Latif, M. Ashraf, and A. H. Gilani, "*Moringa oleifera*: a food plant with multiple medicinal uses," *Phytotherapy Research*, vol. 21, no. 1, pp. 17–25, 2007.

[126] P. Siddhuraju and K. Becker, "Antioxidant properties of various solvent extracts of total phenolic constituents from three different agroclimatic origins of drumstick tree (*Moringa oleifera* Lam.) leaves," *Journal of Agricultural and Food Chemistry*, vol. 51, no. 8, pp. 2144–2155, 2003.

[127] V. Melo, N. Vargas, T. Quirino, and C. M. C. Calvo, "*Moringa oleifera* L.—an underutilized tree with macronutrients for human health," *Emirates Journal of Food and Agriculture*, vol. 25, no. 10, pp. 785–793, 2013.

[128] B. Moyo, P. J. Masika, A. Hugo, and V. Muchenje, "Nutritional characterization of Moringa (*Moringa oleifera* Lam.) leaves," *African Journal of Biotechnology*, vol. 10, no. 60, pp. 12925–12933, 2011.

[129] S. J. S. Flora and V. Pachauri, "Moringa (*Moringa oleifera*) seed extract and the prevention of oxidative stress," in *Nuts & Seeds in Health and Disease Prevention*, pp. 775–785, Elsevier, 2011.

[130] D. Jaiswal, P. Kumar Rai, A. Kumar, S. Mehta, and G. Watal, "Effect of *Moringa oleifera* Lam. leaves aqueous extract therapy on hyperglycemic rats," *Journal of Ethnopharmacology*, vol. 123, no. 3, pp. 392–396, 2009.

[131] R. Gupta, M. Mathur, V. K. Bajaj et al., "Evaluation of antidiabetic and antioxidant activity of *Moringa oleifera* in experimental diabetes," *Journal of Diabetes*, vol. 4, pp. 164–171, 2012.

[132] S. Fakurazi, U. Nanthini, and I. Hairuszah, "Hepatoprotective and antioxidant action of *Moringa oleifera* lam. againsts acetaminophen induced hepatoxicity in rats," *International Journal of Pharmacology*, vol. 4, no. 4, pp. 270–275, 2008.

[133] A. Hannan, J. Kang, M. Mohibbullah et al., "*Moringa oleifera* with promising neuronal survival and neurite outgrowth promoting potentials," *Journal of Ethnopharmacology*, vol. 152, pp. 142–150, 2013.

[134] A. G. Bakre, A. O. Aderibigbe, and O. G. Ademowo, "Studies on neuropharmacological profile of ethanol extract of *Moringa oleifera* leaves in mice," *Journal of Ethnopharmacology*, vol. 149, no. 3, pp. 783–789, 2013.

[135] M. G. Rajanandh, M. N. Satishkumar, K. Elango, and S. Suresh B, "*Moringa oleifera* Lam. A herbal medicine for hyperlipidemia: a preclinical report," *Asian Pacific Journal of Tropical Disease*, pp. 790–795, 2012.

[136] T. J. Marrufo, "Chemical characterization and determination of antioxidant and antimicrobial activities of the leaves of *Moringa oleifera*," *International Network Environmental Management Conflicts*, vol. 2, no. 1, pp. 1–15, 2013.

[137] B. Moyo, P. J. Masika, and V. Muchenje, "Antimicrobial activities of *Moringa oleifera* Lam leaf extracts," *African Journal of Biotechnology*, vol. 11, no. 11, pp. 2797–2802, 2012.

[138] A. Roy, R. V. Geetha, T. Lakshmi, and M. Nallanayagam, "Edible fruits—nature's gift for diabetic patients a comprehensive review," *International Journal of Pharmaceutical Sciences Review and Research*, vol. 9, no. 2, pp. 170–180, 2011.

[139] P. R. Bhandari, "Pomegranate (*Punica granatum* L). Ancient seeds for modern cure? Review of potential therapeutic applications," *International Journal of Nutrition, Pharmacology, Neurological Diseases*, vol. 2, no. 3, pp. 171–184, 2012.

[140] United States Department of Agriculture (USDA), Plants Profile: *Punica granatum* L, 2012, http://plants.usda.gov/java/profile?symbol=PUGR2.

[141] M. N. Al-Muammar and F. Khan, "Obesity: the preventive role of the pomegranate (*Punica granatum*)," *Nutrition*, vol. 28, no. 6, pp. 595–604, 2012.

[142] J. Bekir, M. Mars, J. P. Souchard, and J. Bouajila, "Assessment of antioxidant, anti-inflammatory, anti-cholinesterase and cytotoxic activities of pomegranate (*Punica granatum*) leaves," *Food and Chemical Toxicology*, vol. 55, pp. 470–475, 2013.

[143] J. Jurenka, "Therapeutic applications of pomegranate (*Punica granatum* L.): a review," *Alternative Medicine Review*, vol. 13, no. 2, pp. 128–144, 2008.

[144] M. Aviram, N. Volkova, R. Coleman et al., "Pomegranate phenolics from the peels, arils, and flowers are antiatherogenic: studies *in vivo* in atherosclerotic apolipoprotein E-deficient (E0) mice and *in vitro* in cultured macrophages and lipoproteins," *Journal of Agricultural and Food Chemistry*, vol. 56, no. 3, pp. 1148–1157, 2008.

[145] A. Faria, R. Monteiro, I. Azevedo, and C. Calhau, "Pomegranate juice effects on cytochrome p450s expression: *In vivo* studies," *Journal of Medicinal Food*, vol. 10, no. 4, pp. 643–649, 2007.

[146] K. B. Ajaikumar, M. Asheef, B. H. Babu, and J. Padikkala, "The inhibition of gastric mucosal injury by *Punica granatum* L. (pomegranate) methanolic extract," *Journal of Ethnopharmacology*, vol. 96, no. 1-2, pp. 171–176, 2005.

[147] A. Malik and H. Mukhtar, "Prostate cancer prevention through pomegranate fruit," *Cell Cycle*, vol. 5, no. 4, pp. 371–373, 2006.

[148] J. Mo, P. Panichayupakaranant, N. Kaewnopparat, A. Nitiruangjaras, and W. Reanmongkol, "Topical anti-inflammatory and analgesic activities of standardized pomegranate rind extract in comparison with its marker compound ellagic acid *in vivo*," *Journal of Ethnopharmacology*, vol. 148, pp. 901–908, 2013.

[149] A. L. A. Batista, R. D. A. U. Lins, R. S. Coelho, D. N. Barbosa, N. M. Belém, and F. J. A. Celestino, "Clinical efficacy analysis of the mouth rinsing with pomegranate and chamomile plant extracts in the gingival bleeding reduction," *Complementary Therapies in Clinical Practice*, vol. 20, pp. 93–98, 2013.

[150] S. Abdollahzadeh, R. Y. Mashouf, H. Mortazavi, M. H. Moghaddam, N. Roozbahani, and M. Vahedi, "Antibacterial and antifungal activities of *Punica granatum* peel extracts against oral pathogens," *Journal of Dentistry*, vol. 8, no. 1, pp. 1–6, 2011.

[151] T. S. Mohamed Saleem, C. Madhusudhana Chetty, S. Ramkanth et al., "*Solanum nigrum* Linn.—a review," *Pharmacognosy Reviews*, vol. 3, no. 6, pp. 342–345, 2009.

[152] J. M. Edmonds and J. A. Chweya, *Black Nightshades: Solanum Nigrum L. and Related Species*, International Plant Genetic Resources Institute, Rome, Italy, 1997.

[153] R. Jain, A. Sharma, S. Gupta, I. P. Sarethy, and R. Gabrani, "*Solanum nigrum*: current perspectives on therapeutic properties," *Alternative Medicine Review*, vol. 16, no. 1, pp. 78–85, 2011.

[154] K. R. Kirtikar and B. D. Basu, *Indian Medicinal Plants*, vol. III, Lalit Mohan Basu, Allahabad, India, 2nd edition, 1935.

[155] S. Shanmugam, K. Rajendran, and K. Suresh, "Traditional uses of medicinal plants among the rural people of Sivagangai district of Tamil Nadu, Southern India," *Asian Pacific Journal of Tropical Biomedicine*, vol. 2, no. 1, pp. 429–434, 2012.

[156] H. L. Chou, H. C. Tseng, J. L. Wang, and C. Loa, "Hepatoprotective effects of *Solanum nigrum* L nn extract against CCl4 induced oxidative damage in rats," *Chemico-Biological Interactions*, vol. 171, pp. 283–293, 2008.

[157] H.-Y. Joo, K. Lim, and K.-T. Lim, "Phytoglycoprotein (150 kDa) isolated from *Solanum nigrum* Linne has a preventive effect on dextran sodium sulfate-induced colitis in A/J mouse," *Journal of Applied Toxicology*, vol. 29, no. 3, pp. 207–213, 2009.

[158] X. Ding, F. Zhu, Y. Yang, and M. Li, "Purification, antitumor activity in vitro of steroidal glycoalkaloids from black nightshade (*Solanum nigrum* L.)," *Food Chemistry*, vol. 141, pp. 1181–1186, 2013.

[159] Ding, F. S. Zhu, G. Y. Li, and S. G. Gao, "Purification, antitumour and induction of apoptosis in human hepatoma SMMC-7721 cells by solamargine from *Solanum nigrum* L.," *Food Chemistry*, vol. 139, pp. 599–604, 2012.

[160] S. A. Nirmal, A. P. Patel, S. B. Bhawar, and S. R. Pattan, "Antihistaminic and antiallergic actions of extracts of *Solanum nigrum* berries: possible role in the treatment of asthma," *Journal of Ethnopharmacology*, vol. 142, pp. 91–97, 2012.

[161] S. Sohrabipour, F. Kharazmi, N. Soltani, and M. Kamalinejad, "Effect of the administration of *Solanum nigrum* fruit on blood glucose, lipid profiles, and sensitivity of the vascular mesenteric bed to phenylephrine in streptozotocin-induced diabetic rats," *Medical Science Monitor Basic Research*, vol. 19, pp. 133–140, 2013.

[162] A. Gurib-Fakim, "Small island developing states of the Indian Ocean: towards an action plan for medicinal plants," *Asian Biotechnology and Development Review*, vol. 13, no. 3, pp. 1–5, 2011.

[163] T. N. C. Wells, "Natural products as starting points for future anti-malarial therapies: going back to our roots?" *Malaria Journal*, vol. 10, no. 1, article S3, 2011.

[164] V. Devi, N. Jain, and K. Valli, "Importance of novel drug delivery systems in herbal medicines," *Pharmacognosy Reviews*, vol. 4, no. 7, pp. 27–31, 2010.

[165] A. Annunziata and R. Vecchio, "Consumer perception of functional foods: a conjoint analysis with probiotics," *Food Quality and Preference*, vol. 28, pp. 348–355, 2013.

[166] R. S. Khan, J. Grigor, R. Winger, and A. Win, "Functional food product development—opportunities and challenges for food manufacturers," *Trends in Food Science and Technology*, vol. 30, pp. 27–37, 2013.

[167] B. Wansink, "Helping consumers eat less," *Food Technology*, vol. 61, no. 5, pp. 34–38, 2007.

[168] L. Rodríguez-Fragoso, J. L. Martínez-Arismendi, D. Orozco-Bustos, J. Reyes-Esparza, E. Torres, and S. W. Burchiel, "Potential risks resulting from fruit/vegetable-drug interactions: effects on drug-metabolizing enzymes and drug transporters," *Journal of Food Science*, vol. 76, no. 4, pp. R112–R124, 2011.

[169] K. E. Komperda, "Potential interaction between pomegranate juice and warfarin," *Pharmacotherapy*, vol. 29, no. 8, pp. 1002–1006, 2009.

[170] S. Jarvis, C. Li, and R. G. Bogle, "Possible interaction between pomegranate juice and warfarin," *Emergency Medicine Journal*, vol. 27, no. 1, pp. 74–75, 2010.

[171] S. N. Nivitabishekam, M. Asad, and V. S. Prasad, "Pharmacodynamic interaction of *Momordica charantia* with rosiglitazone in rats," *Chemico-Biological Interactions*, vol. 177, no. 3, pp. 247–253, 2009.

[172] T. Poonam, G. P. Prakash, and L. V. Kumar, "Interaction of *Momordica charantia* with metformin in diabetic rats," *American Journal of Pharmacology and Toxicology*, vol. 8, pp. 102–106, 2013.

[173] J. Smith and E. Charter, *Functional Food Product Development*, Blackwell Publishing, Oxford, UK, 2010.

[174] L. Sanguansri and M. A. Augustin, "Microencapsulation in functional food product development," in *Functional Food Product Development*, J. Smith and E. Charter, Eds., Chapter 1, Blackwell Publishing, Oxford, UK, 2010.

[175] M. Çam, N. C. İçyer, and F. Erdoğan, "Pomegranate peel phenolics: microencapsulation, storage stability and potential ingredient for functional food development," *LWT—Food Science and Technology*, vol. 55, pp. 117–123, 2014.

[176] I. Muqbil, A. Masood, F. H. Sarkar, R. M. Mohammad, and A. S. Azmi, "Progress in nanotechnology based approaches to enhance the potential of chemopreventive agents," *Cancers*, vol. 3, no. 1, pp. 428–445, 2011.

[177] International Symposium: Nanotechnology in the food chain—Opportunities and risks, 2010.

[178] G. Cravotto, L. Boffa, L. Genzini, and D. Garella, "Phytotherapeutics: an evaluation of the potential of 1000 plants," *Journal of Clinical Pharmacy and Therapeutics*, vol. 35, no. 1, pp. 11–48, 2010.

[179] L. Z. Anthony, C. X. Charlie, and H. S. F. Harry, *Integration of Herbal Medicine into Evidence-Based Clinical Practice Current Status and Issues Herbal Medicine: Biomolecular and Clinical Aspects*, Chapter 22, CRC Press, 2nd edition, 2011.

[180] A. L. Zhang, C. C. Xue, and H. H. S. Fong, "Chapter 22 Integration of herbal medicine into evidence-based clinical practice: current status and issues," in *Herbal Medicine: Biomolecular and Clinical Aspects*, I. F. F. Benzie and S. Wachtel-Galor, Eds., CRC Press, Boca Raton, Fla, USA, 2011, http://www.ncbi.nlm.nih.gov/books/NBK92760/#ch22_r32.

[181] M. Serafini, A. Stanzione, and S. Foddai, "Functional foods: traditional use and European legislation," *International Journal of Food Sciences and Nutrition*, vol. 63, no. S1, pp. 7–9, 2012.

21

Embryotoxic and Teratogenic Effects of Norfloxacin in Pregnant Female Albino Rats

Mohamed Aboubakr,[1] Mohamed Elbadawy,[1] Ahmed Soliman,[2] and Mohamed El-Hewaity[3]

[1] Department of Pharmacology, Faculty of Veterinary Medicine, Benha University, Moshtohor, Toukh, Qaliobiya 13736, Egypt
[2] Department of Pharmacology, Faculty of Veterinary Medicine, Cairo University, Giza 12211, Egypt
[3] Department of Pharmacology, Faculty of Veterinary Medicine, University of Sadat City, Minoufiya 32897, Egypt

Correspondence should be addressed to Mohamed Aboubakr; mohamedhafez19@yahoo.com

Academic Editor: Berend Olivier

This study was designed to investigate the possible developmental teratogenicity of norfloxacin in rats. Forty pregnant female rats were divided into four equal groups. Group A received norfloxacin in a dose of 500 mg/kg·b·wt/day orally from 6th to 15th day of gestation. Groups B and C received 1000 and 2000 mg/kg·b·wt/day orally for the same period, respectively; Group D behaved as control and received 0.5 mL distilled water orally for the same period. The dams were killed on 20th day of gestation and their fetuses were subjected to morphological, visceral, and skeletal examinations. Norfloxacin significantly decreased the number of viable fetuses, increased the number of resorbed fetuses, and induced retardation in growth of viable fetuses; some visceral and skeletal defects in these fetuses were seen and these effects were dose dependant. Conclusively, norfloxacin caused some fetal defects and abnormalities, so it is advisable to avoid using this drug during pregnancy.

1. Introduction

Teratology, the study of abnormal prenatal development and congenital malformations induced by exogenous chemical or physical agents, is a growing area of medical research in the quest for the eradication of preventable birth defects. Birth defects are known to occur in huge numbers; roughly 7~10% of all children require extensive medical care to diagnose or treat a birth defect; this compromises the quality of life of millions of people worldwide [1]. Almost all therapeutic agents cross placental barrier and enter fetal circulation. Every agent given during pregnancy therefore has a tendency to produce some sort of structural abnormality in the neonate at birth until proved otherwise [2]. A birth defect or a congenital malformation is a structural abnormality of any type present at birth. It may be macroscopic or microscopic, on the surface or within the body [3]. During the past few decades, it has become increasingly evident that human and animal embryos are subjected to the toxic effects of many drugs, such as the use of some antibiotics in the treatment of serious diseases occurring during pregnancy. Fluoroquinolones are one of the main classes of antimicrobials used in treatment of many infections including urinary, respiratory, gastrointestinal tract, skin, bone, and joint infections [4, 5].

The popularity of fluoroquinolone antibiotics has increased because of their broad antimicrobial spectrum, multiple approved indications, and favorable pharmacokinetics [6]. Norfloxacin is synthetic antimicrobial agent of the fluoroquinolones class. Like other fluoroquinolones, norfloxacin acts principally by inhibition of DNA gyrase, an enzyme required for the proper supercoiling of bacterial chromosomes [7]. Norfloxacin is active mainly against Gram-negative and Gram-positive pathogens. It has a wide spectrum of activity and is rapidly bactericidal at low concentration [8].

Norfloxacin is mainly used for the treatment of urinary tract infections which have high incidence during pregnancy especially in the first trimester. With this objective in view, the present study was done to demonstrate the teratogenic effects of norfloxacin in albino rats.

TABLE 1: Effect of norfloxacin on fetuses obtained from pregnant female rats after repeated oral administration of 500, 1000, and 2000 mg norfloxacin/kg·b·wt from 6th to 15th day of pregnancy once daily ($n = 10$).

Parameters	Control group	500 mg/kg·b·wt (A)	1000 mg/kg·b·wt (B)	2000 mg/kg·b·wt (C)
Number of female rats	10	10	10	10
Number of viable fetuses	91 (100%)	80 (98.88%)	61 (89.71%)	39 (68.42%)
Number of dead fetuses	0	0	2 (2.94%)	7 (12.28%)
Number of resorbed fetuses	0	1 (1.23%)	5 (7.35%)	11 (19.30%)
Total used	91	81	68	57
Fetal body weight (gm)	4.36 ± 0.79	3.71 ± 0.68	3.19 ± 0.54	2.78 ± 0.47
Fetal crown-rump length (cm)	4.29 ± 0.64	3.74 ± 0.71	3.28 ± 0.61	3.01 ± 0.59

%: percent in relation to the total number of examined fetuses.

TABLE 2: Visceral abnormalities in fetuses obtained from pregnant female rats after repeated oral administration of 500, 1000, and 2000 mg norfloxacin per kg·b·wt once daily from 6th to 15th day of pregnancy once daily ($n = 15$).

Parameters	Control group	500 mg/kg·b·wt (A)	1000 mg/kg·b·wt (B)	2000 mg/kg·b·wt (C)
Number of examined fetuses	15	15	15	15
Brain diverticulum	—	8 (53.33%)	9 (60%)	12 (80%)
Thymus hypoplasia	—	6 (40%)	8 (53.33%)	9 (60%)
Lung hypoplasia	—	9 (60%)	9 (60%)	11 (73.33%)
Heart enlargement	—	8 (53.33%)	9 (60%)	12 (80%)
Liver enlargement	—	10 (66.67%)	12 (80%)	14 (93.33%)
Suprarenal gland enlargement	—	7 (46.67%)	8 (53.33%)	11 (73.33%)

%: percent of total abnormalities in relation to the number of examined fetuses.

2. Materials and Methods

2.1. Drug.
Norfloxacin was obtained as an oral solution from ATCO Pharma for pharmaceutical industries, Egypt, under a trade name (Atonor). Each mL contains 300 mg of norfloxacin base.

2.2. Experimental Animals.
Forty mature healthy female albino rats were obtained from department of Laboratory Animal Colonies, Ministry of Public Health, Helwan, Egypt. Animals were kept under hygenic conditions and fed on balanced ration and water *ad libitum*. Female rats were examined periodically using vaginal smear test to ensure that they were always in regular oestrous cycle [9]. They were kept with normal healthy male albino rats allowing one male for two female rats in one cage overnight [10]. The presence of sperms in the vagina next morning was considered as the first day of pregnancy [11]. Pregnancy was confirmed by persistence of diestrus state for 5 days after mating.

2.3. Experimental Design.
The pregnant rats were divided into four groups each of 10 rats. Rats were given norfloxacin orally from 6th to 15th day of gestation.

(i) Group A, received norfloxacin orally at a dose of 500 mg/kg·b·wt/day.

(ii) Group B, received norfloxacin orally at a dose of 1000 mg/kg·b·wt/day.

(iii) Group C, received norfloxacin orally at a dose of 2000 mg/kg·b·wt/day.

(iv) Group D, behaved as control group and received 0.5 mL of distilled water orally for the same period.

The drug was given from 6th to 15th day of gestation during the period of fetal organogenesis. All females were killed on the 20th day of pregnancy and their uteri were dissected in order to examine the position and number of viable, resorbed, or dead fetuses. The surviving fetuses were weighed and the length from crown to rump was measured and examined for any external gross malformations, while others were stained by alizarin red for skeletal examination [12]. Cross-sections through the spinal cord and thoracic vertebrae of fetus at 20th day of gestation were done and stained with haematoxylin and eosin for histopathological examinations [13].

3. Results

Oral administration of norfloxacin in different doses (500, 1000 and 2000 mg/Kg·b·wt) to pregnant female rats from 6th to 15th days of pregnancy induced changes in number of viable, dead, and resorbed fetuses, fetal body weight, and crown-rump length which were recorded in Table 1. Visceral abnormalities of fetuses were recorded (Table 2 and Figures 1(a), 1(b), and 1(c)), while skeletal examination of alizarin red stained fetuses showed different abnormalities (Table 3 and Figures 1(d), 1(e), and 1(f)).

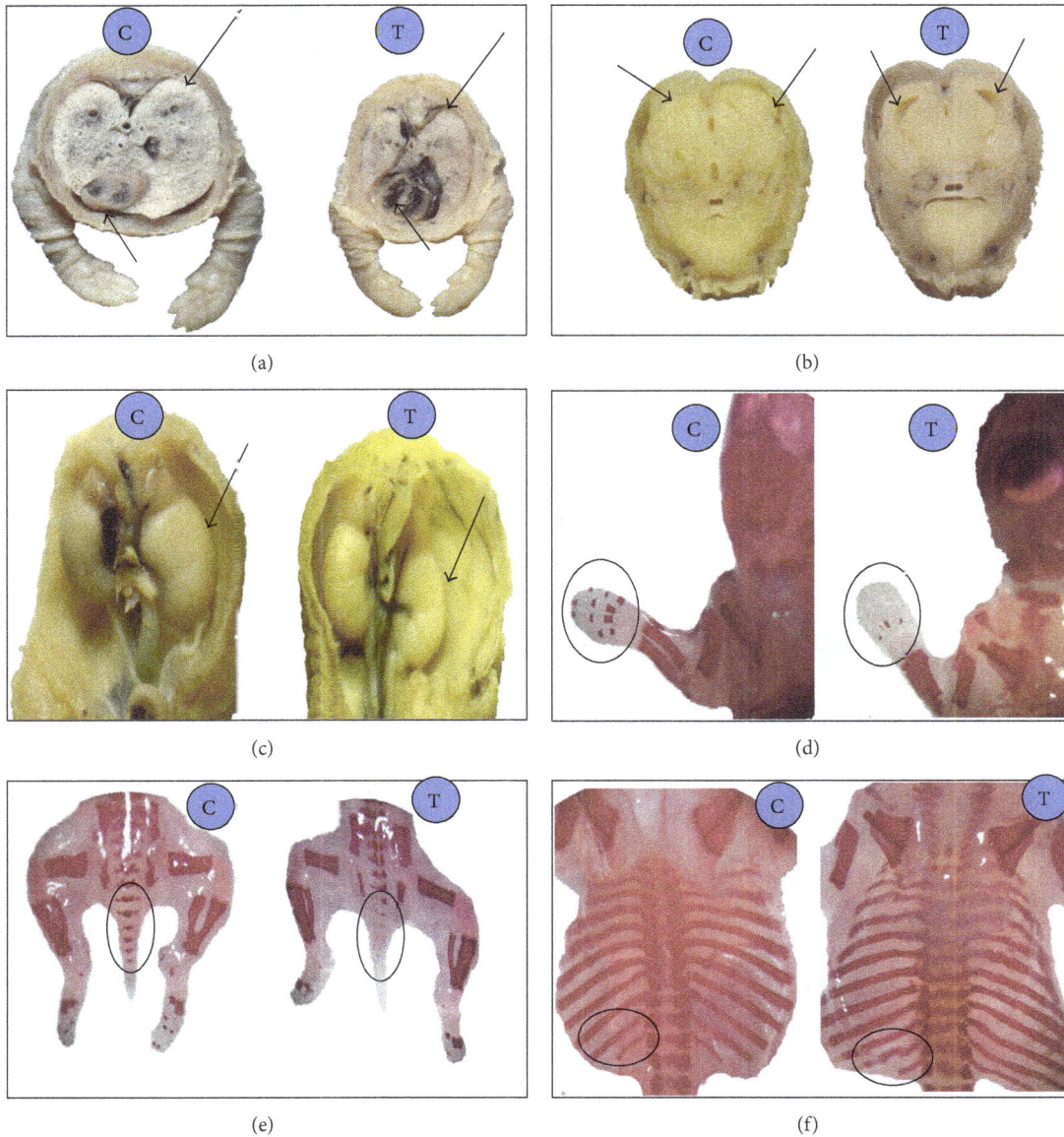

FIGURE 1: (a) Pulmonary hypoplasia with cardiac enlargement, (b) diverticulum dilatation, (c) kidney hypoplasia, (d) absence of digit's bone of fore limb, (e) partial absence of caudal vertebrae, and (f) irregular and short ribs of a fetuses obtained from pregnant rats after repeated oral administration of 2000 mg norfloxacin/Kg·b·wt from 6th to 15th day of pregnancy. C in blue circle represent (control group) and T in blue circle represent (treated group).

Histopathological examination of fetuses bone (spinal cord and thoracic vertebrae) at 20th day of gestation showed absence of ossification especially in treated group (2000 mg/kg·b·wt) in comparison with normal ossification in control group which was shown in Figure 2.

4. Discussion

Oral administration of norfloxacin to female pregnant rats induced decrease in the number of fetuses and increase in the number of resorbed fetuses either early or late when compared with that recorded value of the control group. This result was consistent with the data reported after administration of enrofloxacin, ciprofloxacin, ofloxacin, and norfloxacin to domestic animals, where embryonic losses in female monkeys exposed to very high doses led to decrease in number of the fetuses [14]. The decrease in number of fetuses per mother might be attributed to the lack of oval production or lack of the basic cell constituent as a result of drug administration [15]. Decrease in number of viable fetuses might be explained on the basis of incomplete formation of the placenta and degeneration of the trophoblast and decidual cell, which play an important role in the transmission of nutrients to the embryo [16]. Also, the reduction in number may be due to early embryonic death and an increase in the fetal resorption ratio in the present study.

Administration of norfloxacin to female pregnant rats during the period of organogenesis produced significant

TABLE 3: Skeletal abnormalities in fetuses obtained from pregnant female rats after repeated oral administration of 500, 1000, and 2000 mg norfloxacin/kg·b·wt from 6th to 15th day of pregnancy once daily ($n = 15$).

Parameters	Control group	500 mg/kg·b·wt (A)	1000 mg/kg·b·wt (B)	2000 mg/kg·b·wt (C)
Number of examined fetuses	15	15	15	15
Impairment of skull ossification	—	3 (20%)	5 (33.33%)	8 (53.33%)
Absence or dislocation of sternebrae	—	2 (13.33%)	3 (20%)	5 (33.33%)
Reduction or absence of caudal vertebrae	—	5 (33.33%)	6 (40%)	10 (66.67%)
Absence of digit's bone of fore limb	—	3 (20%)	4 (26.67%)	9 (60%)
Absence of digit's bone of hind limb	—	2 (12.33%)	3 (20%)	7 (46.67%)
Absence of some metatarsal bone	—	3 (20%)	4 (26.67%)	6 (40%)
Absence of some metacarpal bone	—	2 (12.33%)	4 (26.67%)	5 (33.33%)

%: percent of total abnormalities in relation to the number of examined fetuses.

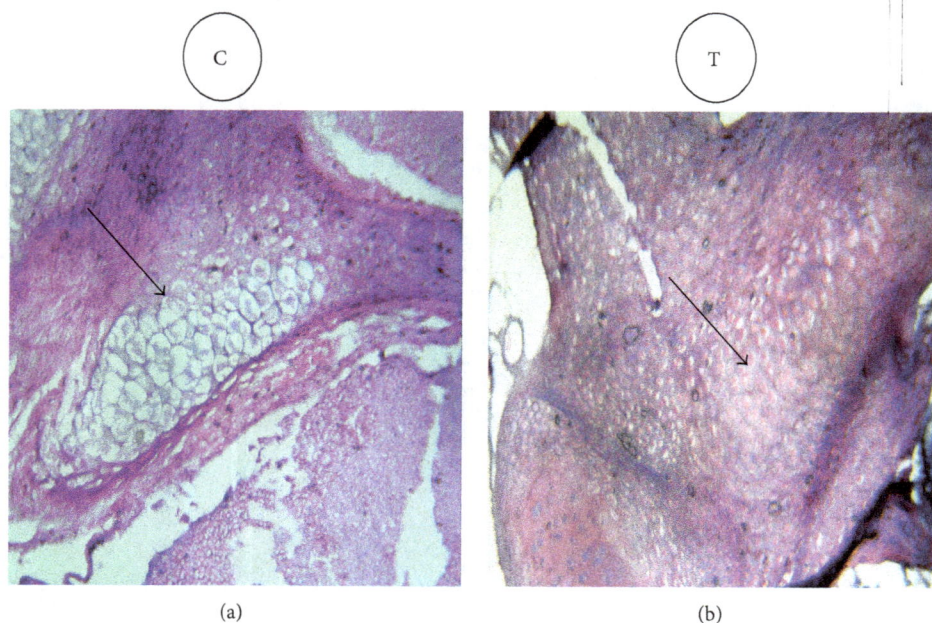

(a)   (b)

FIGURE 2: Cross-section through the spinal cord and thoracic vertebrae of fetuses at 20th day of gestation, showing absence of ossification in treated group (T) (2000 mg norfloxacin/Kg·b·wt from 6th to 15th day of pregnancy) in comparison with normal ossification in control group (C) (×10 H & E).

decrease in both weight and length of fetuses. These results were consistent with those previously reported following administration of ciprofloxacin to albino rats [17]. These changes may be attributed to deficiency of nutritional supply from dam to fetuses because female rats receiving ofloxacin or levofloxacin exhibited soft stool or diarrhea which might be attributed to imbalance in intestinal microflora [18, 19].

Norfloxacin resulted in many visceral abnormalities as diverticulum dilatation in the brain of fetuses which might be attributed to the lack of placental transfusion of amino acid, arginine, metabolism in fetus [15], neurotoxic effect of norfloxacin [20], or some antibacterials that had neurotoxic effect as levofloxacin and ciprofloxacin which easily cross blood brain barrier and compete with gamma-aminobutyric acid receptor [21]. Norfloxacin induced a hypoplasia or absence of thymus gland of fetuses; this fetal abnormality

agreed with the results reported after administration of ciprofloxacin and ofloxacin at a dose of 100 mg/mL, which inhibited the cell growth, while 1000 mg/mL led to cell death [22]. Activity of ciprofloxacin against calf thymus and cultured mammalian cell was studied and this result might be attributed to cytotoxicity of quinolone as ciprofloxacin promotes cell death by converting Topoisomerase II to cellular poison [23]. Norfloxacin induced cardiac hyperplasia. This result agreed with that; animal experiments as well as clinical experience show that the cardiotoxic potentials of sparfloxacin and grepafloxacin are higher than those of the other fluoroquinolones: they cause QT prolongation at rather low doses thus increasing the risk for severe arrhythmia [24]. This lesion might be attributed to ability of fluoroquinolones to block cardiac potassium channel which led to prolonged QT interval with cardiac arrhythmia and consequently cardiac hyperplasia [25]. Pulmonary hypoplasia might be attributed to extensive distribution into lung and achieved higher concentration [26]. Norfloxacin administration induced hypoplasia or atrophy of one or both kidneys. These results agreed with those reported after administration of ofloxacin to rats and rabbits [27].

Oral administration of norfloxacin produced some skeletal malformations such as impairment of skull ossification, absence or dislocation of sternebrae, reduction or absence of caudal vertebrae, and absence of digit's bone of fore- and hindlimb with absence of some metatarsal and metacarpal bone. These skeletal malformations agreed with that recorded by many investigators following administration of ofloxacin to female pregnant rats and rabbits [18]; administration of levofloxacin to rats [19], and administration of fluoroquinolone (DW-116) to the pregnant rats and rabbits, respectively [28, 29]. Fluoroquinolone antibiotics are associated with a wide spectrum of musculoskeletal complications that involve not only tendon but also cartilage, bone, and muscle [30]. Fetal growth retardation could occur as a result of reduction of thickness in proliferative zone of the long bones and absence of the hypertrophic zone. Fluoroquinolone delayed the developmental phase of the epiphyseal growth with growth inhibition [31]. Bone and cartilage damage could be due to fluoride accumulation with repeated fluoroquinolone administration [32]. The fetotoxic effect of ciprofloxacin was observed on skeletal growth as evidenced by decrease of intact bone length in long bones of extremities [17]. The fetotoxicity, high resorption ratio, and fetal loss and malformations could be attributed to the inhibition of DNA transcription in the rapidly divided fetal cells. So fluoroquinolones act as DNA gyrase inhibitors and also mitotic inhibitors. The complete damage of DNA could result in fetal loss or resorption, while partial damage could induce fetal malformation [33].

5. Conclusion

Administration of norfloxacin during pregnancy especially in early stage and at high doses could induce some fetal defects and abnormalities, so it is advisable to avoid using this drug during pregnancy.

Conflict of Interests

The authors declare that there is no conflict of interests regarding the publication of this paper.

Acknowledgment

The authors wish to thank Professor Dr. Mahmoud Gaballah (Department of Pathology, Faculty of Veterinary Medicine, Benha University, Egypt) for his help in histopathological examination.

References

[1] R. O'Rahilly, *Human Embryology & Teratology*, Wiley-Liss, New York, NY, USA, 3rd edition, 2001.

[2] P. N. Schlegel, T. S. K. Chang, and F. F. Marshall, "Antibiotics: potential hazards to male fertility," *Fertility and Sterility*, vol. 55, no. 2, pp. 235–242, 1991.

[3] K. L. Moore, *The Developing Human*, WB Saunder, Philadelphia, Pa, USA, 4th edition, 1988.

[4] P. J. A. Amwayi and G. E. Otiang'a-Owiti, "Use of biometric embryonic growth parameters as indicator of exposure to a teratogen," *East African Medical Journal*, vol. 74, no. 1, pp. 6–11, 1997.

[5] A. Gürbay, C. Garrel, M. Osman, M.-J. Richard, A. Favier, and F. Hincal, "Cytotoxicity in ciprofloxacin-treated human fibroblast cells and protection by vitamin E," *Human and Experimental Toxicology*, vol. 21, no. 12, pp. 635–641, 2002.

[6] A. J. Mehlhorn and D. A. Brown, "Safety concerns with fluoroquinolones," *Annals of Pharmacotherapy*, vol. 41, no. 11, pp. 1859–1866, 2007.

[7] K. S. Wolfson and D. C. Hooper, "Fluoroquinolone antimicrobial agents," *Clinical Microbiology Reviews*, vol. 2, no. 4, pp. 378–424, 1989.

[8] P. B. Fernandes, "Mode of action, and in vitro and in vivo activities of the fluoroquinolones," *Journal of Clinical Pharmacology*, vol. 28, no. 2, pp. 156–168, 1988.

[9] G. L. Hassert, P. J. DeBaecke, J. S. Kulesza, V. M. Traina, D. P. Sinha, and E. Bernal, "Toxicological, pathological, and teratological studies in animals with cephradine," *Antimicrobial Agents and Chemotherapy*, vol. 3, no. 6, pp. 682–685, 1973.

[10] D. J. MacIntyre, H.-H. Chang, and M. H. Kaufman, "Teratogenic effects of amniotic sac puncture: a mouse model," *Journal of Anatomy*, vol. 186, no. 3, pp. 527–539, 1995.

[11] P. Barcellona, O. Fanelli, and A. Campana, "Teratological study of etoperdone in the rat and rabbit," *Toxicology*, vol. 8, no. 1, pp. 87–94, 1977.

[12] A. W. Hayes, *Principles and Method of Toxicology*, Reven Press, New York, NY, USA, 2nd edition, 1988.

[13] R. A. B. Drury and E. A. Wallington, *Carleton's Histological Technique*, Oxford University Press, London, UK, 5th edition, 1980.

[14] P. M. Vancutsem, J. G. Babish, and W. S. Schwark, "The fluoroquinolone antimicrobials: structure, antimicrobial activity, pharmacokinetics, clinical use in domestic animals and toxicity," *The Cornell Veterinarian*, vol. 80, no. 2, pp. 173–186, 1990.

[15] H. Tuchmann, *Drug Effects on Fetus*, ADIS Press, New York, NY, USA, 1975.

[16] M. Kurebe, H. Asaoka, and M. Moriguchi, "Toxicological studies on a new cephamycin, MT-141. IX. Its teratogenicity test in rats and rabbits," *Japanese Journal of Antibiotics*, vol. 37, no. 6, pp. 1186–1210, 1984.

[17] M. A. Siddiqui and S. N. H. Naqvi, "Evaluation of the teratogenic potentials of ciprofloxacin in albino rat," *Journal of Morphological Sciences*, vol. 27, no. 1, pp. 14–18, 2010.

[18] S. Takayama, T. Watanabe, and Y. Akiyama, "Reproductive toxicity of ofloxacin," *Arzneimittel-Forschung*, vol. 36, no. 8, pp. 1244–1248, 1986.

[19] T. Watanabe, K. Fujikawa, S. Harada, K. Ohura, T. Sasaki, and S. Takayama, "Reproductive toxicity of the new quinolone antibacterial agent levofloxacin in rats and rabbits," *Arzneimittel-Forschung A*, vol. 42, no. 3, pp. 374–377, 1992.

[20] L. R. Zhang, Y. M. Wang, B. Y. Chen, and N. N. Cheng, "Neurotoxicity and toxicokinetics of norfloxacin in conscious rats," *Acta Pharmacologica Sinica*, vol. 24, no. 6, pp. 605–623, 2003.

[21] K. Akahane, M. Kato, and S. Takayama, "Involvement of inhibitory and excitatory neurotransmitters in levofloxacin- and

ciprofloxacin-induced convulsions in mice," *Antimicrobial Agents and Chemotherapy*, vol. 37, no. 9, pp. 1764–1770, 1993.

[22] P. Hussy, G. Maass, and B. Tummler, "Effect of 4-quinolones and novobiocin on calf thymus DNA polymerase α primase complex, topoisomerases I and II, and growth of mammalian lymphoblasts," *Antimicrobial Agents and Chemotherapy*, vol. 29, no. 6, pp. 1073–1078, 1986.

[23] S. H. Elsea, P. R. McGuirk, T. D. Gootz, M. Moynihan, and N. Osheroff, "Drug features that contribute to the activity of quinolones against mammalian topoisomerase II and cultured cells: correlation between enhancement of enzyme-mediated DNA cleavage in vitro and cytotoxic potential," *Antimicrobial Agents and Chemotherapy*, vol. 37, no. 10, pp. 2179–2186, 1993.

[24] R. Stahlmann, "Clinical toxicological aspects of fluoroquinolones," *Toxicology Letters*, vol. 127, no. 1–3, pp. 269–277, 2002.

[25] J. Kang, L. Wang, X. Chen, D. J. Triggle, and D. Rampe, "Interactions of a series of fluoroquinolone antibacterial drugs with the human cardiac K+ channel HERG," *Molecular Pharmacology*, vol. 59, no. 1, pp. 122–126, 2001.

[26] E. C. Gilfillan, B. A. Pelak, and J. A. Bland, "Pharmacokinetic studies of norfloxacin in laboratory animals," *Chemotherapy*, vol. 30, no. 5, pp. 288–296, 1984.

[27] G. J. Davis and B. E. McKenzie, "Toxicologic evaluation of ofloxacin," *American Journal of Medicine C*, vol. 87, supplement 6, pp. 43S–46S, 1989.

[28] J. C. Kim, D.-H. Shin, S.-H. Kim et al., "Peri- and postnatal developmental toxicity of the fluoroquinolone antibacterial DW-116 in rats," *Food and Chemical Toxicology*, vol. 42, no. 3, pp. 389–395, 2004.

[29] J. C. Kim, S. H. Kim, D. H. Shin et al., "Developmental toxicity assessment of the new fluoroquinolone antibacterial DW-116 in rabbits," *Journal of Applied Toxicology*, vol. 25, no. 1, pp. 52–59, 2005.

[30] M. M. Hall, J. T. Finnoff, and J. Smith, "Musculoskeletal complications of fluoroquinolones: guidelines and precautions for usage in the athletic population," *Journal of Injury, Function and Rehabilitation*, vol. 3, no. 2, pp. 132–142, 2011.

[31] R. Stahlmann, "Children as a special population at risk-quinolones as an example for xenobiotics exhibiting skeletal toxicity," *Archives of Toxicology*, vol. 77, no. 1, pp. 7–11, 2003.

[32] N. K. Arora, "Are fluoroquinolones safe in children?" *Indian Journal of Pediatrics*, vol. 61, no. 6, pp. 601–603, 1994.

[33] C. W. Jeffry, S. K. Soo, D. R. James et al., "Inhibition of clinically relevant mutant variants of HIV-1 by quinazolinone nonnucleoside reverse transcriptase inhibitors," *Journal of Medicinal Chemistry*, vol. 43, no. 10, pp. 2019–2030, 2000.

22

Response of Bone Resorption Markers to *Aristolochia longa* Intake by Algerian Breast Cancer Postmenopausal Women

Bachir Benarba,[1,2] Boumedienne Meddah,[2] and Aicha Tir Touil[1]

[1] Laboratory of Bioconversion, Microbial engineering and Health Safety, Department of Biology, University of Mascara, 29000 Mascara, Algeria
[2] Laboratory of Research on Biological Systems and Geomatics, University of Mascara, 29000 Mascara, Algeria

Correspondence should be addressed to Bachir Benarba; bachirsb@yahoo.fr

Academic Editor: Thérèse Di Paolo-Chênevert

Aristolochia longa is widely used in traditional medicine in Algeria to treat breast cancer. The aim of the present study was to investigate the response of bone resorption markers to *A. longa* intake by Algerian breast cancer postmenopausal women. According to the *A. longa* intake, breast cancer patients were grouped into *A. longa* group (Al) ($n = 54$) and non-*A. longa* group (non-Al) ($n = 24$). 32 women constituted the control group. Bone resorption markers (from urine) pyridinoline (PYD) and deoxypyridinoline (DPD) were determined by HPLC. Serum and urinary creatinine, uric acid, and urea were measured. 1 g of *A. longa* intake resulted in significant rise of renal serum markers and a pronounced increase of bone resorption markers. The intake of *A. longa* roots is detrimental for kidney function and resulted in high bone resorption, maybe due to the reduction in renal function caused by the aristolochic acids contained in the roots.

1. Introduction

The pyridinium cross-links pyridinoline (PYD) and deoxypyridinoline (DPD) are established markers of bone resorption measured in blood and urine and are used to investigate bone metabolism and manage bone diseases [1]. Deoxypyridinoline (Dpd) distributed mostly in bone collagen has a higher specificity for bone than pyridinoline (pyd), which is excreted in urine, and it is not affected by diet, whereas pyridinoline (Pyd) is abundant in bone and cartilage (Figure 1) [2]. They are inexpensive, sensitive, and useful for the diagnosis of bone metastasis [3].

Aristolochia longa belongs to the genus *Aristolochia* (Aristolochiaceae) consisting of about 500 species mostly distributed along tropical, subtropical, and Mediterranean regions of the world [4]. The plant is widely used in traditional medicine in Algeria [5]. Although plants of the genus *Aristolochia* have been shown to exhibit interesting anticancer activities including cytotoxic and apoptosis-induced, herbal remedies containing plants of *Aristolochia* genus are banned in many countries because of the nephrotoxicity of their aristolochic acid [6, 7].

The aim of the present study was to investigate the response of bone resorption markers to *A. longa* intake by Algerian breast cancer postmenopausal women.

2. Materials and Methods

2.1. Subjects. A total of 110 postmenopausal women were recruited into the study from two hospitals in the State of Mascara (north-west of Algeria). Of these, 32 women (age: 66.4 ± 10.45 years) free from any critical illness or medical problems, constituted the control group and 78 were newly diagnosed with primary breast cancer. Patients with recurrent breast cancer, adjuvant therapy (radiotherapy or chemotherapy) prior to surgery, or a history of previous cancer, renal failure, osteoporosis, connective tissue disease, degenerative bone disease traumatic fracture, early menopause before 40 years of age, and current medication use that may affect

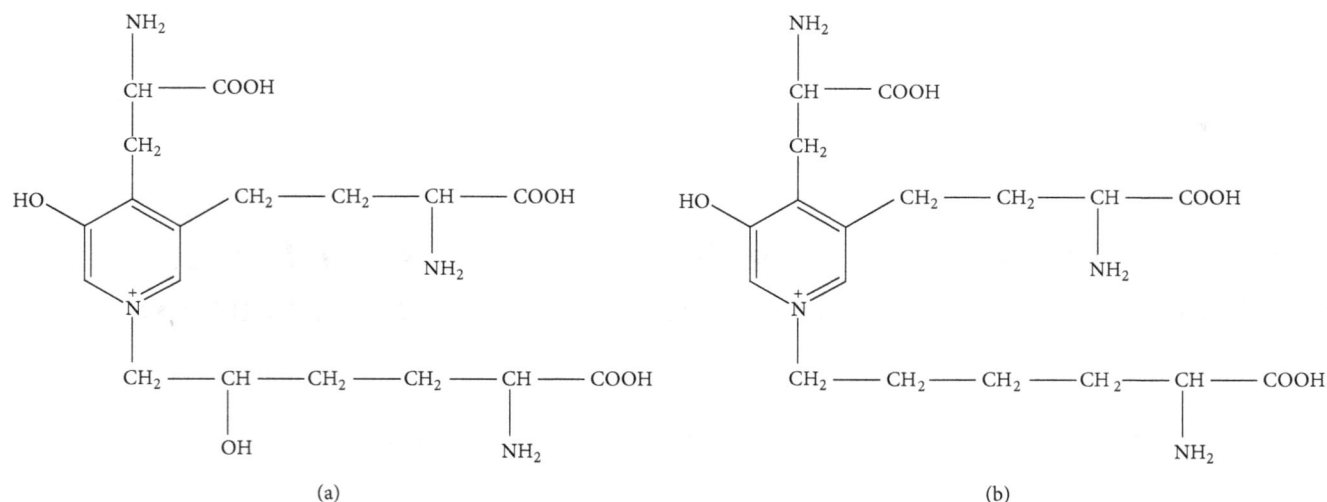

FIGURE 1: Structures of pyridinoline (PYD) and deoxypyridinoline (DPD). Upper: pyridinoline (molecular weight: 429); lower, deoxypyridinoline (molecular weight: 413).

TABLE 1: Age, BMI, and time after menopause of the study population.

	Control ($n = 32$)	Al ($n = 54$)	Non-Al ($n = 24$)
Age (yrs)	66.4 ± 10.45 (49–78)	65.05 ± 10.02 (50–77)	65.87 ± 08.64 (52–80)
BMI (kg/m^2)	24.09 ± 04.32 (21.3–28)	25.21 ± 03.89 (23.43–28.2)	24.77 ± 06.02 (21–27)
Time after menopause (yrs)	15.09 ± 04.11 (5–21)	15.83 ± 05.46 (7–29)	14.98 ± 14 (4–27)

bone density, including hormones, vitamins, and mineral supplements, were excluded from the study.

Aristolochia longa intake was assessed retrospectively using a standardized questionnaire. Subjects were interviewed after diagnosis and before initiating treatment. Breast cancer patients were then grouped into *A. longa* group (Al) ($n = 54$) andnon-*A. longa* group (non-Al) ($n = 24$) (Table 1).

2.2. Specimen Collection. Serum samples separated from antecubital venous blood were centrifuged (1500 g/minute, for 10 minutes). Fresh urine samples were taken at 8–10 AM. Specimens were stored at −20°C until the time of analysis.

2.3. Analysis of Bone Markers. Pyridinoline (PYD) and deoxypyridinoline (DPD) were determined by HPLC. Total urinary PYD and D-PYD were determined as described [8]. In brief, 1 mL urine was hydrolyzed with an equal volume of 12 mol/L HCl at 105°C for 16 h to convert all urinary crosslinks to the peptide-free form. Free urinary PYD and DPD were determined without hydrolysis. After partition chromatography on CFl cellulose, samples and external standards were separated by high performance liquid chromatography (HPLC), and concentrations were determined by fluorometry of the eluent peaks. Standards were derived from standard solution with 249 nmol of PYD and 30 nmol of DPD (a generous gift from Pr Brazier, Clinic pharmacology Lab, University of Amiens, France). To correct for variations in urinary flow, PYD and DPD results were normalized to the urinary creatinine concentration and expressed as nanomoles (PYD, DPD) divided by millimoles creatinine (nM (PYD, DPD)/mM creatinine). Urinary creatinine was measured according to Jaffe method (Fluitest Crea, Biocon Diagnostic, Ref 448, Lot G558, Denmark).

2.4. Statistics. All numeric data were expressed as mean ±SD. Data were analyzed using the student *t*-test. A *P* value ≤ 0.05 was considered significant. Statistical calculations were performed with SPSS version 9.0.

3. Results

One hundred and sixteen women newly diagnosed with primary breast cancer were initially included, of whom 92 women (80%) had used local medicinal plants three months before diagnosis. For 81 women of them, the used plants were known. 24 women did never use medicinal plants. 54 women had consumed 1 ± 0.3 g (0.85–1.5 g)/day/40 days of *A. longa* roots. There was no statistical difference between the three groups (A, B, and control) with regard to age, BMI, and time after menopause. Age, time after menopause, and BMI are shown in Table 1.

According to our results (Table 2), 1 g of *A. longa* intake resulted in significant rise of renal serum markers. In the breast cancer population, mean serum creatinine, urea, and uric acid were significantly higher in patients of Al group than those of non-Al group by 36.63%, 68.36%, and 73.96%, respectively. When compared to controls, they had significantly higher levels of serum creatinine, urea, and uric acid

TABLE 2: Serum creatinine, BUN, and uric acid.

	Control (n = 32)	Al (n = 54)	Non-Al (n = 24)
Creatinine (mg/dL)	0.93 ± 0.1	1.38 ± 0.17[a,b]	1.01 ± 0.09
BUN (mg/dL)	23.89 ± 2.66	42.26 ± 8.13[a,b]	25.10 ± 5.78
Uric acid (mg/dL)	03.87 ± 0.42	07.15 ± 01.89[a,b]	04.11 ± 0.81

[a]High significant value ($P < 0.01$) as compared to controls.
[b]High significant value ($P < 0.01$) as compared to non-Al group.

TABLE 3: Bone resorption markers PYD and DPD concentrations.

	PYD total form (nmol/mmol Cr)	PYD-free form (nmol/mmol Cr)	PYD conjugated form (nmol/mmol Cr)	DPD total form (nmol/mmol Cr)	DPD-free form (nmol/mmol Cr)	DPD conjugated form (nmol/mmol Cr)
Controls	41.2 ± 9.2	32.14 ± 10.4	10.16 ± 8.9	18.9 ± 10.2	8.2 ± 3.11	11.4 ± 6.3
Al	82.63 ± 19.33[a,b]	71.86 ± 15.77[a,b]	25.02 ± 08.47[a,b]	46.55 ± 11.52[a,b]	23.04 ± 04.87[a,b]	30.71 ± 06.89[a,b]
Non-Al	69.40 ± 12.17[a]	39.21 ± 14.92[a]	18.64 ± 05.82[a]	30.21 ± 09.25[a]	13.43 ± 07.76[a]	25.41 ± 11.35[a]

[a]High significant value ($P < 0.01$) as compared to controls.
[b]High significant value ($P < 0.01$) as compared to non-Al group.

(1.38 ± 0.17 versus 0.93 ± 0.1, 42.26 ± 8.13 versus 23.89 ± 2.66, and 07.15 ± 1.89 versus 03.87 ± 0.42, resp.).

Patients newly diagnosed for breast cancer (Al and non-Al patients) had significantly higher concentrations of DPD and PYD (all forms) than controls. Interestingly, the intake of 1 g of *A. longa* by breast cancer patients resulted in a pronounced significant increase of mean concentrations of bone resorption markers. Mean concentrations of DPD (free, conjugated, and total form) increased by 71.55%, 20.85%, and 54.08%, respectively. On the other hand, median concentrations of PYD (free, conjugated, and total form) were significantly higher by 83.26%, 34.22%, and 19.06%, respectively (Table 3).

4. Discussion

A. longa is widely used in anticancer treatment in Algeria [9] and Morocco [10]. We have recently demonstrated that an aqueous extract of *A. longa* induced cell death of Burkitt's lymphoma cell line (BL41) in a dose-dependent manner. The IC_{50} of *A. longa* aqueous extract was estimated at about 15,63 μg/mL. The extract induced apoptosis in Burkitt's lymphoma BL41 cells, by triggering the mitochondrial pathway (disruption of $\Delta\Psi$m, activation of caspases 9 and 3, and PARP cleavage) [11]. To our knowledge, the present study is the first to investigate the effect of *A. longa* intake by breast cancer patients on bone resorption.

Our results showed that intake of 1 g of *A. longa* resulted in marked increasing of serum creatinine, urea, and uric acid levels. Here we give evidence that *A. longa* may be detrimental for kidney function in breast cancer patients. Indeed, many *Aristolochia* plants were reported to cause nephropathy [12, 13]. Our findings support the association established between ingestion of herbal remedies containing aristolochic acids (AAs) and the development of a renal disease, designated as aristolochic acid nephropathy (AAN) [14].

Shibutani et al. [15] concluded that AA-I is solely responsible for the nephrotoxicity associated with AAN, since kidney is the primary target organ for its toxicity. Recently, Cherif et al. [5] isolated and characterized AAI from *A. longa* growing in Algeria. The mechanisms by which AA induces renal interstitial fibrosis are still largely unknown, but defective activation of antioxidative enzymes and mitochondrial damage caused by AA tubular toxicity, impaired regeneration of proximal tubular epithelial cells, and apoptosis secondary to caspase-3 activation may be involved [16].

Measurement of the metabolites of type I collagen, the predominant collagen in bone, like PYD and DPD, has been reported to be useful for monitoring bone turnover in many different disorders, including diseases with bone metastases [17]. Findings of the present study showed that breast cancer patients with 1 g *A. longa* intake were characterized by high bone resorption as assessed by PYD and DPD. Since breast cancer patients included in the present study were newly diagnosed with breast cancer without any chemotherapy, the increased bone resorption may be due to secondary causes of bone loss unrelated to cancer treatment. Secondary causes of bone loss are factors other than menopause and aging that can lead to osteoporosis [18]. Kidney failure is one of the secondary causes of osteoporosis in postmenopausal women. Klawansky et al. [19] found that 85% of women with osteoporosis have some degree of renal compromise. We suggest that in postmenopausal women newly diagnosed with breast cancer, the intake of 1 g of *A. longa* roots could contribute to bone loss, maybe due to the reduction in renal function caused by the aristolochic acids contained in the roots. Our hypothesis may be supported by the relationship demonstrated in many studies between reduction in renal function and increased bone loss [20, 21].

Our study has several limitations. Bone formation markers were not measured. Serum vitamin D and PTH levels which are important mediators in the association between renal function and bone were not assessed.

5. Conclusion

In postmenopausal women newly diagnosed for breast cancer, the intake of *A. longa* roots is detrimental for kidney function and resulted in high bone resorption, maybe due to the reduction in renal function caused by the aristolochic acids contained in the roots.

Conflict of Interests

The authors declare that there is no conflict of interests regarding the publication of this paper.

Acknowledgment

The authors gratefully acknowledge Dr. Kada Righi from Agronomy Department of the University of Mascara for plant identification.

References

[1] H. W. Vesper, C. Audain, A. Woolfitt et al., "High-performance liquid chromatography method to analyze free and total urinary pyridinoline and deoxypyridinoline," *Analytical Biochemistry*, vol. 318, no. 2, pp. 204–211, 2003.

[2] J. H. Chung, M. S. Park, Y. S. Kim et al., "Usefulness of bone metabolic markers in the diagnosis of bone metastasis from lung cancer," *Yonsei Medical Journal*, vol. 46, no. 3, pp. 388–393, 2005.

[3] F. Dane, H. M. Turk, A. Sevinc, S. Buyukberber, C. Camci, and M. Tarakcioglu, "The markers of bone turnover in patients with lung cancer," *Journal of the National Medical Association*, vol. 100, no. 4, pp. 425–428, 2008.

[4] C. Neinhuis, S. Wanke, K. W. Hilu, K. Müller, and T. Borsch, "Phylogeny of Aristolochiaceae based on parsimony, likelihood, and Bayesian analyses of trnL-trnF sequences," *Plant Systematics and Evolution*, vol. 250, no. 1-2, pp. 7–26, 2005.

[5] H. S. Cherif, F. Saidi, H. Boutoumi, A. Rouibi, and C. Chaouia, "Identification et caracterisation de quelques composes chimiques chez *Aristolochia longa* L.," *Agricultura*, vol. 3, pp. 76–82, 2009.

[6] F. D. Debelle, J. L. Nortier, E. G. De Prez et al., "Aristolochic acids induce chronic renal failure with interstitial fibrosis in salt-depleted rats," *Journal of the American Society of Nephrology*, vol. 13, no. 2, pp. 431–436, 2002.

[7] J. L. Nortier, M.-C. M. Martinez, H. H. Schmeiser et al., "Urothelial carcinoma associated with the use of a Chinese herb (*Aristolochia fangchi*)," *The New England Journal of Medicine*, vol. 342, no. 23, pp. 1686–1692, 2000.

[8] B. Meddah, S. Kamel, C. Giroud, and M. Brazier, "Method for the isolation and purification of pyridinoline and deoxypyridinoline crosslinks from bone by liquid chromatographic techniques," *Preparative Biochemistry and Biotechnology*, vol. 29, no. 1, pp. 63–75, 1999.

[9] F. Saidi, H. S. Cherif, H. Lazouri et al., "Determination of the lipid compounds of *Aristolochia Longa* L. from Algeria," *Bulletin UASMV Agricultura*, vol. 66, pp. 17–23, 2009.

[10] G. Benzakour, N. Benkirane, M. Amrani, and M. Oudghiri, "Immunostimulatory potential of *Aristolochia longa* L. induced toxicity on liver, intestine and kidney in mice," *Journal of Toxicology and Environmental Health Sciences*, vol. 3, pp. 214–222, 2011.

[11] B. Benarba, G. Ambroise, A. Aoues, B. Meddah, and A. Vazquez, "*Aristolochia longa* aqueous extract triggers the mitochondrial pathway of apoptosis in BL41 Burkitt's lymphoma cells," *International Journal of Green Pharmacy*, vol. 6, pp. 45–49, 2012.

[12] J. M. Peña, M. Borrás, J. Ramos, and J. Montoliu, "Rapidly progressive interstitial renal fibrosis due to a chronic intake of a herb (*Aristolochia pistolochia*) infusion," *Nephrology Dialysis Transplantation*, vol. 11, no. 7, pp. 1359–1360, 1996.

[13] M.-C. M. Martinez, J. Nortier, P. Vereerstraeten, and J.-L. Vanherweghem, "Progression rate of Chinese herb nephropathy: impact of *Aristolochia fangchi* ingested dose," *Nephrology Dialysis Transplantation*, vol. 17, no. 3, pp. 408–412, 2002.

[14] J. L. Nortier and J. L. Vanherweghem, "Renal interstitial fibrosis and urothelial carcinoma associated with the use of a Chinese herb (*Aristolochia fangchi*)," *Toxicology*, vol. 181-182, pp. 577–580, 2002.

[15] S. Shibutani, H. Dong, N. Suzuki, S. Ueda, F. Miller, and A. P. Grollman, "Selective toxicity of aristolochic acids I and II," *Drug Metabolism and Disposition*, vol. 35, no. 7, pp. 1217–1222, 2007.

[16] A. A. Pozdzik, I. J. Salmon, F. D. Debelle et al., "Aristolochic acid induces proximal tubule apoptosis and epithelial to mesenchymal transformation," *Kidney International*, vol. 73, no. 5, pp. 595–607, 2008.

[17] C. Blomqvist, L. Risteli, J. Risteli, P. Virkkunen, S. Sarna, and I. Elomaa, "Markers of type I collagen degradation and synthesis in the monitoring of treatment response in bone metastases from breast carcinoma," *British Journal of Cancer*, vol. 73, no. 9, pp. 1074–1079, 1996.

[18] P. M. Camacho, A. S. Dayal, J. L. Diaz et al., "Prevalence of secondary causes of bone loss among breast cancer patients with osteopenia and osteoporosis," *Journal of Clinical Oncology*, vol. 26, no. 33, pp. 5380–5385, 2008.

[19] S. Klawansky, E. Komaroff, P. F. Cavanaugh Jr. et al., "Relationship between age, renal function and bone mineral density in the US population," *Osteoporosis International*, vol. 14, no. 7, pp. 570–576, 2003.

[20] S. A. Jamal, V. J. D. Swan, J. P. Brown et al., "Kidney function and rate of bone loss at the hip and spine: The Canadian Multicentre Osteoporosis Study," *American Journal of Kidney Diseases*, vol. 55, no. 2, pp. 291–299, 2010.

[21] K. E. Ensrud, L.-Y. Lui, B. C. Taylor et al., "Renal function and risk of hip and vertebral fractures in older women," *Archives of Internal Medicine*, vol. 167, no. 2, pp. 133–139, 2007.

23

Evaluation of GABAergic Transmission Modulation as a Novel Functional Target for Management of Multiple Sclerosis: Exploring Inhibitory Effect of GABA on Glutamate-Mediated Excitotoxicity

Ankit A. Gilani,[1] Ranjeet Prasad Dash,[2] Mehul N. Jivrajani,[2] Sandeep Kumar Thakur,[2] and Manish Nivsarkar[2]

[1] *Department of Pharmacology and Toxicology, National Institute of Pharmaceutical Education and Research, C/O-B. V. Patel Pharmaceutical Education and Research Development (PERD) Centre, S. G. Highway, Thaltej, Ahmedabad, Gujarat 380054, India*

[2] *Department of Pharmacology and Toxicology, B. V. Patel Pharmaceutical Education and Research Development (PERD) Centre, S. G. Highway, Thaltej, Ahmedabad, Gujarat 380054, India*

Correspondence should be addressed to Manish Nivsarkar; manishnivsarkar@gmail.com

Academic Editor: Berend Olivier

Multiple sclerosis (MS) is an autoimmune inflammatory disease of the central nervous system (CNS) where the communication ability of nerve cells in the brain and spinal cord with each other gets impaired. Some current findings suggest the role of glutamate excitotoxicity in the development and progression of MS. An excess release of glutamate leads to the activation of ionotropic and metabotropic receptors, thus resulting in accumulation of toxic cytoplasmic Ca^{2+} and cell death. However, it has been observed that gamma-aminobutyric acid-A ($GABA_A$) receptors located in the nerve terminals activate presynaptic Ca^{2+}/calmodulin-dependent signaling to inhibit depolarization-evoked Ca^{2+} influx and glutamate release from isolated nerve terminals, which suggest a potential implication of $GABA_A$ receptor in management of MS. With this proof of concept, we tried to explore the potential of selective $GABA_A$ receptor agonists or positive allosteric modulators (diazepam and phenobarbitone sodium) and $GABA_A$ level enhancer (sodium valproate) for management of MS by screening them for their activity in experimental autoimmune encephalomyelitis (EAE) model in rats and cuprizone-induced demyelination model in mice. In this study, sodium valproate was found to show the best activity in the animal models whereas phenobarbitone sodium showed moderate activity. However, diazepam was found to be ineffective.

1. Introduction

Multiple sclerosis (MS) is an autoimmune inflammatory disease of the central nervous system (CNS) where the communication ability of nerve cells in the brain and spinal cord with each other gets impaired [1]. One of the major pathological conditions underlying the development of MS is demyelination of the axons [2]. Some current findings suggest the role of glutamate excitotoxicity in the development and progression of MS. Glutamate is the major excitatory neurotransmitter of the central nervous system, which has been proven to have a central role in a complex communication network established between all residential brain cells [3]. This has been proved from the magnetic resonance spectroscopy studies of MS brains that showed elevated glutamate levels in acute MS lesions [4]. An excess release of glutamate leads to the activation of ionotropic and metabotropic receptors, thus resulting in accumulation of toxic cytoplasmic Ca^{2+} and cell death. However, one interesting finding in this context is that $GABA_A$ receptors located in the nerve terminals activate presynaptic Ca^{2+}/calmodulin-dependent signaling to inhibit depolarization-evoked Ca^{2+} influx and glutamate release from isolated nerve terminals [5], which suggest a potential implication of $GABA_A$ receptor in management of MS. Hence, preventing excitotoxic neuronal damage, by inhibition of glutamate release *via* GABAergic modulation, may serve as an effective approach for the treatment for MS.

This study was focused on evaluating the potential of selective $GABA_A$ receptor agonists or positive allosteric modulators and GABA level enhancers for management of MS in experimental animal models. In particular, diazepam, phenobarbitone sodium, and sodium valproate were screened for their activity in EAE model induced in female *Wistar* rats and cuprizone-induced MS model in C57BL/6 mice. Both diazepam and phenobarbitone sodium are positive allosteric modulators of $GABA_A$ whereas sodium valproate acts as GABA enhancer by inhibiting GABA transaminase that catabolizes GABA or blocks its reuptake into glia and nerve endings [6].

2. Materials and Methods

2.1. Materials. Diazepam, mitoxantrone HCl, and quetiapine fumarate were obtained as gift sample from Intas Pharmaceuticals, Ahmedabad, India. Sodium valproate was obtained as a gift sample from Chemclone Industries, Ahmedabad, India. Phenobarbitone sodium was purchased from Abbott India Ltd., Mumbai, India. Sodium chloride, potassium chloride, glucose, disodium hydrogen phosphate, potassium dihydrogen phosphate, hydrochloric acid, and glacial acetic acid were obtained from Qualigen Fine Chemicals, Mumbai, India. All the reagents and chemicals used for the study were of analytical grade. Paraformaldehyde, percoll, sucrose, disodium EDTA, Tris buffer, HEPES sodium salt, sodium bicarbonate, calcium chloride, magnesium chloride, 4-aminopyridine, glutamate, NAD^+ (oxidized form), cresyl violet acetate stain, and luxol fast blue stain were purchased from Himedia Laboratories Pvt. Ltd., Mumbai, India. Cuprizone, Complete Freund's Adjuvant (CFA), and L-glutamic acid dehydrogenase solution (bovine liver origin) were obtained from Sigma Aldrich, USA. Isoflurane (Raman and Weil Pvt. Ltd., Daman, India) was used for anesthetizing animals. Heparin was purchased from Biological E. Ltd, Hyderabad, India. Deionised water for HPLC was prepared in-house using a Milli-Q integral water purification system (Millipore Elix, Germany).

2.2. Animals. Female *Wistar* rats weighing 150–200 g and male C57BL/6 mice weighing 25 to 30 gm were obtained from the animal house of B. V. Patel PERD Centre, Ahmedabad. Animal housing and handling were performed in accordance with Good Laboratory Practice (GLP) mentioned in CPCSEA guidelines. The animal house is registered with the Committee for the Purpose of Control and Supervision of Experiments on Animals, Ministry of Social Justice and Empowerment, Government of India, vide registration number 1661/PO/a/12/CPCSEA. All experimental protocols were reviewed and accepted by the Institutional Animal Ethics Committee prior to initiation of the experiment.

2.3. Experimental Autoimmune Encephalomyelitis (EAE) Model in Rats

2.3.1. EAE Induction, Drug Treatment, and Clinical Scoring of the Symptoms. To induce EAE, spinal cord was isolated from female *Wistar* rats as previously described by Kennedy et al., 2011 [7]. However, transcardial perfusion of the rats was done according to the method described by Gage et al., 2012 [8], prior to isolation of the spinal cord. Following this, homogenate from the isolated rat spinal cord was prepared following the method reported by Shevach, 2001 [9], with certain modifications. Briefly, one gram of frozen rat spinal cord was homogenized at 13000 rpm on ice in 1 mL of 0.9% w/v NaCl (1:1 ratio) for 3 to 4 min. The homogenate was then emulsified in Complete Freund's Adjuvant by vortexing at high speed to give a final 1:2 (v/v) ratio of spinal cord to CFA (Note: it is very important to add the antigen to the adjuvant and not the other way round). The prepared final emulsion (50 μL) was then injected into each hind footpad (subplantar region) of each rat in all the groups except normal control. The animals were observed daily for weight changes and clinical signs of EAE according to the following scale: 0 = no disease; 0.5 = distal limp tail; 1.0 = flaccid tail; 2 = mild paraparesis; 3 = moderate paraparesis; 3.5 = one hind limb is paralyzed; 4 = weakness of forelimbs with paraparesis or paraplegia and/or atonic bladder; 5 = complete hind limb paralysis; 6 = quadriplegia, moribund state, or death [10].

However, prior to immunization with spinal cord homogenate, animals were divided into 6 different groups of 6 animals each: group I, nonimmunized controls received normal saline; group II (disease control group), immunized and then received normal saline intraperitoneally (vehicle for all the treatments); group III (positive control), immunized and then received mitoxantrone HCl (dose: 0.5 mg/kg body weight intraperitoneally); group IV, immunized and then received diazepam (dose: 2.0 mg/kg body weight intraperitoneally); group V, immunized and then received phenobarbitone sodium (dose: 30.0 mg/kg body weight intraperitoneally), and group VI, immunized and then received sodium valproate (dose: 200.0 mg/kg body weight intraperitoneally). Mitoxantrone was used as a positive control in this experiment as it has been currently approved by FDA for the treatment of MS and has also been reported for reducing the signs and severity of EAE in animals [11]. The doses of diazepam, phenobarbitone sodium, and sodium valproate were the same as those used in some previous reports for their CNS-related activities in rats [12–14]. All the drugs were administered once a day for a period of 21 days.

On day 22, all the animals were euthanized using excess isoflurane anesthesia. This was followed by preparation of cerebrocortical synaptosomes by discontinuous percoll gradient method and glutamate release assay was performed [15].

2.3.2. Preparation of Cerebrocortical Synaptosomes. The frontal cortex was isolated from all the animals and synaptosomes were purified on discontinuous percoll gradients as described previously [16]. Synaptosomes, which sediment between the 10% and 23% percoll bands, were collected and diluted in a final volume of 30 mL of HEPES buffer medium consisting of 140 mM NaCl, 5 mM KCl, 5 mM NaHCO$_3$, 1 mM MgCl$_2$, 1.2 mM Na$_2$HPO$_4$, 10 mM glucose, and 10 mM HEPES, pH 7.4. The resulting sample was then centrifuged at 27,000 ×g for 10 min at 4°C. The pellets formed were thus resuspended in 5 mL of HEPES buffer medium, and the protein content was determined using micro-BCA Protein Assay Reagent Kit (Pierce Cat #23235, Thermo Scientific, Rockford, IL, USA). Subsequently, the glutamate release assay was performed from the synaptosomal pellets. The pellets should be kept on ice and used within 3-4 h.

2.3.3. Glutamate Release Assay. Glutamate release from cerebrocortical synaptosomes was determined using an assay in which exogenous glutamate dehydrogenase and NADP$^+$ are used to couple the oxidative decarboxylation of the released glutamate. This results in the generation of NADPH which was then detected fluorimetrically [17]. Synaptosomal pellets were resuspended in HEPES buffer medium and incubated at 37°C for 3-4 min to facilitate polarization of the plasma membrane. Subsequently, 1 mM NADP$^+$, 50 units/mL glutamate dehydrogenase, and 1.2 mM CaCl$_2$ were added. The resulting sample was then incubated for 5 min, following which 3 mM 4-AP (4-amino pyridine) was added to stimulate the glutamate release. Fluorescence was then measured using spectrofluorometer (SL174, Systronics India Ltd.) at excitation and emission wavelengths of 359 nm and 468 nm, respectively. Data points were obtained at 10 sec intervals. 4-AP (potassium channel blocker) was used in this study to destabilize the plasma membrane potential of the synaptosomes, which subsequently results in an increase in the cytoplasmic free Ca^{2+} concentration through the opening of voltage-gated Ca^{2+} channels. Finally, this leads to generation of spontaneous action potentials which are capable of triggering the exocytotic release of glutamate [15].

2.4. Cuprizone-Induced Demyelination in Mice

2.4.1. Model Development and Treatment. Thirty-six male C57BL/6 mice ($n = 6$) were used in the study. Experimental group, route of administration, and treatment protocol were the same as those of EAE model. However, the doses of the drugs were as follows: diazepam, 1.0 mg/kg body weight; phenobarbitone, 20.0 mg/kg body weight; and sodium valproate, 150.0 mg/kg body weight. The doses of diazepam, phenobarbitone sodium, and sodium valproate were the same as those used in some previous reports for their CNS-related activities in mice [13, 18, 19]. Acute demyelination was induced by feeding the animals a diet containing 0.2% cuprizone (bis(cyclohexanone)oxaldihydrazone) mixed into a ground standard rodent chow *ad libitum* for a period of 4 weeks. The food was freshly prepared as cuprizone is an unstable compound. Control animals received normal pellet diet. Diazepam, phenobarbitone sodium, and sodium valproate were administered daily for 28 days starting from the same day as of cuprizone treatment. Quetiapine fumarate (dose: 10 mg/kg bodyweight) was used as a positive control since it has been reported that chronic administration of

quetiapine attenuates myelin breakdown in the cerebral cortex of cuprizone-exposed mice [20]. All the drugs were administered once a day for a period of 28 days.

2.4.2. Tissue Preparation, Staining, and Microscopy. On day 29, tissue evaluation was performed. All the animals were anaesthetized using isoflurane anaesthesia and perfused transcardially with 10 U/mL heparin in phosphate buffer saline (pH 7.4) followed by 4% w/v paraformaldehyde. The brains were isolated and 5 μm sectioning of the coronal sections was done using a rotary microtome (Model 0126, Yorco, India). The slides were then stained with luxol fast blue and incubated overnight at 60°C followed by secondary staining with cresyl violet acetate for 5 min. Tissue sections were observed for all possible changes in the anatomy under Olympus IX51 optical microscope (Olympus Optical Co. Ltd., Tokyo, Japan). The photographs were taken with an Olympus TL4 camera. The observations were compared to detect the extent of demyelination.

3. Results

3.1. Clinical Scoring of the Symptoms in EAE Model. The clinical symptoms of EAE in different animal groups are shown in Figure 1. The clinical scores for the phenobarbitone sodium and sodium valproate treated animals were significantly less ($P \leq 0.05$) as compared to the diseased group animals. Moreover, the inhibition pattern of clinical symptoms of the above mentioned treatment groups was similar to positive control group. However, no significant inhibition of EAE symptoms was found in the diazepam treated animals as compared to the disease control group, indicating that it may not be effective in preventing the disease progression.

3.2. Glutamate Release Assay in EAE Model. The amount of glutamate released (nmol/mg protein) at different time intervals from the synaptosomes of animals of all the groups is shown in Figure 2. The results showed an excessive release of glutamate from the synaptosomes of the diseased control group (indicating the occurrence of glutamate excitotoxicity) whereas the levels of glutamate released from the synaptosomes of the animals of normal control and positive control groups were significantly low ($P \leq 0.05$). However, no significant difference was observed in the glutamate release profiles of the animals treated with diazepam and phenobarbitone when compared to the diseased control group. This indicates that they did not produce any inhibition of glutamate release. Sodium valproate treated animals showed a glutamate release profile much similar to that of normal and positive control groups and was also significantly different ($P \leq 0.05$) as compared to the diseased animals.

3.3. Histological Observation in Cuprizone-Induced Demyelination in Mice. Luxol fast blue stained coronal sections observed under 40x magnification are shown in Figure 3 where myelinated axons were stained blue while nonmyelinated axons were stained pink. The confirmation of successful

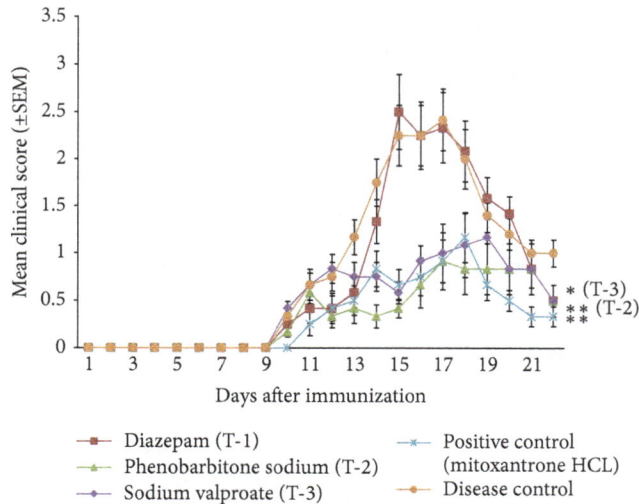

FIGURE 1: Changes in neurological/clinical signs of EAE with days after immunization. Significant difference was found in the mean clinical scores (±SEM), [n = 6] of animals of phenobarbitone (T-2) and sodium valproate (T-3) groups as compared to the diseased control group, [$^*P \leq 0.05$ by one way ANOVA (Dunnett's multiple comparisons test)].

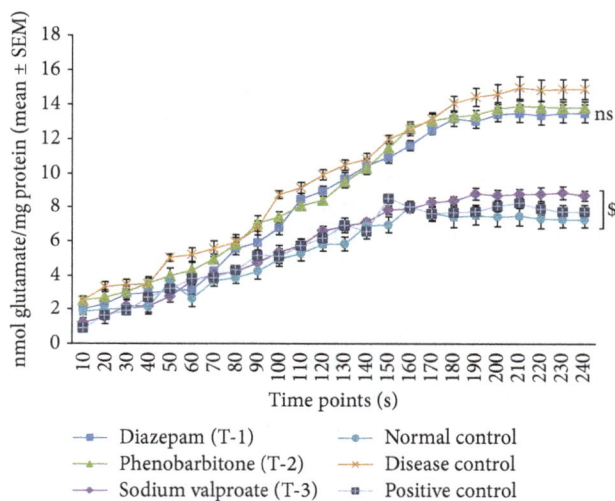

FIGURE 2: Glutamate released from the synaptosomes at different time points detected fluorimetrically. Diazepam and phenobarbitone did not show any inhibition in the glutamate release. Glutamate release from the synaptosomes of the animals of sodium valproate group (T-3) group was significantly lower than the diseased control group [n = 6], [$^*P \leq 0.05$ by one way ANOVA (Dunnett's multiple comparisons test)]. * indicates that the observed neurological/clinical signs of EAE in animals of T-2 and T-3 group were significantly different ($P \leq 0.05$) from that of disease control animals.

model development was confirmed from prominent demyelination in the region of corpus callosum of diseased control group. However, tissue sections of normal and positive control animals showed blue colored bands which indicate the presence of myelinated axons. In this experiment, it was observed that sodium valproate inhibited demyelination, as

majority of the axons in corpus callosum stained blue while few others stained pink. However, phenobarbitone showed moderate protection against cuprizone-induced demyelination (thin and less intense bands of blue colored myelinated fibers in the sections). The images revealed a prompt demyelination in the diazepam treated animals, thus indicating that diazepam was not able to inhibit demyelination induced by cuprizone.

4. Discussion

Previous studies have shown that the concentration of GABA and the glutamate decarboxylase activity in blood are reduced in EAE and MS [21, 22]. Based on these findings, an attempt was made to explore the potential of selective $GABA_A$ receptor agonists or positive allosteric modulators and GABA level enhancers for treatment of MS. In the present study, diazepam, phenobarbitone sodium, and sodium valproate were screened for their activity against MS in EAE model in rats and cuprizone-induced demyelination model in mice. In context to the EAE model, it was observed that phenobarbitone sodium and sodium valproate inhibited the clinical symptoms of EAE; however, diazepam failed to control these EAE symptoms. Although both diazepam and phenobarbitone are positive allosteric modulators of the $GABA_A$ receptors, the probable reason for the difference in their observed activity may be the difference in their binding sites [23]. Phenobarbitone sodium and diazepam acts independently, by binding to the beta subunit and benzodiazepine binding site of $GABA_A$ receptor, respectively. Diazepam has only GABA facilitatory action whereas phenobarbitone has GABA facilitatory as well as GABA mimetic effect [23]. This means that it not only enhances the action of GABA but also causes opening of the Cl^- ion channels. Moreover, phenobarbitone also blocks calcium channels, thus resulting in inhibition of excitatory transmitter release. Sodium valproate is an inhibitor of GABA transaminase and increases GABA levels which may be responsible for inhibition of glutamate excitotoxicity and hence demyelination in EAE animals.

However, in context to the glutamate release assay, sodium valproate was found to be the most effective amongst all the three drugs. It significantly inhibited both clinical signs and glutamate release which may be attributed to its ability to enhance the inhibitory effect of GABA on glutamate release and thus preventing glutamate excitotoxicity. It was observed that although phenobarbitone inhibited the clinical signs of EAE, it failed to inhibit glutamate release. Although the reason for this finding is still unclear, it may be presumed that some other pathway is involved in its mechanism of action.

In the cuprizone-induced demyelination in C57BL/6 mice, it was observed that diazepam did not produce any inhibition of demyelination while sodium valproate inhibited demyelination to good extent which was comparable with that of positive control. The animals treated with phenobarbitone sodium showed moderate inhibition of demyelination.

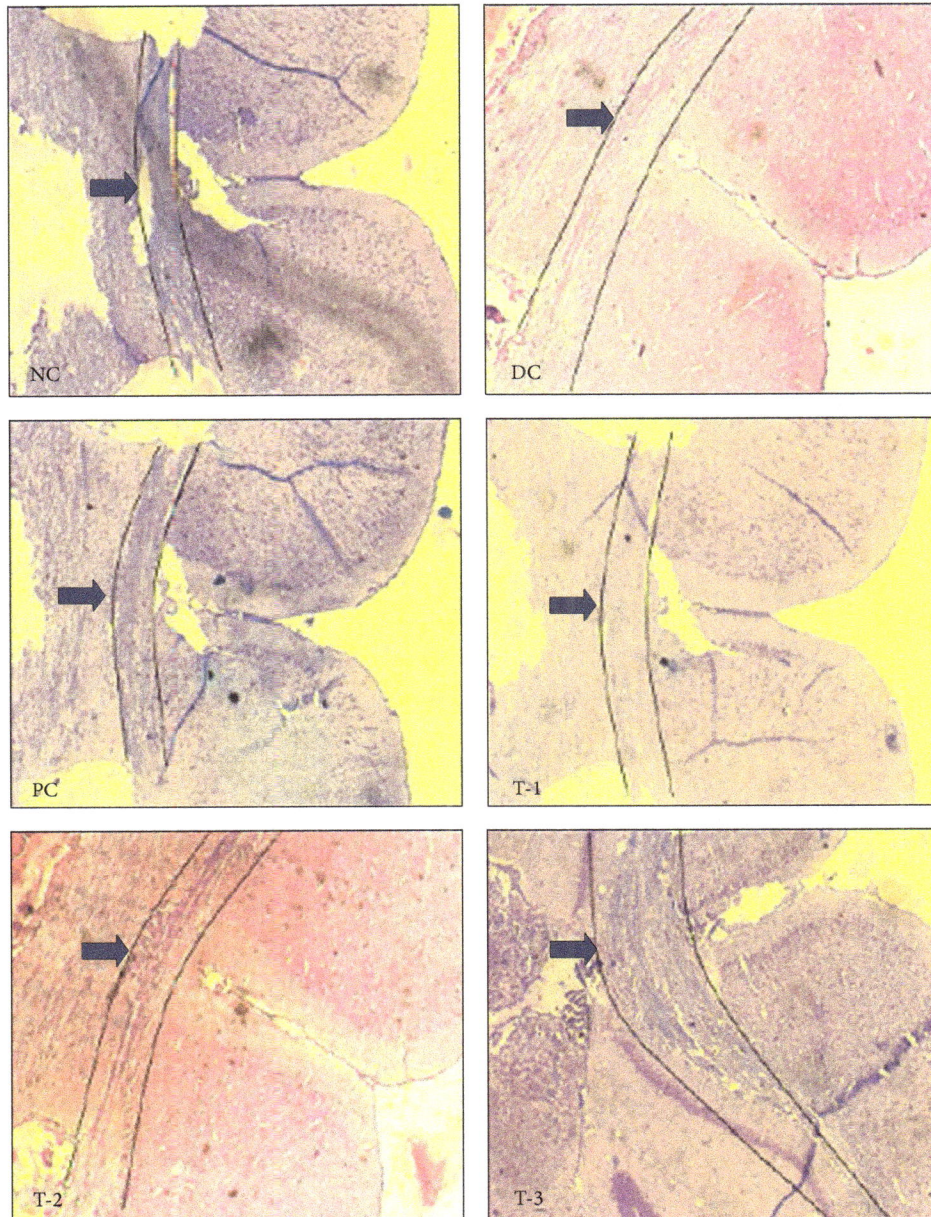

FIGURE 3: Luxol fast blue stained coronal sections of C57BL/6 mice brains observed under 40x magnification. The region of corpus callosum is highlighted and indicated by the arrow. Blue colour indicates presence of myelin. (NC: normal control; DC: disease control; PC: positive control; T-1: diazepam treatment; T-2: phenobarbitone sodium treatment; T-3: sodium valproate treatment.)

Cuprizone induces alterations of mitochondrial morphology and it is also speculated that the neurotoxic properties of this copper-chelating compound are due to a disturbance of cellular respiration which is a key function of mitochondria. Moreover, it appears that the activity of a set of enzymes is disturbed prior to myelin loss during the first days or weeks of cuprizone exposure [24]. However, no reports are available with respect to the activity of sodium valproate and phenobarbitone sodium on cellular response of mitochondria. Thus, further mechanistic studies are required to understand the exact reason underlying these findings and elucidate the pathway by which these drugs showed their pharmacological activity in this model.

5. Conclusion

The findings of this study indicate that sodium valproate may serve as a potential drug for management of MS. However, this is only a preliminary finding and further extensive studies are required in this context. Moreover, new drug candidates selectively acting by GABAergic system may be designed and screened for their activity against MS.

Conflict of Interests

The authors declare that they have no conflict of interests to disclose.

Acknowledgments

The authors wish to acknowledge NIPER, Ahmedabad, Submission No. NIPERA330913, for providing all the facilities to carry out this work; Intas Pharmaceuticals, Ahmedabad, India, for providing diazepam, mitoxantrone HCl, and quetiapine fumarate as gift samples; and Chemclone Industries, Ahmedabad, India, for providing sodium valproate as gift sample.

References

[1] A. Compston and A. Coles, "Multiple sclerosis," *The Lancet*, vol. 359, no. 9313, pp. 1221–1231, 2002.

[2] A. Compston and A. Coles, "Multiple sclerosis," *The Lancet*, vol. 372, no. 9648, pp. 1502–1517, 2008.

[3] S. A. Lipton and P. A. Rosenberg, "Excitatory amino acids as a final common pathway for neurologic disorders," *The New England Journal of Medicine*, vol. 330, no. 9, pp. 613–622, 1994.

[4] R. Srinivasan, N. Sailasuta, R. Hurd, S. Nelson, and D. Pelletier, "Evidence of elevated glutamate in multiple sclerosis using magnetic resonance spectroscopy at 3T," *Brain*, vol. 128, no. 5, pp. 1016–1025, 2005.

[5] P. Long, A. Mercer, R. Begum, G. J. Stephens, T. S. Sihra, and J. N. Jovanovic, "Nerve terminal GABAA receptors activate Ca^{2+} / calmodulin-dependent signaling to inhibit voltage-gated Ca^{2+} influx and glutamate release," *The Journal of Biological Chemistry*, vol. 284, no. 13, pp. 8726–8737, 2009.

[6] J. Lazo, K. Parker, and L. Bruton, *Goodman and Gilman's: The Pharmacological Basis of Therapeutics*, McGraw-Hill, New York, NY, USA, 10th edition, 2007.

[7] H. S. Kennedy, F. Puth, M. Van Hoy, and C. Le Pichon, "A method for removing the brain and spinal cord as one unit from adult mice and rats," *Lab Animal*, vol. 40, no. 2, pp. 53–57, 2011.

[8] G. J. Gage, D. R. Kipke, and W. Shain, "Whole animal perfusion fixation for rodents," *Journal of Visualized Experimentation*, no. 65, Article ID e3564, 2012.

[9] E. M. Shevach, "Animal models for autoimmune and inflammatory disease," in *Current Protocols in Immunology*, pp. 15.2.1–15.2.4, John Wiley & Sons, Oxford, UK, 2001.

[10] C. Beeton, A. Garcia, and A. G. Chandy, "Induction and clinical scoring of chronic-relapsing experimental autoimmune encephalomyelitis," *Journal of Visualized Experiments*, no. 5, article e224, 2007.

[11] S. C. Ridge, A. E. Sloboda, and R. A. McReynolds, "Suppression of experimental allergic encephalomyelitis by mitoxantrone," *Clinical Immunology and Immunopathology*, vol. 35, no. 1, pp. 35–42, 1985.

[12] R. Farooq, D. J. Haleem, and M. A. Haleem, "Dose related anxiolytic effects of diazepam: relation with serum electrolytes, plasma osmolality and Systolic Blood Pressure (SBP) in rats," in *Pakistan Journal of Pharmacology*, vol. 25, pp. 37–42, 2008.

[13] W. Loscher and D. Honack, "Comparison of the anticonvulsant efficacy of primidone and phenobarbital during chronic treatment of amygdala-kindled rats," *European Journal of Pharmacology*, vol. 162, no. 2, pp. 309–322, 1989.

[14] F. Bosetti, J. M. Bell, and P. Manickam, "Microarray analysis of rat brain gene expression after chronic administration of sodium valproate," *Brain Research Bulletin*, vol. 65, no. 4, pp. 331–338, 2005.

[15] M. P. Cid, A. A. Vilcaes, L. L. Rupil, N. A. Salvatierra, and G. A. Roth, "Participation of the GABAergic system on the glutamate release of frontal cortex synaptosomes from Wistar rats with experimental autoimmune encephalomyelitis," *Neuroscience*, vol. 189, pp. 337–344, 2011.

[16] P. R. Dunkley, J. W. Heath, S. M. Harrison, P. E. Jarvie, P. J. Glenfield, and J. A. P. Rostas, "A rapid Percoll gradient procedure for isolation of synaptosomes directly from an S1 fraction: homogeneity and morphology of subcellular fractions," *Brain Research*, vol. 441, no. 1-2, pp. 59–71, 1988.

[17] A. A. Vilcaes, G. Furlan, and G. A. Roth, "Inhibition of Ca^{2+}-dependent glutamate release from cerebral cortex synaptosomes of rats with experimental autoimmune encephalomyelitis," *Journal of Neurochemistry*, vol. 108, no. 4, pp. 881–890, 2009.

[18] S. E. File and L. J. Wilks, "Effects of sodium phenobarbital on motor activity and exploration in the mouse: development of tolerance and incidence of withdrawal responses," *Pharmacology Biochemistry and Behavior*, vol. 35, no. 2, pp. 317–320, 1990.

[19] A. K. Rehni and N. Singh, "Reversal of pentylenetetrazole-induced seizure activity in mice by nickel chloride," *Indian Journal of Pharmacology*, vol. 41, no. 1, pp. 15–18, 2009.

[20] Y. Zhang, H. Xu, W. Jiang et al., "Quetiapine alleviates the cuprizone-induced white matter pathology in the brain of C57BL/6 mouse," *Schizophrenia Research*, vol. 106, no. 2-3, pp. 182–191, 2008.

[21] Z. Gottesfeld, D. Teitelbaum, C. Webb, and R. Arnon, "Changes in the GABA system in experimental allergic encephalomyelitis induced paralysis," *Journal of Neurochemistry*, vol. 27, no. 3, pp. 695–699, 1976.

[22] E. V. Demakova, V. P. Korobov, and L. M. Lemkina, "Determination of gamma-aminobutyric acid concentration and activity of glutamate decarboxylase in blood serum of patients with multiple sclerosis," *Klinicheskaia Laboratornaia Diagnostika*, no. 4, pp. 15–17, 2003.

[23] R. E. Twyman, C. J. Rogers, and R. L. Macdonald, "Differential regulation of γ-aminobutyric acid receptor channels by diazepam and phenobarbital," *Annals of Neurology*, vol. 25, no. 3, pp. 213–220, 1989.

[24] S. Arnold and C. Beyer, "Neuroprotection by estrogen in the brain: the mitochondrial compartment as presumed therapeutic target," *Journal of Neurochemistry*, vol. 110, no. 1, pp. 1–11, 2009.

24

Effects of Methanol Extract of Breadfruit (*Artocarpus altilis*) on Atherogenic Indices and Redox Status of Cellular System of Hypercholesterolemic Male Rats

Oluwatosin Adekunle Adaramoye and Olubukola Oyebimpe Akanni

Drug Metabolism and Toxicology Research Laboratories, Department of Biochemistry, College of Medicine, University of Ibadan, Ibadan 20005, Nigeria

Correspondence should be addressed to Oluwatosin Adekunle Adaramoye; aoadaramoye@yahoo.com

Academic Editor: Neal Davies

We investigated the effects of methanol extract of *Artocarpus altilis* (AA) on atherogenic indices and redox status of cellular system of rats fed with dietary cholesterol while Questran (QUE) served as standard. Biochemical indices such as total cholesterol (TC), triglycerides (TG), low- and high-density lipoproteins-cholesterol (LDL-C and HDL-C), aspartate and alanine aminotransferases (AST and ALT), lactate dehydrogenase (LDH), reduced glutathione, glutathione-s-transferase, glutathione peroxidase (GPx), catalase (CAT), superoxide dismutase (SOD), and lipid peroxidation (LPO) were assessed. Hypercholesterolemic (HC) rats had significantly increased relative weight of liver and heart. Dietary cholesterol caused a significant increase ($P < 0.05$) in the levels of serum, hepatic, and cardiac TC by 110%, 70%, and 85%, LDL-C by 79%, 82%, and 176%, and TG by 68%, 96%, and 62%, respectively. Treatment with AA significantly reduced the relative weight of the organs and lipid parameters. There were beneficial increases in serum and cardiac HDL-C levels in HC rats treated with AA. In HC rats, serum LDH, ALT, and AST activities and levels of LPO were increased, whereas hepatic and cardiac SOD, CAT, and GPx were reduced. All biochemical and histological alterations were ameliorated upon treatment with AA. Extract of AA had protective effects against dietary cholesterol-induced hypercholesterolemia.

1. Introduction

Recent studies have demonstrated that increased formation of free radicals/reactive oxygen species (ROS) contributes to cardiovascular disease (CVD) progression [1]. Generation of large amounts of ROS can overwhelm the intracellular antioxidant defense, causing lipid peroxidation, protein modification, and DNA breaks [2]. It is known that ROS-induced depletion of antioxidants is a key factor for the initiation of atherosclerosis and the development of CVD [3]. Hypercholesterolemia, characterized by the presence of high levels of cholesterol in the blood [4], is a form of hyperlipidemia and hyperlipoproteinemia. Hyperlipidemia has also been found to induce oxidative stress in various organs of the body [5]. Although several factors, such as life style, a diet rich in cholesterol, and age, have been reported to cause heart failure [6, 7], high levels of cholesterol, particularly LDL-cholesterol, are mainly responsible for hypercholesterolemia [8]. Drugs that lower cholesterol such as fibrates and bile acid sequestrants were used for several decades, but the high prevalence of adverse effects led to the introduction of statins (HMG-CoA inhibitors) [9]. Although the adverse effect of statins is relatively low, one rare effect called rhabdomyolysis can be very serious with statins [9]. In view of these adverse effects, the quest for natural products with hypolipidemic potential and minimal side effect is warranted.

Breadfruit (*Artocarpus altilis*) is a flowering tree in the mulberry family. The fruit can be eaten once cooked or can be further processed into a variety of other foods. It is an excellent source of fiber, calcium, copper, iron, magnesium, potassium, thiamine, niacin, carbohydrates, and vitamins and very low in fat [10]. In herbal homes, leaves of this plant are used for the treatment of liver disorders, hypertension, and diabetes [11, 12]. *In vitro* studies by Nwokocha et al. [13] supported the folkloric use of this plant. However, little information is available with respect to *in vivo* studies on its ethnomedicinal uses. This study was designed to evaluate the effects of *Artocarpus altilis* on atherogenic indices and redox status of cellular system of hypercholesterolemic rats.

2. Materials and Methods

2.1. Chemicals. Questran (Bristol-Myers Squibb, Hounslow, UK) was purchased from a local chemist in Ibadan, Nigeria. Dietary cholesterol and thiobarbituric acid (TBA) were procured from Aldrich Chemical Co. (Milwaukee, WI, USA). Glutathione, hydrogen peroxide, 5,5′-dithio-bis-2-nitrobenzoic acid (DNTB), and epinephrine were purchased from Sigma Chemical Co., Saint Louis, MO, USA. Trichloroacetic acid (TCA) and thiobarbituric acid (TBA) were purchased from British Drug House (BDH) Chemical Ltd., Poole, UK. Other reagents were of analytical grade and the purest quality available.

2.2. Collection and Extraction of Artocarpus altilis. The stem bark of *Artocarpus altilis* was collected in Ibadan (Oyo State) and authenticated at the Botanical Garden of the University of Ibadan. The stem bark of *Artocarpus altilis* was air-dried and crushed into fine powder. The powdered part was extracted with n-hexane and methanol using soxhlet extractor and the extract was concentrated in vacuum at 40°C with rotary evaporator and water bath to dryness. The yield of the extraction was 5.7%.

2.3. Determination of Total Phenolic Contents. The total phenolic content of the extract was determined using the method of Singleton et al. [14] with slight modifications. Folin-C reagent (1 mL) was added to 1 mL of extract or standard. After 3 minutes, 1 mL of 15% Na_2CO_3 was added and the solution was made up to 5 mL with distilled water. The reaction mixture was kept in the dark for 90 minutes with intermittent shaking or placed in a water bath at 40°C for 20 minutes. The absorbance was measured by a Beckman DU (70) Spectrophotometer at 760 nm. All experiments were done in triplicate. A standard curve was plotted with catechin and the phenolic content expressed as CE (catechin equivalent) per mg dry weight of the extract.

2.3.1. DPPH—Radical Scavenging Activity. The radical scavenging activity of the extract was measured as described by Mensor et al. [15]. The stable 2,2-diphenyl-1-picrylhydrazyl (DPPH) radical was used for the determination of free radical scavenging activities of the extracts. A portion (1 mL) of each of the different concentrations (10–1000 μg/mL) of the extracts or standard (catechin) was added to 1 mL of 1 mM DPPH in methanol. The mixtures were vortexed and incubated in a dark chamber for 30 minutes after which the absorbance was measured at 517 nm against a DPPH control containing only 1 mL of methanol in place of the extract. All

calculations were carried out in triplicates. The inhibition of DPPH was calculated as a percentage using the expression

$$I\% = \frac{A_{\text{control}} - A_{\text{sample}}}{A_{\text{control}}} \times 100, \qquad (1)$$

where $I\%$ is the percentage inhibition of the DPPH radical, A_{control} is the absorbance of the control, and A_{sample} is the absorbance of the test compound.

2.4. Animals. Inbred male Wistar rats weighing between 150 and 180 g were purchased from the animal house of the Department of Veterinary Physiology, Biochemistry, and Pharmacology, University of Ibadan, Nigeria. Animals were kept in ventilated cages at room temperature (28–30°C) and maintained on normal laboratory chow (Ladokun Feeds, Ibadan, Nigeria) and water *ad libitum*. Rats handling and treatments conform to guidelines of the National Institute of Health (NIH publication 85-23, 1985) for laboratory animal care and use. The study was approved by the Faculty of Basic Medical Sciences, University of Ibadan Animal Ethics Committee.

2.5. Study Design. Thirty-five male rats were randomly divided into seven groups of five rats each. The first group (control) received drug vehicle (corn oil), the second group (HC) received dietary cholesterol at 30 mg/0.3 mL [16], the third group (HC + AA1) received dietary cholesterol and *Artocarpus altilis* (100 mg/kg), the fourth group (HC + AA2) received dietary cholesterol and *Artocarpus altilis* (200 mg/kg), the fifth group (HC + QUE) received dietary cholesterol and Questran (0.26 g/kg) [16], the sixth group (QUE) received questran alone, and the seventh group (AA) received *Artocarpus altilis* at a dose of 200 mg/kg body weight.

2.6. Preparation of Tissues. Rats were fasted overnight and sacrificed 24 hours after the last dose of drugs. Liver and heart were quickly removed and washed in ice-cold 1.15% KCl solution, dried, and weighed. A section of liver and aorta samples were fixed in 10% formalin for histological examination. The remaining parts of liver and heart were homogenized in 4 volumes of 50 mM phosphate buffer, pH 7.4, and centrifuged at 10,000 g for 15 minutes to obtain post-mitochondrial supernatant fraction (PMF). All procedures were carried out at temperature of 0–4°C.

2.6.1. Preparation of Serum. Blood was collected from the heart of the animals into plain centrifuge tubes and was allowed to stand for 1 hour. Serum was prepared by centrifugation at 3,000 g for 15 minutes in a Beckman bench centrifuge. The clear supernatant was used for the estimation of serum lipid profile and enzymes.

2.7. Biochemical Assays. Protein contents of the samples were assayed by the method of Lowry et al. [17] using bovine serum albumin as standard. The activities of alanine and aspartate aminotransferases (ALT and AST) were assayed by the combined methods of Mohun and Cook [18] and Reitman

TABLE 1: Changes in the body weight and relative weight of organs of hypercholesterolemic rats treated with methanol extract of *Artocarpus altilis* for nine weeks.

Treatment	Body weight (g)		Weight of organs (g)			Relative weight of organs		
	Initial	Final	Liver	Kidney	Heart	Liver	Kidney	Heart
Control	151.00 ± 4.94	194.00 ± 23.02	5.38 ± 0.49	1.03 ± 0.11	0.53 ± 0.09	2.77 ± 0.75	0.53 ± 0.05	0.27 ± 0.04
HC	160.00 ± 3.10	198.00 ± 29.03	6.89 ± 0.89	1.09 ± 0.14	0.69 ± 0.06	$3.48 \pm 0.23^*$	0.55 ± 0.03	$0.39 \pm 0.02^*$
HC + AA1	159.00 ± 5.48	196.00 ± 37.15	5.12 ± 1.22	1.09 ± 0.20	0.55 ± 0.08	$2.61 \pm 0.13^{**}$	0.56 ± 0.04	$0.28 \pm 0.03^{**}$
HC + AA2	167.00 ± 6.04	185.00 ± 45.00	5.20 ± 1.24	1.09 ± 0.20	0.52 ± 0.09	$2.81 \pm 0.15^{**}$	0.59 ± 0.06	$0.28 \pm 0.04^{**}$
HC + QUE	173.00 ± 4.74	202.50 ± 5.00	5.39 ± 1.05	1.19 ± 0.07	0.55 ± 0.01	$2.66 \pm 0.43^{**}$	0.59 ± 0.05	$0.27 \pm 0.01^{**}$
QUE	188.00 ± 3.95	225.00 ± 20.41	5.06 ± 1.21	1.17 ± 0.05	0.51 ± 0.49	2.24 ± 0.41	0.52 ± 0.07	0.23 ± 0.04
AA2	192.00 ± 8.34	235.00 ± 22.36	5.19 ± 0.55	1.21 ± 0.11	0.62 ± 0.06	2.21 ± 0.17	0.52 ± 0.04	0.26 ± 0.03

Values are means ± SD of 5 animals per group; HC: cholesterol at 30 mg/0.3 mL.
AA1: *Artocarpus altilis* at 100 mg/kg, AA2: *Artocarpus altilis* at 200 mg/kg, and QUE: Questran at 0.26 g/kg.
*Significantly different from control ($P < 0.05$), **significantly different from HC ($P < 0.05$).

and Frankel [19]. Serum total cholesterol level was assayed by the method of Richmond [20]. The method involved enzymatic hydrolysis and oxidation of cholesterol with the formation of quinoneimine (an indicator) from hydrogen peroxide and 4-aminoantipyrine in the presence of phenol and peroxide. The serum level of triglyceride was determined by Jacobs and van Demark [21] and Koditschek and Umbreit [22]; this was based on the hydrolysis of triglycerides with the formation of glycerol which is substrate for other enzymes with the subsequent formation of hydrogen peroxide. This then reacts with 4-aminophenazone and 4-chlorophenol in the presence of peroxidase to give quinoneimine which is measured spectrophotometrically at 500 nm.

The lipoproteins (measured using the enzymatic colorimetric method), very low-density lipoprotein (VLDL) and low-density lipoprotein (LDL), were precipitated by the addition of phosphotungstic acid and magnesium chloride. After centrifugation at 3,000 g for 10 minutes at 25°C, the clear supernatant contained HDL fraction, which was assayed for cholesterol with the Randox diagnostic kit. The low-density lipoprotein (LDL) was calculated using the formula of Friedewald et al. [23]. Lipid peroxidation level was assayed by the reaction between 2-thiobarbituric acid (TBA) and malondialdehyde (MDA), an end product of lipid peroxides as described by Buege and Aust [24].

The activity of lactate dehydrogenase (LDH) was determined by the method of Zimmerman and Weinstein [25], while tissue superoxide dismutase (SOD) activity was measured by the nitro blue tetrazolium (NBT) reduction method of McCord and Fridovich [26]. Catalase (CAT) activity was assayed spectrophotometrically by measuring the rate of decomposition of hydrogen peroxide at 240 nm as described by Aebi [27]. Reduced glutathione level was measured by the method of Beutler et al. [28]; this method is based on the development of a relatively stable (yellow) colour when 5',5'-dithiobis-(2-nitrobenzoic acid) (Ellman's reagent) is added to sulfhydryl compounds. The chromophoric product resulting from the reaction of Ellman's reagent with the reduced glutathione (2-nitro-5-thiobenzoic acid) possesses a molar absorption at 412 nm which is proportion to the level of reduced glutathione in the test sample. The glutathione peroxidase (GPx) activity was assessed by the method of Rotruck

et al. [29], while glutathione-S-transferase (GST) activity was determined according to Habig et al. [30]; the principle is based on the fact that all of known GST demonstrates a relatively high activity with 1-chloro-2,4-dinitrobenzene as the second substrate. When this substance is conjugated with reduced glutathione, its absorption maximum shifts to a longer wavelength 340 nm and the absorption increase at this wavelength provides a direct measurement of the enzymatic reaction.

2.7.1. Determination of Antiatherogenic, Cardioprotective, and Coronary Risk Indices. Cardioprotective index (CPI) was estimated in terms of HDL-C to LDL-C ratio [31, 32], whereas antiatherogenic (AAI) and coronary risk indices (CRI) were calculated by the following formulae [33, 34]:

$$
AAI = 100 \times \frac{[\text{HDL-C}]}{[\text{Total cholesterol} - \text{HDL-C}]},
$$
$$
CRI = \frac{\text{Total cholesterol}}{\text{HDL-cholesterol}}. \tag{2}
$$

2.8. Histopathology of Tissues. Tissues fixed in 10% formalin were dehydrated in 95% ethanol and then cleared in xylene before embedded in paraffin. Microsections (about 4 μm) were prepared and stained with haematoxylin and eosin (H&E) dye and were examined under a light microscope by a histopathologist who was ignorant of the treatment groups.

2.9. Statistical Analysis. All values were expressed as the mean ± SD of five animals per group. Data were analyzed using one-way ANOVA followed by the post hoc Duncan multiple range test for analysis of biochemical data using SPSS (10.0). Values were considered statistically significant at $P < 0.05$.

3. Results

3.1. Phenolic and Flavonoids Contents and Effects of Artocarpus altilis on Body Weight and Relative Weight of Organs of Hypercholesterolemic (HC) Rats. In Table 1, there were significant increases ($P < 0.05$) in the relative weight of liver

TABLE 2: The total phenolic contents and scavenging activity of *Artocarpus altilis* on 2,2-diphenyl-1-picrylhydrazyl radical (DPPH) *in vitro*.

Conc.	% Scavenging activity		Phenolic content
(μg/mL)	Catechin	AA	(μg CE/mg)
100	42.2 ± 4.4	22.7 ± 5.9	0.18 ± 0.02
300	47.6 ± 1.6	50.4 ± 3.1	0.39 ± 0.03
500	63.1 ± 5.1	51.1 ± 2.3	0.52 ± 0.07
750	67.8 ± 3.9	62.5 ± 8.5	0.68 ± 0.05

Data are expressed as mean ± SD ($n = 4$).
AA: *Artocarpus altilis*.

and heart of HC rats when compared with the control, while treatment with AA (100 and 200 mg/kg) significantly reduced the relative weight of heart and liver of HC rats to values that were statistically similar ($P > 0.05$) to the control. Similar reduction was obtained in questran-treated HC rats. The total phenolic contents (TPC) of AA expressed in μg catechin equivalent per mg dry weight of the extract increased with increase in concentration (Table 2). At 750 μg/mL, the TPC of AA was 0.68 ± 0.05 μg CE/mg. There were significant ($P < 0.05$) and dose-dependent increases in scavenging activity of AA on DPPH radicals (Table 2). At 100 μg/mL and 750 μg/mL, the percentage DPPH radical scavenging activities of AA were 42.2% and 67.8%, respectively.

3.2. Effects of Artocarpus altilis on Antioxidant Parameters and Marker Enzymes in Hypercholesterolemic (HC) Rats.

Administration of dietary cholesterol significantly increased ($P < 0.05$) serum, hepatic, and cardiac lipid peroxidation (LPO) products measured as thiobarbituric acid reactive substances (TBARS) by 265%, 83%, and 80%, respectively (Table 3). However, treatment with AA completely ameliorated dietary cholesterol-induced increase in LPO. In HC rats, the activities of hepatic, and cardiac SOD and CAT as well as cardiac GPx decreased significantly relative to the control (Table 4). Specifically, hepatic SOD and CAT decreased by 54% and 45%, while cardiac SOD, CAT, and GPx decreased by 67%, 59%, and 36%, respectively. Also, activities of phase II and antioxidant enzyme (GST) in the liver of HC rats were significantly reduced when compared to controls (Figure 5). Administration of AA (200 mg/kg) reversed the adverse effect of high dietary cholesterol by normalizing these enzymic antioxidant indices. In HC rats, serum ALT, AST and LDH were significantly increased by 2.3-, 1.7-, and 2.4-fold, respectively, while cardiac LDH activity was decreased by 3.0-fold relative to controls (Table 5 and Figures 3 and 4). However, the observed elevations in the activities of these serum enzymes in HC rats were reversed following treatment with AA and quetsran.

3.3. Effects of Artocarpus altilis on the Lipid Profile of Hypercholesterolemic Rats.

Feeding rats on high dietary cholesterol for nine consecutive weeks significantly ($P < 0.05$) increased the serum, hepatic, and cardiac total cholesterol levels by 110%, 70%, and 85%, respectively (Table 6 and Figures 1 and 2). Furthermore, serum, hepatic, and cardiac triglycerides increased by 68%, 96%, and 62%, while serum LDL-C

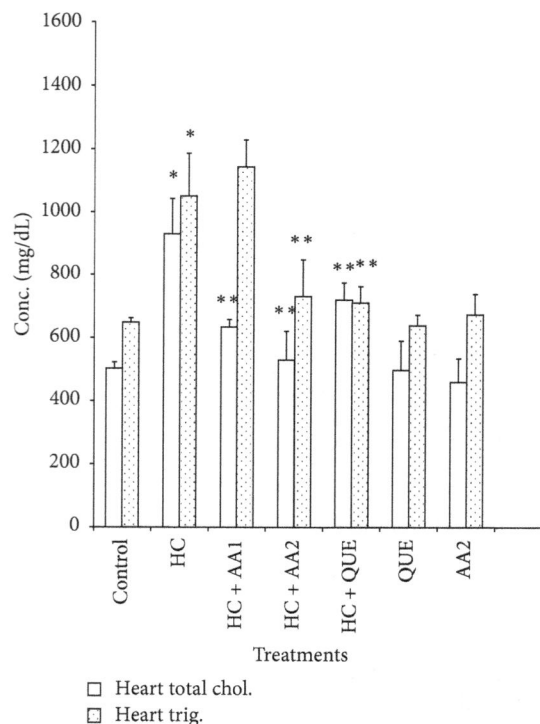

FIGURE 1: Effects of methanol extract of *Artocarpus altilis* and Questran on cardiac total cholesterol and triglyceride levels of hypercholesterolemic rats. *Significantly different from control ($P < 0.05$), **significantly different from HC ($P < 0.05$). HC: Hypercholesterolemic rats, AA1: *Artocarpus altilis* at 100 mg/kg, AA2: *Artocarpus altilis* at 200 mg/kg, and QUE: Questran at 0.26 g/kg.

increased by 79%, respectively, in HC rats relative to controls. In addition, HC rats had significantly lower HDL-C values when compared to the control (Table 6). Administration of AA at 200 mg/kg attenuated the elevated levels of these lipid indices to near normal in the tissues of HC rats. The protective effect of AA at 200 mg/kg seems better than the standard hypolipidemic drug (Questran). Furthermore, AA increased serum antiatherogenic index in HC rats, while coronary risk index was decreased (Table 7).

3.4. Effects of Artocarpus altilis on the Histology of Aorta and Liver.

The histology of liver slide showed marked portal congestion, severe periportal cellular infiltration by mononuclear cells, and mild diffuse vacuolar degeneration of hepatocytes (Figure 6), while aorta from HC rats revealed large focal area of myofibril necrosis with severe hemorrhages and fibrous connective tissue laid down (Figure 7). Treatment with AA (200 mg/kg) reversed the adverse effect of high dietary cholesterol on the histological architecture of the aorta and liver of the rats. The histological results further corroborated the biochemical findings indicating the beneficial effects of AA in hypercholesterolemic rats.

4. Discussion

It is generally known that elevation of serum LDL-C and total cholesterol (TC) can lead to CVD, especially atherosclerosis.

TABLE 3: Changes in the levels of lipid peroxidation in hypercholesterolemic rats treated with methanol extract of *Artocarpus altilis* for nine weeks.

Treatments	Liver (μmol MDA/mg protein)	Heart (μmol MDA/mg protein)	Serum (μmol MDA/mg protein)
Control	0.06 ± 0.01	0.15 ± 0.02	1.32 ± 0.24
HC	0.11 ± 0.02*	0.27 ± 0.03*	4.82 ± 0.68*
HC + AA1	0.08 ± 0.03**	0.13 ± 0.03**	2.63 ± 0.56**
HC + AA2	0.07 ± 0.02**	0.14 ± 0.03**	2.04 ± 0.35**
HC + QUE	0.08 ± 0.02	0.15 ± 0.02	2.85 ± 0.77
QUE	0.05 ± 0.01	0.16 ± 0.07	1.82 ± 0.60
AA2	0.07 ± 0.01	0.15 ± 0.02	1.16 ± 0.33

Values are means ± SD of 5 animals per group; HC: cholesterol at 30 mg/0.3 mL.
AA1: *Artocarpus altilis* at 100 mg/kg, AA2: *Artocarpus altilis* at 200 mg/kg, and QUE: Questran at 0.26 g/kg.
*Significantly different from control ($P < 0.05$), **significantly different from HC ($P < 0.05$).

TABLE 4: Changes in the levels of hepatic and cardiac antioxidant parameters in hypercholesterolemic rats treated with methanol extract of *Artocarpus altilis* for nine weeks.

Treatment	Liver				Heart			
	GSH	GPx	SOD	CAT	GSH	GPx	SOD	CAT
	(mg/g tissue)		(U/mg protein)		(mg/g tissue)		(U/mg protein)	
Control	0.85 ± 0.15	5.55 ± 0.83	7.36 ± 1.01	5.57 ± 1.08	21.06 ± 1.11	145.74 ± 5.74	0.03 ± 0.01	5.37 ± 0.81
HC	0.73 ± 0.01	4.92 ± 0.08	3.40 ± 0.69*	3.04 ± 0.05*	19.25 ± 0.99	92.82 ± 2.87*	0.01 ± 0.01*	2.19 ± 0.65*
HC + AA1	0.92 ± 0.26	4.98 ± 0.06	7.26 ± 1.00**	5.43 ± 1.71**	19.35 ± 0.85	108.43 ± 2.87	0.01 ± 0.01	2.99 ± 0.74
HC + AA2	0.96 ± 0.25	5.73 ± 1.50	7.43 ± 0.71**	5.55 ± 1.59**	20.38 ± 1.11	137.47 ± 3.01**	0.03 ± 0.00**	4.03 ± 0.80**
HC + QUE	0.85 ± 0.12	5.37 ± 0.99	5.95 ± 0.24	5.32 ± 3.90	21.21 ± 3.10	147.50 ± 4.81	0.03 ± 0.01	5.65 ± 0.74
QUE	0.79 ± 0.08	4.55 ± 0.69	5.39 ± 0.86	4.90 ± 0.59	20.24 ± 1.66	130.64 ± 3.39	0.02 ± 0.00	4.55 ± 0.90
AA2	0.88 ± 0.04	5.24 ± 0.12	6.03 ± 0.56	5.11 ± 0.04	20.46 ± 0.77	144.46 ± 3.83	0.03 ± 0.01	3.92 ± 0.91

Values are means ± SD of 5 animals per group; HC: cholesterol at 30 mg/0.3 mL.,
AA1: *Artocarpus altilis* at 100 mg/kg, AA2: *Artocarpus altilis* at 200 mg/kg, and QUE: Questran at 0.26 g/kg.
*Significantly different from control ($P < 0.05$), **significantly different from HC ($P < 0.05$).

Reducing LDL-C and TC can prevent the risk of CVD, a leading cause of mortality worldwide [35]. Appropriate lifestyle changes and pharmacologic approaches have both demonstrated their effectiveness in lowering LDL-C and TC [36], but the negative side effects of the pharmacological intervention have been a major setback. Lifestyle changes to include decreased saturated fats and increased soluble fibre in the diet, weight loss and regular physical activity are primary strategy for preventing CVD. Regular consumption of dietary supplements or functional foods that have demonstrated positive effects on plasma lipid values in randomised placebo-controlled clinical studies can also be considered as part of this CVD prevention strategy [37]. On this basis, we investigated the effects of methanol extract of AA on atherogenic indices and redox status of cellular system in hypercholesterolemic (HC) rats.

The present study clearly shows that feeding rats on high cholesterol diets for nine weeks caused significant increase in relative weight of heart and liver of the rats. This observation is consistent with the findings of Adaramoye et al. [16] and Yuji et al. [38]. However, treatment with AA (100 and 200 mg/kg) and Questran significantly reduced the relative weight of liver and heart of the HC rats. In this study, HC rats had high serum, hepatic, and cardiac

TC, TG, and LDL-C when compared to controls. Similar observations on hypercholesterolemic rats were observed by Yuji et al. [38], Adaramoye et al. [39], and, Kamesh and Sumathi [40]. Furthermore, a decrease in serum HDL-C levels was also observed in HC rats, which actually reflects the lower cholesterol transports by HDL-C in blood from peripheral tissues to liver for its metabolism and excretion [41]. The elevated serum and tissues levels of TC, TG, and LDL-C and lower levels of HDL-C provide a high risk for the development of atherosclerosis and other CVD [42]. In the study, extract of AA significantly decreased the levels of TC, TG, and LDL-C and increased HDL-C in the HC rats as compared to controls. The lipoproteins, especially LDL-C are involved in depositing TC and TG on walls of coronary arteries and initiate the process of atherosclerotic plaques [43]. Reduced serum and tissues levels of TC, TG, and LDL-c found in HC rats treated with doses (100 and 200 mg/kg) of AA are among the beneficial aspects of this current research and proved the antiatherosclerotic potential of this extract. The crucial risk factor for CVD includes a low level of HDL-C and high level of LDL-C. The association between a low level of HDL-C and an increased risk of CVD has been well established through epidemiological and clinical studies [44]. Since low level of HDL-C plays a direct role in the

TABLE 5: Changes in the activities of serum, hepatic, and cardiac alanine and aspartate aminotransferases in hypercholesterolemic rats treated with methanol extract of *Artocarpus altilis* for nine weeks.

Treatments	Liver (U/L)		Heart (U/L)		Serum (U/L)	
	AST	ALT	AST	ALT	AST	ALT
Control	610.6 ± 16.3	70.2 ± 5.4	552.2 ± 24.2	317.3 ± 12.3	218.0 ± 18.0	52.0 ± 7.6
HC	662.5 ± 19.3	72.7 ± 9.5	586.8 ± 21.2	330.2 ± 19.5	362.8 ± 11.0*	121.8 ± 10.5*
HC + AA1	642.8 ± 13.7	69.4 ± 8.8	549.4 ± 17.8	341.0 ± 15.0	243.8 ± 17.0**	73.3 ± 4.3**
HC + AA2	641.3 ± 19.5	67.93 ± 7.2	571.2 ± 25.3	309.4 ± 15.6	258.7 ± 13.0**	70.8 ± 4.8**
HC + QUE	642.2 ± 15.0	66.9 ± 01.8	558.7 ± 18.2	282. ± 24.8	263.5 ± 11.0**	63.5 ± 8.5
QUE	617.5 ± 15.3	69.3 ± 10.5	569.1 ± 13.54	274.0 ± 11.3	211.0 ± 9.6	60.4 ± 7.6
AA2	617.0 ± 10.6	67.0 ± 7.9	533.0 ± 22.5	312.2 ± 17.4	229.4 ± 16.5	64.0 ± 6.6

Values are means ± SD of 5 animals per group; HC: cholesterol at 30 mg/0.3 mL.
AA1: *Artocarpus altilis* at 100 mg/kg, AA2: *Artocarpus altilis* at 200 mg/kg, and QUE: Questran at 0.26 g/kg.
*Significantly different from control ($P < 0.05$), **significantly different from HC ($P < 0.05$).

TABLE 6: Changes in serum lipid profile of hypercholesterolemic rats treated with methanol extract of *Artocarpus altilis* for nine weeks.

Treatment	Total chol.	Triglyceride (mg/dL)	LDL-C	HDL-C
Control	325.07 ± 7.71	416.51 ± 24.92	211.40 ± 9.03	242.13 ± 29.55
HC	680.81 ± 16.42*	701.77 ± 18.63*	376.55 ± 13.71*	150.39 ± 32.49*
HC + AA1	511.19 ± 13.99**	521.44 ± 15.13**	366.04 ± 14.21	110.15 ± 14.00
HC + AA2	464.07 ± 16.65**	484.88 ± 11.03**	257.39 ± 16.50**	228.52 ± 16.67**
HC + QUE	378.71 ± 12.59	452.46 ± 13.17	308.28 ± 10.95	223.01 ± 14.67
QUE	411.33 ± 16.72	409.51 ± 14.08	298.72 ± 16.19	176.19 ± 51.72
AA2	345.54 ± 11.01	438.69 ± 18.63	228.18 ± 10.21	242.78 ± 17.18

Values are means ± SD of 5 animals per group; HC: cholesterol at 30 mg/0.3 mL.
AA1: *Artocarpus altilis* at 100 mg/kg, AA2: *Artocarpus altilis* at 200 mg/kg, and QUE: Questran at 0.26 g/kg,
*Significantly different from control ($P < 0.05$).
**Significantly different from HC ($P < 0.05$).

TABLE 7: Changes in antiatherogenic, coronary risk, and cardioprotective indices of hypercholesterolemic rats treated with methanol extract of *Artocarpus altilis* and Questran for nine weeks.

Treatment	Serum		
	AAI (%)	CRI	CPI
Control	292.1 ± 21.2	1.34 ± 0.03	1.15 ± 0.05
HC	28.0 ± 3.7*	4.53 ± 0.25*	0.40 ± 0.06*
HC + AA1	27.2 ± 2.7*	4.65 ± 0.43*	0.30 ± 0.05*
HC + AA2	116.1 ± 17.3**	1.86 ± 0.17**	0.89 ± 0.15**
HC + QUE	143.0 ± 21.8**	1.70 ± 0.22**	0.72 ± 0.08**
QUE	149.1 ± 12.1	1.67 ± 0.26	0.83 ± 0.10
AA2	233.0 ± 22.7	1.43 ± 0.22	1.06 ± 0.41

HC: cholesterol at 30 mg/0.3 mL, AA1: *Artocarpus altilis* at 100 mg/kg,
AA2: *Artocarpus altilis* at 200 mg/kg, QUE: questran at 0.26 g/kg,
antiatherogenic index (AAI): 100 × [HDL-C/total cholesterol−HDL-C],
coronary risk index (CRI): total cholesterol/HDL-C,
cardioprotective index (CPI): HDL-C/LDL-C.
*Significantly different from control ($P < 0.05$), **significantly different from HC ($P < 0.05$).

atherogenic process, therapeutic intervention to raise HDL-C together with other risk factors is widely encouraged. In this study, treatment with AA led to significant elevation of HDL-C, indicating its promising protective role against CVD. The protective roles of HDL-C from CVD have been suggested to occur in various ways [45]. HDL exerts part of its antiatherogenic effect by counteracting LDL oxidation and studies also showed that HDL promotes the reverse cholesterol transport pathway, by inducing an efflux of excess accumulated cellular cholesterol, and prevents the generation of an oxidatively modified LDL [46]. Furthermore, HDL not only inhibits the oxidation of LDL by transition metal ions but also prevents 12-lipoxygenase-mediated formation of lipid hydroperoxides [45]. On the basis of our results, AA may probably plays an antiatherogenic role through the inhibition of lipids oxidation, due to its antilipoperoxidative effect

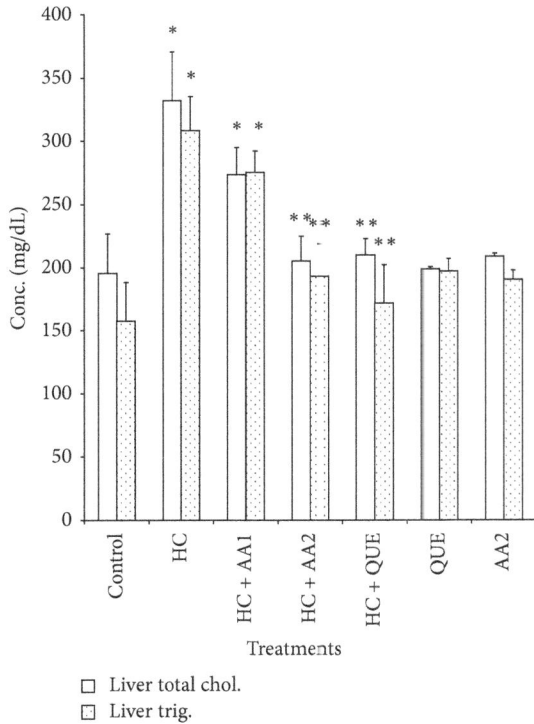

□ Liver total chol.
□ Liver trig.

FIGURE 2: Effects of methanol extract of *Artocarpus artilis* and Questran on hepatic total cholesterol and triglyceride levels of hypercholesterolemic rats. *Significantly different from control ($P <$ 0.05), **significantly different from HC ($P < 0.05$). HC: hypercholesterolemic rats, AA1: *Artocarpus altilis* at 100 mg/kg, AA2: *Artocarpus altilis* at 200 mg/kg, and QUE: Questran at 0.26 g/kg.

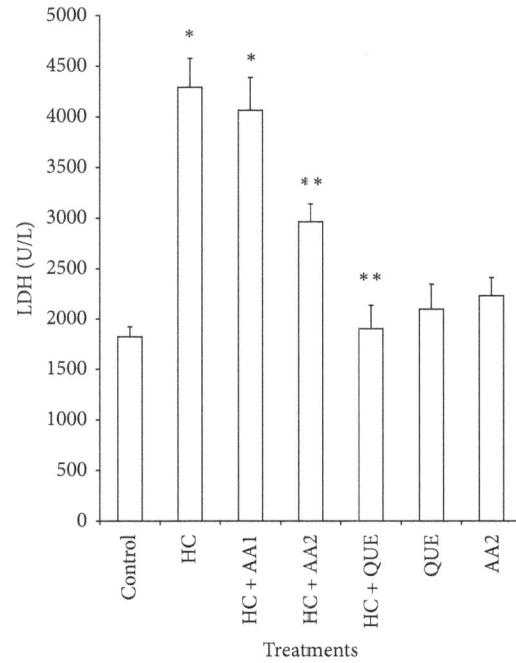

FIGURE 3: Effects of methanol extract of *Artocarpus artilis* on the activities of serum lactate dehydrogenase (LDH) of hypercholesterolemic rats. *Significantly different from control ($P < 0.05$), **significantly different from HC ($F < 0.05$). HC: hypercholesterolemic rats, AA1: *Artocarpus altilis* at 100 mg/kg, AA2: *Artocarpus altilis* at 200 mg/kg, and QUE: Questran at 0.26 g/kg.

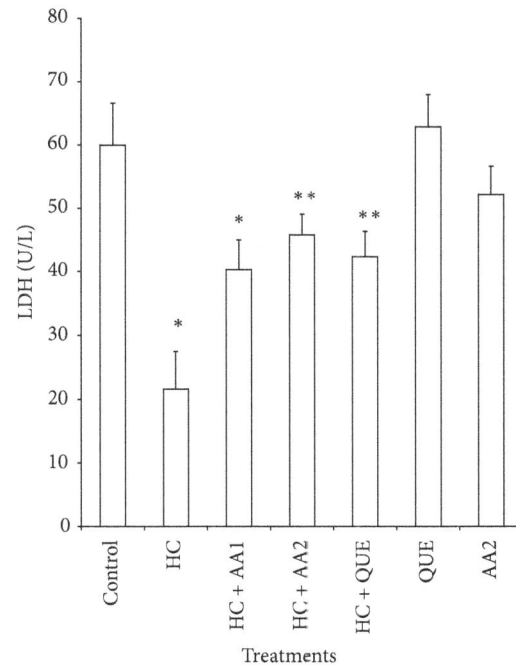

FIGURE 4: Effects of methanol extract of *Artocarpus artilis* on the activities of cardiac lactate dehydrogenase (LDH) of hypercholesterolemic rats. *Significantly different from control ($P < 0.05$), **significantly different from HC ($F < 0.05$). HC: hypercholesterolemic rats, AA1: *Artocarpus altilis* at 100 mg/kg, AA2: *Artocarpus altilis* at 200 mg/kg, and QUE: Questran at 0.26 g/kg.

observed in this study as well as the elevation of HDL-C. LDL-C, another primary target of CVD risk reduction therapy [41]. In this study, AA administered at a dose of 200 mg/kg lowered LDL-C levels of hypercholesterolemic rats. It is known that excess of LDL can be deposited on the blood vessel walls and becomes a major component of atherosclerotic plaque lesions. Therefore, serum LDL-C level has been used to monitor treatment of patients with elevated blood cholesterol levels. In view of our results, AA elicited beneficial effects by lowering serum total cholesterol including low-density lipoprotein of the hypercholesterolemic rats. In addition, hypocholesterolemic and hypotriglyceridemic effects of AA may probably be due to the inhibition of rate-limiting enzyme 3-hydroxy-3-methyl glutaryl CoA reductase (HMG-CoA reductase) of cholesterol biosynthesis. The experimentally obtained hypotriglyceridemic effect of AA may also be due to the improvement in lipolysis by reducing the activity of hormone-sensitive lipase [42]. To further support the lipid lowering potential of AA, the antiatherogenic index (AAI) was also evaluated and found to increase in HC rats treated with AA as compared to controls. Similarly, improvement was also observed in cardioprotective index (CPI) of HC rats treated with AA in terms of HDL-C/LDL-C ratio relative to controls. Out of the risk indices considered, HDL-C/LDL-C ratio (CPI) was found ideal in the present study. It has been reported that a decrease in HDL-C/LDL-C ratio is

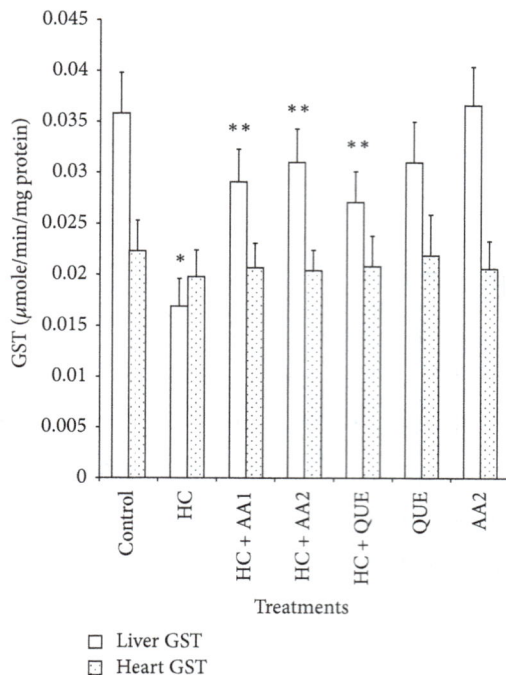

FIGURE 5: Effects of methanol extract of *Artocarpus artilis* on the activities of hepatic and cardiac glutathione-s-transferase (GST) of hypercholesterolemic rats. *Significantly different from control ($P < 0.05$), **significantly different from HC ($P < 0.05$). HC: hypercholesterolemic rats, AA1: *Artocarpus altilis* at 100 mg/kg, AA2: *Artocarpus altilis* at 200 mg/kg, and QUE: Questran at 0.26 g/kg.

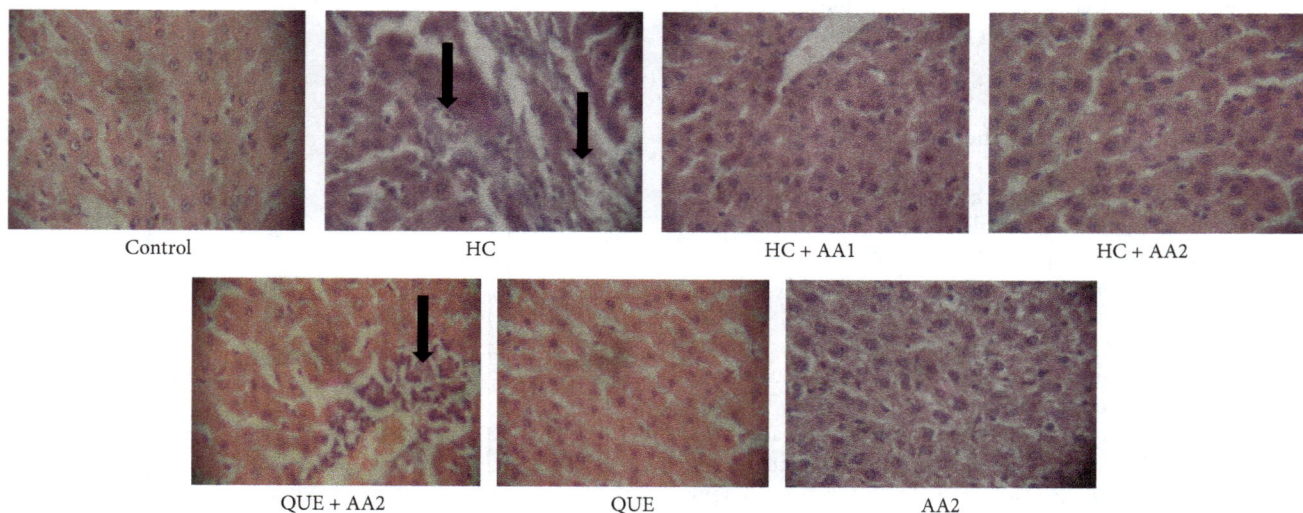

FIGURE 6: Changes in histology of liver samples of hypercholesterolemic rats treated with *Artocarpus altilis* and Questran for nine consecutive weeks (M ×400). HC: cholesterol at 30 mg/0.3 mL, AA1: *Artocarpus altilis* at 100 mg/kg, AA2: *Artocarpus altilis* at 200 mg/kg, and QUE: Questran at 0.26 g/kg. Black arrow shows portal congestion, periportal cellular infiltration, and vacuolar degeneration of hepatocytes.

good predictor of CVD in subjects [47]. Similarly, coronary risk index (CRI) in terms of TC/HDL-C ratio significantly decreased in AA-treated HC rats, which further strengthen the beneficial effects of AA.

Serum AST and ALT are the reliable markers for liver function, while serum LDH may give information on the state of the cardiac tissue. It is established that AST can be found in the liver, cardiac muscle, skeletal muscle, and so forth, whereas ALT is predominantly present in the liver [48]. The increased levels of serum AST and ALT in HC rats indicate an increased permeability and damage and/or necrosis of hepatocytes. Similar results were reported by Suk et al. [49] and Mohd Esa et al. [50] in which ALT and AST activities were elevated in HC rats. In our study, we found that extract

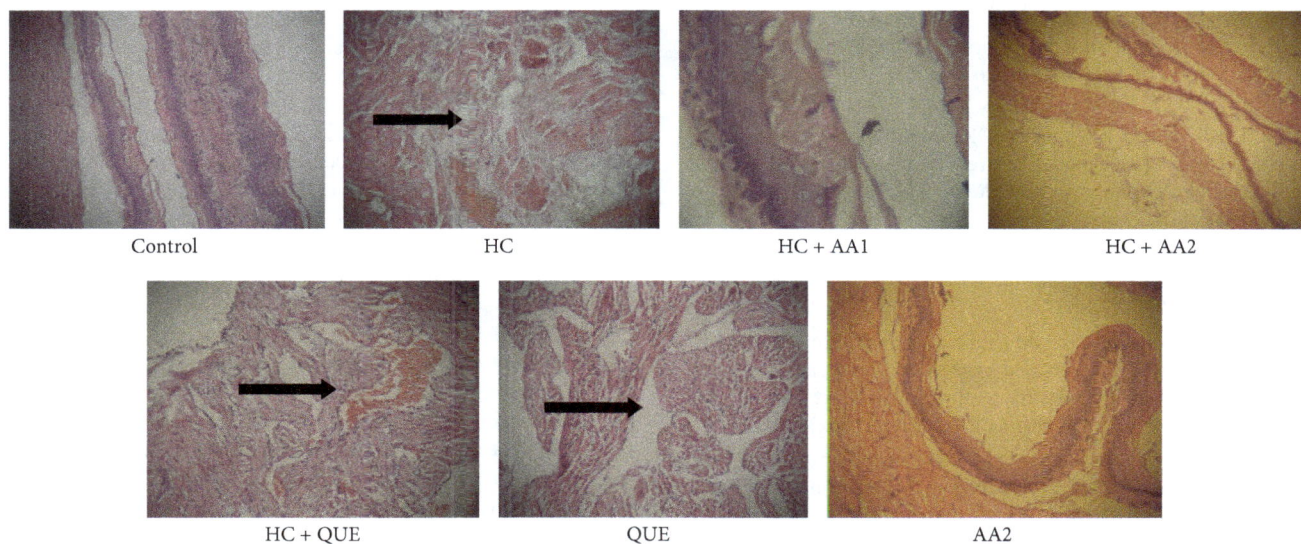

FIGURE 7: Changes in histology of aorta from hypercholesterolemic rats treated with *Artocarpus altilis* and Questran for nine consecutive weeks (M ×400). HC: cholesterol at 30 mg/0.3 mL, AA1: *Artocarpus altilis* at 100 mg/kg, AA2: *Artocarpus altilis* at 200 mg/kg, and QUE: Questran at 0.26 g/kg. Black arrows shows myofibril necrosis, severe hemorrhages, and fibrous connective tissue laid down.

of AA at a dose of 200 mg/kg caused a significant reduction in the activities of serum AST, ALT, and LDH, which further supports the beneficial effects of the extract of AA in HC rats.

Oxidative stress, defined as a disruption of the balance between oxidative and antioxidative processes, plays an important role in the pathogenesis of atherosclerosis [51]. Studies in animal models and human clinical trials have established a relationship between hypercholesterolemia and lipid peroxidation [50]. In agreement with these findings, our results show increased levels of MDA in the serum and tissues of HC rats when compared to controls. On the other hand, treatment with AA caused a significant reduction in the levels of MDA in these organs. This protective effect is probably based on the antioxidant activity of AA, which reduced the oxidative damage by blocking the production of free radicals and thus inhibited lipid peroxidation. In this study, we also observed a significant decrease in the activities of free radical scavenging enzymes, SOD and CAT, which are the first line of defence against oxidative injury. The inhibition of antioxidant system (SOD and CAT) may cause the accumulation of H_2O_2 or products of its decomposition [52]. SOD catalyzes the conversion of superoxide anion into H_2O_2. The primary role of CAT is to scavenge H_2O_2 that has been generated by free radical or by SOD. Importantly, administration of AA restored the activities of enzymatic antioxidants (SOD and CAT) in liver and heart of HC rats. AA may therefore act as an effective antioxidant of great importance against diseases and degenerative processes caused by oxidative stress. Our results showed that the extract of AA at 750 µg/mL produced 63% inhibition of DPPH radical relative to catechin (68%). The antioxidant property of AA may be linked to high polyphenolic compounds in this plant as shown in our results. From these findings, AA positively modulates the antioxidant redox status of HC rats, in addition to its beneficial effects on the lipid profile.

5. Conclusion

The present study suggests that *Artocarpus altilis* has potent blood and tissues lipid-lowering capability. In addition, it has significant antiatherogenic effect and also improves antioxidant system of hypercholesterolemic rats. Further studies are required to identify the active component(s) and mechanism(s) underlying the beneficial effects of this plant.

Conflict of Interests

The authors declare that they have no conflict of interests.

Acknowledgments

This research was partly supported by Senate Research Grants from University of Ibadan, Nigeria Oluwatosin Adekunle given to Dr. Oluwatosin Adekunle Adaramoye (SRG/COM/2010/7A).

References

[1] P. Kresanov, M. Ahotupa, T. Vasankari et al., "The associations of oxidized high-density lipoprotein lipids with risk factors for atherosclerosis: the cardiovascular risk in young finns study," *Free Radical Biology and Medicine C*, vol. 65, pp. 1284–1290, 2013.

[2] K. Kovács, K. Erdélyi, C. Hegedűs et al., "Poly(ADP-ribosyl)ation is a survival mechanism in cigarette smoke-induced and hydrogen peroxide-mediated cell death," *Free Radical Biology and Medicine*, vol. 53, no. 9, pp. 1680–1688, 2012.

[3] G. Sikka, D. Pandey, A. K. Bhuniya et al., "Contribution of arginase activation to vascular dysfunction in cigarette smoking," *Atherosclerosis*, vol. 231, no. 1, pp. 91–94, 2013.

[4] M. Füzi, Z. Palicz, J. Vincze et al., "Fluvastatin-induced alterations of skeletal muscle function in hypercholesterolaemic rats," *Journal of Muscle Research and Cell Motility*, vol. 32, no. 6, pp. 391–401, 2012.

[5] N. A. Salem and E. A. Salem, "Renoprotective effect of grape seed extract against oxidative stress induced by gentamicin and hypercholesterolemia in rats," *Renal Failure*, vol. 33, no. 8, pp. 824–832, 2011.

[6] T. Rantanen, "Midlife fitness predicts less burden of chronic disease in later life," *Clinical Journal of Sport Medicine*, vol. 23, no. 6, pp. 499–500, 2013.

[7] J. A. Borke and P. C. Wyer, "Eating a larger number of high-salt foods is not associated with short-term risk of acute decompensation in patients with chronic heart failure," *The Journal of Emergency Medicine*, vol. 44, no. 1, pp. 36–45, 2013.

[8] R. Schekman, "Discovery of the cellular and molecular basis of cholesterol control," *Proceedings of the National Academy of Sciences of the United States of America*, vol. 110, no. 37, pp. 14833–14836, 2013.

[9] C. A. Miller, "Update on statins and other lipid-lowering drugs," *Geriatric Nursing*, vol. 22, no. 5, pp. 276–277, 2001.

[10] A. M. Rincón, L. B. Rached, L. E. Aragoza, and F. Padilla, "Effect of acetylation and oxidation on some properties of Breadfruit (*Artocarpus altilis*) seed starch," *Archivos Latinoamericanos de Nutricion*, vol. 57, no. 3, pp. 287–294, 2007.

[11] N. J. C. Zerega, D. Ragone, and T. J. Motley, "Systematics and species limits of breadfruit (*Artocarpus moraceae*)," *Systematic Botany*, vol. 30, no. 3, pp. 603–615, 2005.

[12] C. A. Lans, "Ethnomedicines used in Trinidad and Tobago for urinary problems and diabetes mellitus," *Journal of Ethnobiology and Ethnomedicine*, vol. 2, pp. 45–56, 2006.

[13] C. R. Nwokocha, D. U. Owu, M. McLaren et al., "Possible mechanisms of action of the aqueous extract of *Artocarpus altilis* (breadfruit) leaves in producing hypotension in normotensive Sprague-Dawley rats," *Pharmaceutical Biology*, vol. 50, no. 9, pp. 1096–1102, 2012.

[14] V. L. Singleton, R. Orthofer, and R. M. Lamuela-Raventós, "Analysis of total phenols and other oxidation substrates and antioxidants by means of folin-ciocalteu reagent," *Methods in Enzymology*, vol. 299, no. 1, pp. 152–178, 1998.

[15] L. I. Mensor, F. S. Menezes, G. G. Leitao et al., "Screening of Brazilian plant extracts for antioxidant activity by the use of DPPH free radical method," *Phytotherapy Research*, vol. 15, no. 2, pp. 127–130, 2001.

[16] O. A. Adaramoye, V. O. Nwaneri, K. C. Anyanwo, E. O. Farombi, and G. O. Emerole, "Possible anti-atherogenic effect of kolaviron (a *Garcinia kola* seed extract) in hypercholesterolaemic rats," *Clinical and Experimental Pharmacology and Physiology*, vol. 32, no. 1-2, pp. 40–46, 2005.

[17] O. H. Lowry, N. J. Rosebrough, A. L. Farr, and R. J. Randall, "Protein measurement with the Folin phenol reagent," *The Journal of Biological Chemistry*, vol. 193, no. 1, pp. 265–275, 1951.

[18] A. F. Mohun and I. J. Cook, "Simple methods for measuring serum levels of the glutamic-oxalacetic and glutamic-pyruvic transaminases in routine laboratories," *Journal of Clinical Pathology*, vol. 10, no. 4, pp. 394–399, 1957.

[19] S. Reitman and S. Frankel, "A colorimetric method for the determination of serum glutamic oxalacetic and glutamic pyruvic transaminases," *American Journal of Clinical Pathology*, vol. 28, no. 1, pp. 56–63, 1957.

[20] W. Richmond, "Preparation and properties of a cholesterol oxidase from *Nocardia sp.* and its application to the enzymatic assay of total cholesterol in serum," *Clinical Chemistry*, vol. 19, no. 12, pp. 1350–1356, 1973.

[21] N. J. Jacobs and P. J. van Demark, "The purification and properties of the α-glycerophosphate-oxidizing enzyme of Streptococcus faecalis 10C1," *Archives of Biochemistry and Biophysics*, vol. 88, no. 2, pp. 250–255, 1960.

[22] L. K. Koditschek and W. W. Umbreit, "Alpha-glycerophosphate oxidase in *Streptococcus faecium* F 24," *Journal of Bacteriology*, vol. 98, no. 3, pp. 1063–1068, 1969.

[23] W. T. Friedewald, R. I. Levy, and D. S. Fredrickson, "Estimation of the concentration of low-density lipoprotein cholesterol in plasma, without use of the preparative ultracentrifuge," *Clinical Chemistry*, vol. 18, no. 6, pp. 499–502, 1972.

[24] J. A. Buege and S. D. Aust, "Microsomal lipid peroxidation," *Methods in Enzymology*, vol. 52, pp. 302–310, 1978.

[25] H. J. Zimmerman and H. G. Weinstein, "Lactic dehydrogenase activity in human serum," *The Journal of Laboratory and Clinical Medicine*, vol. 48, no. 2, pp. 607–609, 1956.

[26] J. M. McCord and I. Fridovich, "Superoxide dismutase. An enzymic function for erythrocuprein (hemocuprein)," *The Journal of Biological Chemistry*, vol. 244, no. 22, pp. 6049–6055, 1969.

[27] H. Aebi, "Catalase estimation," in *Methods of Enzymatic Analysis*, H. V. Bergmeyer, Ed., pp. 673–684, Verlag Chemic, New York, NY, USA, 1974.

[28] E. Beutler, O. Duron, and B. M. Kellin, "Improved method for the determination of blood glutathione," *The Journal of Laboratory and Clinical Medicine*, vol. 61, pp. 882–888, 1963.

[29] J. T. Rotruck, A. L. Pope, H. E. Ganther, A. B. Swanson, D. G. Hafeman, and W. G. Hoekstra, "Selenium: biochemical role as a component of glatathione peroxidase," *Science*, vol. 179, no. 4073, pp. 588–590, 1973.

[30] W. H. Habig, M. J. Pabst, and W. B. Jakoby, "Glutathione S transferases. The first enzymatic step in mercapturic acid formation," *The Journal of Biological Chemistry*, vol. 249, no. 22, pp. 7130–7139, 1974.

[31] P. Barter, A. M. Gotto, J. C. LaRosa et al., "HDL cholesterol, very low levels of LDL cholesterol, and cardiovascular events," *The New England Journal of Medicine*, vol. 357, no. 13, pp. 1301–1310, 2007.

[32] H.-T. Kang, J.-K. Kim, J.-Y. Kim, J. A. Linton, J.-H. Yoon, and S.-B. Koh, "Independent association of TG/HDL-C with urinary albumin excretion in normotensive subjects in a rural Korean population," *Clinica Chimica Acta*, vol. 413, no. 1-2, pp. 319–324, 2012.

[33] A. A. Adeneye and J. A. Olagunju, "Preliminary hypoglycaemic and hypolipidemic activities of the aqueous seed extract of *Carica papaya* Linn. in Wistar rats," *Biology and Medicine*, vol. 1, no. 1, pp. 1–10, 2009.

[34] M. A. Waqar and Y. Mahmmod, "Anti-platelet, anti-hypercholesterolemia and anti-oxidant effects of Ethanolic extract of *Brassica oleracea* in high fat diet provided rats," *World Applied Sciences Journal*, vol. 8, no. 1, pp. 107–112, 2010.

[35] S. Paolillo, G. L. Della Ratta, A. Vitagliano et al., "New perspectives in cardiovascular risk reduction: focus on HDL," *Archives for Chest Disease*, vol. 80, no. 1, pp. 27–30, 2013.

[36] S. C. Smith Jr., E. J. Benjamin, R. O. Bonow et al., "AHA/ACCF secondary prevention and risk reduction therapy for patients with coronary and other atherosclerotic vascular disease," *Circulation*, vol. 124, no. 22, pp. 2458–2473, 2011.

[37] Ž. Reiner, A. L. Catapano, G. de Backer et al., "ESC/EAS Guidelines for the management of dyslipidaemias," *European Heart Journal*, vol. 32, no. 14, pp. 1769–1818, 2011.

[38] K. Yuji, H. Sakaida, T. Kai et al., "Effect of dietary blueberry (*Vaccinium ashei* Reade) leaves on serum and hepatic lipid levels in rats," *Journal of Oleo Science*, vol. 62, no. 2, pp. 89–96, 2013.

[39] O. A. Adaramoye, O. Akintayo, J. Achem, and M. A. Fafunso, "Lipid-lowering effects of methanolic extract of *Vernonia amygdalina* leaves in rats fed on high cholesterol diet," *Vascular Health and Risk Management*, vol. 4, no. 1, pp. 235–241, 2008.

[40] V. Kamesh and T. Sumathi, "Antihypercholesterolemic effect of *Bacopa monniera* linn. on high cholesterol diet induced hypercholesterolemia in rats," *Asian Pacific Journal of Tropical Medicine*, vol. 5, no. 12, pp. 949–955, 2012.

[41] P. O. Kwiterovich Jr., "The metabolic pathways of high-density lipoprotein, low-density lipoprotein, and triglycerides: a current review," *American Journal of Cardiology*, vol. 86, no. 12, pp. 5–10, 2000.

[42] M. L. Bishop, E. P. Fody, and L. Schoeff, *Clinical Chemistry: Principles, Procedures, Correlations*, Lippincott Williams & Wilkins, 6th edition, 2010.

[43] S. A. Qureshi, M. Kamran, M. Asad, A. Zia, T. Lateef, and M. B. Azmi, "A preliminary study of *Santalum album* on serum lipids and enzymes," *Global Journal of Pharmacology*, vol. 4, no. 2, pp. 71–74, 2010.

[44] T. D. Filippatos and M. S. Elisaf, "High density lipoprotein and cardiovascular diseases," *World Journal of Cardiology*, vol. 5, no. 7, pp. 210–214, 2013.

[45] J.-R. Nofer, B. Kehrel, M. Fobker, B. Levkau, G. Assmann, and A. V. Eckardstein, "HDL and arteriosclerosis: beyond reverse cholesterol transport," *Atherosclerosis*, vol. 161, no. 1, pp. 1–16, 2002.

[46] T. Yokozawa, E. J. Cho, S. Sasaki, A. Satoh, T. Okamoto, and Y. Sei, "The protective role of Chinese prescription Kangen-karyu extract on diet-induced hypercholesterolemia in rats," *Biological and Pharmaceutical Bulletin*, vol. 29, no. 4, pp. 760–765, 2006.

[47] T. Marotta, B. F. Russo, and L. A. Ferrara, "Triglyceride-to-HDL-cholesterol ratio and metabolic syndrome as contributors to cardiovascular risk in overweight patients," *Obesity*, vol. 18, no. 8, pp. 1608–1613, 2010.

[48] R. Rej, "Liver diseases and the clinical laboratory—the twentieth Arnold O. Beckman conference in clinical chemistry," *Clinical Chemistry*, vol. 43, no. 8, pp. 1473–1475, 1997.

[49] F.-M. Suk, S.-Y. Lin, C.-H. Chen et al., "Taiwanofungus camphoratus activates peroxisome proliferator-activated receptors and induces hypotriglyceride in hypercholesterolemic rats," *Bioscience, Biotechnology and Biochemistry*, vol. 72, no. 7, pp. 1704–1713, 2008.

[50] N. Mohd Esa, K. K. Abdul Kadir, Z. Amom, and A. Azlan, "Antioxidant activity of white rice, brown rice and germinated brown rice (in vivo and in vitro) and the effects on lipid peroxidation and liver enzymes in hyperlipidaemic rabbits," *Food Chemistry*, vol. 141, no. 2, pp. 1306–1312, 2013.

[51] A. V. Rzheshevsky, "Fatal, "triad": lipotoxicity, oxidative stress, and phenoptosis," *Biochemistry*, vol. 78, no. 9, pp. 991–1000, 2013.

[52] C. E. Cross, A. van der Vliet, C. A. O'Neill, S. Louie, and B. Halliwell, "Oxidants, antioxidants, and respiratory tract lining fluids," *Environmental Health Perspectives*, vol. 102, no. 10, pp. 185–191, 1994.

25

Trapa bispinosa Roxb.: A Review on Nutritional and Pharmacological Aspects

Prafulla Adkar,[1,2] Amita Dongare,[1] Shirishkumar Ambavade,[1] and V. H. Bhaskar[3]

[1] *Department of Pharmacology, JSPM's Jayawantrao Sawant College of Pharmacy and Research, Hadapsar, Pune, Maharashtra 411028, India*

[2] *Post Graduates Department of Pharmacology and Toxicology, JSPM's Jayawantrao Sawant College of Pharmacy and Research, Handewadi Road, Hadapsar, Pune, Maharashtra 411028, India*

[3] *Department of Pharmaceutical Medicinal Chemistry, Gahlot Institute of Pharmacy Plot No. 59, Sector No. 14, Koparkhairane, Navi Mumbai, Maharashtra 400709, India*

Correspondence should be addressed to Prafulla Adkar; prafi.phd@gmail.com

Academic Editor: Robert Gogal

Trapa bispinosa Roxb. which belongs to the family Trapaceae is a small herb well known for its medicinal properties and is widely used worldwide. *Trapa bispinosa* or *Trapa natans* is an important plant of Indian Ayurvedic system of medicine which is used in the problems of stomach, genitourinary system, liver, kidney, and spleen. It is bitter, astringent, stomachic, diuretic, febrifuge, and antiseptic. The whole plant is used in gonorrhea, menorrhagia, and other genital affections. It is useful in diarrhea, dysentery, ophthalmopathy, ulcers, and wounds. These are used in the validated conditions in pitta, burning sensation, dipsia, dyspepsia, hemorrhage, hemoptysis, diarrhea, dysentery, strangely, intermittent fever, leprosy, fatigue, inflammation, urethrrorhea, fractures, erysipelas, lumbago, pharyngitis, bronchitis and general debility, and suppressing stomach and heart burning. Maybe it is due to photochemical content of *Trapa bispinosa* having high quantity of minerals, ions, namely, Ca, K, Na, Zn, and vitamins; saponins, phenols, alkaloids, H-donation, flavonoids are reported in the plants. Nutritional and biochemical analyses of fruits of *Trapa bispinosa* in 100 g showed 22.30 and 71.55% carbohydrate, protein contents were 4.40% and 10.80%, a percentage of moisture, fiber, ash, and fat contents were 70.35 and 7.30, 2.05 and 6.35, 2.30 and 8.50, and 0.65 and 1.85, mineral contents of the seeds were 32 mg and 102.85 mg calcium, 1.4 and 3.8 mg Iron, and 121 and 325 mg phosphorus in 100 g, and seeds of *Trapa bispinosa* produced 115.52 and 354.85 Kcal of energy, in fresh and dry fruits, respectively. Chemical analysis of the fruit and fresh nuts having considerable water content citric acid and fresh fruit which substantiates its importance as dietary food also reported low crude lipid, and major mineral present with confirming good amount of minerals as an iron and manganese potassium were contained in the fruit. Crude fiber, total protein content of the water chestnut kernel, *Trapa bispinosa* are reported. In this paper, the recent reports on nutritional, phytochemical, and pharmacological aspects of *Trapa bispinosa* Roxb, as a medicinal and nutritional food, are reviewed.

1. Introduction

Trapa bispinosa Roxb(water chestnut) is an annual, floating-leaved aquatic plant (Figure 1) found in freshwater wetlands, lakes, ponds, and sluggish reaches of rivers in India [1, 2]. *Trapa bispinosa* is an aquatic floating herb which belongs to the family Trapaceae [3]. It has flexuose stem, ascending in the water; the submerged parts are furnished with numerous opposite pairs of green root-like spreading pectinate organs. Leaves are alternate, crowded on the upper part of the stem;

3.8–5 cm long, rhomboid, somewhat truncate at the base, irregularly inciso-serrate, reddish-purple beneath; petiole dilated near the apex. Flowers are few, auxiliary, solitary, pure white. Fruits obovoid, angular, 2.2–5 cm long, and broad, with a spreading flattened very sharp spinous horn at either side.

Trapa bispinosa is commonly grown throughout India and locally known as water chestnut [4]. In addition to being important for aquatic ecosystems, *Trapa bispinosa* species are also food for humans and animals in India, China, and Southeast Asia. It is grown throughout Asia and tropical

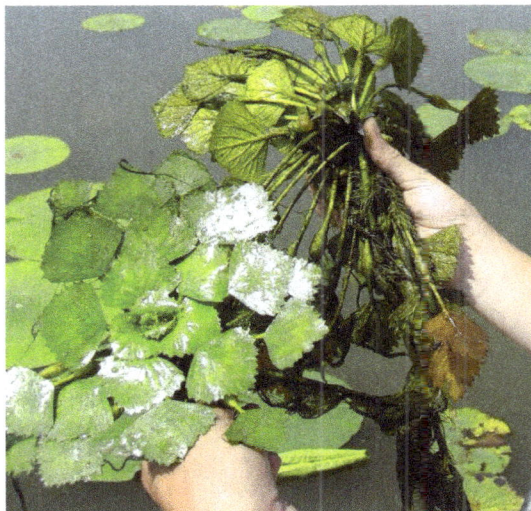

FIGURE 1: Whole plant *Trapa bispinosa*.

Africa in lakes and ponds and is often cultivated for its edible fruit. The medicinal values of the whole herb and fruit have long been recognized in folklore medicine as a cure for various diseases [5].

Trapa bispinosa is an annual aquatic plant found in tropical and subtropical and temperate zones of the world. Their natural range of growth includes Southern Europe, Africa and Asia. It has been grown in Europe since Neolithic times. It is commonly used as food by ancient Europeans as an easy growing plant; it has become neutralized in part of USA since it was first introduced into North America in 1874. It was found in slow moving rivers, ponds, lakes, and damps and is widely cultivated in Asia. It favors nutrient rich water with pH range between 6.7 and 8.2 and the alkalinity between 12 and 128 mg/L of calcium carbonate [6].

2. Historical Perspectives

Trapa bispinosa had been introduced from Europe as an ornamental plant. Dispersal is limited because of the large, sinking nuts, but water chestnut has persisted and spread in the Northeastern states. In the Chinese Zhou Dynasty, water caltrop was an important food for worship as prayer offerings. The rites of Zhou (2nd century BC) mentioned that a worshipper should use a bamboo basket containing dried water caltrops. In India it is known as singhara or paniphal (eastern India) and is widely cultivated in fresh water lakes. The fruits are eaten raw or boiled. When the fruit has been dried, it is ground to a flour called singhare ka atta which is used in many religious rituals and can be consumed as a *Phalahar* diet on the Hindu fasting days, in Indian traditional festival "*Navratri*" [7].

The *Trapa bispinosa* is native to Eurasia. It was first introduced to North America in the 1870s, where it is known to have been grown in a botanical garden at Harvard University in 1877. The plant had escaped cultivation and was found growing in the Charles River by 1879.

3. Habitat

Trapa bispinosa Roxb. (Family: Trapaceae) is native to India. The fruit is commonly known as "Paniphal." It grows abundantly in the lakes of Kashmir, India. The plant is commercially cultivated in tropical parts of the world such as Pakistan, Sri Lanka, Ceylon, Indonesia, and Africa. The plant is also abundant in Indonesia, southeast Asia, and the Southern part of China and in the eutrophic waters of Japan, Italy, and tropical America. It has become naturalized in a few places in the Eastern United States [9]. It is commercially cultivated across different parts of India for its consumable seasonal fruit commonly known as singhara which is a good source of nutrition having considerable amount of carbohydrate, protein, and vitamins. *Trapa bispinosa* Roxb plant floats just beneath the water surface and thus forms a thick mat in the water column. Only its upper leaves float over water surface in an artistic radial pattern with swollen, air-filled petioles that keep the upper part of the plant afloat [9].

Trapa bispinosa Roxb was first observed in North America, growing "luxuriantly" in Sanders Lake, Schenectady, New York, in 1884. The plant subsequently spread to many other areas in the Northeastern United States including Connecticut, Delaware, Maryland, Massachusetts, New Hampshire, Pennsylvania, Vermont, Virginia, and Washington D.C. The plant is now present in the Great Lakes Basin and recently has been found in Quebec, Canada.

4. Cultivation and Collection

Trapa bispinosa seedlings are transplanted in May/June in a perennial pond. These plants make use of the available organic matter for their growth. Stock of 800 (50 g) common carp fingerlings is maintained in September-October. *Trapa bispinosa* fruits ripen in winter and are harvested from November to January [4].

5. Botanical Description

See Figure 2.

6. Pharmacognostic Characters

Trapa bispinosa contains a great quantity of nonnutritional antioxidants, such as flavonoids, flavones, and total phenol contents. Flavonoids are present in plant tissues, such as fruits, vegetables, nuts, seeds, and leaves, in relatively high concentrations. Flavonoids act as natural antioxidants. Phytochemical screening of seed extract of *Trapa bispinosa* fruits reveals the presence of carbohydrates, saponins, phytosterols, fixed oils, and fat, while the pericarp extract of the fruits of *Trapa bispinosa* revealed the presence of tannins, flavonoids and glycosides alkaloids, saponins, steroids, and phenolic compound (Table 3) [10]. The literature reveals the presence of saponins, tannins, flavonoids, and glycosides in the pericarp extract of fruit [6]. The kernel is delicious and contains carbohydrates, proteins, and essential minerals. It also contains plentiful B vitamins (including B1, B2, B5,

Botanical description

Common names

English: water chest nut

Hindi: singhara; singhada

Marathi: shingade

Sanskrit: smgtakah; jalphala

Biogeography and ecology

Kingdom: Plantae

Subkingdom: Tracheobionta
Family: Trapaceae
Genus: *Trapa*
Species: *Trapa natans* L

Botanical description

It is an annual aquatic floating herb found in lakes and ponds. Floating leaves are rhomboid in shape, 2–6.5 cm in diameter, dark green above and reddish purple beneath, broader than long, denticulate, dentate, serrate or incised with entire base, apex acute red, and densely pubescent or villous beneath. The reddish green leaves are villous on the dorsal side, are about 5 to 8 cm long, and have hairy petioles from 10 to 15 cm in length. The submerged leaves are laterally dissected into capillary segments.

Flowers

are axillary, white in color, and with a solitary peduncle. They open above the surface of the water towards the afternoon. After pollination, the flowers submerge to facilitate fruit formation.

Fruit

It is obovoid, triangular with two horns and is about 2 cm in diameter. One seeded nut, has very unequal cotyledons and a top-shaped drupe. The fleshy pericarp covers a large 2–4 horned, stony endocarp. (Karmakar et al., 2011). It is green in fresh condition, but after drying it becomes blackish; pulp of the fruit is whitish, sweet in taste.

Stem

The stem anchors into the mud by numerous branched roots and extends upward to the surface of the water. Cord like stems are spongy and buoyant and can reach lengths of up to approximately five meters (16 feet).

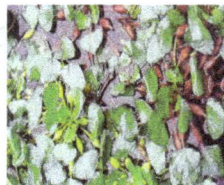

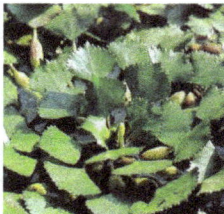

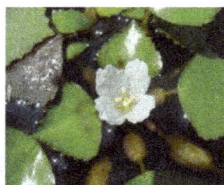

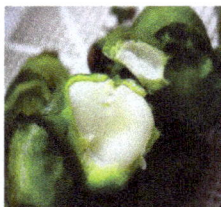

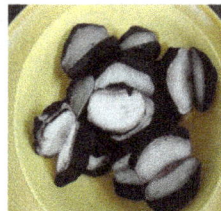

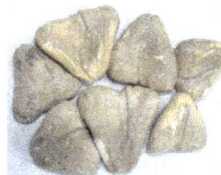

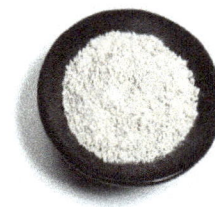

FIGURE 2: Botanical description of plant *Trapa bispinosa* Roxb [32].

and B6), E, A, and C vitamins. Seeds also contain thiamine [4].

6.1. Growth Response.

Dry weight per plant, percent cover, rosette number and rosette diameter of *Trapa bispinosa* increased significantly in all the five treatments during the experiment ($P < 0.01$ in all cases). At the first harvest before removal, the maximum value of dry weight per plant was obtained in the T9 treatment which differed markedly from the other four treatments ($P = 0.006$). Furthermore, dry weights per plant of *Trapa bispinosa* in the monocultures (T7, T8, and T9) were always higher than those in mixed-species treatments (T5 and T6). At the final harvest, the removal of *N. peltata* had a positive impact on dry weights of *Trapa bispinosa*. Mean dry weight per plant of *Trapa bispinosa* individuals was much higher in the *N. peltata* removed aquaria (the T5 treatment) than those in the control aquaria (the T6 treatment). However, the removal of *Trapa bispinosa* did not facilitate the growth of remaining individual plants of *Trapa bispinosa*. There were no significant differences in dry weight of *Trapa bispinosa* between the T7 and the T8. Similarly, at the 12th week, a clear difference was observed in percent cover among the +ve treatments ($P < 0.001$). In the T5 treatment, the cover of *T. bispinosa* reached 62% at the 12th week which was significantly high [10].

6.2. Photosynthetic Response and Carboxylation Activity.

Trapa bispinosa plant often develops a large scale root system in natural waters. The roots are green colored with chlorophyll and capable of photosynthesis using light energy coming through the water. The production of this plant depends solely on the photosynthesis of these roots until leaves expand on and above the water surface to function in photosynthesis. Interestingly, photosynthesis in this plant is carried out fewer than two different environments, by roots in water and by leaves in the atmosphere. The researchers investigated photosynthetic features of green roots in terms of 0, evolution response, and activity of photosynthetic enzymes. Leaf photosynthesis exhibited a C3 type trait, but in roots photosynthetic system was comparative to that of the submerged type (SUM) showing an increased activity in phosphoenolpyruvate carboxylase (PEP Case) and malate accumulation in root cells at night [11].

7. Phytochemistry

Trapa bispinosa (singhara) contains many organic and inorganic constituents which are mentioned below.

7.1. Inorganic Constituents (Table 2).

Acids, minerals, calcium, phosphorus, iron, copper, manganese, magnesium, sodium and potassium [12], and the physico-chemical characteristics of *Trapa bispinosa* are shown in Table 1.

Biochemical analyses of fruits of *Trapa bispinosa* in 100 g showed 22.30 and 71.55% carbohydrate in fresh and dry fruits, respectively. The protein contents were 4.40% and 10.80% in fresh and dry fruits, respectively. The percentage of moisture, fiber, ash, and fat contents was 70.35 and 7.30, 2.05 and 6.35,

TABLE 1: Physicochemical Characteristics of *Trapa bispinosa*.

Constituent	Percentage (wet basis)
Moisture	81.12 ± 0.5
Total soluble solids (°Brix)	7.2 ± 0.2
Total acidity	0.142 ± 0.03
Crude lipids	0.36 ± 0.02
Total ash	1.33 ± 0.04
Crude fiber	0.72 ± 0.02
Total proteins	1.87 ± 0.03

TABLE 2: Mineral composition of *Trapa bispinosa* on concentration basis (ppm).

Minerals	Content in *Trapa bispinosa*
Ca	365 ± 0.23
K	98.2 ± 1.23
Na	37.24 ± 0.36
Zn	6.926 ± 0.12
Ba	0.482 ± 0.32
Cr	0.106 ± 0.02

2.30 and 8.50, and 0.65 and 1.85, in fresh and dry fruits, respectively. The mineral contents of the seeds were 32 mg and 102.85 mg calcium, 1.4 and 3.8 mg iron and 121 and 325 mg phosphorus in 100 g, in fresh and dry fruits, respectively (Table 1). In 100 g fresh and dried seeds of *Trapa bispinosa* produced 115.52 and 354.85 Kcal of energy, respectively [13].

7.2. Chemical Composition of Water Chestnut Kernel.

Chemical analysis of the fruit showed that the moisture content of *Trapa bispinosa* kernel was 81.12% (wet basis). Fresh nuts having considerable water content are taken at breakfasts and are believed to suppress stomach and heart burning. The total soluble solids content of the fruit was 7.2%. The total acid in terms of citric acid present was 0.142%. Negligible amount of fat content was noticed in the fruit as 0.36% which substantiates its importance as dietary food. Also reported low crude lipid content in Chinese water chestnut was 0.06%. Total ash content obtained in fruit was 1.33% confirming good amount of minerals contained in the fruit. The potassium content of 0.41% has been reported as the major mineral present with iron and manganese contents which were 0.21 and 0.08%, respectively, being the minor minerals present [12]. Crude fiber content of the water chestnut kernel was found to be 0.72% slightly higher than reported in Chinese *Trapa bispinosa* [12] as 0.60%. The total protein content calculated in the fruit was 1.87%. Low protein content has been earlier reported in *Trapa bispinosa*.

Previously isolated classes of constituents, ascorbic acid, amylase, and amylopectin were isolated from the fruits of *Trapa bispinosa* [14].

TABLE 3: Total Phenolic and total flavonoids content of extracts of *Trapa bispinosa*.

Extract	Total phenolic content (μg GAE/mg extract)	Total flavonoids content (μg GAE/mg extract)
Acetone DCM : MeOH	$7.924 \pm 0.03 : 743.38 \pm 0.35$	$3.924 \pm 0.01 : 491.37 \pm 0.56$

7.3. Organic Constituents. It contains carbohydrates and vitamins, namely, Vitamin B-complex (thiamine, riboflavin, pantothenic acid, pyridoxine, nicotinic acid), vitamin-C, vitamin-A, D-amylase, amylase, and considerable amount of phosphorylase [12]. Cycloeucalenol, ursolic acid, and $2\beta,3\alpha,23$-trihydroxyurs-12-en-28-oic acid [29].

The phytochemical content of *Trapa bispinosa* showed high quantity of saponins ($36.92 \pm 0.67\%$). Alkaloids present in the plants function as spasmolytic, anticholinergic, and anesthetic agents. The alkaloid content in *Trapa bispinosa* was found to be $0.775 \pm 0.33\%$. Reports suggest that phenols antioxidant activity is due to their redox properties, H-donation, prevention of chain initiation by donating electrons or by binding transition metal ion catalysts, and singlet oxygen quenchers. Flavonoids are important for their pharmacological activities as scavengers. Flavonoids prevent platelet stickiness and hence platelet aggregation. Colorimetric study of the two extracts of *Trapa bispinosa* showed that acetone solvent system was able to extract more phytochemicals in comparison to DCM : Me OH.

7.4. Chemical Constituents. See Figure 3.

8. Ethnopharmacology

Actions are aphrodisiac, astringent, appetizer, anti-pyretic, constipating, diuretic, haemostatic, refrigerant, nutritive, anti-diarrheal, and tonic [30].

Indications are dyspepsia, diarrhea, dysentery, strangury, intermittent fevers, leprosy, pharyngitis, lumbago, bronchitis, sore throat, hemorrhage, generalized debility, leucorrhea, threatened abortion, dysuria, and inflammation [12, 30]. The fruits are used as intestinal astringent, aphrodisiac, and antiinflammatory, and in leprosy, urinary discharges, fractures, sore throat, and anemia [14].

In Kashmir the water nuts form a staple farinaceous food. Fruit or nut or seed contains manganese and starch. It is nutritive, sweet, tonic, and cooling. Fresh fruits are edible, raw, and cooked; dried ones are baked and eaten. They are also grated into flour and made into cakes. The nutritive value of the kernels is shown by analysis to be equal to that of rice. Fruits are refrigerant and useful in diarrhea and bilious affections with diarrhea. The upper portion of the stem was used in poultices as a discutient and the expressed juice in eye diseases [31].

8.1. Uses in Unani Medicine. It is used in cases of sexual debility, spermatorrhea, general debility, fatigue, tuberculosis, intermittent fevers, dysentery, dry cough bilious affections

[32], bleeding disorders, anal fissure, lumbago, dental caries [32], and sore throat.

8.2. Uses during Pregnancy, Sexual Transmitted Disease and Fertility. If there is itching on her lower abdomen, thigh or, breast, take water chestnut (*Trapa bispinosa*) lotus [31].

Water chestnut fruits with milk are used in nervous and general debility, seminal weakness and leucorrhoea, as confection made of it is given in 2 to 4 doctor doses. In menorrhagia hakims prescribe it as a compound powder thus; Take of *Trapa bispinosa*, kamarkas (kino) and white sugar. Divide them into 7 parts and take 1 part every day [31].

9. Nutritional Aspects

Biochemical composition of fruits of *Trapa bispinosa* was studied and concluded that *Trapa bispinosa* could be important sources of carbohydrate, protein, and minerals, which is suitable for incorporation in human diet [13].

Nutrient composition of water chestnuts revealed moisture 62.5, ash 1.04, crude fiber 2.13%, total soluble sugar 0.92%, reducing sugar 0.33%, nonreducing sugar 0.59%, starch 8.7%, lipid 0.84%. One hundred gram of green variety contained water soluble protein 0.275 mg, beta-carotene 60 microg, vitamin-C 1.1 mg, and total phenol 0.5 mg. The minerals contents of green variety were potassium 5.22%, sodium 0.64%, calcium 0.25%, phosphorus 6.77%, sulphur 0.38%, and iron, copper, manganese, and zinc 200, 430, 90, and 600 ppm, respectively. The red variety contained moisture 62.7%, ash 1.30%, crude fiber 2.27%, total soluble sugar 0.90%, reducing sugar 0.30%, nonreducing sugar 0.60%, starch 8.2%, and lipid 0.83%. The red variety contained water soluble protein 0.251 mg, beta-carotene 92 microg, vitamin-C 0.9 mg, and total phenol 0.60 mg per 100 g. The red variety contained potassium 5.32%, sodium 0.59%, calcium 0.26% phosphorus 6.77%, sulphur 0.32%, iron 200 ppm, copper 450 ppm, manganese 110 ppm, and zinc 650 ppm. The free amino acids, glutamic acid, tryptophan, tyrosine, alanine, lysine, and leucine were commonly found in both varieties. In addition, green and red varieties contained cysteine, arginine and proline, and glutamine and asparagines, respectively. Thus, the present study sheds light on the nutrient contents of the two varieties of water chestnuts and suggests that water chestnuts may play a crucial role in human nutrition [33].

10. Pharmacology (Table 4)

10.1. Acute Oral Toxicity Study. Acute oral toxicity study of *Trapa bispinosa* was carried out in albino rats. The animals were divided into eight groups of six in each. The animals

Name of constituents	Chemical structure
Riboflavin (vitamin B$_2$)	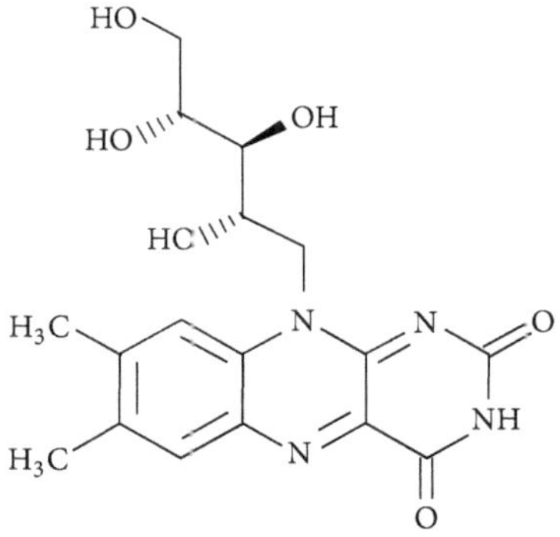
Nicotinic acid/Niacin (vitamin B$_3$)	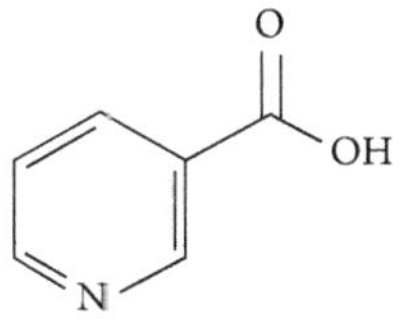
Thiamine (vitamin B$_1$)	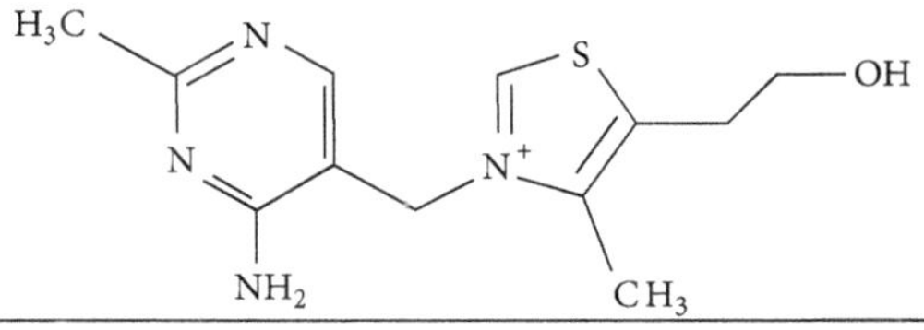
Pantothenic acid (vitamin B$_5$)	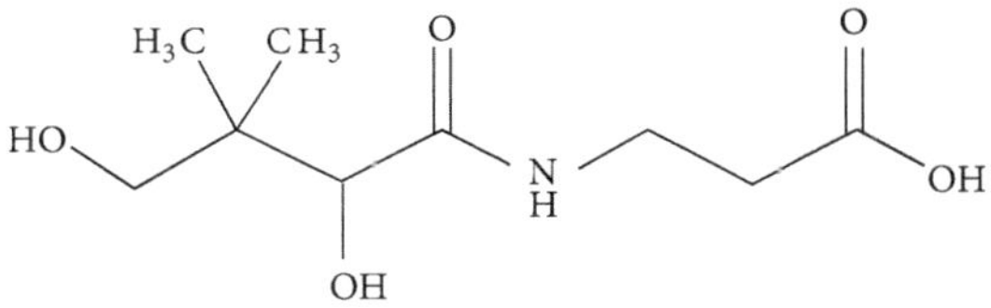
Flavonoids	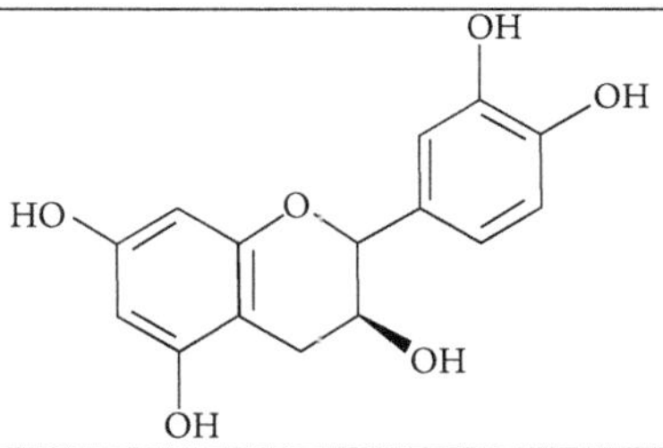
Alkaloids	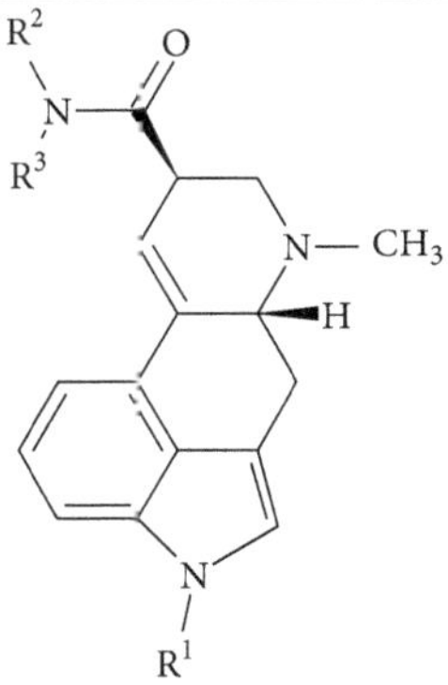
Pyridoxine (vitamin B$_6$)	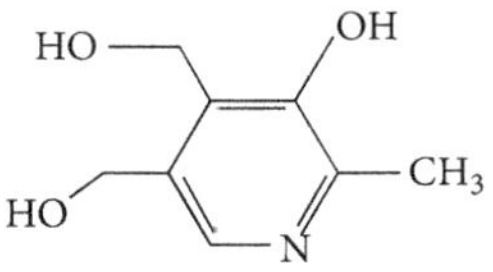

(a)

FIGURE 3: Continued.

Ascorbic acid (vitamin C)	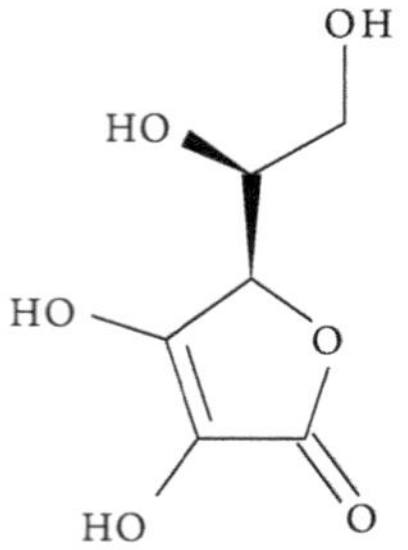
Retinol (vitamin A)	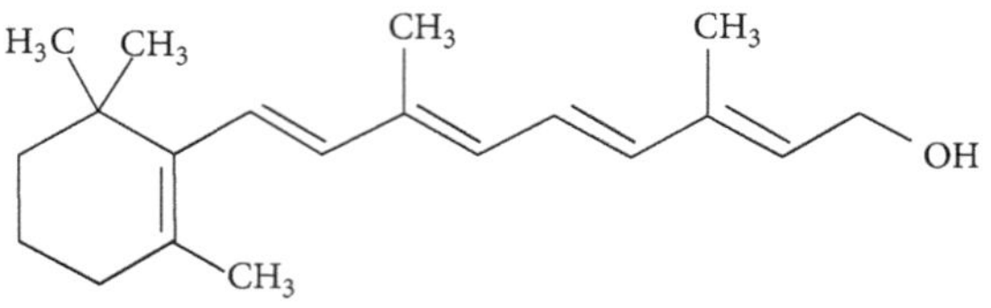
Triterpenoids (ursolic acid)	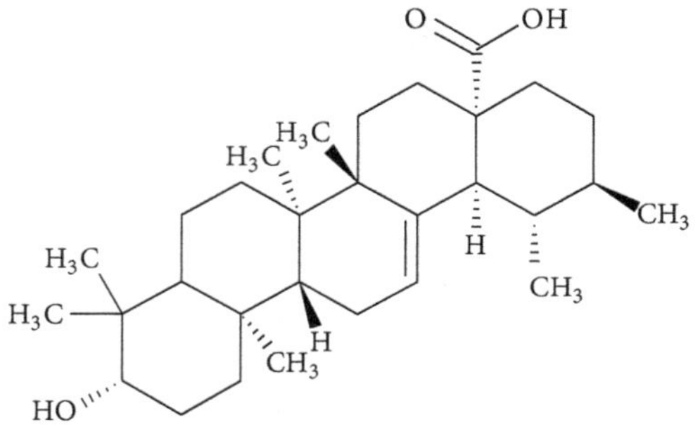
Triterpenoids (cycloeucalenol)	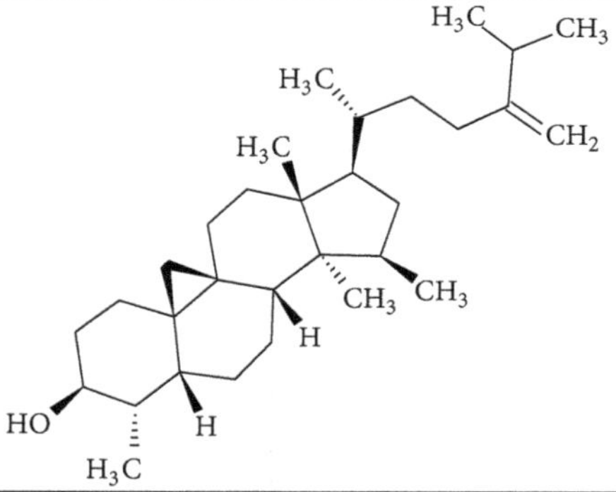
(2β, 3α)-2,3-Dihydroxy-urs-12-en-28-oic acid	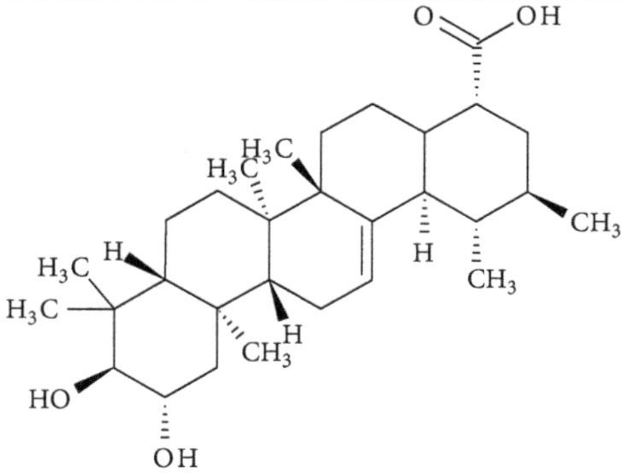

(b)

FIGURE 3: Chemical constituents present in the plant of *Trapa bispinosa*.

TABLE 4: A summary of reported pharmacological activity of *Trapa bispinosa* Roxb.

Species/method used	Property	Source
	Immunomodulator	[10]
	Nootropic, neuroprotective	[15]
Rats	Antiulcer	[16]
	Analgesic	[17]
	Antidiabetic	[18]
Female Swiss albino mice	Neuroprotective	[19]
	Antifungal	[20]
Fungi	Antifungal peptides	[21]
	Antimicrobial and enzymatic activity	[22]
	Antimicrobial activity and cytotoxicity	[14]
On starch-chitosan edible films	Antimicrobial properties	[22]
Staphylococcus aureus, *Bacillus subtilis*, *Bacillus megaterium*, *Sarcinallutea*, and *Bacillus cereus*	Antibacterial Activity	[20]
Yeast leavened breads	Physical and sensory properties of starch	[23]
	Starch as pharmaceutical, binder in solid dosage form	[4]
	Nutritional, photochemical and antioxidant	[24]
	Characteristics of starch	[25]
	Stabilizer	[26]
	Starch as excipient in tablet manufacturing	[27]
	Yogurt as a stabilizer	[26]
	Antioxidantactivity	[8]
In vitro methods	Anticancer activity	[28]
	Enzymatic activity	[22]

were fasted overnight prior to the acute experimental procedure. Karber's method was used to determine the dose; acacia gum (2% w/v) was used as vehicle to suspend the extracts and administered intraperitoneally. The control group received 2 mL/kg of the vehicle intraperitoneally. The other group received the extract as test drug in one of the following doses: 100, 200, 400, 800, 1000, 2000, and 3000 mg/kg in a similar manner. Immediately after dosing, the animals were observed continuously for first four hours for behavioral changes and for mortality at the end of 24 hrs, and 48 hrs and 72 hrs, respectively. The toxicity study showed that the hydroethanol extract of drug at a minimum dose of 200 mg/kg onwards shows the reaction in experimental animals. However, no mortality was reported even after 72 hours. This indicates that the hydroethanol extract is safe up to a single dose of 3 g/kg body weight [17].

10.2. Analgesic Activity. Analgesic activity of the methanolic extract of the *T. bispinosa* root at a dose of 200 mg/kg and 400 mg/kg was evaluated against the standard drug pentazocine at a dose of 30 mg/kg. Adult Swiss albino mice of either sex of six numbers in each group were undertaken for study and evaluated by tail flick and tail immersion method.

Both doses of *T. bispinosa* roots methanolic extract were found to produce significant ($P < 0.01$) analgesic activity. In tail flick method, the extract at 200 mg/kg showed significant activity ($P < 0.01$) after 45 minutes, but in tail immersion method, the extract showed significant activity at all tested dose levels after 30-minute interval. The results showed significant analgesic activity against stimuli [17].

10.3. Antidiabetic Activity. To evaluate the antidiabetic activity of methanol extract of *T. natans* fruit peels (METN) in Wistar rats, the effect of METN on oral glucose tolerance and its effect on normoglycemic rats were studied. Diabetes was induced in rats by single intraperitonial injection of streptozotocin. Three days after STZ induction, the hyperglycemic rats were treated with METN orally at the dose of 100 and 200 mg/kg body weight daily for 15 days.

METN at the dose of 100 and 200 mg/kg orally significantly ($P < 0.001$) and dose dependently improved oral glucose tolerance exhibited hypoglycaemic effect in normal rats and antidiabetic activity in STZ-induced diabetic rats by reducing and normalizing the elevated fasting blood glucose levels as compared to those of STZ control group [34].

10.4. Antiulcer Activity. The antiulcer activity of the fruits of *Trapa bispinosa* was studied on Wistar rats. The antiulcer activity of 50% ethanolic extract at two dose levels was evaluated by using pyloric ligation and aspirin plus pyloric ligation models. The tests extract revealed significant antiulcer activity, which might be due to increase in total carbohydrate content and alter state of mucosal barrier of the stomach. The results indicate that the ethanolic extract of fruits of *Trapa bispinosa* is endowed with potential antiulcer activity [16].

10.5. Neuropharmacological Activity. The different doses (100, 250, 500 mg/kg, p.o) of hydroalcoholic extract of *Trapa bispinosa* were administered in laboratory animals. The effects of extract on various parameters, like motor coordination, spontaneous locomotor activity, object recognition, transfer latency, anxiolytic activity, and sodium nitrite induced respiratory arrest and hypoxic stress, and so forth, were studied. The *Trapa bispinosa* (250 & 500 mg/kg) was found to decrease time required to occupy the central platform (transfer latency) in the elevated plus maze and to increase discrimination index in the object recognition test, indicating nootropic activity. *Trapa bispinosa* (250 & 500 mg/kg) showed significant increase in reaction time in hot plate analgesic activity. Moreover, it also showed significant reduction in spontaneous locomotory activity and latency memory which may be due to enhanced cholinergic function. It also showed significant analgesic activity [19].

10.6. Nootropic Activity. *Trapa bispinosa* extract showed significant facilitatory effect and aversively investigated for its nootropic activity using various experimental paradigms of learning and memory, namely, transfer latency (TL) on elevated plus maze, passive avoidance response (PAS) and object recognition test. The investigation reported that *Trapa bispinosa* 500 mg/kg significantly reduced the TL on 2nd and 9th day while *Trapa bispinosa* 250 mg/kg was found effective on 9th day. *Trapa bispinosa* 250 and 500 mg/kg significantly increased the step-down latency in the PAS at acquisition and retention test, 250 and 500 mg/kg motivated learning and memory in mice as well as improvement of memory in absence of cognitive deficit. From the above experiment it was proved that the hydroalcoholic extract of *Trapa bispinosa* had significant nootropic activity [7].

10.7. Neuroprotective Activity. Effect of hydroalcoholic extract of *Trapa bispinosa* was studied on fluorescence product and biochemical parameters like lipid peroxidation, catalase activity, and glutathione peroxidase activity in brain of female albino mice. Ageing was accelerated by the treatment of 0.5 mL 5%D-galactose for 15 days. This resulted in increased fluorescence product, increased lipid peroxidation and decreased antioxidant enzyme like glutathione peroxidase and catalase in cerebral cortex. After cotreatment with hydroalcoholic extract of *Trapa bispinosa* (500 mg/kg, p.o) there was decrease in fluorescence product in cerebral cortex. Moreover, *T. bispinosa* inhibited increased lipid peroxidation and restored glutathione peroxidase and catalase activity in cerebral cortex as compared to ageing accelerated control group [15].

10.8. Immunomodulatory Activity. In a study, the immunomodulatory potential of aqueous extract of fruits of *T. bispinosa* was scrutinized in experimental animals. The immunomodulatory effect was assessed in rats against sheep red blood cells as antigen by studying cell-mediated delayed type hypersensitivity reaction, humoral immunity response, and percent change in neutrophil count. Macrophage phagocytosis assay was carried out by carbon clearance method in mice. Oral administration of TBAE dose dependently increased immunostimulatory response. Delayed type hypersensitivity reaction was found to be augmented significantly ($P < 0.05$) by increasing the mean foot pad thickness at 48 hr and production of circulatory antibody titer (humoral antibody response) was significantly ($P < 0.05$) increased in response to SRBC as an antigen. In addition, immune stimulation was counteracted by upregulating macrophage phagocytosis in response to carbon particles. Immunostimulatory property of TBAE further confirmed by elevated neutrophil counts was significantly ($P < 0.01$) compared to control values. The result of this study suggests that aqueous extract of fruits of *T. bispinosa* could stimulate the cellular and humoural response in animals [15].

10.9. Antifungal and Antimicrobial Activity. In recent years, attempts have been made to investigate indigenous drugs against infectious disease. *Trapa bispinosa* can be used as antimicrobial agent [20] which has evaluated antifungal activity of fruit extracts of different water chestnut varieties. A strong antifungal activity of ethanol and petroleum extract was found against the treated fungi resulting in remarkable inhibition zone in comparison to both dithane-Mfungicide and control. It was also evident that wild variety of water chestnut was comparatively more efficient in respect to antifungal activity compared to the red and green varieties of the same plant [5]. It was mentioned that the extracts of *Trapa bispinosa* showed interesting antimicrobial activity against Gram-positive and Gram-negative test organisms and significant cytotoxic activity [20].

10.10. Antibacterial Activity. Antibacterial activities of the fruit extract of two varieties (green and red) of water chestnut by the disc diffusion method from methanol extract were studied. The extract of red variety of water chestnut showed high antibacterial potential (31 mm) against *Bacillus subtilis* with the concentration of 600 micron. On the other hand, green variety showed highest antibacterial activities (12 mm) against both *Staphylococcus aureus* and *Shigellasonnei* with the concentration of 600 microgram Kanamycin used as standard. In this disc diffusion assay, the methanol extract of red variety was found to have a significant antibacterial efficiency compared to the extract of green variety of water chestnut. These findings pinpoint the efficiency of these extracts to inhibit microbial growth [20].

10.11. ABTS Scavenging Activity. ABTS scavenging assay is applicable for screening both lipophilic and hydrophilic antioxidants which shows the percentage inhibition of ABTS radical by *Trapa bispinosa* extracts and standard trolox. Acetone extract (IC50 = 5 ± 0.24 mg/mL) and DCM: Me OH (IC50 = 7 ± 0.76 mg/mL) showed less scavenging than that of standard trolox (IC50 = 1 ± 0.01 mg/mL). There was significant difference ($P < 0.05$) in ABTS scavenging activity of both the extracts (Gupta et al., 2012).

10.12. Enzymatic Activity. The activities of some enzyme like amylase, cellulose, invertase, lipase, and protease were studied in locally available two varieties (green and red) of water chestnuts, Asian aquatic fruits popular for its nutritive value and medicinal properties. All the tested enzyme activities were found slightly higher in green variety than in red variety. The amylase, cellulase, invertase, lipase, and protease activities were 0.3532, 0.1922, 0.0587, 0.0234, and 0.0548 mg/mL/min, respectively, in green variety and 0.2514, 0.1221, 0.0520, 0.0204, and 0.0515 mg/mL/min, respectively, in red variety. From the enzyme activity assay it was found that water chestnuts might be used as a source of some enzymes such as amylase, cellulase, invertase, lipase, and protease. These enzyme activities could be major factor for determining the nutritive and medicinal value of the water chestnuts.

11. Pharmaceutical Uses

11.1. Excipients. Starch obtained from *Trapa bispinosa* has comparable physicochemical and binding activities compared to official starches. Physicochemical property of water chestnut starch (WCS) was comparatively evaluated with official potato and maize starch. The granule shape is round to oval with the particle size diameter 18–130 *um*. The powder characteristics are nearby similar to the official starches. Hydration and swelling capacity of WCS is approximately similar which make this potential excipient in pharmaceutical formulation development. Thus, it has potential to be used as binder industrial [35].

11.2. Metal Chelation Activity. Lipid peroxidation by the Fenton reactions is initiated by ferrous iron. Thus, minimizing Fe^{+2} concentrations in Fenton reactions by metal chelation affords protection against oxidative damage. The chelating of Fe^{+2} ions by the extracts was estimated by the method of Dinis. In this assay, both extracts interfered with the formation of ferrous and ferrozine complex in an almost similar manner, suggesting that they have chelating activity and capture Fe^{+2} ion before ferrozine.

11.3. Freeze Thaw Stabilization. Among the four gums tested, GG was effective in increasing freeze thaw stability, when 0.2% gum was added; while at 0.3%, gum ACA was more effective than GG. It was noted that the addition of salts increases the stability of the gel towards low temperature. The addition of NaCl at 0.5%, 1%, and 2% showed maximum

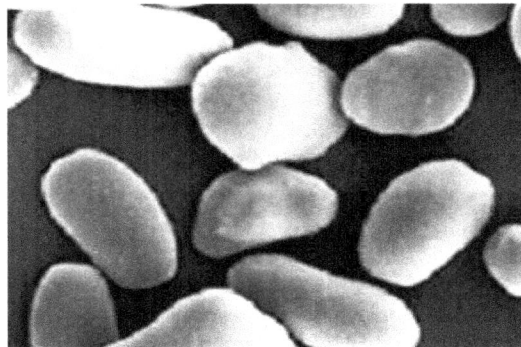

stability compared to other salts due to the hydrophilic nature of the sodium chloride enhanced water-holding ability of the starch pastes thereby limiting amount of water exuded but the reduced stability was observed in the presence of $CaCl_2$. The addition of salts increased the stability of the mixtures against the freeze thawing at varying concentrations [27].

11.4. Starch as Additive in Pharmaceuticals. The appearances of native *Trapa bispinosa* starches are shown in Figure 4. The surfaces of the granules of all samples are smooth with no evidence of cracks. Some granules appeared to be either round or oval in shape with "horn(s)" protruding from the surface [32]. The physicochemical properties of the starch extracted from krajub *Trapa bispinosa* were investigated. Scanning electron microscopy of the starch granules showed that they were either oval or round in shape with small horn(s) protruding from the surface Amylose content of the krajub starch was 29.62% (dry weight basis dwb). The pasting temperatures of 6–8% starch suspension were 81–83°C. Brabender amylogram showed no peak viscosity and very low breakdown, indicating high heat and shear stability of the starch suspension. The starch pastes highly retrograded and formed an opaque gel. The X-ray diffraction patterns of the starch revealed a C-type crystallite. The starch granules were more resistant to acid hydrolysis (2.2 NHCl at ambient temperature) than mung bean starch (C-type crystallite) [36].

12. Analytical Evaluation

12.1. Yoghurt Stabilizer. Enriched yoghurt with *Trapa bispinosa* starch at different levels was studied with physicochemical and sensory analysis. Yoghurt prepared by incorporation of *Trapa bispinosa* starch at concentration of 0.5%, 0.75%, 1%, and 1.25% was compared for these characteristics to the yoghurt containing stabilizer gelatin 0.5% w/w. Physiochemical parameters (fat, pH, acidity, synergies, water holding capacity, viscosity, protein, etc.) sensory evaluation, and microbial analysis (total viable count and coli form test) were studied. Use of *Trapa bispinosa* starch produced better results in terms of lowering synergies and increasing water holding capacity, viscosity, and overall acceptability for all sensory attributes. Addition of *Trapa bispinosa* starch did not influence the taste and overall acceptability. *Trapa bispinosa* starch 1.25% gave most excellent results for water holding capacity, synergies, and viscosity and *Trapa bispinosa* starch 0.75% gave most excellent results for all sensory attributes. Yoghurt shelf life was increased up to 25 days [26].

12.2. Molecular Identification. Reference [37] developed two marker systems for the molecular identification of three *Trapa* species based on the length variation of nuclear AP2 and trnL-F chloroplast intergenic spacer region and concluded that that nucleotide sequence variations can serve as a fast, reliable, and reproducible tool for molecular genotyping and examining the natural hybrid of water chestnut species.

12.3. Characterization and Antimicrobial Properties of Starch-Chitosan Edible Films. The characterization and antimicrobial properties of water chestnut starch-chitosan (WSC) films containing *Cornus* officinal are fruit extract (COE 1% w/w), glycerol monolaurate (GML 1% w/w), nisin (10,000 IU/g), and pine needle essential oil (PNEO 0.35% v/v), and their combinations were evaluated. Incorporation of COE decreased pH value of the film-forming solution, the moisture content, and the water absorption expansion ability (WAEA). GML-incorporated film had lower WAEA, tensile strength, elongation, and puncture strength. However, films with nisin displayed good mechanical properties. All the treated films were less transparent and higher in water vapour permeability values. For film microstructure, the presence of PNEO caused discontinuities with lipid droplets or holes embedded in a continuous network and the incorporation of GML led to abaisse-like structures. The COE, GML, nisin, PNEO and their combinations incorporated in the WSC films are effective in inhibiting the growth of *Escherichia coli* O157:H7, *Staphylococcus aureus*, and *Listeria monocytogenes* at different levels. The results showed that WSC films containing COE and GML, GML and nisin, and COE and nisin were able to reduce the number of *E. coli* O157:H7, *S. aureus*, and *L. monocytogenes*. This research has potential applications to the extension of the shelf life of food products [22].

12.4. Rheological Character of High-Amylose Starch. The molecular structure and rheological properties of high-amylose water caltrop (*Trapa bispinosa* Roxb) starch cultivated in Vietnam were investigated. The water caltrop starch had 47.1% amylose and its molecular weight (Mw) was $(4.77 \pm 0.27) \times 10^6$ g/mol, whereas the Mw was $(2.07 \pm 0.10) \times 10^7$ g/mol for amylopectin an extremely high storage modulus up to approximately 1,200 Pa. High-amylose water caltrop starch paste had an extremely high final viscosity compared to that of other cereal starches. These rheological behaviors may have been due to the extremely high amylose content [38].

12.5. Rapid Biosynthesis of Silver Nanoparticles. Trapa bispinosa has high reducing capacity to synthesize monodispersed silver nanoparticles (SNPs) within 120 seconds at 30°C which is the shortest tenure reported for SNP synthesis using plants. Moreover, we also instigated impact of different pH values on fabrication of SNPs using visible spectroscopy with respect to time. Percentage of conversion of Ag^+ ions into $Ag^°$ was calculated using ICP-AES analysis and was found to be 97% at pH = 7. To investigate the reduction of Ag^+ ions to SNPs, cyclic voltammetry (CV) and open circuit potential (OCP) using 0.1 $MKNO_3$ were performed. There was prompt reduction in cathodic and anodic currents after addition of the peel extract which indicates the reducing power of *T. bispinosa* peel. Stability of the SNPs was studied using flocculation parameter (FP) which was found to be the least at all the pH values. FP was found to be indirectly proportional to stability of the nanoparticles [25].

13. Conclusion

The systematic review of Unani, Ayurvedic literature indicates that *Trapa bispinosa* has immense potential in the treatment of conditions such as diarrhoea, strangury, dysuria, polyuria, sexual debility, general debility, sore throat, and lumbago. The recent pharmacological studies reveal that this has important analgesic, antibiotic, antidiabetic and immunomodulatory activities. The global interest toward traditional medicines is increasing due to the safe and time tested remedies with lesser side effects. This review directs *Trapa bispinosa* as a potentially safe and effective plant that has immense medicinal and nutritional values and benefits.

Conflict of Interests

The authors declare that there is no conflict of interests regarding the publication of this paper.

Acknowledgments

The authors are thankful to Professor T. J. Sawant Founder Secretary of JSPM and Dr. V. I. Hukkeri Principal, for providing all necessary facilities to carry out the present review. Authors are also thankful to National Informatics Centre (NIC), Pune, India, Botanical Survey of India (BSI), Pune, and University of Pune, Pune, India, for contribution in this review. The authors thank Professor S. Tushar and Dr. S. V. Renke, Faculty of Pharmacology for their kind help and suggestion during research.

References

[1] R. P. Rodrigues, C. Aggarwal, and N. K. Saha, "Canning of water chestnut (Singhara) (*Trapa bispinosa* Roxb.)," *Journal of Food Science and Technology*, vol. 1, pp. 28–31, 1964.

[2] Rodrigues, R. Agarwal PC, and N. K. Saha, "Canning of water chestnut (*Trapa bispinosa*) Roxb," *Journal of Food Science and Technology*, vol. 1, pp. 28–31, 1964.

[3] R. Kirtikar and B. D. Basu, *Indian Medicinal Plants*, 2nd edition, 1993.

[4] G. Singh, S. Singh, N. Jindal et al., "Environment friendly antibacterial activity of water chestnut fruits," *Journal of Biodiversity and Environmental Sciences*, vol. 1, no. 1, pp. 26–34, 2011.

[5] M. M. Rahman, M. I. Wahed, M. H. Biswas, G. M. Sadik, and M. E. Haque, "*In vitro* antibacterial activity of *Trapa bispinosa* Roxb," *Science*, vol. 1, pp. 214–246, 2001.

[6] S. Bhatiwal, A. Jain, and J. Chaudhary, "*Trapa natans* (Water Chestnut): an overview," *International Research Journal of Pharmacy*, vol. 3, no. 6, pp. 31–33, 2012.

[7] M. Chandana, R. Mazumder, and G. S. Chakraborthy, "A review on potential of plants under Trapa species," *International Journal of Research in Pharmacy and Chemistry*, vol. 3, no. 2, pp. 502–508, 2013.

[8] N. Malviya, S. Jain, A. Jain, S. Jain, and R. Gurjar, "Evaluation of in vitro antioxidant potential of aqueous extract of *Trapa natans* L. fruits," *Acta Poloniae Pharmaceutica*, vol. 67, no. 4, pp. 391–396, 2010.

[9] U. K. Karmakar, K. S. Rahman, N. N. Biswas et al., "Antidiarrheal, analgesic and antioxidant activities of *Trapa bispinosa* Roxb. fruits," *Research Journal of Pharmacy and Technology*, vol. 4, no. 2, pp. 111–115, 2011.

[10] S. Patel, D. Banji, O. J. F. Banji, M. M. Patel, and K. K. Shah, "Scrutinizing the role of aqueous extract of *Trapa bispinosa* as an immunomodulator in experimental animals," *International Journal of Research in Pharmaceutical Sciences*, vol. 1, no. 1, pp. 13–19, 2010.

[11] K. Ishimaru, F. Kubota, K. Saitou, and M. Nakayama, "Photosynthetic response and carboxylation activity of enzymes in leaves and roots of water chestnut, *Trapa bispinosa* Roxb," *Journal of the Faculty of Agriculture, Kyushu University*, vol. 41, no. 1-2, pp. 57–65, 1996.

[12] C. P. Khare, *Indian Medicinal Plants: An Illustrated Dictionary*, Springer, Berlin, Germay, 2007.

[13] M. A. Alfasane, K. Moniruzzaman, and M. M. Rahman, "Biochemical composition of the fruits of water chestnut (*Trapa bispinosa* Roxb)," *Dhaka University Journal of Biological Sciences*, vol. 20, no. 1, pp. 95–98, 2011.

[14] M. M. Rahman, M. A. Mosaddik, M. I. I. Wahed, and M. E. Haque, "Antimicrobial activity and cytotoxicity of *Trapa bispinosa*," *Fitoterapia*, vol. 71, no. 6, pp. 704–706, 2000.

[15] D. B. Ambikar, U. N. Harle, R. A. Khandare, V. V. Bore, and N. S. Vyawahare, "Neuroprotective effect of hydroalcoholic extract of dried fruits of *Trapa bispinosa* roxb on lipofuscinogenesis and fluorescence product in brain of d-galactose induced ageing accelerated mice," *Indian Journal of Experimental Biology*, vol. 48, no. 4, pp. 378–382, 2010.

[16] D. Kar, L. Maharana, S. C. Si, M. K. Kar, and D. Sasmal, "Anti-ulcer activity of ethanolic extract of fruit of *Trapa bispinosa* Roxb. in animals," *Der Pharmacia Lettre*, vol. 2, no. 2, pp. 190–197, 2010.

[17] A. K. Agrahari, M. Khaliquzzama, and S. K. Panda, "Evaluation of analgesic activity of methanolic extract of *Trapa natans* l.var. Bispinosa roxb. Roots," *Journal of Current Pharmaceutical Research*, vol. 1, pp. 8–11, 2010.

[18] M. M. Rahman, M. A. Mosaddik, M. I. I. Wahed, and M. E. Haque, "Antimicrobial activity and cytotoxicity of *Trapa bispinosa*," *Fitoterapia*, vol. 71, no. 6, pp. 704–706, 2000.

[19] N. S. Vyawahare and D. B. Ambikar, "Evaluation of neuropharmacological activity of hydroalcoholic extract of fruits of *Trapa bispinosa* in laboratory animals," *International Journal of Pharmacy and Pharmaceutical Sciences*, vol 2, no. 2, pp. 32–35, 2010.

[20] M. A. Razvy, O. F. Mohammad, and A. Mohammad Hoque, "Environment friendly antibacterial activity of water chestnut fruits," *Journal of Biodiversity and Environmental Sciences*, vol. 1, no. 1, pp. 26–34, 2011.

[21] S. M. Mandal, L. Migliolo, O. L. Franco, and A. K. Ghosh, "Identification of an antifungal peptide from *Trapa natans* fruits with inhibitory effects on *Candida tropicalis* biofilm formation," *Peptides*, vol. 32, no. 8, pp. 1741–1747, 2011.

[22] J. Mei, Y. Yuan, Q. Guo, Q. Wu, Y. Li, and H. Yu, "Characterization and antimicrobial properties of water chestnut starch-chitosan edible films," *International Journal of Biological Macromolecules*, vol. 61, pp. 169–174, 2013.

[23] R. Nawale and S. Poojari, "Review on chemical constituents and parts of plants as immunomodulator," *Research Journal of Pharmaceutical, Biological and Chemical Sciences*, vol. 4, no. 1, pp. 76–89, 2012.

[24] S. Mann, D. Gupta, V. Gupta, and R. K. Gupta, "Evaluation of nutritional, phytochemical and antioxidant potential of *Trapa bispinosa* roxb. Fruits," *International Journal of Pharmacy and Pharmaceutical Sciences*, vol. 4, no. 1, pp. 432–436, 2012.

[25] S. Pandey, A. Mewada, M. Thakur et al., "Rapid biosynthesis of silver nanoparticles by exploiting the reducing potential of *Trapa bispinosa* peel extract," *Journal of Nanoscience*, vol. 2013, Article ID 516357, 9 pages, 2013.

[26] A. H. Malik, M. Faqir, S. Ayesh, I. Muhammad, and S. Muhammad, "Extraction of starch from Water Chestnut (*Trapa bispinosa* Roxb) and its application in yogurt as a stabilizer," *Pakistan Journal of Food Sciences*, vol. 22, no. 4, pp. 209–218, 2012.

[27] Z. Lutfi and A. Hasnain, "Effect of different hydrocolloids on pasting behavior of native water chestnut (*Trapa bispinosa*) starch," *Agriculturae Conspectus Scientificus*, vol. 74, no. 2, pp. 111–114, 2009.

[28] C. Majee, R. Mazumder, and G. Chakraborthy, "A Review on potential of plants under Trapa Species," *International Journal for Radiation Physics and Chemistry*, vol. 3, no. 2, pp. 502–508, 2013.

[29] M. C. Song, D. Y. Lee, E. M. Ahn et al., "Triterpenoids from *Trapa pseudoincisa*," *Journal of Applied Biological Chemistry*, vol. 50, no. 4, pp. 259–263, 2007.

[30] A. Chatterjee and S. Prakash, *The Treatise on Indian Medicinal Plants*, vol. 4, NISCAIR, New Delhi, India, 1995.

[31] K. M. Nadkarni, *Indian Materia Medica*, vol. 1, Popular Prakashan, Mumbai, India, 2nd edition, 2007.

[32] A. Ghani, S. S. Haq, F. A. Masoodi, A. A. Broadway, and A. Gani, "Physico-chemical, Morphological and pasting properties of starches extracted from water chestnuts (*Trapa natans*) from three lakes of Kashmir, India," *Brazilian Archives of Biology and Technology*, vol. 53, no. 3, pp. 731–740, 2010.

[33] M. O. Faruk, M. Z. Amin, N. K. Sana, R. K. Shaha, and K. K. Biswas, "Biochemical analysis of two varieties of water chestnuts (Trapa sp.)," *Pakistan Journal of Biological Sciences*, vol. 15, no. 21, pp. 1019–1026, 2012.

[34] P. K. Das, S. Bhattacharya, J. N. Pandey, and M. Biswas, "Antidiabetic activity of *Trapa natans* fruit peel extract against streptozotocin induced diabetic rats," *Global Journal of Pharmacology*, vol. 5, no. 3, pp. 186–190, 2010.

[35] A. V. Singh, A. Singh, L. K. Nath, and N. R. Pani, "Evaluation of *Trapa bispinosa* Roxb. starch as pharmaceutical binder in solid dosage form," *Asian Pacific Journal of Tropical Biomedicine*, vol. 1, no. 1, pp. S86–S89, 2011.

[36] V. Tulyathan, K. Boondee, and T. Mahawanich, "Characteristics of starch from water chestnut (*Trapa bispinosa* Roxb.)," *Journal of Food Biochemistry*, vol. 29, no 4, pp. 337–348, 2005.

[37] C. Kim, H. R. Na, and H.-K. Choi, "Molecular genotyping of *Trapa bispinosa* and *T. japonica* (Trapaceae) based on nuclear AP2 and chloroplast DNA trnL-F region," *American Journal of Botany*, vol. 97, no. 12, pp. e149–e152, 2010.

[38] L. T. Phuong, L. Jin-Sil, and P. Kwan-Hwa, "Molecular structure and rheological character of high-amylose water caltrop (*Trapa bispinosa* Roxb.) starch," *Food Science and Biotechnology*, vol. 22, no. 4, pp. 979–985, 2013.

26

Attenuation of Carcinogenesis and the Mechanism Underlying by the Influence of Indole-3-carbinol and Its Metabolite 3,3′-Diindolylmethane: A Therapeutic Marvel

V. L. Maruthanila, J. Poornima, and S. Mirunalini

Department of Biochemistry and Biotechnology, Faculty of Science, Annamalai University, Annamalainagar, Tamilnadu 608 002, India

Correspondence should be addressed to S. Mirunalini; mirunasankar@gmail.com

Academic Editor: Masahiro Oike

Rising evidence provides credible support towards the potential role of bioactive products derived from cruciferous vegetables such as broccoli, cauliflower, kale, cabbage, brussels sprouts, turnips, kohlrabi, bok choy, and radishes. Many epidemiological studies point out that *Brassica* vegetable protects humans against cancer since they are rich sources of glucosinolates in addition to possessing a high content of flavonoids, vitamins, and mineral nutrients. Indole-3-carbinol (I3C) belongs to the class of compounds called indole glucosinolate, obtained from cruciferous vegetables, and is well-known for tits anticancer properties. In particular, I3C and its dimeric product, 3,3′-diindolylmethane (DIM), have been generally investigated for their value against a number of human cancers *in vitro* as well as *in vivo*. This paper reviews an in-depth study of the anticancer activity and the miscellaneous mechanisms underlying the anticarcinogenicity thereby broadening its therapeutic marvel.

1. Introduction

Plant materials present in the human diet contain a large number of naturally occurring compounds that may be useful to protect the body against cancer development. Recently, many candidates have been assayed to identify the presence of anticarcinogens in their diet [1]. Recognition of diet as a primary causative factor to overcome cancer risk has directed much research attention towards the chemoprotective role of certain compounds in foods [2]. Technological progress in manipulating plant metabolism and metabolites, combined with the explosive growth of the "functional food" industry, has led to many attempts to enhance the concentration of these health-promoting compounds in specific plant-based foods [2].

The anticancer properties of cruciferous vegetables are primarily documented by the Roman statesman, Cato and Elder (234-149 BC), who in his study of drug wrote "if a cancerous ulcer appears on the breasts, apply a crushed cabbage leaf and it will make it well [3]." It is now well set up that cruciferous vegetables contain a forerunner phytochemical openly glucosinolate that undergoes hydrolysis by the plant enzyme myrosinase, yielding a bioactive compound known as I3C [3]. It is rapidly converted to many condensation products as it is chemically unbalanced in aqueous and gastric acidic environment. The dietary indoles, I3C and DIM, occur naturally as glucosinolate conjugates in *Brassica* vegetables and are released upon hydrolysis [3]. The cancer-protecting properties of *Brassica* (i.e., broccoli, cauliflower, kale, cabbage, brussels sprouts, bok choy, radishes, turnips, and kohlrabi) utilization are most likely mediated through "bioactive compounds" that induce a variety of physiological process including direct or indirect antioxidant action, detoxifying enzymes, inducing apoptosis, and cell cycle regulation [4].

DIM is readily detected in the livers and feces of rodents fed I3C, whereas the parent I3C compound has not been detected in tissues of these rodents [5]. Thus, the natural effects of I3C are attributable to DIM, which show evidence of antitumorigenic activities *in vivo* and *in vitro* by reducing the growth of prostate, colon, and breast cancer cells [6, 7]. I3C and its derivatives also suppress cell propagation and induce apoptosis in colon cancer cells [8], as well as in other types of cancer cells including prostate [9], breast [7], bladder [10], pancreas [11], and hepatoma [12]. This review mainly focuses on the role of I3C and DIM against various types of malignancy and underlying mechanisms.

2. Cruciferous Vegetables and Their Derivatives

Glucosinolates are a class of organic compounds that give pungent smell and piquant taste in the cruciferous vegetables and some condiments, such as wasabi and mustard. The main function of glucosinolates in plants is that it acts as natural pesticides and accelerates the resistance against herbivores [13].

The central carbon of all glucosinolates is bound 6 to a thioglucose group to a sulfate group via the nitrogen molecule [22]. The central carbon of each glucosinolate is bound to a side group and this makes each glucosinolate unique [22]. Glucosinolates are classified as aliphatic (e.g., alkenyl, alkyl, hydroxyalkenyl, or w-methylthioalkyl), aromatic (e.g., benzyl, substituted benzyl), or heterocyclic with the R-group of the aliphatic glucosinolates being derived from alanine, methionine, leucine, or valine and those of aromatic and heterocyclic glucosinolates being derived from phenylalanine or tyrosine or tryptophan [14] (Figure 1(a)). Although glucosinolates are related to inhibition of carcinogenesis, it is actually their hydrolysis products, not the glucosinolates themselves that are biologically active. Hydrolysis of glucosinolates is catalyzed by the enzyme myrosinase, also known as β-thioglucoside glucohydrolase [13]. In a low pH environment, I3C is converted into polymeric products and DIM is the main one. DIM is a major in vivo acid catalyzed condensation product of I3C [23] (Figures 1(b) and 1(c)). They are no more natural products from DIM. Maciejewska et al. synthesized a series of DIM derivatives bearing fluoro, bromo, iodo, and nitro substituents in indole or benzene rings and tested for cytotoxicity against human melanoma cell lines after characterizing their structure [23]. These derivatives were found to cause 50% inhibition of the viability of ME18 and ME18/R cell lines at concentrations ranging between 9.7 and 17.3 mM [23]. These finding clearly suggested that synthetic analog of DIM has potential role in cancer therapy in the near future once their systemic toxicity studies have been determined [23].

3. Bioavailability of I3C and DIM

Reed et al. [24] in his extensive article of pharmacokinetic studies reported that women received oral doses of 400, 600, 800, 1,000, and 1,200 mg I3C and these serial plasma samples were analyzed by high-performance liquid chromatography-mass spectrometry method for the detection and quantitation of the I3C and DIM. I3C itself is not detectable in plasma [24]. The only detectable I3C-derived product is DIM. High initial value, plasma DIM for all subjects, decreased to near

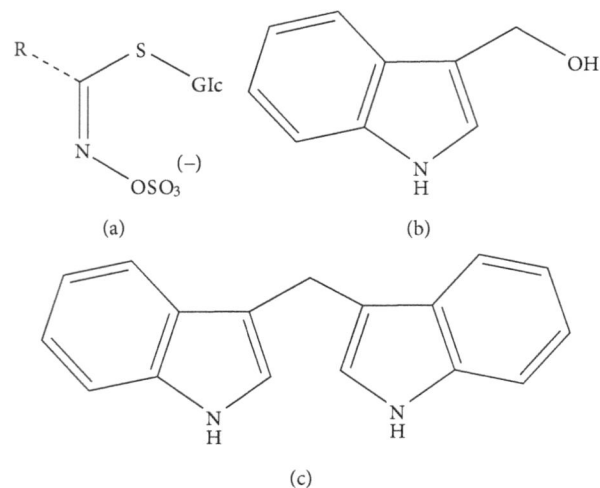

FIGURE 1: Structures of (a) glucosinolates, (b) I3C, and (c) DIM.

or below the limit of quantitation within the 12 h sampling period [24]. Physiologically based pharmacokinetic (PBPK) model is developed using plasma and tissue (brain, heart, liver, kidneys, and lungs) concentration data for DIM to compare the pharmacokinetic properties and biodistribution of pure crystalline and a novel formulation (BioResponse-DIM (BR-DIM)) of DIM after oral administration to mice [25]. I3C is hard to develop as a drug because it is highly unstable and can transform into many other derivatives such as DIM, 5,6,11,12,17,18-hexahydrocyclonona[1,2-b:4,5-b':7,8-b''] triindole (CTr), indolo [3,2-b] carbazole (ICZ), N-methoxyindole-3-carbinol (NI3C), two tetramers, one linear (LTET) and one cyclic (CTET), and 1-(3-hydroxymethyl) indolylmethane (HI-IM). Anderton et al. reported oral doses of I3C to female CD-1 mice, and studied the disposition of I3C and its acid condensation products DIM, ICZ, LTr(1), and HI-IM in blood, liver, kidney, lung, heart, and brain. I3C was rapidly absorbed, distributed, and eliminated from plasma and tissues, falling below the limit of detection by 1 h [5]. The major acid condensation product of I3C, DIM, has proven very stable in acidic conditions during prolonged exposure to high temperature and humidity [4]. Another report BR-DIM has proven very stable and it is not converted into other forms [4]. Based on these outcomes authors suggested that one could exploit further development of DIM as a potential therapeutic agent.

4. Metabolism and Distribution

Under the acidic conditions of the gastric tract, I3C undergoes condensation to form several oligomeric products, particularly DIM [23]. The tissue distribution of I3C has been determined in mice by radio-labelled I3C [26]. Both I3C and DIM have been detected in kidneys, lungs, heart, liver, plasma, and brain samples of mice treated with 250 mg/kg of I3C as early as 15 mins after administration [26]. These results suggest that I3C is rapidly absorbed and spread to a number of well-perfused tissues, where it is transformed to DIM to perform its anticancer actions [26].

5. Epidemiological Studies

For more than 25 years, the interdependence between nutrition and the development and progression of cancer have been recognized [27]. The key challenge is to identify the specific components responsible for contributing to this relationship [27]. In the United States, cancers of the lungs, colon, rectum, breast, and prostate account for almost half of the total cancer incidence [27]. Cohen et al. [28] examined the association of fruit and vegetable intake and prostate cancer risk among newly diagnosed men residing in the Seattle, WA, area. With each 10 g of cruciferous vegetables consumed per day, one could expect an 8% decrease in risk for colorectal cancer.

Several recent case-control studies in the US, Sweden, and China found that measures of cruciferous vegetable intake are significantly lower in women diagnosed with breast cancer than in cancer-free control groups [29]. High intake of cruciferous vegetables has been associated with lower risk of lung and colorectal cancer in some epidemiological studies, but there is evidence that genetic polymorphisms may influence the effectiveness of cruciferous vegetables on human cancer risk [30]. Epidemiological studies show that consumption of large quantities of fruits and vegetables, particularly cruciferous vegetables, is associated with a reduced occurrence of cancer [30].

6. Experimental Studies

Studies in various experimental models have shown that I3C can alter the metabolism of carcinogens and provide protection against chemically induced carcinogenesis [31]. When administered before or at the same time as the carcinogen, oral I3C has been originated to inhibit the spreading out of cancer in a variety of animal models and tissues, including cancers of the mammary gland (breast) [7], colon [8], stomach [31], lung [26], and liver [32]). However, a number of studies have found that I3C actually promoted or enhanced the development of cancer when administered chronically after the carcinogen [32].

The cancer promoting effects of I3C is first reported in a trout model of liver cancer [32]. However, I3C also has been found to promote cancer of the thyroid, liver, colon, and uterus in rats [33]. Although the long-term effects of I3C supplementation on cancer risk in humans are not known, but the contradictory results of animal studies have led some to caution against the widespread use of I3C and DIM supplements in humans until their potential risks and benefits are better understood [33].

7. Therapeutic Action of Indole Glucosinolates

7.1. Apoptosis. Apoptosis or programmed cell death is a highly regulated process that involves activation of a series of molecular events, leading to cell death that is characterized by cellular morphological change chromatin condensation, and apoptotic bodies which are associated with DNA cleavage into ladders [34]. The nuclear factor kappa B (NF-κB) signaling plays critical roles in regulating cell proliferation,

survival, tumor invasion, metastasis, drug resistance, and stress response [35]. We confirmed that NF-κB activity is significantly upregulated by docetaxel, gemcitabine or oxaliplatin treatment and that the NF-κB inducing activity of these agents was completely abrogated in cells pretreated with DIM [36]. We found that DIM, or the formulated BR-DIM treatment, could restrict its nuclear localization and inactivate NF-κB DNA-binding activity in prostate [14], breast [15], and pancreatic cancer cells [36], resulting in the inhibition of transcriptional downregulation of several NF-κB downstream genes causing inhibition of cell growth and inducing apoptotic cell death. Collectively, these results clearly suggest that DIM pretreatment, which inactivates NF-κB activity, along with other cellular effects of DIM, may contribute to enhanced cell growth inhibition and apoptosis with suboptimal doses of cytotoxic chemotherapeutic agents with minimal side effects (Figure 2).

I3C trigger the stress-induced MAP-kinases p38 and C-jun N-terminal kinase (JNK) in prostate cancer cells and to inhibit constitutively active STAT3, a transcription factor, in pancreatic cancer cells [18]. Irrespective of the cell type I3C suppressed NF-κB activation induced by various agents [18]. NF-κB inhibition correlated with suppression of inhibitor of kappa B kinase (IKK) and IκBα phosphorylation, ubiquitination, degradation with p65 phosphorylation, nuclear translocation, and acetylation [20]. I3C also downregulated NF-κB α regulated reporter gene transcription and gene products involved in cell proliferation, antiapoptosis, and invasion [20]. This led to the potentiation of apoptosis induced by cytokines and chemotherapeutic agents [20]. Collectively, the concerted effects on those proapoptotic components underlie the ability of I3C/DIM to induce mitochondrial dependent apoptosis in tumor cells [20].

7.2. Regulation of Redox Status. Reactive oxygen species (ROS) including H_2O_2 can cause different combinations of apoptosis, necrosis, and autophagy in a cell line dependent and stimulus-dependent manner [37]. The capacity of I3C to form adducts with electrophiles or free radicals appears too autonomous on their chemical reactivity hence the scavenging ability of I3C is compatible with the adduct formation [38]. Arnao et al. [38] investigate the ability of I3C to trap a metastable synthetic-free radical and inhibition of carcinogenesis. This induction may be produced by I3C itself and/or I3C derived polymerization products such as DIM and others [39].

According to Benabadji et al. [40], they reported that DIM and 6-methoxy-DIM in DPPH model, their IC_{50}, were 50% and 40% smaller than that of vitamin E, due to their hydrogen-donating ability with the presence of two N–H groups as an H-donating group necessary to react with free radical and slightly less potent than the standard phenolic antioxidant BHA in β-carotene model with IC_{50} 4% and 9% smaller for DIM and 6-methoxy-DIM.

7.3. Anti-Inflammatory Effect. The effect of DIM on inflammatory responses and its molecular mechanisms of DIM have been examined using lipopolysaccharide (LPS) stimulated

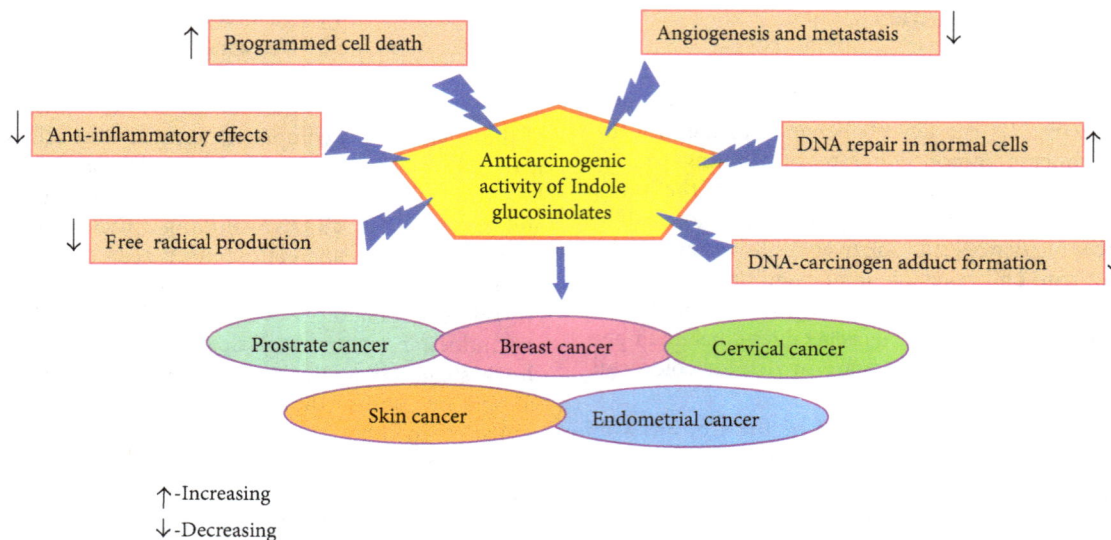

↑-Increasing
↓-Decreasing

FIGURE 2: Sources of anticancer effect of indole glucosinolates (I3C and DIM) and its mode of action.

RAW264.7 murine macrophages [16]. DIM inhibits LPS-induced increases in protein levels of inducible nitric oxide synthase (iNOS), which are accompanied by decreased iNOS mRNA levels and transcriptional activity [16]. In addition, DIM suppresses LPS-induced NF-κB transcriptional and DNA-binding activity, translocation of p65 (RelA) to the nucleus, and degradation of inhibitor of kappa B alpha (IκBα) [16]. Also the results of RT-PCR analysis exposed that LPS augmented the steady-state levels of proinflammatory cytokines such as TNF-α, IL-1β, PLA2, and interleukin-6 (IL-6) transcripts, which are substantially suppressed by DIM treatment [16]. DIM pretreatment significantly repressed LPS-induced phosphorylation of SAPK/JNK, whereas the phosphorylation of other MAPK family proteins (p38 or ERK-1/2) is unaltered by DIM pretreatment [41].

7.4. Cell Cycle Arrest. Cell cycle arrest is defined as the halt of the cell cycle. I3C is reported to inhibit cyclin dependent kinase 2 (CDK2) kinase activities in MCF-7 cells through selective alterations in cyclin E composition, size distribution, and subcellular localization of the CDK2 protein complex [42]. Cell-cycle arrest involves the upregulation of the CDK inhibitors p21 WAF1 and p27 KIP1 and the concurrent downregulation of cyclin D1, cyclin E, and CDKs 2, 4, and 6 attributable to the effect of I3C and DIM on regulating SP1-promoter binding activity [19]. Inhibition of CDK4/6 cyclin D1 and CDK2 cyclin E activities led to decreased Rb phosphorylations, which cause the Rb protein to bind to the E2F transcription factor [43]. This E2F sequestration blocks the transcription of S phase genes resulting in G_1 arrest; also the involvement of p53 and cell cycle arrest in the I3C-mediated effect has been studied in various cancer cells [44].

Treatment of I3C betters the expression of p53 (Ser 15) and CDKIs such as p21 and p27, while cyclin D1 expression is suppressed and cyclin E is not altered [45]. Collectively, the data for the cell cycle analysis, the Plk-1 assay, and the western

blot of p53 and CDKIs explain that I3C augments the expression of p53 and CDKIs and that I3C induced cell cycle arrest at G_0/G_1 in A549 cells [45]. In addition, cotreatment with I3C and wortmannin prevents both phosphorylation of p53 at Ser 15 and p21 expression. Hence it is clear that A549 cell arrest by I3C is involved in the PI3 K and p53 signal pathways [45].

7.5. Angiogenesis. Angiogenesis is the physiological process through which new blood vessels form from preexisting vessels. This is distinct from vasculogenesis, which is the *de novo* formation of endothelial cells from mesoderm cell precursors [46]. Dysregulated angiogenesis that consists of the unbalanced production of pro- and antiangiogenic factors is linked to a number of pathological situations [21]. For example, the overexpression of angiogenic factors, including vascular endothelial growth factor (VEGF), IL-6, and matrix metalloproteinases (MMP-9) is closely associated with the development of cancers and metastasis [21]. The effect of I3C on LPS-activated macrophage-induced tube formation and its associated factors in endothelial EAhy926 cells are investigated [21]. LPS significantly enhanced the capillary-like structure of endothelial cells (ECs) cocultured with macrophages, but no such effect was observed in single-cultured ECs [21]. I3C, on the other hand, suppressed such enhancement in concert with decreased secretions of VEGF, NO, IL-6, and MMPs [21]. The results obtained from cultivating ECs with conditioned medium (CM) collected from macrophages suggested that both ECs and macrophages were inactivated by I3C [21].

7.6. Detoxification. Detoxification is the physiological or medicinal removal of toxic substances from living organisms [47]. Both the Phase I and Phase II detoxification centers in the liver and the intestinal epithelial cells can be accelerated by some minor exogenous agent like I3C [47]. Many

TABLE 1: Modulation of genes involved in various mechanisms by the influence of I3C and DIM.

Mechanisms involved	Upregulated genes (↑) modulated by I3C and DIM	Downregulated genes (↓) modulated by I3C and DIM	References
Apoptosis	JNK/SAPK and Bax	Bcl-xl, Bcl-2, surviving, and NF-κB	[14–16]
Xenobiotic metabolism	CYP, CYP 1A1, CYP 1A2, and CYP 1B1	—	[17]
Antioxidant	GSH and GST	—	[4]
Transcription factor	Nrf2 and ATF3	NF-κB and STAT3	[4, 18]
Cell cycle	p21 WAF1, and p27 KIP1	Cyclin D1, E, CDK2, and CDK6	[19]
Inflammation	NAG-1	NF-κB and MMP-9	[16, 20]
Angiogenesis	VEGF, IL-6, and MMP-9	—	[21]

researchers indicate that the ability of cruciferous vegetables to motivate Phase I and Phase II detoxification, particularly their I3C content, is a primary factor in which these nutrients are related to reduce cancer risk in humans [48]. Animals are exposed to or injected with carcinogens; the animals receiving the cruciferous vegetables or the I3C in their food supply have a significantly lower tumor incidence than the animals fed the same diet, but without cruciferous vegetables or I3C fortification [48]. Table 1 showed the genes modulated by I3C and DIM in the above mechanisms.

8. Anticancer Effects of I3C and DIM

DIM inhibits proliferation of human breast cancer cells at concentrations achievable through oral supplementation with I3C (10–50 μM) [49]. Recently a report by Fan et al. [50] demonstrated that DIM protects cancer cells and normal epithelial cells against ROS in a breast cancer type 1 susceptibility protein (BRCA1-)dependent manner. Moreover I3C inhibits DMBA initiated and TPA promoted mouse skin tumour formation [51]. I3C also exhibits inhibitory and preventive effects on prostate tumors in mice [9]. Other investigators reported that this activity of I3C is associated with its action as a nonspecific inducer of powerful cytochrome enzymes responsible for "Phase I" detoxification metabolism, the efficiency of I3C to inhibit prostate tumor growth [52]. The anticancer efficacy of I3C is well proven including the reduction of cervical intraepithelial neoplasia (CIN) and its progression to cervical cancer [53]. It is perceived that the diminished phosphatase and tensin homolog protein (PTEN) expression is observed during the progression from low-grade to high-grade cervical dysplasia in humans and in a mouse model for cervical cancer the K14HPV16 transgenic mice promoted with estrogen [53]. PTEN could impede tumor progression by inhibiting proliferation and by increasing tumor cell apoptosis [53]. This is supported by the previous findings that I3C decreased proliferating cell nuclear antigen- (PCNA-)positive cells and increased TdT-mediated dUTP nick-end labeling- (TUNEL-)positive cells in abnormal cervical epithelium of HPV16 mice [54].

9. Drug Resistance

While a number of therapeutic options are available for the cure of various cancers, a major clinical problem is the development of drug resistance [55]. Intrinsic and acquired resistances are the two broad classifications of resistance to anticancer drugs. Natural compounds, such as indoles, which induce apoptosis in human cancer cells without causing unwanted toxicity in normal cells, can be useful in combination with conventional chemotherapeutic agents for the treatment of human malignancies with diminished toxicity and higher efficacy [55].

10. Conclusion

As seen throughout the review, cruciferous vegetables impart several mechanisms of action to develop its outsized number of function. The experimental studies as described above suggest that I3C and DIM, the components of cruciferous vegetables, have therapeutic potential both for prevention and for treatment of cancer. Moreover the future research can focus on the advantageous effect of I3C and DIM in various clinical studies to overcome the cancer epidemic among the population by the application of diverse technologies.

Conflict of Interests

The authors declare that they have no conflict of interests.

References

[1] L. W. Wattenberg, "Inhibition of carcinogenesis by minor anutrient constituents of the diet," *Proceedings of the Nutrition Society*, vol. 49, no. 2, pp. 173–183, 1990.

[2] J. W. Finley, "Proposed criteria for assessing the efficacy of cancer reduction by plant foods enriched in carotenoids, glucosinolates, polyphenols and selenocompounds," *Annals of Botany*, vol. 95, no. 7, pp. 1075–1096, 2005.

[3] C. A. de Kruif, J. W. Marsman, J. C. Venekamp et al., "Structure elucidation of acid reaction products of indole-3-carbinol: detection *in vivo* and enzyme induction *in vitro*," *Chemico-Biological Interactions*, vol. 80, no. 3, pp. 303–315, 1991.

[4] S. Banerjee, D. Kong, Z. Wang, B. Bao, G. G. Hillman, and F. H. Sarkar, "Attenuation of multi-targeted proliferation-linked signaling by 3,3′-diindolylmethane (DIM): from bench to clinic," *Mutation Research*, vol. 728, no. 1-2, pp. 47–66, 2011.

[5] M. J. Anderton, M. M. Manson, R. D. Verschoyle et al., "Pharmacokinetics and tissue disposition of indole-3-carbinol and its acid condensation products after oral administration to

mice," *Clinical Cancer Research*, vol. 10, no. 15, pp. 5233–5241, 2004.

[6] D. J. Kim, D. H. Shin, B. Ahn et al., "Chemoprevention of colon cancer by Korean food plant components," *Mutation Research*, vol. 523-524, pp. 99–107, 2003.

[7] K. M. W. Rahman and F. H. Sarkar, "Inhibition of nuclear translocation of nuclear factor-κB contributes to 3,3'-Diindolylmethane-induced apoptosis in breast cancer cells," *Cancer Research*, vol. 65, no. 1, pp. 364–371, 2005.

[8] S. Chintharlapalli, R. Smith III, I. Samudio, W. Zhang, and S. Safe, "1,1-Bis(3'-indolyl)-1-(p-substitutedphenyl)methanes induce peroxisome proliferator-activated receptor γ-mediated growth inhibition, transactivation, and differeatiation markers in colon cancer cells," *Cancer Research*, vol. 64, no. 17, pp. 5994–6001, 2004.

[9] M. Nachshon-Kedmi, S. Yannai, A. Haj, and F. A. Fares, "Indole-3-carbinol and 3,3'-diindolylmethane induce apoptosis in human prostate cancer cells," *Food and Chemical Toxicology*, vol. 41, no. 6, pp. 745–752, 2003.

[10] W. Kassouf, S. Chintharlapalli, M. Abdelrahim, G. Nelkin, S. Safe, and A. M. Kamat, "Inhibition of bladder tumor growth by 1,1-bis(3'-indolyl)-1-(p- substitutedphenyl)methanes: a new class of peroxisome proliferator-activated receptor γ agonists," *Cancer Research*, vol. 66, no. 1, pp. 412–418, 2006.

[11] M. Abdelrahim, K. Newman, K. Vanderlaag, I. Samudio, and S. Safe, "3,3'-Diindolylmethane (DIM) and its derivatives induce apoptosis in pancreatic cancer cells through endoplasmic reticulum stress-dependent upregulation of DR5," *Carcinogenesis*, vol. 27, no. 4, pp. 717–728, 2006.

[12] Y. Gong, G. L. Firestone, and L. F. Bjeldanes, "3,3'-Diindolylmethane is a novel topoisomerase IIα catalytic inhibitor that induces S-phase retardation and mitotic delay in human hepatoma HepG2 cells," *Molecular Pharmacology*, vol. 69, no. 4, pp. 1320–1327, 2006.

[13] A.-S. Keck and J. W. Finley, "Cruciferous vegetables: cancer protective mechanisms of glucosinolate hydrolysis products and selenium," *Integrative Cancer Therapies*, vol. 3, no. 1, pp. 5–12, 2004.

[14] Y. Li, S. R. Chinni, and F. H. Sarkar, "Selective growth regulatory and pro-apoptotic effects of DIM is mediated by Akt and NF-kappaB pathways in prostate cancer cells," *Frontiers in Bioscience*, vol. 10, no. 1, pp. 236–243, 2005.

[15] K. M. W. Rahman, S. Banerjee, S. Ali et al., "3,3'-diindolylmethane enhances taxotere-induced apoptosis in hormone-refractory prostate cancer cells through survivin downregulation," *Cancer Research*, vol. 69, no. 10, pp. 4468–4475, 2009.

[16] H. J. Cho, M. R. Seon, Y. M. Lee et al., "3,3'-Diindolylmethane suppresses the inflammatory response to lipopolysaccharide in murine macrophages," *The Journal of Nutrition*, vol. 138, no. 1, pp. 17–23, 2008.

[17] M. Yoshida, S. Katashima, J. Ando et al., "Dietary indole-3-carbinol promotes endometrial adenocarcinoma development in rats initiated with N-ethyl-N/ -nitro-N-nitrosoguanidine, with induction of cytochrome P450s in the liver and consequent modulation of estrogen metabolism," *Carcinogenesis*, vol. 25, no. 11, pp. 2257–2264, 2004.

[18] J. P. Lian, B. Word, S. Taylor, G. J. Hammons, and B. D. Lyn-Cook, "Modulation of the constitutive activated STAT3 transcription factor in pancreatic cancer prevention effects of indole-3-carbinol (I3C) and genistein," *Anticancer Research*, vol. 24, no. 1, pp. 133–137, 2004.

[19] C. Hong, G. L. Firestone, and L. F. Bjeldanes, "Bcl-2 family-mediated apoptotic effects of 3,3'-diindolylmethane (DIM) in human breast cancer cells," *Biochemical Pharmacology*, vol. 63, no. 6, pp. 1085–1097, 2002.

[20] Y. Takada, M. Andreeff, and B. B. Aggarwal, "Indole-3-carbinol suppresses NF-κB and IκBα kinase activation, causing inhibition of expression of NF-κB-regulated antiapoptotic and metastatic gene products and enhancement of apoptosis in myeloid and leukemia cells," *Blood*, vol. 106, no. 2, pp. 641–649, 2005.

[21] K. Kunimasa, T. Kobayashi, K. Kaji, and T. Ohta, "Antiangiogenic effects of indole-3-carbinol and 3,3'-diindolylmethane are associated with their differential regulation of ERK1/2 and Akt in tube-forming HUVEC," *The Journal of Nutrition*, vol. 140, no. 1, pp. 1–6, 2010.

[22] J. D. Hayes, M. O. Kelleher, and I. M. Eggleston, "The cancer chemopreventive actions of phytochemicals derived from glucosinolates," *European Journal of Nutrition*, vol. 47, no. 2, pp. 73–88, 2008.

[23] D. Maciejewska, M. Rasztawicka, I. Wolska, E. Anuszewska, and B. Gruber, "Novel 3,3'-diindolylmethane derivatives: Synthesis and cytotoxicity, structural characterization in solid state," *European Journal of Medicinal Chemistry*, vol. 44, no. 10, pp. 4136–4147, 2009.

[24] G. A. Reed, D. W. Arneson, W. C. Putnam et al., "Single-dose and multiple-dose administration of indole-3-carbinol to women: pharmacokinetics based on 3,3'-diindolylmethane," *Cancer Epidemiology Biomarkers and Prevention*, vol. 15, no. 12, pp. 2477–2481, 2006.

[25] M. J. Anderton, M. M. Manson, R. Verschoyle et al., "Physiological modeling of formulated and crystalline 3,3'-diindolylmethane pharmacokinetics following oral administration in mice," *Drug Metabolism and Disposition*, vol. 32, no. 6, pp. 632–638, 2004.

[26] F. Kassie, L. B. Anderson, R. Scherber et al., "Indole-3-carbinol inhibits 4-(methylnitrosamino)-1-(3-pyridyl)-1-butanone plus benzo(a)pyrene-induced lung tumorigenesis in A/J mice and modulates carcinogen-induced alterations in protein levels," *Cancer Research*, vol. 67, no. 13, pp. 6502–6511, 2007.

[27] G. Murillo and R. G. Mehta, "Cruciferous vegetables and cancer prevention," *Nutrition and Cancer*, vol. 41, no. 1-2, pp. 17–28, 2001.

[28] J. H. Cohen, A. R. Kristal, and J. L. Stanford, "Fruit and vegetable intakes and prostate cancer risk," *Journal of the National Cancer Institute*, vol. 92, no. 1, pp. 61–68, 2000.

[29] C. B. Ambrosone, S. E. McCann, J. L. Freudenheim, J. R. Marshall, Y. Zhang, and P. G. Shields, "Breast cancer risk in premenopausal women is inversely associated with consumption of broccoli, a source of isothiocyanates, but is not modified by GST genotype," *The Journal of Nutrition*, vol. 134, no. 5, pp. 1134–1138, 2004.

[30] J. V. Higdon, B. Delage, D. E. Williams, and R. H. Dashwood, "Cruciferous vegetables and human cancer risk: epidemiologic evidence and mechanistic basis," *Pharmacological Research*, vol. 55, no. 3, pp. 224–236, 2007.

[31] L. W. Wattenberg and W. D. Loub, "Inhibition of polycyclic aromatic hydrocarbon-induced neoplasia by naturally occurring indoles," *Cancer Research*, vol. 38, no. 5, pp. 1410–1413, 1978.

[32] S. Hendrich and L. F. Bjeldanes, "Effects of dietary cabbage, Brussels sprouts, Illicium verum, Schizandra chinensis and alfalfa on the benzo[a]pyrene metabolic system in mouse liver," *Food and Chemical Toxicology*, vol. 21, no. 4, pp. 479–486, 1983.

[33] B. M. Lee and K.-K. Park, "Beneficial and adverse effects of chemopreventive agents," *Mutation Research*, vol. 523-524, pp. 265–278, 2003.

[34] Y.-C. Chen, S.-Y. Lin-Shiau, and J.-K. Lin, "Involvement of p53 and HSP70 proteins in attenuation of UVC-induced apoptosis by thermal stress in hepatocellular carcinoma cells," *Photochemistry and Photobiology*, vol. 70, no. 1, pp. 73–86, 1999.

[35] M. Karin and F. R. Greten, "NF-κB: linking inflammation and immunity to cancer development and progression," *Nature Reviews, Immunology Cancer Cell*, vol. 5, no. 10, pp. 749–759, 2005.

[36] S. Banerjee, Z. Wang, D. Kong, and F. H. Sarkar, "3,3′-diindolylmethane enhances chemosensitivity of multiple chemotherapeutic agents in pancreatic cancer," *Cancer Research*, vol. 69, no. 13, pp. 5592–5600, 2009.

[37] Y. Chen, E. McMillan-Ward, J. Kong, S. J. Israels, and S. B. Gibson, "Oxidative stress induces autophagic cell death independent of apoptosis in transformed and cancer cells," *Cell Death and Differentiation*, vol. 15, no. 1, pp. 171–182, 2008.

[38] M. B. Arnao, J. Sanchez-Bravo, and M. Acosta, "Indole-3-carbinol as a scavenger of free radicals," *Biochemistry and Molecular Biology International*, vol. 39, no. 6, pp. 1125–1134, 1996.

[39] S. Sun, J. Han, W. M. Ralph et al., "Endoplasmic reticulum stress as a correlate of cytotoxicity in human tumor cells exposed to diindolylmethane *in vitro*," *Cell Stress and Chaperones*, vol. 9, pp. 76–87, 2004.

[40] S. H. Benabadji, R. Wen, J.-B. Zheng, X.-C Dong, and S.-G. Yuan, "Anticarcinogenic and antioxidant activity of diindolylmethane derivatives," *Acta Pharmacologica Sinica*, vol. 25, no. 5, pp. 666–671, 2004.

[41] M. Karin, "Inflammation-activated protein kinases as targets for drug development," *Proceedings of the American Thoracic Society*, vol. 2, no. 4, pp. 386–390, 2005.

[42] H. H. Garcia, G. A. Brar, D. H. H. Nguyen, L. F. Bjeldanes, and G. L. Firestone, "Indole-3-carbinol (I3C) inhibits cyclin-dependent kinase-2 function in human breast cancer cells by regulating the size distribution, associated cyclin E forms, and subcellular localization of the CDK2 protein complex," *The Journal of Biological Chemistry*, vol. 280, no. 10, pp. 8756–8764, 2005.

[43] S. Safe, S. Papineni, and S. Chintharlapalli, "Cancer chemotherapy with indole-3-carbinol, bis(3′-indolyl)methane and synthetic analogs," *Cancer Letters*, vol. 269, no. 2, pp. 326–338, 2008.

[44] C.-Y. Chen, Y.-L. Hsu, Y.-C. Tsai, and P.-L. Kuo, "Kotomolide A arrests cell cycle progression and induces apoptosis through the induction of ATM/p53 and the initiation of mitochondrial system in human non-small cell lung cancer A549 cells," *Food and Chemical Toxicology*, vol. 46, no. 7, pp. 2476–2484, 2008.

[45] G. L. Firestone and L. F. Bjeldanes, "Indole-3-carbinol and 3-3′-diindolylmethane antiproliferative signaling pathways control cell-cycle gene transcription in human breast cancer cells by regulating promoter-Sp1 transcription factor interactions," *The Journal of Nutrition*, vol. 133, no. 7, pp. 2448S–2455S, 2003.

[46] W. Risau and I. Flamme, "Vasculogenesis," *Annual Review of Cell and Developmental Biology*, vol. 11, pp. 73–91, 1995.

[47] W. D. Loub, L. W. Wattenberg, and D. W. Davis, "Aryl hydrocarbon hydroxylase induction in rat tissues by naturally occurring indoles of cruciferous plants," *Journal of the National Cancer Institute*, vol. 54, no. 4, pp. 985–988, 1975.

[48] R. McDanell, A. E. M. McLean, and A. B. Hanley, "Differential induction of mixed-function oxidase (MFO) activity in rat liver and intestine by diets containing processed cabbage: correlation with cabbage levels of glucosinolates and glucosinolate hydrolysis products," *Food and Chemical Toxicology*, vol. 25, no. 5, pp. 363–368, 1987.

[49] I. Chen, A. McDougal, F. Wang, and S. Safe, "Aryl hydrocarbon receptor-mediated antiestrogenic and antitumorigenic activity of diindolylmethane," *Carcinogenesis*, vol. 19, no. 9, pp. 1631–1639, 1998.

[50] S. Fan, Q. Meng, T. Saha, F. H. Sarkar, and E. M. Rosen, "Low concentrations of diindolylmethane, a metabolite of indole-3-carbinol, protect against oxidative stress in a BRCA1-dependent manner," *Cancer Research*, vol. 69, no. 15, pp. 6083–6091, 2009.

[51] B. Srivastava and Y. Shukla, "Antitumour promoting activity of indole-3-carbinol in mouse skin carcinogenesis," *Cancer Letters*, vol. 134, no. 1, pp. 91–95, 1998.

[52] L. W. Wattenberg and W. D. Loub, "Inhibition of polycyclic aromatic hydrocarbon-induced neoplasia by naturally occurring indoles," *Cancer Research*, vol. 38, no. 5, pp. 1410–1413, 1978.

[53] D.-Z. Chen, M. Qi, K. J. Auborn, and T. H. Carter, "Indole-3-carbinol and diindolylmethane induce apoptosis of human cervical cancer cells and in murine HPV16-transgenic preneoplastic cervical epithelium," *The Journal of Nutrition*, vol. 131, no. 12, pp. 3294–3302, 2001.

[54] B. Davidson, I. Goldberg, and J. Kopolovic, "Angiogenesis in uterine cervical intraepithelial neoplasia and squamous cell carcinoma: An immunohistochemical study," *International Journal of Gynecological Pathology*, vol. 16, no. 4, pp. 335–338, 1997.

[55] G. Szakács, J. K. Paterson, J. A. Ludwig, C. Booth-Genthe, and M. M. Gottesman, "Targeting multidrug resistance in cancer," *Nature Reviews Drug Discovery*, vol. 5, no. 3, pp. 219–234, 2006.

27

Beneficial Effect of *Cissus quadrangularis* Linn. on Osteopenia Associated with Streptozotocin-Induced Type 1 Diabetes Mellitus in Male Wistar Rats

Srinivasa Rao Sirasanagandla,[1] Sreedhara Ranganath Pai Karkala,[2] Bhagath Kumar Potu,[3] and Kumar M.R. Bhat[4]

[1] *Department of Anatomy, Melaka Manipal Medical College, Manipal University, Madhav Nagar, Manipal, Karnataka 576104, India*
[2] *Department of Pharmacology, Manipal College of Pharmaceutical Sciences, Manipal University, Manipal, Karnataka 576104, India*
[3] *Department of Anatomy, College of Medicine and Medical Sciences, Arabian Gulf University, P.O. Box 26671, Bahrain*
[4] *Department of Anatomy, Kasturba Medical College, Manipal University, Manipal, Karnataka 576104, India*

Correspondence should be addressed to Kumar M.R. Bhat; kummigames@yahoo.com

Academic Editor: Antonio Ferrer-Montiel

Petroleum ether fraction of *Cissus quadrangularis* (*PECQ*) impact on the development of osteopenia in type 1 diabetic rat model has been evaluated. Diabetic rats were treated orally with two doses of *PECQ*. Another group of diabetic rats were treated with subcutaneous injection of synthetic human insulin. The cortical and trabecular bone thickness and bone strength were significantly decreased in diabetic rats. Treatment with two doses of *PECQ* significantly prevented these changes in diabetic rats. However, *PECQ* treatment (two doses) did not alter the glycemic levels in these diabetic rats. Increased levels of serum alkaline phosphatase (ALP), tartrate-resistant acid phosphatase (TRAP), and hydroxyproline were noted in diabetic rats when compared to normal control rats. The two doses of *PECQ* treatment further improved the serum ALP levels and significantly decreased the serum levels of TRAP and hydroxyproline. The effects of *PECQ* treatment on histological, biomechanical, and biochemical parameters are comparable to those of insulin. Since *PECQ* improves the bone health in hyperglycemic conditions by enhancing the cortical and trabecular bone growth and altering the circulating bone markers, it could be used as an effective therapy against diabetes-associated bone disorders.

1. Introduction

Diabetes mellitus (DM) is a combination of metabolic disorders characterized by impaired metabolism of carbohydrates, proteins, and fat resulting from insulin deficiency [1]. Skeletal disorders are common in diabetic patients, namely, reduced bone mineral content [2, 3], deranged calcium and phosphate levels, and altered bone metabolism [3–6]. Osteopenia [7], increased risk of fractures [8], and delayed fracture healing [9] are evident in these patients. Earlier, animal models have proved the association between osteopenic/osteoporotic changes and type 1 DM [10–15]. It has been demonstrated that the adverse effects of DM on bone tissue could be due to insulinopenia, bone microangiopathy, impaired regulation

of mineral metabolism, and alterations in local factors that regulate bone remodeling [16, 17]. Dimensions of the femur such as weight, length, and diaphyseal width were found to be decreased in diabetic rats [18]. Furthermore, experimental studies have demonstrated that the mechanical strength of bones is reduced in diabetic rats [19–21]. Diabetes is also found to delay fracture healing and treatment with synthetic calcium phosphate or hydroxyapatite has been shown to have a positive effect on fracture healing [22–24]. It was also shown that the treatment with either insulin or 17-b estradiol (E2) can reverse the altered architecture of bones in diabetic rats and their effects were found to be similar [25]. Verhaeghe et al. have observed the positive effect of E2 against the metaphyseal trabecular bone damage in ovariectomized diabetic rats, when compared to nontreated control rats [26].

Cissus quadrangularis (*CQ*) is a climbing shrub, which belongs to the Vitaceae family. It is usually seen in hot climate in various states of India, Sri Lanka, Malaya, Java, and West Africa [27]. In Ayurveda, its usage in the treatment of bone fractures and swelling has been mentioned [28]. *CQ* has been shown to have an ability to accelerate the healing of bone fracture [29]. Experimental animal models have proved the antiosteoporotic potential of ethanol, petroleum ether, and hexane fractions of the *CQ* [27, 30, 31]. A pharmacological study on *CQ* has shown the presence of phytoestrogen steroids [32]. Recently, the phytoestrogen-rich fraction separated from the *CQ* has been shown to have potent antiosteoporotic activity [33]. *In vitro* study has shown that the petroleum ether fraction of *CQ* (PECQ) enhances the proliferation and differentiation of rat bone marrow mesenchymal stem cells [34]. Previously in our laboratory, the protective effect of *PECQ* on defective fetal skeletal ossification in maternal diabetes has been studied (ahead of print). Though the pharmacological effect of *CQ* on bone health has been studied extensively, no attempt has been made to study the efficacy of *CQ* on osteopenia associated with DM. In the presented study, we evaluated the effect of *CQ* against bone histology, biomechanical changes, and circulating bone markers in type 1 diabetic rats.

2. Material and Methods

2.1. Preparation of Plant Extract. The fresh stems of *CQ* were air-dried and grinded into powder. Using a soxhlet apparatus, 1.3 kg *CQ* powder was subjected to extraction with 95% ethyl alcohol. The ethanol extract obtained (125 g) was further suspended in water. Then, it was partitioned with petroleum ether (b.p. 60–90°C) solvent. The total yield (9.1% w/w) of *PECQ* was stored at 4°C until use. Every day fresh suspension of *PECQ* was prepared by using carboxymethyl cellulose (CMC).

2.2. Animals. In the present study, 3-month-old male Wistar rats (180–220 g weight) were used. After obtaining approval from the Institutional Animal Ethical Committee, rats were placed in the Central animal research facility of Manipal University according to guidelines of the Committee for the Purpose of Control and Supervision of Experiments on Animals (CPCSEA). Proper ventilation with temperature control was maintained on a 12 hr dark and 12 hr light schedule throughout the experiment. Rats were fed a standard balanced diet and water.

2.3. Induction of Diabetes and Treatments. After one week male Wistar rats were induced diabetes with streptozotocin (STZ) injection intraperitoneally (40 mg/kg body weight), which was dissolved in 0.1 M citrate buffer, pH 4.5. Control rats were injected 0.1 M citrate buffer. The blood glucose levels were analyzed seven days after injection using Glucometer (AccuChek Active). Animals demonstrating hyperglycemia (>250 mg/dL) were treated orally with *PECQ* at daily doses of

500 mg/kg and 750 mg/kg body weight. The dose was selected based on the previous study [30]. The diabetic rats in another group were injected subcutaneously twice daily with human synthetic insulin (INS) (Actrapid, Novo Nordisk India Pvt. Ltd., India), at a dose of 10 U/kg body weight. Treatment continued for 45 days.

2.4. Experimental Design. Experimental rats ($n = 30$) were allocated to 5 groups each containing 6 rats. Rats in normal control (NC) Group A received 0.5% CMC; Group B, diabetic control group (DC), received 0.5% CMC; Group C, the diabetic + CQ1 group (DC + CQ1), received 500 mg/kg body weight dose of *PECQ*; Group D, the diabetic + CQ2 group (DC + CQ2), received 750 mg/kg body weight dose of *PECQ*; and Group E, the diabetic + INS group (DC + INS), rats received INS. The blood glucose levels were analyzed at regular intervals of the experimental period. Following the completion of experiment, the animals were sacrificed under anesthesia by cervical dislocation. Before sacrificing the animals, blood was collected for estimation of serum ALP, TRAP, and hydroxyproline. Right femora were collected for histomorphometrical analysis of trabecular bone and cortical bone. Left femora were stored at −70°C for testing the biomechanical properties. Right tibia was collected for measuring the dry weight.

2.5. Histomorphometrical Analysis. Left femora were dissected and the soft tissue separated. Tissues were fixed in the PLP fixative for 24 hr at 4°C. Then, the femora were subjected to decalcification using EDTA-glycerine solution. After 20 days of complete decalcification, tissues were dehydrated and placed in paraffin wax. The longitudinal sections (5 μm thickness) of the lower end of the femur were taken on rotary microtome and then processed for eosin and hematoxylin staining. The stained sections were used for analysis of the thickness of trabecular bone in the metaphyseal and epiphyseal regions, by using Olympus Cellsens Imaging Software (1.6 version, USA).

2.6. Measurement of Biomechanical Properties. The maximum flexor load was measured by a three-point bending test, using a Universal testing 3366 machine (Instron Corp, UK). Briefly, the left femora were brought to room temperature from −70°C and wiped with tissue paper. In the material testing machine, the bone was placed horizontally on two supports and load was applied in the middle of the shaft, at a speed of 5 mm/min until the bone was fractured.

2.7. Biochemical Analysis of Serum Bone Markers. ALP and TRAP levels were estimated by spectrophotometric method, using commercially available kits (Agappe diagnostics). Serum hydroxyproline levels were analyzed by Neuman and Logan method [35].

2.8. Dry Weight of the Tibia. Right tibia were collected and dissected free of soft tissue. Bone tissues were kept in a hot-air oven at 110°C for 48 hr and were weighed in digital balance as described previously [36].

TABLE 1: Effect of *PECQ* on blood glucose levels (mg/dL) in diabetic rats.

Groups	Day 0	Day 5	Day 15	Day 25	Day 35	Day 45
NC	89 ± 5.71	97.16 ± 5.02	92.5 ± 3.51	95.5 ± 4.58	99.83 ± 4.86	105.33 ± 5.14
DC	294.5 ± 9.66[***]	351.16 ± 23.5[***]	390 ± 18.44[***]	394 ± 19.52[***]	398 ± 26.51[***]	381 ± 21.59[***]
DC + CQ1	305 ± 13.8	342.66 ± 21.12	374.5 ± 14.49	379.5 ± 19.97	372.83 ± 23.65	375 ± 25.91
DC + CQ2	308.66 ± 13.48	346.33 ± 14.25	364.66 ± 22.08	365 ± 19.81	379 ± 26.61	378.5 ± 17.49
DC + INS	292.66 ± 9.05	102.83 ± 6.35[$$$]	109.5 ± 6.14[$$$]	99.16 ± 4.63[$$$]	117.16 ± 5.31[$$$]	103.83 ± 6.1[$$$]

[***]$P < 0.001$ when compared to NC group. [$$$]$P < 0.001$ when compared to DC group.

2.9. Statistical Analysis. Results were expressed as the mean ± standard error of mean. Data was analyzed by using Graphpad Prism (version 5.1). One-way ANOVA followed by Bonferroni's multiple comparison test was used to evaluate differences between groups. Statistical significance was considered at $P < 0.05$.

3. Results

3.1. Effect of PECQ on Blood Glucose Levels. DC rats had hyperglycemia (>250 mg/dL) throughout the experiment. The two doses of *PECQ* treatment did not alter the blood glucose levels in diabetic rats when compared to diabetic nontreated rats ($P > 0.05$; Table 1). However, insulin treatment significantly decreased the blood glucose levels, when compared to DC group ($P < 0.001$; Table 1).

3.2. Effect of PECQ on Trabecular Bone in Epiphyseal Region. DC rats had thinner trabeculae in the epiphyseal region ($P < 0.001$; Figures 1(a) and 1(b)) when compared to NC rats suggesting that the hyperglycemia affects the normal bone architecture and leads to bone loss in the epiphyseal region. Treatment with *PECQ* significantly improved the trabecular bone thickness in the DC + CQ1 ($P < 0.01$; Figures 1(a) and 1(b)) and DC + CQ2 ($P < 0.001$; Figures 1(a) and 1(b)) groups when compared to DC rats. On the other hand, metabolic control with INS significantly prevented the bone loss in diabetic rats ($P < 0.001$; Figures 1(a) and 1(b)) when compared to DC rats.

3.3. Effect of PECQ on Trabecular Bone in Metaphyseal Region. Thinner trabeculae were observed in the DC rats ($P < 0.001$; Figures 2(a) and 2(b)) when compared to NC rats, suggesting that hyperglycemia also affects the bone growth in the metaphyseal region. Treatment with two doses of *PECQ* significantly improved the trabecular bone thickness in DC + CQ1 and DC + CQ2 groups ($P < 0.01$; Figures 2(a) and 2(b)) when compared to diabetic nontreated rats. INS treatment also significantly improved the bone thickness in DC + INS rats ($P < 0.001$; Figures 2(a) and 2(b)) when compared to diabetic nontreated rats.

3.4. Effect of PECQ on Cortical Bone. The thickness of cortical bone significantly decreased in the DC group ($P < 0.001$; Figures 3(a) and 3(b)) when compared to NC rats, indicating the effect of hyperglycemia on cortical bone loss. *PECQ* treatment significantly improved the cortical bone thickness

TABLE 2: Effects of *PECQ* on serum bone markers in diabetic rats.

Groups	ALP (U/L)	TRP (U/L)	Hydroxyproline (μg/mL)
NC	96.45 ± 5.93	6.40 ± 0.29	0.233 ± 0.008
DC	188.7 ± 7.02[***]	8.52 ± 0.19[***]	0.285 ± 0.007[**]
DC + CQ1	217.3 ± 9.4[***]	6.90 ± 0.24[$]	0.250 ± 0.007[$]
DC + CQ2	223.3 ± 13.21[***]	6.74 ± 0.40[$$]	0.249 ± 0.009[$]
DC + INS	229.1 ± 9.75[***]	6.57 ± 0.37[$$]	0.239 ± 0.009[$$]

[***]$P < 0.001$, [**]$P < 0.01$ when compared to NC group. [$$]$P < 0.01$, [$]$P < 0.05$ when compared to DC group.

in the DC + CQ1 ($P < 0.01$; Figures 3(a) and 3(b)) and DC + CQ2 ($P < 0.001$; Figures 3(a) and 3(b)) groups when compared to DC rats. INS treatment also significantly improved the cortical bone thickness in diabetic rats ($P < 0.001$; Figures 3(a) and 3(b)) when compared to diabetic nontreated rats.

3.5. Effect of PECQ on Biomechanical Strength. Mean maximum flexor load (N) required to produce break in the femur of NC, DC, DC + CQ1, DC + CQ2, and DC + INS groups was 96.53 ± 5.37, 53.2 ± 5.03, 76.47 ± 4.4, 81.42 ± 6.24, and 91.53 ± 4.79 newtons, respectively. Mean maximum flexor load was significantly less in the diabetic nontreated rats ($P < 0.001$; Figure 4), when compared to nondiabetic control rats. Further, mean maximum flexor load was significantly more in DC + CQ1 ($P < 0.05$), DC + CQ2 ($P < 0.01$), and DC + INS ($P < 0.001$) groups when compared to DC rats (Figure 4).

3.6. Effect of PECQ on Dry Weight of Tibia. Dry weight of the tibia measured in NC, DC, DC + CQ1, DC + CQ2, and DC + INS groups was 0.42 ± 0.019, 0.26 ± 0.017, 0.35 ± 0.013, 0.36 ± 0.021, and 0.39 ± 0.022 grams, respectively. Bone weight was significantly decreased in the DC rats ($P < 0.001$; Figure 5), when compared to NC rats. Dry weight was significantly increased in all the treated groups, DC + CQ1 ($P < 0.05$), DC + CQ2 ($P < 0.05$), and DC + INS ($P < 0.001$), when compared to DC rats (Figure 5).

3.7. Effect of PECQ on ALP, TRAP, and Hydroxyproline. Serum ALP levels were significantly increased in diabetic nontreated animals ($P < 0.001$; Table 2) when compared to NC group. Increased ALP levels confirm that diabetes induces bone damage. Serum ALP levels further increased

(a)

(b)

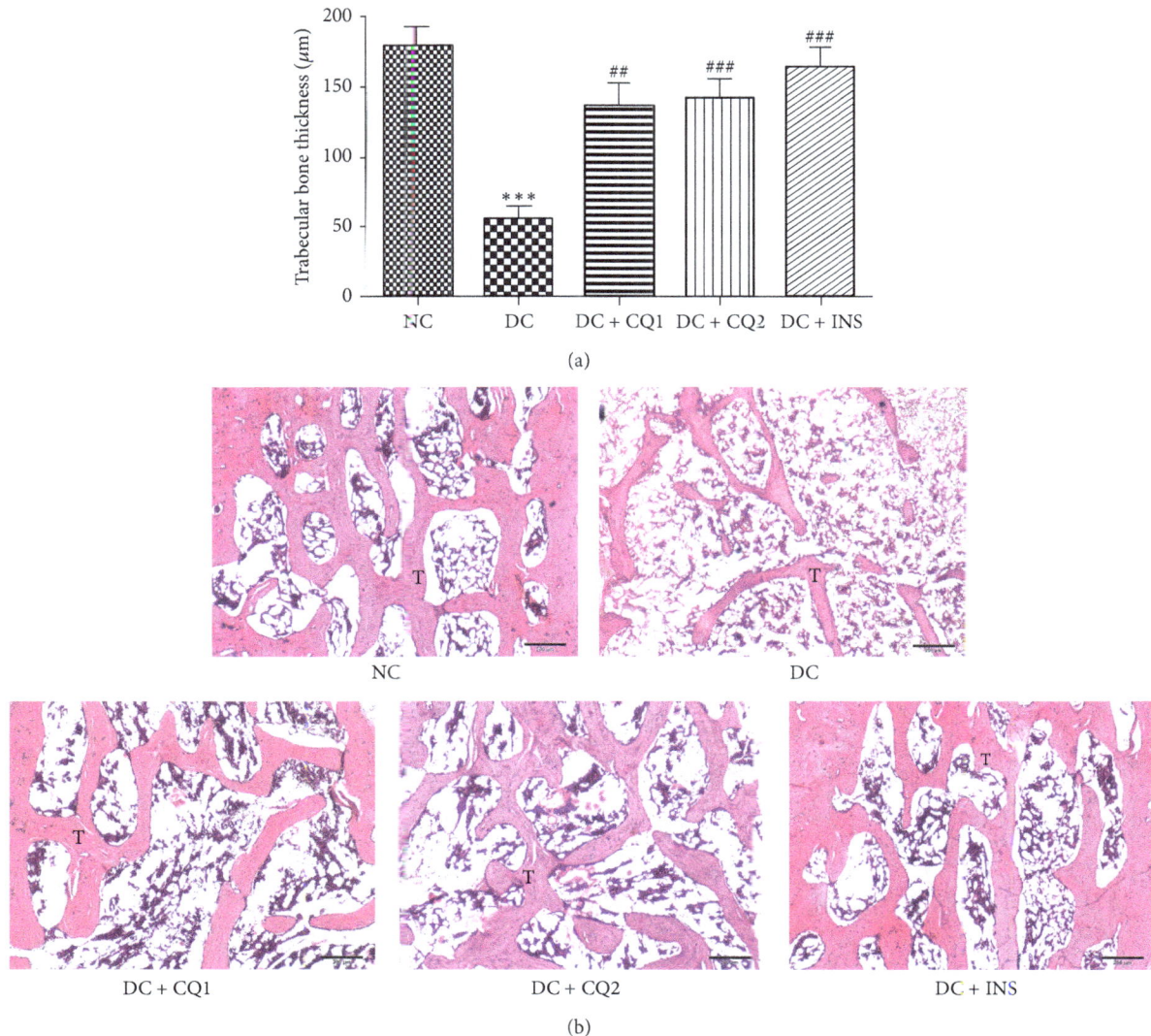

FIGURE 1: (a) Effect of *PECQ* on mean thickness of trabecular bone in the epiphyseal region. Significant decrease in the thickness of the trabecular bone was observed in the diabetic control (DC) rats when compared to normal control (NC) rats. However, diabetic rats treated with two different doses of *PECQ* (DC + CQ1 & DC + CQ2) or with insulin (DC + INS) showed a significant increase in bone thickness. *** $P < 0.001$ when compared to NC group; ### $P < 0.001$, ## $P < 0.01$ when compared to DC group. (b) Photomicrographs of trabecular bone in epiphyseal region. Thinner and reduced number of trabeculae can be seen in the diabetic control group (DC) when compared to normal control group (NC). Further treatment with two doses of *PECQ* (DC + CQ1, DC + CQ2) and insulin (DC + INS) improved the trabecular bone thickness. T: trabecular bone; H and E staining, scale bar: 200 μm.

in DC + CQ1 ($P < 0.001$), DC + CQ2 ($P < 0.001$), and DC + INS ($P < 0.001$) groups when compared to NC group (Table 2). This result shows that both *PECQ* and metabolic control with INS enhance the bone formation and mineralization process in hyperglycemic conditions. When compared to NC group, serum levels of TRAP ($P < 0.001$; Table 2) and hydroxyproline ($P < 0.01$; Table 2) were significantly increased in diabetic rats. Serum TRAP is a biomarker of osteoclast activity and hydroxyproline is considered as an end product of collagen degradation. The increased levels of these two proteins indicate the excessive bone resorption in the diabetic rats. Further, all the treatments significantly decreased the serum TRAP activity in the DC + CQ1 ($P < 0.05$),

DC + CQ2 ($P < 0.01$), and DC + INS ($P < 0.01$) groups in comparison to diabetic nontreated rats (Table 2). Similarly, the hydroxyproline levels were also significantly decreased in the DC + CQ1 ($P < 0.05$), DC + CQ2 ($P < 0.05$), and DC + INS ($P < 0.01$) groups in comparison to DC group (Table 2).

4. Discussion

Results of the present study showed that *PECQ* treatment is effective against type 1 DM- induced histological, biomechanical, and biochemical changes in the bone. Further, these

(a)

NC

DC

DC + CQ1

DC + CQ2

DC + INS

(b)

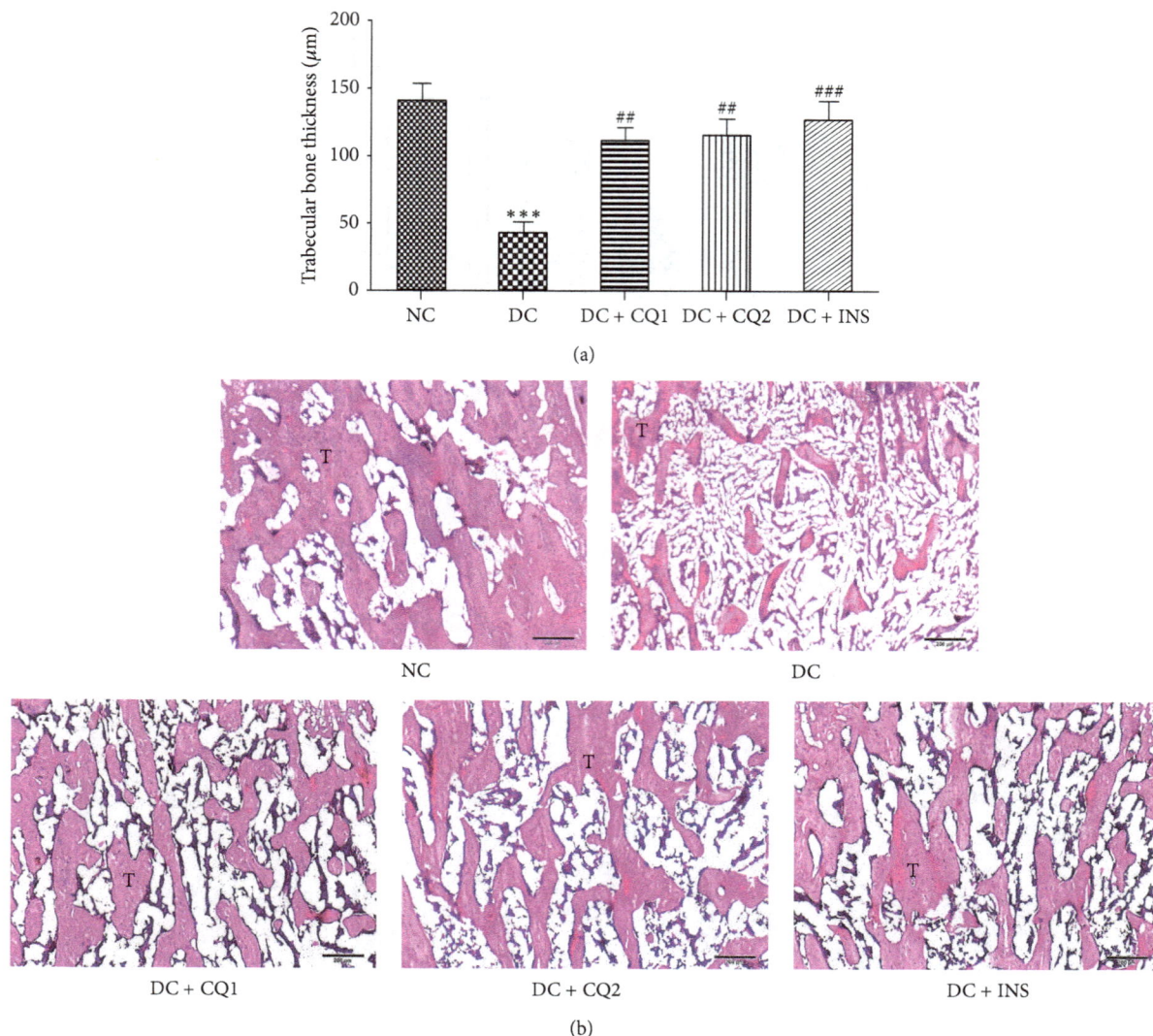

FIGURE 2: (a) Effect of *PECQ* on mean thickness of trabecular bone in the metaphyseal region. Thickness of the trabecular bone significantly decreased in diabetic control (DC) rats when compared to normal control (NC) rats. However, treatment with two different doses of *PECQ* (DC + CQ1 and DC + CQ2) or with insulin (DC + INS) showed a significant increase in the bone thickness, when compared to diabetic nontreated rats. ***$P < 0.001$ when compared to NC group; ###$P < 0.001$, ##$P < 0.01$ when compared to DC group. (b) Photomicrographs of the trabecular bone in metaphyseal region. Thinner, disrupted, and reduced number of trabeculae were observed in the diabetic control group (DC) when compared to the normal control group (NC). Further treatment with two doses of *PECQ* (DC + CQ1, DC + CQ2) and insulin (DC + INS) improved the trabecular bone growth. T: trabecular bone; H and E staining, scale bar: 200 μm.

results are comparable to the effects of insulin treatment. Unlike insulin, *PECQ* did not reduce the blood glucose levels in the diabetic rats indicating that *PECQ* has shown its effect through mechanisms other than the glycemic control.

The association between type 1 DM and osteoporosis has been accepted widely both experimentally [37, 38] and clinically [16, 39]. Based on the existing data, it is uncertain that reduced bone mass in diabetic rats is either due to defective bone formation or due to reduced bone growth [40]. Previous studies have reported the histological changes in both cortical bone [13, 41, 42] and trabecular bone [43, 44] in diabetic animals. Our results are consistent with those of earlier studies wherein the diabetic rats showed a marked

reduction in the thickness of both cortical and trabecular bones. The diabetic rats also had decreased dry weight of the bone compared to healthy animals. Bone strength depends on the integrity of the two components of bone: cortical and trabecular bone. Previous studies on the effect of diabetes on bone strength have reported conflicting data. In few reports bone strength is increased [20, 21]; meanwhile it is reduced in others [13, 42]. Our results indicate that diabetic rats seem to have lower bone strength.

It has been hypothesized that inflammation plays a role in the pathology of diabetes- induced bone complications [45]. Cytokines such as IL-6, IL-1β, and TNF-α are known for their involvement in the process of bone loss in diabetes

(a)

(b)

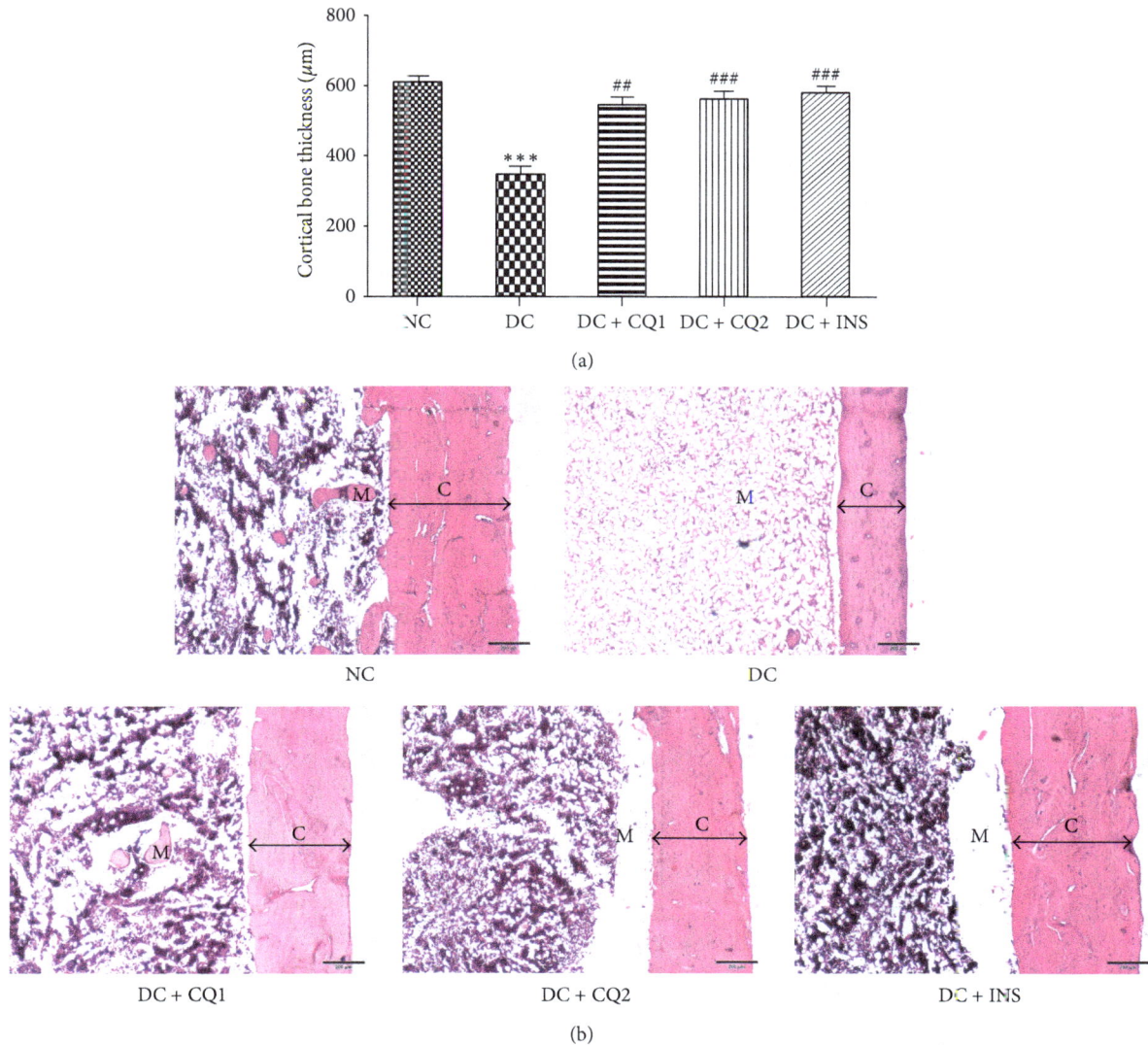

FIGURE 3: (a) Effect of *PECQ* on mean thickness of cortical bone. Thickness of the cortical bone significantly decreased in diabetic control (DC) rats when compared to normal control (NC) rats. Treatment with two different doses of *PECQ* (DC + CQ1 and DC + CQ2) or with insulin (DC + INS) significantly increased the bone thickness in diabetic rats when compared to nontreated diabetic rats. $^{***}P < 0.001$ when compared to NC group; $^{###}P < 0.001$, $^{##}P < 0.01$ when compared to DC group. (b) Photomicrographs of cortical bone. Thickness of the cortical bone was significantly less in the diabetic control group (DC) when compared to normal control group (NC). Further treatment with two doses of the *PECQ* (DC + CQ1, DC + CQ2) and insulin (DC + INS) improved the cortical bone growth. C: cortical bone; M: medullary cavity; H and E staining, scale bar: 200 μm.

[46]. LT-β, IL-6, IFN-γ, and TNF-α were found to increase in the diabetic bone [45]. Anti-inflammatory activity of *CQ* has been shown by previous studies [47, 48]. Ethanol fraction of *CQ* has been shown to decrease the serum levels of the proinflammatory cytokines TNF-α, IL-1β, and IL-6 in ovariectomized mice [48]. The positive effect of *PECQ* on bone loss in the diabetic state could be due to its anti-inflammatory property. However, experimental evidence is required to confirm effect of *PECQ* on both bone and serum cytokines levels in diabetic state.

Hyperglycemia is known to alter the antioxidant defense by increasing the polyol pathway flux, rate of formation of the ROS, and glucose-derived advanced glycosylation end products [49]. Previous studies have confirmed the association between oxidative stress and the development of osteopenia in DM [50, 51]. ROS is known to stimulate bone resorption by altering the function of osteoclasts [52]. Bai et al., have observed that oxidative stress can inhibit the differentiation of osteoblast cells [53]. Previous studies have demonstrated antioxidant and free radical scavenging potential of *CQ* both *in vitro* and *in vivo* [54, 55]. Hence, beneficial effects of *PECQ* against bone damage in diabetic rats can be correlated to its antioxidant properties.

Endocrine factor such as insulin-like growth factor-1 (IGF-1) signaling is found to be downregulated in both humans and animal models with type I DM [56, 57].

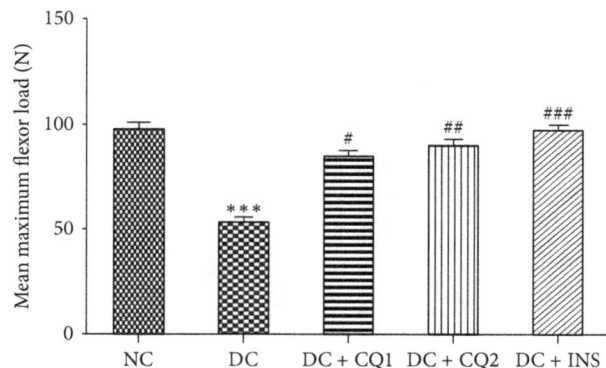

FIGURE 4: Effect of *PECQ* on mean maximum flexor load of femur. Mean maximum flexor load significantly decreased in diabetic control (DC) rats when compared to normal control (NC) rats. Treatment with two different doses of *PECQ* (DC + CQ1 and DC + CQ2) or with insulin (DC + INS) significantly increased the mean maximum flexor load in diabetic rats when compared to DC rats. ***$P < 0.001$ when compared to NC group; ###$P < 0.001$, ##$P < 0.01$, and #$P < 0.05$ when compared to DC group.

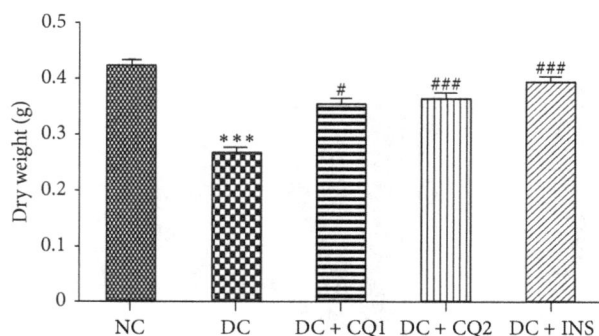

FIGURE 5: Effect of *PECQ* on dry weight of the tibia. Dry weight of the tibia significantly decreased in diabetic control (DC) rats when compared to normal control (NC) rats. Treatment with two different doses of *PECQ* (DC + CQ1 and DC + CQ2) or with insulin (DC + INS) significantly increased the dry weight in diabetic rats when compared to DC rats. ***$P < 0.001$ when compared to NC group; ###$P < 0.001$, #$P < 0.05$ when compared to DC group.

Decreased bone mineral density and altered osteoblast differentiation are seen with low serum levels of IGF-1 [58, 59]. Further, it has been demonstrated that improving the serum IGF-1 levels can prevent bone loss in diabetic rats [60]. Muthusami et al. studied the effect of ethanol extract *CQ* on IGF system components and found that *CQ* can enhance the mRNA expression of IGF-IR, IGF-I, and IGF-II [61]. Based on the above facts, we hypothesize that *PECQ* could have prevented the bone loss in diabetic rats by increasing the expression of IGF system components. However, further studies are required to confirm the effect of the *PECQ* on IGF system components in hyperglycemic conditions.

Earlier studies have demonstrated the beneficial effect of synthetic estrogen E2 against the bone loss in hyperglycemic state [25, 26]. The positive effect of *PECQ* on bone changes in diabetic rats observed in the present study could be due to

the phytoestrogen steroids present in it [32, 33], which may increase the bone formation and/or accelerate bone growth. Alterations in the mineral metabolism and bone remodeling factors are claimed to be the possible mechanism of diabetes-induced osteoporosis [17]. It has been observed that altered bone turnover in diabetes is usually associated with the changes in serum ALP, TRAP, and hydroxyproline activities [25]. In the present study, ALP levels were significantly increased in diabetic rats. Serum ALP is considered as a biomarker of osteoblast activity. The increased ALP levels in the diabetic rats indicate the compensatory mechanism of the body against diabetes-induced bone damage. Administration of two doses of *PECQ* and INS showed further increase in the ALP levels compared to diabetic group. This result indicates that *PECQ* enhances osteoblast proliferation and thus facilitates the bone formation. An *in vitro* study has demonstrated the stimulatory effect of E2 on differentiation of bone marrow mesenchymal stem cells, in hyperglycemic conditions [62]. The beneficial effect of *PECQ* on ALP activity could be due to estrogen-mimicking action of phytoestrogen steroids present in it [32, 33].

Compared to normal control group, serum TRAP levels are significantly increased in diabetic animals. Serum TRAP is a biomarker of osteoclast activity. The increased levels of this protein indicate that the reduced bone mass in the diabetic rats is also due to excessive bone resorption. With respect to serum TRAP activity, our results are consistent with previous findings [25]. However, Waud et al. have observed normal TRAP activity in the experimental diabetic animals [37]. In another study on patients with type I diabetes, TRAP activity was found to be low [63]. Administration of *PECQ* and INS significantly decreased the TRAP levels compared to diabetic animals. The observed effect of the *PECQ* on the TRAP activity could be due to the direct action of the phytoestrogen steroids present in it [32, 33]. This can be explained based on the fact that estrogen can accelerate the apoptosis of matured osteoclast cells [64].

Serum hydroxyproline is a breakdown product of collagen. In the present study, the hydroxyproline levels were significantly increased in the diabetic rats indicating the inhibitory effect of diabetes on bone collagen. This result is consistent with that of the previous study [25]. Treatment with *PECQ* and INS significantly decreased the serum hydroxyproline levels. Gopalakrishnan et al. in their *in vitro* study demonstrated the positive effect of E2 on mineralization and histochemical staining for collagen in the bone marrow stromal cells [62]. The positive effect of the *PECQ* could be due to the estrogen-like action of phytoestrogen steroids [32, 33] on collagen formation.

5. Conclusion

Preliminary results of the present study indicate that *PECQ* is effective in improving histological, biomechanical, and biochemical changes of bone in diabetic rats. Though exact mechanism of action of *PECQ* has not been ascertained, the observed effect of *PECQ* could be due to its osteogenic, antioxidant, and anti-inflammatory properties.

However, in this context, extensive studies are required to confer the exact mechanism of *PECQ* on bone cells in hyperglycemic conditions.

Conflict of Interests

The authors declare that there is no conflict of interests regarding the publication of this paper.

References

[1] B. Balkau, M. A. Charles, and E. Eschwege, "Discussion épidémiologique des nouveaux critères de diabète," *Médecine Thérapeutique Endocrinologie & Reproduction*, vol. 2, no. 3, pp. 229–234, 2000.

[2] J. V. Santiago, W. H. McAlister, S. K. Ratzan et al., "Decreased cortical thickness and osteopenia in children with diabetes mellitus," *The Journal of Clinical Endocrinology and Metabolism*, vol. 45, no. 4, pp. 845–848, 1977.

[3] M. E. Levin, V. C. Boisseau, and L. V. Avioli, "Effects of diabetes mellitus on bone mass in juvenile and adult onset diabetes," *The New England Journal of Medicine*, vol. 294, no. 5, pp. 241–245, 1976.

[4] I. de Leeuw and R. Abs, "Bone mass and bone density in maturity-type diabetics measured by the ^{125}I photon-absorption technique," *Diabetes*, vol. 26, no. 12, pp. 1130–1135, 1977.

[5] H. Heath III, P. W. Lambert, F. J. Service, and S. B. Arnaud, "Calcium homeostasis in diabetes mellitus," *The Journal of Clinical Endocrinology and Metabolism*, vol. 49, no. 3, pp. 462–466, 1979.

[6] P. McNair, S. Madsbad, C. Christiansen, O. K. Faber, I. Transbol, and C. Binder, "Osteopenia in insulin treated diabetes mellitus. Its relation to age at onset, sex and duration of disease," *Diabetologia*, vol. 15, no. 2, pp. 87–90, 1978.

[7] Y. Seino and H. Ishida, "Diabetic osteopenia: pathophysiology and clinical aspects," *Diabetes/Metabolism Reviews*, vol. 11, no. 1, pp. 21–35, 1995.

[8] J. Levy, I. Reid, L. Halstad, J. R. Gavin III, and L. V. Avioli, "Abnormal cell calcium concentrations in cultured bone cells obtained from femurs of obese and noninsulin-dependent diabetic rats," *Calcified Tissue International*, vol. 44, no. 2, pp. 131–137, 1989.

[9] L. Cozen, "Does diabetes delay fracture healing?" *Clinical Orthopaedics and Related Research*, vol. 82, pp. 134–140, 1972.

[10] R. Shires, S. L. Teitelbaum, M. A. Bergfeld, M. D. Fallon, E. Slatopolsky, and L. V. Avioli, "The effect of streptozotocin-induced chronic diabetes mellitus on bone and mineral homeostasis in the rat," *Journal of Laboratory and Clinical Medicine*, vol. 97, no. 2, pp. 231–240, 1981.

[11] K. Suzuki, N. Miyakoshi, T. Tsuchida, Y. Kasukawa, K. Sato, and E. Itoi, "Effects of combined treatment of insulin and human parathyroid hormone(1–34) on cancellous bone mass and structure in streptozotocin-induced diabetic rats," *Bone*, vol. 33, no. 1, pp. 108–114, 2003.

[12] J. J. Tomasek, S. W. Meyers, J. B. Basinger, D. T. Green, and R. L. Shew, "Diabetic and age-related enhancement of collagen-linked fluorescence in cortical bones of rats," *Life Sciences*, vol. 55, no. 11, pp. 855–861, 1994.

[13] J. Verhaeghe, A. M. Suiker, T. A. Einhorn et al., "Brittle bones in spontaneously diabetic female rats cannot be predicted by bone mineral measurements: studies in diabetic and ovariectomized rats," *Journal of Bone and Mineral Research*, vol. 9, no. 10, pp. 1657–1667, 1994.

[14] J. Verhaeghe, A. M. Suiker, B. L. Nyomba et al., "Bone mineral homeostasis in spontaneously diabetic BB rats. II. Impaired bone turnover and decreased osteocalcin synthesis," *Endocrinology*, vol. 124, no. 2, pp. 573–582, 1989.

[15] J. Verhaeghe, E. van Herck, W. J. Visser et al., "Bone and mineral metabolism in BB rats with long-term diabetes: decreased bone turnover and osteoporosis," *Diabetes*, vol. 39, no. 4, pp. 477–482, 1990.

[16] S. A. G. Kemink, A. R. M. M. Hermus, L. M. J. W. Swinkels, J. A. Lutterman, and A. G. H. Smals, "Osteopenia in insulin-dependent diabetes mellitus: prevalence and aspects of pathophysiology," *Journal of Endocrinological Investigation*, vol. 23, no. 5, pp. 295–303, 2000.

[17] D. T. Ward, S. K. Yau, A. P. Mee et al., "Functional, molecular, and biochemical characterization of streptozotocin-induced diabetes," *Journal of the American Society of Nephrology*, vol. 12, no. 4, pp. 779–790, 2001.

[18] P. K. Dixit and R. A. Ekstrom, "Retardation of bone fracture healing in experimental diabetes," *Indian journal of medical research*, vol. 85, pp. 426–435, 1987.

[19] H. A. Beam, J. R. Parsons, and S. S. Lin, "The effects of blood glucose control upon fracture healing in the BB Wistar rat with diabetes mellitus," *Journal of Orthopaedic Research*, vol. 20, no. 6, pp. 1210–1216, 2002.

[20] J. R. Funk, J. E. Hale, D. Carmines, H. L. Gooch, and S. R. Hurwitz, "Biomechanical evaluation of early fracture healing in normal and diabetic rats," *Journal of Orthopaedic Research*, vol. 18, no. 1, pp. 126–132, 2000.

[21] G. K. Reddy, L. Stehno-Bittel, S. Hamade, and C. S. Enwemeka, "The biomechanical integrity of bone in experimental diabetes," *Diabetes Research and Clinical Practice*, vol. 54, no. 1, pp. 1–8, 2001.

[22] J. Griffet, A. Chevallier, E. Accorsi, T. El Hayek, G. Odin, and B. Pebeyre, "Osteosynthesis of diaphyseal fracture by Ossatite experimental study in rat," *Biomaterials*, vol. 20, no. 6, pp. 511–515, 1999.

[23] S. Pramanik, A. K. Agarwal, K. N. Rai, and A. Garg, "Development of high strength hydroxyapatite by solid-state-sintering process," *Ceramics International*, vol. 33, no. 3, pp. 419–426, 2007.

[24] J. R. Woodard, A. J. Hilldore, S. K. Lan et al., "The mechanical properties and osteoconductivity of hydroxyapatite bone scaffolds with multi-scale porosity," *Biomaterials*, vol. 28, no. 1, pp. 45–54, 2007.

[25] V. Gopalakrishnan, J. Arunakaran, M. M. Aruldhas, and N. Srinivasan, "Effects of streptozotocin-induced diabetes mellitus on some bone turnover markers in the vertebrae of ovary-intact and ovariectomized adult rats," *Biochemistry and Cell Biology*, vol. 84, no. 5, pp. 728–736, 2006.

[26] J. Verhaeghe, J. S. Thomsen, R. van Bree, E. van Herck, R. Bouillon, and L. Mosekilde, "Effects of exercise and disuse on bone remodeling, bone mass, and biomechanical competence in spontaneously diabetic female rats," *Bone*, vol. 27, no. 2, pp. 249–256, 2000.

[27] A. Shirwaikar, S. Khan, and S. Malini, "Antiosteoporotic effect of ethanol extract of *Cissus quadrangularis* Linn. on ovariectomized rat," *Journal of Ethnopharmacology*, vol. 89, no. 2-3, pp. 245–250, 2003.

[28] E. M. Williamson, *Major Herbs of Ayuraveda*, Churchill Living-stone, London, UK, 2002.

[29] S. J. Stohs and S. D. Ray, "A review and evaluation of the efficacy and safety of *Cissus quadrangularis* extracts," *Phytotherapy Research*, vol. 27, no. 8, pp. 1107–1114, 2013.

[30] B. K. Potu, M. S. Rao, G. K. Nampurath, M. R. Chamallamudi, S. R. Nayak, and H. Thomas, "Anti-osteoporotic activity of the petroleum ether extract of *Cissus quadrangularis* Linn. in ovariectomized wistar rats," *Chang Gung Medical Journal*, vol. 33, no. 3, pp. 252–257, 2010.

[31] T. Pathomwichaiwata, W. Suvitayavatb, A. Sailasutac, P. Piy-achaturawatd, N. Soonthornchareonnone, and S. Prathantu-raruga, "Antiosteoporotic effect of sequential extracts and freezedried juice of *Cissus quadrangularis* L. in ovariectomized mice," *Asian Biomedicine*, vol. 6, no. 3, pp. 377–384, 2012.

[32] G. C. Prasad and K. N. Udupa, "Pathways and site of action of a phytogenic steroid from *Cissus quadrangularis*," *Journal of Research in Indian Medicine*, vol. 4, article 132, 1972.

[33] U. M. Aswar, V. Mohan, and S. L. Bodhankar, "Antiosteoporotic activity of phytoestrogen-rich fraction separated from ethanol extract of aerial parts of *Cissus quadrangularis* in ovariec-tomized rats," *Indian Journal of Pharmacology*, vol. 44, no. 3, pp. 345–350, 2012.

[34] B. K. Potu, K. M. Bhat, M. S. Rao et al., "Petroleum ether extract of *Cissus quadrangularis* (linn.) enhances bone marrow mesenchymal stem cell proliferation and facilitates osteoblasto-genesis," *Clinics*, vol. 64, no. 10, pp. 993–998, 2009.

[35] R. E. Neuman and M. A. Logan, "The determination of collagen and elastin in tissues," *The Journal of Biological Chemistry*, vol. 186, no. 2, pp. 549–556, 1950.

[36] N. P. Reddy, M. Lakshmana, and U. V. Udupa, "Antiosteoporotic activity of OST-6(Osteocare), a herbomineral preparation in calcium deficient ovariectomized rats," *Phytotherapy Research*, vol. 18, no. 1, pp. 25–29, 2004.

[37] C. E. Waud, S. C. Marks Jr., R. Lew, and D. T. Baran, "Bone mineral density in the femur and lumbar vertebrae decreases after twelve weeks of diabetes in spontaneously diabetic-prone BB/Worcester rats," *Calcified Tissue International*, vol. 54, no. 3, pp. 237–240, 1994.

[38] S. Herrero, O. M. Calvo, C. García-Moreno et al., "Low bone density with normal bone turnover in ovariectomized and streptozotocin-induced diabetic rats," *Calcified Tissue Interna-tional*, vol. 62, no. 3, pp. 260–265, 1998.

[39] T. Miazgowski and S. Czekalski, "A 2-year follow-up study on bone mineral density and markers of bone turnover in patients with long-standing insulin-dependent diabetes mellitus," *Osteo-porosis International*, vol. 8, no. 5, pp. 399–403, 1998.

[40] M. J. Silva, M. D. Brodt, M. A. Lynch et al., "Type 1 diabetes in young rats leads to progressive trabecular bone loss, cessation of cortical bone growth, and diminished whole bone strength and fatigue life," *Journal of Bone and Mineral Research*, vol. 24, no. 9, pp. 1618–1627, 2009.

[41] P. K. Dixit and R. A. Ekstrom, "Decreased breaking strength of diabetic rat bone and its improvement by insulin treatment," *Calcified Tissue International*, vol. 32, no. 3, pp. 195–199, 1980.

[42] T. A. Einhorn, A. L. Boskey, C. M. Gundberg, V. J. Vigorita, V. J. Devlin, and M. M. Beyer, "The mineral and mechanical properties of bone in chronic experimental diabetes," *Journal of Orthopaedic Research*, vol. 6, no. 3, pp. 317–323, 1988.

[43] T. Tsuchida, K. Sato, N. Miyakoshi et al., "Histomorphometric evaluation of the recovering effect of human parathyroid hor-mone (1–34) on bone structure and turnover in streptozotocin-induced diabetic rats," *Calcified Tissue International*, vol. 66, no. 3, pp. 229–233, 2000.

[44] W. G. Goodman and M. T. Hori, "Diminished bone formation in experimental diabetes. Relationship to osteoid maturation and mineralization," *Diabetes*, vol. 33, no. 9, pp. 825–831, 1984.

[45] K. J. Motyl, S. Botolin, R. Irwin et al., "Bone inflammation and altered gene expression with type I diabetes early onset," *Journal of Cellular Physiology*, vol. 218, no. 3, pp. 575–583, 2009.

[46] R. Blakytny, M. Spraul, and E. B. Jude, "Review: the diabetic bone: a cellular and molecular perspective," *The International Journal of Lower Extremity Wounds*, vol. 10, no. 1, pp. 16–32, 2011.

[47] A. M. Bhujade, S. Talmale, N. Kumar et al., "Evaluation of *Cissus quadrangularis* extracts as an inhibitor of COX, 5-LOX, and proinflammatory mediators," *Journal of Ethnopharmacology*, vol. 141, no. 3, pp. 989–996, 2012.

[48] J. Banu, E. Varela, A. N. Bahadur, R. Soomro, N. Kazi, and G. Fernandes, "Inhibition of bone loss by *Cissus quadrangularis* in mice: a preliminary report," *Journal of Osteoporosis*, vol. 2012, Article ID 101206, 10 pages, 2012.

[49] T. Oyama, Y. Miyasita, H. Watanabe, and K. Shirai, "The role of polyol pathway in high glucose-induced endothelial cell damages," *Diabetes Research and Clinical Practice*, vol. 73, no. 3, pp. 227–234, 2006.

[50] K. Ding, Z. Wang, M. W. Hamrick et al., "Disordered osteoclast formation in RAGE-deficient mouse establishes an essential role for RAGE in diabetes related bone loss," *Biochemical and Biophysical Research Communications*, vol. 340, no. 4, pp. 1091–1097, 2006.

[51] Y. Hamada, S. Kitazawa, R. Kitazawa, H. Fujii, M. Kasuga, and M. Fukagawa, "Histomorphometric analysis of diabetic osteopenia in streptozotocin-induced diabetic mice: a possible role of oxidative stress," *Bone*, vol. 40, no. 5, pp. 1408–1414, 2007.

[52] I. R. Garrett, B. F. Boyce, R. O. Oreffo, L. Bonewald, J. Poser, and G. R. Mundy, "Oxygen-derived free radicals stimulate osteoclastic bone resorption in rodent bone *in vitro* and *in vivo*," *The Journal of Clinical Investigation*, vol. 85, no. 3, pp. 632–639, 1990.

[53] X.-C. Bai, D. Lu, J. Bai et al., "Oxidative stress inhibits osteoblas-tic differentiation of bone cells by ERK and NF-κB," *Biochemical and Biophysical Research Communications*, vol. 314, no. 1, pp. 197–207, 2004.

[54] M. Jainu and C. S. Devi, "*In vitro* and *in vivo* evaluation of free-radical scavenging potential of *Cissus quadrangularis*," *African Journal of Biomedical Research*, vol. 8, no. 2, pp. 95–99, 2005.

[55] K. N. C. Murthy, A. Vanitha, M. M. Swamy, and G. A. Ravishankar, "Antioxidant and antimicrobial activity of *Cissus quadrangularis* L," *Journal of Medicinal Food*, vol. 6, no. 2, pp. 99–105, 2003.

[56] R. G. Clark, "Recombinant human insulin-like growth factor I (IGF-I): risks and benefits of normalizing blood IGF-I concen-trations," *Hormone Research in Paediatrics*, vol. 62, supplement 1, pp. 93–100, 2004.

[57] P. M. Jehle, D. R. Jehle, S. Mohan, and B. O. Böhm, "Serum levels of insulin-like growth factor system components and relationship to bone metabolism in type 1 and type 2 diabetes mellitus patients," *The Journal of Endocrinology*, vol. 159, no. 2, pp. 297–306, 1998.

[58] C. J. Rosen, C. L. Ackert-Bicknell, M. L. Adamo et al., "Congenic mice with low serum IGF-I have increased body fat, reduced

bone mineral density, and an altered osteoblast differentiation program," *Bone*, vol. 35, no. 5, pp. 1046–1058, 2004.

[59] M. Zhang, S. Xuan, M. L. Bouxsein et al. "Osteoblast-specific knockout of the insulin-like growth factor (IGF) receptor gene reveals an essential role of IGF signaling in bone matrix mineralization," *The Journal of Biological Chemistry*, vol. 277, no. 46, pp. 44005–44012, 2002.

[60] J. Verhaeghe, A. M. Suiker, W. J. Visser, E. van Herck, R. van Bree, and R. Bouillon, "The effects of systemic insulin, insulin-like growth factor-I and growth hormone on bone growth and turnover in spontaneously diabetic BB rats," *The Journal of Endocrinology*, vol. 134, no. 3, pp. 485–492, 1992.

[61] S. Muthusami, I. Ramachandran, S. Krishnamoorthy, R. Govindan, and S. Narasimhan, "*Cissus quadrangularis* augments IGF system components in human osteoblast like SaOS-2 cells," *Growth Hormone and IGF Research*, vol. 21, no. 6, pp. 343–348, 2011.

[62] V. Gopalakrishnan, R. C. Vignesh, J. Arunakaran, M. M. Aruldhas, and N. Srinivasan, "Effects of glucose and its modulation by insulin and estradiol on BMSC differentiation into osteoblastic lineages," *Biochemistry and Cell Biology*, vol. 84, no. 1, pp. 93–101, 2006.

[63] M. M. C. Pastor, P. J. López-Ibarra, F. Escobar-Jiménez, M. D. Serrano Pardo, and A. García-Cervigón, "Intensive insulin therapy and bone mineral density in type 1 diabetes mellitus: a prospective study," *Osteoporosis International*, vol. 11, no. 5, pp. 455–459, 2000.

[64] D. E. Hughes, A. Dai, J. C. Tiffee, H. H. Li, G. R. Munoy, and B. F. Boyce, "Estrogen promotes apoptosis of murine osteoclasts mediated by TGF-β," *Nature Medicine*, vol. 2, no. 10, pp. 1132–1136, 1996.

Permissions

List of Contributors

Prafulla P. Adkar
Department of Pharmacology, JSPM's Jayawantrao Sawant College of Pharmacy and Research, University of Pune, Pune, Maharashtra 411028, India
Vinayaka Missions University, Sankari Main Road, NH-47, Ariyanoor, Salem, Tamil Nadu 636308, India

V. H. Bhaskar
Department of Pharmaceutical Medicinal Chemistry, Gahlot Institute of Pharmacy, Plot No. 59, Sector No. 14, Kopar khairane, Navi Mumbai, Maharashtra 400709, India

Muhammad Aslam
Department of Basic Medical Sciences, Faculty of Pharmacy, Ziauddin University, Karachi 75600, Pakistan

Ali Akbar Sial
Department of Pharmaceutics, Faculty of Pharmacy, Ziauddin University, Karachi 75600, Pakistan

Doa'a Anwar Ibrahim
Department of Pharmacology, Faculty of Pharmacy, University of Science and Technology, Sana'a, Yemen

Rowida Noman Albadani
Department of Pharmacognosy, Faculty of Pharmacy, University of Science and Technology, Sana'a, Yemen

Ritu Singh, Jyoti Sharma and P. K. Goyal
Radiation & Cancer Biology Laboratory, Department of Zoology, University of Rajasthan, Jaipur 302 004, India

Davood Oliaee
Student Research Committee, Mashhad University of Medical Sciences, Mashhad 9137503645, Iran

Mohammad Taher Boroushaki
Pharmacological Research Center of Medicinal Plants, School of Medicine, Mashhad University of Medical Sciences, Mashhad 9177948564, Iran
Department of Pharmacology, School of Medicine, Mashhad University of Medical Sciences, Mashhad 9177948564, Iran

Naiime Oliaee and Ahmad Ghorbani
Pharmacological Research Center of Medicinal Plants, School of Medicine, Mashhad University of Medical Sciences, Mashhad 9177948564, Iran

Candice Pullen, Fiona R. Coulson and Andrew Fenning
School of Medical and Applied Sciences, CQ University, Rockhampton, Australia

Mohamed El-Hewaity
Department of Pharmacology, Faculty of Veterinary Medicine, University of El-Sadat City, Minoufiya 32897, Egypt

Elio A. Soria, Patricia L. Quiroga and Claudia Albrecht
Facultad de Ciencias Médicas, Universidad Nacional de Córdoba, INICSA-CONICET/UNC, Enrique Barros S/N, 5014 Córdoba, Argentina

Sabina I. Ramos Elizagaray
Consejo Interuniversitario Nacional, Pacheco de Melo 2084, 1126 Ciudad Autónoma de Buenos Aires, Argentina

Juan J. Cantero
Facultad de Agronomía y Veterinaria, Universidad Nacional de Río Cuarto, IMBIV-CONICET/UNC, Ruta 36 Km 601, 804 Río Cuarto, Argentina

Guillermina A. Bongiovanni
Facultad de Ciencias Agrarias, Universidad Nacional del Comahue, PROBIEN-CONICET/UNCO, CP 8300, Neuquén, 1400 Buenos Aires, Argentina

Manish Kumar, Satyendra K. Prasad, Sairam Krishnamurthy and Siva Hemalatha
Pharmacognosy Research Laboratory, Department of Pharmaceutics, Indian Institute of Technology, Banaras Hindu University, Varanasi 221005, India

Carene M. N. Picot, A. Hussein Subratty and M. Fawzi Mahomoodally
Department of Health Sciences, Faculty of Science, University of Mauritius, 230 Réduit, Mauritius

Alejandra Herrera Herrera, Luis Fang and Antonio Díaz Caballero
Grupo de Investigaciones GITOUC, Facultad de Odontología, Universidad de Cartagena, Campus de la Salud, Cartagena, Colombia

Luis Franco Ospina
Grupo de Evaluación Biológica de Sustancias Promisorias, Facultad de Ciencias Farmacéuticas, Universidad de Cartagena, Campus de la Salud, Cartagena, Colombia

Yalda Shokoohinia
Novel Drug Delivery Research Center, School of Pharmacy, Kermanshah University of Medical Sciences, Kermanshah 6734667149, Iran
Department of Pharmacognosy and Biotechnology, School of Pharmacy, Kermanshah University of Medical Sciences, Kermanshah 6734667149, Iran

Leila Hosseinzadeh
Novel Drug Delivery Research Center, School of Pharmacy, Kermanshah University of Medical Sciences, Kermanshah 6734667149, Iran

Maryam Alipour
Students Research Committee, School of Pharmacy, Kermanshah University of Medical Sciences, Kermanshah 6734667149, Iran

Ali Mostafaie and Hamid-RezaMohammadi-Motlagh
Medical Biology Research Center, Kermanshah University of Medical Sciences, Kermanshah 6734667149, Iran

Xingjiang Hu, Mingzhu Huang, Jian Liu, Junchun Chen and Jianzhong Shentu
Research Center for Clinical Pharmacy, State Key Laboratory for Diagnosis and Treatment of Infectious Diseases, First Affiliated Hospital, Zhejiang University, Qingchun Road 79, Hangzhou 310003, China

Arthur T. Kopylov and Ksenia G. Kuznetsova
Institute of Biomedical Chemistry, 10 Pogodinskaya Street, Moscow 119121, Russia

Olga M. Mikhailova, Andrey G. Moshkin, Vladimir V. Turkin and Andrei A. Alimov
Institute of Applied Biochemistry JSC "Biochimmash," 4 KlaraTsetkin Street, Moscow 127299, Russia

Chibueze Peter Ihekwereme and Edward Chieke Nwanegbo
Department of Pharmacology and Toxicology, Faculty of Pharmaceutical Sciences, Nnamdi Azikiwe University, Awka 420281, Nigeria

Charles Okechukwu Esimone
Department of Pharmaceutical Microbiology and Biotechnology, Faculty of Pharmaceutical Sciences, Nnamdi Azikiwe University, Awka 420281, Nigeria

Azam Bakhtiarian, Farahnaz Jazaeri and Vahid Nikoui
Department of Pharmacology, School of Medicine, Tehran University of Medical Sciences, Pour Sina Street, Qods Street, Keshavarz Boulevard, Tehran 1417613151, Iran

Nasrin Takzare
Department of Anatomy, School of Medicine, Tehran University of Medical Sciences, Tehran 1417613146, Iran

Mehdi Sheykhi
School of Medicine, Tehran University of Medical Sciences, Tehran 1417613110, Iran

Narges Sistany
Department of Neurosurgery, Shariati Hospital, Tehran University of Medical Sciences, Tehran, Iran

Mario Giorgi
Department of Veterinary Sciences, University of Pisa, San Piero a Grado, Pisa 56122, Italy

Amang André Perfusion
Department of Animal Biology & Physiology, Faculty of Science, P.O. Box 812, University of Yaoundé I, Yaoundé, Cameroon
Department of Biological Sciences, Faculty of Science, P.O. Box 46, University of Maroua, Maroua, Cameroon

Paul V. Tan
Department of Animal Biology & Physiology, Faculty of Science, P.O. Box 812, University of Yaoundé I, Yaoundé, Cameroon

Nkwengoua Ernestine and Nyasse Barthélemy
Department of Organic Chemistry, Faculty of Science, P.O. Box 812, University of Yaoundé I, Yaoundé, Cameroon

Florent Duval, Jorge E. Moreno-Cuevas, Maria Teresa González-Garza and Delia Elva Cruz-Vega
Catedra de Terapia Celular, Escuela de Medicina, Tecnológico de Monterrey, Avenida Morones Prieto 3000 Pte., 64710 Monterrey, NL, Mexico

Carlos Rodríguez-Montalvo
Centro de Enfermedades Hepáticas-Digestivas y Nutrición, Hospital San José, Avenida Morones Prieto 3000, 64710 Monterrey, NL, Mexico

Vijay K. Bharti
Division of Physiology and Climatology, Indian Veterinary Research Institute (IVRI), Izatnagar, Uttar Pradesh 243122, India
Nutrition and Toxicology Laboratory, Defence Institute of High Altitude Research (DIHAR), Defence Research and Development Organization (DRDO), Ministry of Defence, C/o- 56 APO, Leh 194101, India

R. S. Srivastava, S. Bag, A. C. Majumdar and G. Singh
Division of Physiology and Climatology, Indian Veterinary Research Institute (IVRI), Izatnagar, Uttar Pradesh 243122, India

H. Kumar
Division of Animal Reproduction, Indian Veterinary Research Institute (IVRI), Izatnagar, Uttar Pradesh 243122, India

S. R. Pandi-Perumal
Somnogen Inc., College Street, Toronto, ON, Canada M6H 1C5

Gregory M. Brown
Department of Psychiatry, Faculty of Medicine, University of Toronto and Centre for Addiction and Mental Health, 250 College Street, Toronto, ON, Canada M5T 1R8

Nelvana Ramalingum and M. FawziMahomoodally
Department of Health Sciences, Faculty of Science, University of Mauritius, 230 Réduit, Mauritius

Mohamed Aboubakr and Mohamed Elbadawy
Department of Pharmacology, Faculty of Veterinary Medicine, Benha University, Moshtohor, Toukh, Qaliobiya 13736, Egypt

Ahmed Soliman
Department of Pharmacology, Faculty of Veterinary Medicine, Cairo University, Giza 12211, Egypt

Mohamed El-Hewaity
Department of Pharmacology, Faculty of Veterinary Medicine, University of Sadat City, Minoufiya 32897, Egypt

Bachir Benarba
Laboratory of Bioconversion, Microbial engineering and Health Safety, Department of Biology, University of Mascara, 29000 Mascara, Algeria
Laboratory of Research on Biological Systems and Geomatics, University of Mascara, 29000 Mascara, Algeria

Boumedienne Meddah
Laboratory of Research on Biological Systems and Geomatics, University of Mascara, 29000 Mascara, Algeria

Aicha Tir Touil
Laboratory of Bioconversion, Microbial engineering and Health Safety, Department of Biology, University of Mascara, 29000 Mascara, Algeria

Ankit A. Gilan
Department of Pharmacology and Toxicology, National Institute of Pharmaceutical Education and Research, C/O-B. V. Patel Pharmaceutical Education and Research Development (PERD) Centre, S. G. Highway, Thaltej, Ahmedabad, Gujarat 380054, India

Ranjeet Prasad Dash, Mehul N. Jivrajani, Sandeep Kumar Thakur and Manish Nivsarkar
Department of Pharmacology and Toxicology, B. V. Patel Pharmaceutical Education and Research Development (PERD) Centre, S. G. Highway, Thaltej, Ahmedabad, Gujarat 380054, India

Oluwatosin Adekunle Adaramoye and Olubukola Oyebimpe Akanni
Drug Metabolism and Toxicology Research Laboratories, Department of Biochemistry, College of Medicine, University of Ibadan, Ibadan 20005, Nigeria

Prafulla Adkar
Department of Pharmacology, JSPM's Jayawantrao Sawant College of Pharmacy and Research, Hadapsar, Pune, Maharashtra 411028, India

Amita Dongare and Shirishkumar Ambavade
Department of Pharmacology, JSPM's Jayawantrao Sawant College of Pharmacy and Research, Hadapsar, Pune, Maharashtra 411028, India
Post Graduates Department of Pharmacology and Toxicology, JSPM's Jayawantrao Sawant College of Pharmacy and Research, Handewadi Road, Hadapsar, Pune, Maharashtra 411028, India

V. H. Bhaskar
Department of Pharmaceutical Medicinal Chemistry, Gahlot Institute of Pharmacy Plot No. 59, Sector No. 14, Koparkhairane, Navi Mumbai, Maharashtra 400709, India

V. L. Maruthanila, J. Poornima and S. Mirunalini
Department of Biochemistry and Biotechnology, Faculty of Science, Annamalai University, Annamalainagar, Tamilnadu 608 002, India

Srinivasa Rao Sirasanagandla
Department of Anatomy, Melaka Manipal Medical College, Manipal University, Madhav Nagar, Manipal, Karnataka 576104, India

Sreedhara Ranganath Pai Karkala
Department of Pharmacology, Manipal College of Pharmaceutical Sciences, Manipal University, Manipal, Karnataka 576104, India

Bhagath Kumar Potu
Department of Anatomy, College of Medicine and Medical Sciences, Arabian Gulf University, P.O. Box 26671, Bahrain

Kumar M.R. Bhat
Department of Anatomy, Kasturba Medical College, Manipal University, Manipal, Karnataka 576104, India

www.ingramcontent.com/pod-product-compliance
Lightning Source LLC
Chambersburg PA
CBHW080522200326
41458CB00012B/4301